Medical Management of HIV Infection
2005-2006 Edition

John G. Bartlett, M.D.
Professor of Medicine and Epidemiology
Chief, Division of Infectious Diseases,
Director, Johns Hopkins AIDS Service,
Department of Medicine,
Johns Hopkins University School of Medicine

Joel E. Gallant, M.D., M.P.H.
Associate Professor of Medicine and Epidemiology
Associate Director, Johns Hopkins AIDS Service
Division of Infectious Diseases,
Department of Medicine,
Johns Hopkins University School of Medicine

Published by Johns Hopkins Medicine
Health Publishing Business Group
Baltimore, Maryland
United States of America

 Roche

Stanley Kassimir B.S.M.S.R.Ph
HIV Specialist

Roche Laboratories Inc.
340 Kingsland Street
Nutley, New Jersey 07110-1199
Voice Mail 1(800)LA-ROCHE Ext 8002293
Mobile 917-763-2976
E-Mail stanley.kassimir@roche.com

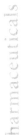
Pharmaceuticals

i

Some of the information contained in this book may cite the use of a particular drug in a dosage, for an indication, or in a manner other than recommended or FDA-approved. Therefore, the manufacturers' package inserts should be consulted for complete prescribing information.

ISBN: 0-9755326-2-6

Address of the publisher:
   2005-2006 MMHIV
   Johns Hopkins Medicine
   Health Publishing Business Group
   100 N. Charles Street, 5th Floor
   Baltimore, MD 21201

Acknowledgements

We thank our Johns Hopkins colleagues for their consultation and content review:

Richard Ambinder, M.D., Ph.D., Department of Oncology: HIV-associated Malignancies.

Jean R. Anderson, M.D., Department of Gynecology and Obstetrics: Pregnancy and PAP Smears

Richard E. Chaisson, M.D., The Johns Hopkins Center for Tuberculosis Research: Mycobacterial Disease

Joseph Cofrancesco, Jr., M.D., Johns Hopkins AIDS Service: Wasting and Lipodystrophy

Douglas Jabs, M.D., Department of Ophthalmology: CMV Retinitis

Brooks Jackson, M.D., Department of Pathology: HIV Laboratory Testing

Gregory M. Lucas, M.D., Division of Infectious Diseases, Department of Medicine

Ciro Martins, M.D., Department of Dermatology: Dermatology

Justin McArthur, M.B., B.S., M.P.H., Department of Neurology: Peripheral Neuropathy and CNS

Mark Sulkowski, M.D., The Johns Hopkins Hepatitis Center: Hepatitis B and C Detection and Management

Glenn Treisman, M.D., Ph.D. and Andrew F. Angelino, M.D., Department of Psychiatry: Mental Health

Project director: Steve Libowitz

Editorial director: Eileen O'Brien

Review: Paul Pham, Pharm.D.

Design: WorldComp, Sterling, Virginia

Typesetting: PR Graphics, Timonium, Maryland

Printed in the U.S.A. by PMR Printing, Sterling, Virginia

Note

This book is provided as a resource for physicians and other health care professionals in providing care and treatment to patients with HIV/AIDS. Every possible effort is made to ensure the accuracy and reliability of material presented in this book; however, recommendations for care and treatment change rapidly, and opinion can be controversial. Therefore, physicians and other healthcare professionals are encouraged to consult other sources and confirm the information contained within this book. The author, reviewers, and production staff will not be held liable for errors, omissions, or inaccuracies in information or for any perceived harm to users of this book. It is up to the individual physician or other health care professional to use his/her best medical judgment in determining appropriate patient care or treatment because no single reference or service can take the place of medical training, education, and experience.

Neither The Johns Hopkins University, The Johns Hopkins Health System Corporation, nor the authors and reviewers are responsible for deletions or inaccuracies in information or for claims of injury resulting from any such deletions or inaccuracies. Mention of specific drugs or products within this book does not constitute endorsement by the authors, The Johns Hopkins University Division of Infectious Diseases, or The Johns Hopkins University School of Medicine. With regard to specific drugs or products, physicians are advised to consult their normal resources before prescribing to their patients.

Additional sources of information include the websites of the Johns Hopkins University Division of Infectious Diseases:

The Johns Hopkins AIDS Service: **http://www.hopkins-aids.edu**

The Hopkins Antibiotic-Guide: **http://www.hopkins-abxguide.org**

The Johns Hopkins Center for Tuberculosis Research:
  http://www.hopkins-tb.org

Foreword

The 2005-2006 edition of *Medical Management of HIV Infection* reflects substantial changes in the treatment of patients with HIV infection and AIDS since the previous edition was published in July 2004. This edition was completed in October 2005, so new developments in treatment guidelines occurring after that time do not appear in this edition. Updates are available on the Johns Hopkins Aids Service Web site, **http://www.hopkins-aids.edu**.

The 2004 edition was distributed to approximately 40,000 readers in more than 60 countries and accessed by more than 10,000 additional readers online. The book has been translated into Portuguese, Chinese and Russian.

This edition includes more than 140 tables and more than 300 new references to publications or presentations made in 2004 and 2005, reflecting the authors' efforts to keep abreast of new developments by attendance at major scientific conferences and by systematic review of 42 relevant journals. Recommendations presented here are based largely on federal guidelines for antiretroviral therapy for adults, pregnancy management, opportunistic infection prophylaxis, management of occupational exposure, management of TB co-infection, management of HCV co-infection, prevention of transmission, and management of sexually transmitted infections. Based on recent advances there has been substantial expansion of and change in sections dealing with adverse reactions and treatment options following virologic failure. The authors have provided recommendations based on available data and personal experiences and opinions, as well as guidelines from authoritative sources.

As always, comments and suggestions are welcome.

John G. Bartlett, M.D.

Contents

Medical Management of HIV Infection: Contents

Medical Management of HIV Infection

1 I Natural History and Classification

Stages

The natural history of untreated HIV infection is divided into the following stages:

Viral transmission $\xrightarrow{\text{2-3 wks}}$ Acute retroviral syndrome $\xrightarrow{\text{2-3 wks}}$ Recovery + seroconversion $\xrightarrow{\text{2-4 wks}}$ Asymptomatic chronic HIV infection $\xrightarrow{\text{Avg. 8 yrs}}$ Symptomatic HIV infection/AIDS $\xrightarrow{\text{Avg. 1.3 yrs}}$ Death

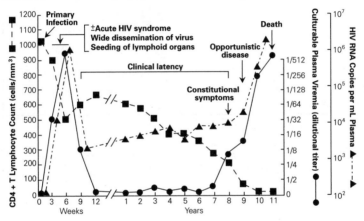

■ FIGURE 1-1: **Natural history of HIV infection in an average patient without antiretroviral therapy from the time of HIV transmission to death at 10-11 years.** The initial event is the acute retroviral syndrome (Table 1-2, p. 3), which is accompanied by a precipitous decline in CD4 cell counts (closed squares) and high concentrations of HIV RNA in plasma (closed triangles). Clinical recovery is accompanied by a reduction in plasma viremia, reflecting development of cytotoxic T-cell (CTL) response. The CD4 cell count decreases are due to HIV-induced cell death (*J Exp Med* 2001;194:1277). This may be due to a high state of CD8 and CD4 cell stimulation producing "T cell exhaustion" and cell death. (Papagno L, *PLoS Biol* 2004;2:E20). The slope of the CD4 cell decline depends on the viral load; in one study the median rate of decline was 4%/year for each $\log_{10}$ HIV RNA/mL (*J Infect Dis* 2002;185:905). The slope increases in late stage disease. HIV RNA concentrations in plasma show an initial "burst" during acute infection and then decline to a "set point" as a result of seroconversion and immune response. With continued infection, HIV RNA levels gradually increase (*J Infect Dis* 1999;180:1018). Late-stage disease is characterized by a CD4 count <200 cells/mm³ and the development of opportunistic infections, selected tumors, wasting, and neurologic complications (Table 1-2, p. 2). In an untreated patient, the median survival after the CD4 count has fallen to <200 cells/mm³ is 3.7 years; the median CD4 count at the time of the first AIDS-defining complication is 60-70 cells/mm³; the median survival after an AIDS-defining complication is 1.3 years. (Figure reprinted with permission from *Ann Intern Med* 1996;124:654).

Natural History and Classification

■ TABLE 1-1: **Correlation of Complications With CD4 Cell Counts (see *Arch Intern Med* 1995;155:1537)**

CD4 Cell Count*	Infectious Complications	Noninfectious† Complications
>500/mm³	■ Acute retroviral syndrome ■ Candidal vaginitis	■ Persistent generalized lymphadenopathy (PGL) ■ Guillain-Barré syndrome ■ Myopathy ■ Aseptic meningitis
200-500/mm³	■ Pneumococcal and other bacterial pneumonia ■ Pulmonary tuberculosis ■ Herpes zoster ■ Oropharyngeal candidiasis (thrush) ■ Cryptosporidiosis, self-limited ■ Kaposi's sarcoma ■ Oral hairy leukoplakia	■ Cervical intraepithelial neoplasia ■ Cervical cancer ■ B-cell lymphoma ■ Anemia ■ Mononeuronal multiplex ■ Idiopathic thrombocytopenic purpura ■ Hodgkin's lymphoma ■ Lymphocytic interstitial pneumonitis
<200/mm³	■ *Pneumocystis carinii* pneumonia‡ ■ Disseminated histoplasmosis and coccidioidomycosis ■ Miliary/extrapulmonary TB ■ Progressive multifocal leuko-encephalopathy (PML)	■ Wasting ■ Peripheral neuropathy ■ HIV-associated dementia ■ Cardiomyopathy ■ Vacuolar myelopathy ■ Progressive polyradiculopathy ■ Non-Hodgkin's lymphoma
<100/mm³	■ Disseminated herpes simplex ■ Toxoplasmosis ■ Cryptococcosis ■ Cryptosporidiosis, chronic ■ Microsporidiosis ■ Candidal esophagitis	
<50/mm³	■ Disseminated cytomegalovirus (CMV) ■ Disseminated *Mycobacterium avium* complex	■ Central nervous system (CNS) lymphoma

* Most complications occur with increasing frequency at lower CD4 cell counts.

† Some conditions listed as "noninfectious" are probably associated with transmissible microbes. Examples include lymphoma (Epstein-Barr virus [EBV]) and cervical cancer (human papillomavirus [HPV]).

‡ Preferred name is now *P. jiroveci* pneumonia; PCP is the accepted abbreviation. See p. 49.

Natural History and Classification

Primary HIV Infection

DIAGNOSIS: HIV RNA >10,000 c/mL + indeterminant or negative HIV serology or recent seroconversion (*Ann Intern Med* 2001;134:25).

■ TABLE 1-2: **Primary HIV Infection: Signs and Symptoms (Department of Health and Human Services [DHHS] Guidelines [*Ann Intern Med* 2002;137:381])**

Fever – 96%	Myalgias – 54%	Hepatosplenomegaly – 14%
Adenopathy – 74%	Diarrhea – 32%	Weight loss – 13%
Pharyngitis – 70%	Headache – 32%	Thrush – 12%
Rash* – 70%	Nausea & vomiting – 27%	Neurologic symptoms[†] – 12%

* Rash – erythematous maculopapular rash on face and trunk, sometimes extremities, including palms & soles. Some have mucocutaneous ulceration involving mouth, esophagus, or genitals.

[†] Aseptic meningitis, meningoencephalitis, peripheral neuropathy, facial palsy, Guillain-Barré syndrome, brachial neuritis, cognitive impairment, or psychosis.

■ TABLE 1-3: **AIDS Surveillance Case Definition for Adolescents and Adults: 1993**

	Clinical Categories		
	A	**B**	**C***
CD4 Cell Categories	Asymptomatic, or PGL, or Acute HIV Infection	Symptomatic[†] (not A or C)	AIDS Indicator Condition (1987)
>500/mm³ (≥29%)	A1	B1	C1
200 to 499/mm³ (14% to 28%)	A2	B2	C2
<200/mm³ (<14%)	A3	B3	C3

* All patients in categories A3, B3, and C1-3 are defined as having AIDS based on the presence of an AIDS-indicator condition (Table 1-4, p. 4) and/or a CD4 cell count <200/mm³.

[†] Symptomatic conditions not included in Category C that are a) attributed to HIV infection or indicative of a defect in cell-mediated immunity or b) considered to have a clinical course or management that is complicated by HIV infection. Examples of B conditions include, but are not limited to, bacillary angiomatosis; thrush; vulvovaginal candidiasis that is persistent, frequent, or poorly responsive to therapy; cervical dysplasia (moderate or severe); cervical carcinoma *in situ*; constitutional symptoms such as fever (38.5°C) or diarrhea >1 month; oral hairy leukoplakia; herpes zoster involving two episodes or >1 dermatome; idiopathic thrombocytopenic purpura (ITP); listeriosis; pelvic inflammatory disease (PID) (especially if complicated by a tubo-ovarian abscess); and peripheral neuropathy.

Natural History and Classification

■ TABLE 1-4: **Indicator Conditions in Case Definition of AIDS (Adults) – 1997***

Candidiasis of esophagus, trachea, bronchi, or lungs – 3,846 (16%)
Cervical cancer, invasive[†][‡] – 144 (0.6%)
Coccidioidomycosis, extrapulmonary[†] – 74 (0.3%)
Cryptococcosis, extrapulmonary – 1,168 (5%)
Cryptosporidiosis with diarrhea >1 month – 314 (1.3%)
CMV of any organ other than liver, spleen, or lymph nodes; eye – 1,638 (7%)
Herpes simplex with mucocutaneous ulcer >1 month or bronchitis, pneumonitis, esophagitis – 1,250 (5%)
Histoplasmosis, extrapulmonary[†] – 208 (0.9%)
HIV-associated dementia[†]: Disabling cognitive and/or other dysfunction interfering with occupation or activities of daily living – 1,196 (5%)
HIV-associated wasting[†]: Involuntary weight loss >10% of baseline plus chronic diarrhea (≥2 loose stools/day ≥30 days) or chronic weakness and documented enigmatic fever ≥30 days – 4,212 (18%)
Isoporosis with diarrhea >1 month[†] – 22 (0.1%)
Kaposi's sarcoma in patient under 60 yrs (or over 60 yrs)[†] – 1,500 (7%)
Lymphoma, Burkitt's – 162 (0.7%), immunoblastic – 518 (2.3%), primary CNS – 170 (0.7%)
Mycobacterium avium, disseminated – 1,124 (5%)
Mycobacterium tuberculosis, pulmonary – 1,621 (7%), extrapulmonary – 491 (2%)
Pneumocystis carinii pneumonia – 9,145 (38%)
Pneumonia, recurrent-bacterial (≥2 episodes in 12 months)[†][‡] – 1,347 (5%)
Progressive multifocal leukoencephalopathy – 213 (1%)
Salmonella septicemia (nontyphoid), recurrent[†] – 68 (0.3%)
Toxoplasmosis of internal organ – 1,073 (4%)

* Indicates frequency as the AIDS-indicator condition among 23,527 reported cases in adults for 1997. The AIDS diagnosis was based on CD4 count in an additional 36,643 or 61% of the 60,161 total cases. Numbers indicate sum of definitive and presumptive diagnosis for stated condition. The number in parentheses is the percentage of all patients reported with an AIDS-defining diagnosis; these do not total 100% because some had a dual diagnosis.

† Requires positive HIV serology.

‡ Added in the revised case definition, 1993.

Natural History and Classification

2 | Laboratory Tests

Laboratory tests recommended for initial evaluation and follow-up of all patients are summarized in Table 2-16, p.38.

HIV Types and Subtypes

HIV infection is established by detecting antibodies to the virus, viral antigens, viral RNA/DNA, or by culture (*Lancet* 1996;348:176). The standard test is serology for antibody detection. There are two HIV types: HIV-1 and HIV-2, which show 40% to 60% amino acid homology. HIV-1 accounts for nearly all cases except a minority of strains that originate in West Africa. HIV-1 is divided into subtypes designated A to K (collectively referred to as "M subtypes") and O. There are now also Circulating Recombinant Forms. The major ones are CRF01_AE (a mosaic with sequences from clades A and E), and CRF02_AG. Subtype O shows 55% to 70% homology with the M subtypes. A new group of viruses labeled "N" for "new" was reported in 1998 (*Nat Med* 1998;4:1032; *Science* 2000;287:607). Over 98% of HIV-1 infections in the United States are caused by subtype B; most non-B subtypes in the United States were acquired in other countries (*J Infect Dis* 2000;181:470); the relatively rare O and N subtypes are found primarily in West Africa.

■ TABLE 2-1: **HIV-1 Subtype Distribution** (*J Acquir Immune Defic Syndr 2002;29:184*)

Predominant Subtypes	Regions
A	W. Africa, E. Africa, Central Africa, East Europe, Russia, Mideast
B	N. America, Europe, Mideast, E. Asia, Latin America
C	S. Africa, S. Asia, Ethiopia, Brazil
D	E. Africa
E	S.E. Asia
CRF02_AG	West and West Central Africa, Spain, Russia

HIV-2

HIV-2 is another human retrovirus that causes immune deficiency due to depletion of CD4 cells. It is found primarily in West Africa.*

---

* Endemic areas in West Africa – Benin, Burkina Faso, Cape Verde, Cote d'Ivoire, Gambia, Ghana, Guinea Guinea-Bissau, Liberia, Mali, Mauritania, Niger, Nigeria, São Tome, Senegal, Sierra Leone, and Togo; other African countries – Angola and Mozambique (*MMWR* 1992;4[RR-12]:1).

CLINICAL FEATURES: Compared with HIV-1, HIV-2 is less transmissible (5- to 8-fold less efficient than HIV-1 in early-stage disease and rarely the cause of vertical transmission), is associated with a lower viral load, and is associated with a slower rate of both CD4 cell decline and clinical progression (*Lancet* 1994;344:1380; *AIDS* 1994;8 [suppl 1]:585; *J Infect Dis* 1999;180:1116; *J Acquir Immune Defic Syndr* 2000;24:257; *Arch Intern Med* 2000;160:3286; *AIDS* 2000;14:441; *J Infect Dis* 2002;185:905). Nevertheless, mortality rates for HIV-1 and HIV-2 infection are similar when adjusted for viral load (*J Acquir Immune Defic Syndr* 2005;38:335). HIV-2 shows reduced homology with HIV-1 compared with HIV-1 subtypes (*Nature* 1987;328:543), and 20% to 30% have negative antibody tests depending on which enzyme immunosorbent assay (EIA) is used. Western blots (WBs) for HIV-2 are neither well standardized nor FDA approved (*Ann Intern Med* 1993;118:211; *JAMA* 1992;267:2775).

Issues affecting the management of HIV-2-infected patients:

1) Many patients are co-infected with HIV-1 (*AIDS* 2002;16:1775).

2) There are currently no treatment guidelines for HIV-2; it is suggested that the same clinical, viral load and CD4 count criteria should be used (*J Acquir Immun Defic Syndr* 2005;38:335).

3) HIV-2 is not susceptible to NNRTIs and may have multiple PI-associated resistance mutations, suggesting possible PI resistance (*J Clin Microbiol* 2000;38:1370; *NEJM* 2000;342:1758; *JAIDS* 2000;25:11; *AIDS* 2004;18:495; *Antivir Ther* 2004;9:57; *J Clin Microbiol* 2005;43:484).

4) Laboratory confirmation of infection may be difficult (see below).

5) There are no commercially available viral load assays for HIV-2 or resistance (*Arch Intern Med* 2000;160:3286), although these tests can be performed by some specialty laboratories (*J Virol Methods* 2000;88:81; *Clin Infect Dis* 2004;38:1771; *J Acquir Immun˙Defic Syndr* 2000;24:257; see www.phls.co.uk).

SEROLOGY: An HIV-2 EIA was licensed by the FDA in 1990 and became mandatory for screening blood donors in 1992. Some commercial labs now use combination EIA screening assays to detect HIV-1 and HIV-2 simultaneously, although this is not recommended by the CDC for routine testing (*MMWR* 1992;41[RR-12]:1). Of the FDA-approved rapid tests OraQuick detects HIV-1 and -2, and Multispot distinguishes HIV-1 and -2. Reveal G2 and UniGold Recombigen are approved for detection of only HIV-1. For information on the Multispot HIV-1/HIV-2 Rapid Test: 1-800-224-6723 and www.medcompare.com/itemdetails .asp?itemd=35295.

PREVALENCE: There were 78 persons diagnosed with HIV-2 infection in the United States between 1987 and January 1998; 52 were born in West Africa, and most of the rest had either traveled there, had a sexual partner from that region, or had incomplete data (*MMWR* 1995;44:603;

The CDC recommends that HIV-2 serology be included in serologic testing of 1) natives of endemic areas,* 2) needle-sharing and sex partners of persons from an endemic area,* 3) sex partners or needle-sharing partners of persons with HIV-2 infection, 4) persons who received transfusions or nonsterile injections in endemic areas,* and 5) children of women with risk for HIV-2 infection. Contact CDC for HIV-2 serologic testing.

HIV Serology

Indications
(Primary care guidelines, IDSA, *Clin Infect Dis* 2004;39:609)

- Adults in populations with an estimated prevalence >1%
- Pregnant women
- Sexual assault victims
- Occupational exposure
- Anyone who requests the test

Standard Test

The standard serologic test consists of a screening EIA followed by a confirmatory WB. EIA screening requires a "repeatedly reactive" test, which is the criterion for WB testing. WB detects antibodies to HIV-1 proteins, including core (p17, p24, p55), polymerase (p31, p51, p66), and envelope (gp41, gp120, gp160). WB testing should always be coupled with EIA screening due to a 2% rate of false positives. Results (*Am J Med* 2000;109:568) of WB are interpreted as follows:

- **Negative:** No bands.
- **Positive:** Reactivity to gp120/160 plus either gp41 or p24.
- **Indeterminate:** Presence of any band pattern that does not meet criteria for positive results.

ACCURACY: Standard serologic assays (EIA and WB or immuno-fluorescent assay) show sensitivity in patients with established disease (>3 months after transmission) of 99.5% (CI 98-99.9%) and a specificity of 99.994 (*N Engl J Med* 2005;352:570; *JAMA* 1991;266:2861; *Am J Med* 2000;109:568). Positive tests should be confirmed with repeat tests or with corroborating clinical or laboratory data.

FALSE-NEGATIVE RESULTS: False-negative results are usually due to testing in the "window period." The rate of false negatives ranges from 0.3% in a high-prevalence population (*J Infect Dis* 1993;168:327) to <0.001% in low-prevalence populations (*N Engl J Med* 1991;325:593). Causes of false-negative results include:

---

* Endemic areas in West Africa – Benin, Burkina Faso, Cape Verde, Cote d'Ivoire, Gambia, Ghana, Guinea Guinea-Bissau, Liberia, Mali, Mauritania, Niger, Nigeria, São Tome, Senegal, Sierra Leone, and Togo; other African countries – Angola and Mozambique (*MMWR* 1992;4[RR-12]:1).

7

- **Window period:** The time delay from infection to positive EIA averages 10 to 14 days with newer test reagents (*Clin Infect Dis* 1997;25:101; *Am J Med* 2000;109:568). Some do not seroconvert for 3 to 4 weeks, but virtually all patients seroconvert within 6 months (*Am J Med* 2000;109:568).

- **Seroreversion:** Rare patients serorevert in late-stage disease (*JAMA* 1993;269:2786; *Ann Intern Med* 1988;108:785). Seroreversion has also been reported in patients who achieve prolonged immune reconstitution due to highly active antiretroviral therapy (HAART) (*N Engl J Med* 1999;340:1683).

- **"Atypical host response"** accounts for rare cases and is largely unexplained (*AIDS* 1995;9:95; *MMWR* 1996;45:181; *Clin Infect Dis* 1997;25:98).

- **Agammaglobulinemia**

- **Type N or O strains or HIV-2:** Standard serologic tests detect M subtypes (subtypes A-K) of HIV-1, and some detect HIV-1 and -2. EIA screening tests may fail to detect the O and N subtypes (*Lancet* 1994;343:1393; *Lancet* 1994;344:1333; *MMWR* 1996;45:561). Only two patients with strain O HIV infection were detected in the United States through July 2000 (*MMWR* 1996;45:561; *Emerg Infect Dis* 1996;2:209; *AIDS* 2002;18:269). The N group is another rare variant that causes false-negative EIA screening tests but may be positive by WB (*Nat Med* 1998;4:1032). There have been no recognized infections with the N strain in the United States through March 2000 (*J Infect Dis* 2000;181:470). Standard EIA screening tests are falsely negative in 20% to 30% of patients infected with HIV-2. Detection may require tests specifically for HIV-2. Risks for HIV-2 are summarized above (pp. 5-6).

- **Technical or clerical error**

FALSE-POSITIVE RESULTS: The frequency of false-positive HIV serology (both EIA and WB) was reported to range from 0.0004% to 0.0007% (*JAMA* 1998;280:1080; *Arch Intern Med* 2003;163:1857; *Arch Intern Med* 2000;160:2386) Important clues to possible false positive tests are lack of risk factors, undetectable viral load, and normal CD4 count (*Arch Intern Med* 2003;163:1857). The serologic test should be repeated in patients without other laboratory evidence of infection. Causes of false-positive results include:

- **Autoantibodies:** A single case was reported in which a false-positive serology was ascribed to autoantibodies in a patient with lupus erythematosus and end-stage renal disease (*N Engl J Med* 1993;328:1281). However, a subsequent report indicated that this patient did have HIV infection as verified by positive cultures (*N Engl J Med* 1994;331:881). Another patient with two positive tests and two indeterminate WB tests was found to be uninfected, with a negative HIV culture and PCR (*Clin Infect Dis* 1992;15:707).

Laboratory Tests

- **HIV vaccines:** HIV vaccines are the most common cause of false-positive HIV serology. In an analysis of 266 healthy volunteers in HIV vaccine studies, 68% had positive EIA tests, and 0% to 44% had positive WB, depending on the antigen used in the vaccine (*Ann Intern Med* 1994;121:584).

- **Factitious HIV infection:** This refers to patients who report a history of a positive test that is erroneous, due to either misunderstanding or an intent to deceive (*Ann Intern Med* 1994;121:763). It is important to confirm anonymous tests and to repeat laboratory reports that cannot be verified, using either repeat serology or viral load testing. [Note that 2% to 9% of viral load tests are falsely positive, usually with low viral titers (*Ann Intern Med* 1999;130:37)].

- **Technical or clerical error** (*Arch Intern Med* 2003;163:1857)

INDETERMINATE RESULTS: Indeterminate test results account for 4% to 20% of WB assays with positive bands for HIV-1 proteins. Causes of indeterminate results include:

- **Serologic tests in the process of seroconversion**; anti-p24 is usually the first antibody to appear.

- **Late-stage HIV infection**, usually with loss of core antibody.

- **Cross-reacting nonspecific antibodies**, as seen with collagen-vascular disease, autoimmune diseases, lymphoma, liver disease, injection drug use, multiple sclerosis, parity, or recent immunization.

- **Infection with O strain or HIV-2**

- **HIV vaccine recipients** (see above)

- **Technical or clerical error**

The most important factor in evaluating indeterminate results is risk assessment. Patients in low-risk categories with indeterminate tests are almost never infected with either HIV-1 or HIV-2; repeat testing often continues to show indeterminate results, and the cause of this pattern is infrequently established (*N Engl J Med* 1990;322:217). For this reason, such patients should be reassured that HIV infection is extremely unlikely, although follow-up serology at 3 months is recommended to provide absolute assurance. Patients with indeterminate tests who are in the process of seroconversion usually have positive WBs within 1 month. Repeat tests at 1, 2, and 6 months are generally advocated, along with appropriate precautions to prevent viral transmission in the interim (*J Gen Intern Med* 1992;7:640; *J Infect Dis* 1991;164:656; *Arch Intern Med* 2000; 160:2386; *J Acquir Immune Defic Syndr* 1998;17:376).

FREQUENCY OF TESTING: Periodic tests are recommended for patients who practice high-risk behavior. The frequency is arbitrary, but most suggest annual testing for high risk patients (*MMWR* 2002;51:736;

MMWR 2002;57[RR-6]:7). Annual seroconversion rates are estimated as follows: general population – 0.001%, military recruits – 0.04%, MSM – 0.5% to 2% (higher among younger MSM), and injection drug users in areas with high seroprevalence – 0.7% to 6% (*Am J Epidemiol* 1991;134:1175; *J Acquir Immune Defic Syndr* 1993;6:1049; *Arch Intern Med* 1995;155:1305; *Am J Public Health* 1996;86:642; *Am J Public Health* 2000;90:352; *MMWR* 2001;50:440).

Alternative HIV Serologic Tests (Table 2-4, p. 13)

IFA: This is another method to detect HIV antibodies using patient serum reacted with HIV infected cells. A fluorochrome is used as the indicator method.

HOME KITS: *Home Access Express Test* (Home Access Health Corp., Hoffman Estates, III; 800-HIV-TEST) is the only available home kit. This test is sold in retail and online pharmacies for approximately $49.99 for routine mailing with results in 7 days or for $59.99 for *Federal Express* transport with results in 3 days. Blood is obtained by lancet, and a filter strip with blotted blood is mailed in a protected envelope using an anonymous code. Home Access' tests use a double EIA with a confirmatory IFA. Sensitivity and specificity approach 100%. Callers learn of a negative test through a prerecorded message, but the patient can access a representative to discuss results if desired. Callers with positive results receive counseling and referral for medical and social services from a database of 19,000 organizations. In a study of 174,316 HIV home sample collection tests in 1996 to 1997, 0.9% were positive and 97% of users called for their results. The company sells approximately 60,000 tests/year, and the number positive continued to be about 0.9% in 2003. Nearly 60% of all users and 49% of HIV-positive persons had never previously been tested (*JAMA* 1998;280:1699). Merits of this type of home testing are debated (*N Engl J Med* 1995;332:1296).

RAPID TESTS: There are four FDA-approved rapid serologic tests which show variations in the specimen type and CLIA category as follows (www.cdc.gov/hiv/rapid_testing):

Test	Source	Specimen*	CLIA**	Sens. %	Spec. %	Comment
OraQuick	OraSure Technologies www.orasure.com	Blood	Waived	99.6	99.8	HIV-1&2
		Plasma		99.6	99.8	20 min
		Oral Fluid		99.6	99.7	20-40 min
UniGold Recombigen	Trinity BioTech www.trinitybiotech.com/en/index.asp	Blood	Waived	100	99.7	HIV-1
		Plasma		100	99.8	10 min
		Serum		100	99.8	
Reveal G$_2$	MedMira Inc. www.medmira.com	Plasma	Mod Complex	99.8	99.1	HIV-1
						5 min
		Serum		99.8	98.6	
Multispot HIV-1/HIV-2 HIV-2	Bio-Rad Labs 1-800-224-6723 www.medcompare.com/itemdetails.asp?itemid=35295	Serum	Mod Complex	100	99.9	Distinguishes HIV-2 & 2
		Serum		100		15 min

*Whole blood avoids the need for a centrifuge or any other equipment.

**CLIA requirements include registration with CLIA and compliance with their standards for testing, inspection, etc.

Performance of these tests is regulated by the Clinical Laboratory Improvement Amendment of 1988 (CLIA). The tests are categorized as CLIA "waived" or "moderate complexity." OraQuick and Uni-Gold are CLIA waived tests, which means no federal restrictions for personnel, quality assessment or proficiency testing. The tests can be done in laboratories, clinical settings, mobile vans, physicians' offices, etc. The requirement is to obtain a certificate of waiver and follow manufacturers instructions (see: www.phppo.cdc.gov/clia/regs/toc/aspx). Reveal and Multispot HIV-1/HIV-2 are "moderately complex," which requires registering with CLIA, and satisfying CLIA standards for personnel, quality assessment, proficiency testing and inspections. Reveal and Multispot require plasma or serum, and thus a centrifuge. For all four tests:

- persons tested must receive a "Subject Information pamphlet" provided with the test;

- a negative test is a definitive negative unless tested in the "window period" (first 3 months post exposure);

- positive tests are considered preliminary positive results and should be confirmed with a Western blot or IFA. Note that confirmation tests done only with EIA have yielded false negative results (*MMWR* 2004;53:221);

- indeterminate tests should be repeated in 1 month.

Laboratory Tests

2

Sensitivity and specificity of these rapid tests is consistently >99% (*J Acquir Immune Defic Syndr* 1993;6:115; *Am J Emerg Med* 1991; 9:416; *Am Intern Med* 1996;125:471; *J Human Virol* 2001;4:278; *Internat J STD AIDS* 2002;13:171; *J Clin Microbiol* 2003;41:3868; *J Lab Med* 2003;27:288), but the positive predictive value is dependent on HIV prevalence, an observation that emphasized the need for a confirmatory test as shown in Table 2-3. Rapid tests are recommended for general use but may be especially useful where rapid results are important as with occupational exposure (*MMWR* 2001;50[RR-11]:1; *Infect Control Hosp Epidemiol* 2001;22:289) for women who present in labor without prior testing (*JAMA* 2004;292:219), and for patients who are unlikely to return for test results including emergency rooms and STD clinics (*MMWR* 1998;47:215). With provider-read (CLIA) tests the average turnaround time is 45 minutes (www.cdc.gov/hiv/rapid_testing).

■ TABLE 2-3: **Positive Predictive Value of a Single Test***

HIV prevalence	Predictive Value, positive test		
	Ora-Quick	Unigold	Single EIA
10%	99%	97%	98%
2%	95%	87%	91%
1%	91%	77%	83%
0.5%	83%	63%	71%
0.1%	50%	25%	33%
Specificity	99.9%	99.7%	99.8%

*Branson B www.cdc.gov/hiv/rapid_testing (posted Jan. 20, 2005)

SALIVA TEST: *OraSure* (OraSure Technologies, Inc.; Bethlehem, Pa; 800-672-7873; www.orasure.com), is an FDA-approved device for collecting saliva and concentrating IgG for application of EIA tests for HIV antibody. The *OraSure* test system consists of a specimen collection device, the bioMérieux *Vironostika* HIV-1 antibody screen, and the WB confirmatory assay, at a cost of $24.15 per test. It is available for testing in public health departments, physicians' offices, community-based service organizations, and AIDS Service organizations. *OraSure* testing is also available by calling 800-Ora-Sure or 800-672-7873. The test may be anonymous or confidential. Results are available by phone or fax within 3 days. The test consists of a specially treated pad used to swab the gums; the swab is then inserted into a vial for 20 minutes and read at 20 to 40 minutes. The amount of IgG obtained from saliva is far higher than in plasma and is well above the 0.5 mg/L level necessary for detection of HIV antibodies. Specimens saved from 3,570 subjects showed correct results compared with standard serology in 672 of 673 (99.9%) positives and 2,893 of 2,897 (99%) negatives (*JAMA* 1997;277:254). Potential advantages over standard serologic testing are the ease of collecting specimens, reduced cost, and better patient acceptance.

URINE TEST: *Calypte* HIV-1 Urine EIA (Calypte Biomedical Corp; Alameda, Calif; 877-225-9783; www.calypte.com) is an FDA-approved screening EIA. This test can be administered only by a physician, and positive results require confirmation by a standard serologic test with WB. Reported sensitivity is 99% (88/89), specificity is 94% (49/52) (*Lancet* 1991;337:183; *Clin Chem* 1999;45:1602). The supplier has included a pretest counseling form, which should be read to and initialed by the patient prior to administration. The assay is sold as a 192-test kit at $816 or a 480-test kit at $1,920. The cost per test is $4.00.

VAGINAL SECRETIONS: HIV antibodies can be detected in vaginal secretions with IgG EIA (*Wellcozyme* HIV-1&2, Gracelisa Murex Diagnostics Ltd., Dartford, UK). This test is recommended by the CDC for victims of rape because HIV IgG antibodies are in semen (*MMWR* 1985;34:75S; *J Clin Microbiol* 1994;32:1249).

Viral Detection

Other methods to establish HIV infection include techniques to detect DNA (HIV-1 DNA PCR) or RNA (HIV-1 RNA by bDNA or RT-PCR (Table 2-4, p. 13). HIV-1 DNA PCR is the most sensitive and can detect 1 to 10 copies of HIV proviral DNA, but the reagents are not well standardized or FDA-approved. None of these tests is considered to be more accurate than routine serology, but some may be useful in patients with confusing serologic test results, and for HIV detection when routine serologic tests are likely to be misleading, as in patients with agammaglobulinemia, acute retroviral infection, neonatal HIV infection, and patients in the window period following viral exposure. In most cases, confirmation of positive serology is accomplished simply by repeat serology. None of these tests should replace serology to circumvent the informed consent process.

■ TABLE 2-4: **Tests for HIV-1**

Assay	Sensitivity	Comments
Routine serology	99.7%	Readily available and inexpensive. Sensitivity >99.7% and specificity >99.9% (*MMWR* 1990;39:380; *N Engl J Med* 1988;319:961; *JAMA* 1991;266:2861).
Rapid test See p.10 and Table 2-2.	>99%	Results are available in 20 min. Advantages with CLIA-waived tests (Ora-Quick and UniGold Recombigen) are that results are available in ≤20 minutes and interpretation may be done by the provider. Negative tests are a definitive negative; positive tests must be confirmed with a western blot. Table 2-2 lists the for FDA-approved rapid tests in the U.S. (www.cdc.gov/hiv/rapid–testing). Other rapid tests are available but are not FDA-approved (*Int J STD AIDS* 1997;8:192; *Vox Sang* 1997;72:11; *J Hum Virol* 2001;4:278).

(continued)

2 Laboratory Tests

Assay	Sensitivity	Comments
Salivary test (*OraSure* Test System)	99.6%	Salivary collection device to collect IgG for EIA and WB. Advantage is avoidance of phlebotomy. Sensitivity and specificity are comparable with standard serology (*JAMA* 1997;227:254).
Urine test (*Calypte HIV-1 Test*)	>99%	Used for EIA test only, so positive results must be verified by serology. Must be administered by a physician. Cost is low – about $4 per test.
PBMC culture	95% to 100%	Viral isolation by co-cultivation of patient's PBMC with phytohemagglutinin-stimulated donor PBMC with IL-2 over 28 days. Expensive and labor-intensive. May be qualitative or quantitative. Main use of qualitative technique is viral isolation for further analysis such as sequence analysis. Studies prior to availability of quantitative HIV RNA PCR showed quantitative culture results correlated with stage: Mean titer was $2000/10^6$ cells in patients with AIDS (*N Engl J Med* 1989;321:1621).
DNA PCR assay	>99%	Qualitative DNA PCR is used to detect cell-associated proviral DNA, including HIV reservoirs in peripheral CD4 cells in patients responding to HAART with a sensitivity of about 5 copies/10^6 cells (*J Virol Methods* 2005;124:157). This is not considered sufficiently accurate for diagnosis without confirmation and is not FDA approved (*Ann Intern Med* 1996;124:803) although it is occasionally used with disputed or indeterminate serologic tests.
HIV RNA PCR	95% to 98%	False positive tests in 2% to 9%, usually at low titer (<10,000 c/mL). Sensitivity depends on viral load, threshold of assay, and status of antiretroviral therapy. Sensitivity approaches 100% with acute HIV infection; specificity is 97% but nearly 100% with viral load >10,000 c/mL.
p24 antigen	30% to 90%	Sometimes used as an alternative to HIV RNA test to detect acute HIV infection due to reduced cost. Specificity is 100%, but sensitivity is about 90% – less than quantitative HIV RNA tests (*Ann Intern Med* 2001;134:25). Another use is for a low cost viral load testing in resource limited countries (*J CLin Micro* 2005;43:506).

Quantitative Plasma HIV RNA (Viral Load)

TECHNIQUES (see Table 2-4, p. 13)

- **HIV RNA PCR** (*Amplicor HIV-1 Monitor Test* version 1.5, Roche; 800-526-1247).

- **Branched chain DNA or bDNA** (*Versant HIV-1 RNA 3.0 Assay*, Bayer; 800-434-2447.

- **Nucleic acid sequence-based amplification (NABSA)** or *NucliSens* HIV-1 QT (bioMérieux), 800-682-2666.

REPRODUCIBILITY: Commercially available assays vary based on the lower level of detection and dynamic ranges, as shown in Table 2-4 (*J Clin Microbiol* 1996;34:3016; *J Med Virol* 1996;50:293; *J Clin Microbiol* 1996;34:1058; *J Clin Microbiol* 1998;36:3392). Two standard deviations (95% confidence limits) with this assay are 0.3 to 0.5 $\log_{10}$ (2- to 3-fold) (*J Infect Dis* 1997;175:247; *AIDS* 1999;13:2269). This means that the 95% confidence limit for a value of 10,000 c/mL ranges from 3,100 to 32,000 c/mL. Quantitative results with the *Amplicor* (Roche) assay version 1.5 and bDNA assay (*Versant* 3.0) shows results that are comparable except at the low end of the linear range (<1,500 c/mL) (*J Clin Microbiol* 2000;38:2837; *J Clin Microbiol* 2000;38:1113). Comparative testing for the *NucliSens* (bioMérieux) assay is less extensive but appears comparable (*J Clin Microbiol* 2000;38:3882; *J Clin Microbiol* 2000;38:2837).

SUBTYPES: *Versant* 3.0 (Bayer) and *Amplicor* 1.5 (Roche) assays show reasonable accuracy, comparability, and reproducibility for subtypes A-G, although one comparative trial favored the bDNA (Bayer) assay (*J Acquir Immune Defic Syndr* 2002;29:330).

SEX DIFFERENCE: There appears to be a modest difference in viral load that averages 0.23 $\log_{10}$ c/mL (about 2-fold) lower in women compared with men according to a meta-analysis of 12 reports (*J Acquir Immune Defic Syndr* 2002;31:11). However, these differences disappear at CD4 counts <300 cells/mm^3 and are therefore unlikely to affect treatment decisions (*J Acquir Immune Defic Syndr* 2000;24:218; *J Infect Dis* 1999;180:666; *Clin Infect Dis* 2002;35:313; *Lancet* 1998;352:1510; *N Engl J Med* 2001;344:720).

COST: $100 to $150 per assay (Medicare reimbursement $111 to $130).

INDICATIONS: Quantitative HIV RNA is useful for diagnosing acute HIV infection, for predicting probability of transmission, predicting the rate of progression in chronically infected patients, and for therapeutic monitoring (*Ann Intern Med* 1995;122:573; *N Engl J Med* 1996;334:426; *J Infect Dis* 1997;175:247; *J Infect Dis* 2002;185:905).

- **Acute HIV infection:** Plasma HIV RNA is commonly used to disagnose the acute retroviral syndrome prior to seroconversion. Most studies show high levels of virus (10^5 to 10^6 c/mL). Note that 2% to 9% of persons without HIV infection have false-positive results, virtually always with low HIV RNA titers (<10,000 c/mL) (*Ann Intern Med* 1999;130:37; *J Clin Microbiol* 2000;38:2837; *Ann Intern Med* 2001;134:25). The alternative is the HIV p24 antigen assay, which is less expensive ($20 vs $100) and highly specific but only 89% sensitive (*Ann Intern Med* 2001;134:25).

- **Prognosis:** Viral load correlates with the rate of CD4 decline (CD4 slope) and serves as an important prognostic indicator in early stage disease (*J Infect Dis* 2002;185:908). The most comprehensive study to assess the association between viral load and natural history is the analysis of stored sera from the Multicenter AIDS Cohort Study (MACS), which showed a strong association between "set point" and rate of progression that was independent of the baseline CD4 count (*Ann Intern Med* 1995;122:573; *Science* 1996;272:1167; *J Infect Dis* 1996;174:696; *J Infect Dis* 1996;174:704; *AIDS* 1999;13: 1305; *N Engl J Med* 2001;349,720; *AIDS* 2002;16:2455; *Lancet* 2003;362:679; *J Acquir Immun Defic Syndr* 2005;38:289). Some studies show baseline viral load predicts long-term outcome with HAART (*J Infect Dis* 2003;188:1421), but this depends on the potency of the regimen (*J Infect Dis* 2004;190:280).

- **Risk of opportunistic infection:** The viral load appears to predict opportunistic infections independently of CD4 count when counts are <200 cells/mm³ (*JAMA* 1996;276:105; *AIDS* 1999;13:341; *AIDS* 1999;13:1035; *J Acquir Immune Defic Syndr* 2001;27:44). The only prospective study examining this association was ACTG 722, which showed that the failure to decrease viral load by ≥1 $\log_{10}$ c/mL in patients with a baseline CD4 count of <150 cells/mm³ increased the risk of an opportunistic infection 15-fold (*J Acquir Immune Defic Syndr* 2002;30:154). A retrospective review of over 12,000 patients showed CD4 counts were the best method to predict progression defined as an AIDS-defining complication (*Lancet* 2002;360:119), but the viral load (VL) predicts the rate of CD4 decline (*J Infect Dis* 2002;185:908).

- **Probability of transmission:** The probability of HIV transmission with nearly any type of exposure is directly correlated with viral load (*N Engl J Med* 2000;342:921; *J Acquir Immune Defic Syndr* 1996;12:427; *J Acquir Immune Defic Syndr* 1998;17:42; *J Acquir Immune Defic Syndr* 1999;21:120; *J Infect Dis* 2002;185:428; *Lancet* 2001;357:1149; *AIDS* 2001;15:621; *Clin Infect Dis* 2002;34:391).

- **Therapeutic monitoring:** Following initiation of therapy, there is a rapid initial decline in HIV RNA level over 1 to 4 weeks (alpha slope), reflecting activity against free plasma HIV virions and HIV in acutely infected CD4 cells. This is followed by a second decline (beta slope) that is longer in duration (months) and more modest in degree (see quantitation, below, under "Frequency and therapeutic monitoring"). The beta slope reflects activity against HIV infected macrophages and HIV released from other compartments, especially those trapped in follicular dendritic cells of lymph follicles. The maximum antiviral effect is expected by 4 to 6 months. Most authorities now believe that HIV RNA levels are the most important barometer of therapeutic response, although CD4 count best predicts clinical progression (*N Engl J Med* 1996;335:1091; *Ann Intern Med* 1996;124:984; *J Infect Dis* 2002;185:178). Important support for the long-term benefit of achieving a VL <50 c/mL are clonal sequence analyses showing no viral evolution with resistance mutations at that VL level (*J Infect Dis* 2004;189:1452; *J Infect Dis* 2004;189:1444).

- **Unexpectedly low viral load:** Aberrant results should be repeated. The RT-PCR assay (Roche) version 1.0 uses primers designed primarily for detection of clade B strains of HIV, but version 1.5 RT-PCR (Roche), bDNA (Bayer), and the *NucliSens* (bioMérieux) assay all quantitate the M subtypes A-G. None is accurate for the non-M subtypes (N or O) or HIV-2 strains (*J Acquir Immune Defic Syndr* 2003;33:1).

- **Reservoirs:** HIV resides in some anatomical sites that may be differently affected by antiretroviral drugs and may be the source of archived strains resistant to these drugs. The major sources are the latent CD4 cells; others are the CNS and genital tract (*AIDS* 2002;16:39; *J Clin Microbiol* 2000;38:1414).

RECOMMENDATIONS: Adapted from the International AIDS Society–USA (*JAMA* 2002;288:222) and DHHS Guidelines (*MMWR* 2002;51 [RR-7]:1; *Ann Intern Med* 2002;137:381).

- **Quality assurance:** Assays on individual patients should be obtained at times of clinical stability, at least 4 weeks after immunizations or intercurrent infections, and with use of the same lab and same technology over time.

- **Frequency and therapeutic monitoring:** Tests should be performed at baseline (x 2) and followed by routine testing at 3- to 4-month intervals according to guidelines from DHHS and IAS-USA (*Clin Infect Dis* 2001;33:1060). With new therapy and changes in therapy, assays should be obtained at 1 to 4 weeks (alpha slope), at 12 to 16 weeks, and at 16 to 24 weeks. An expected response to therapy is a decrease of 0.75-1.0 $\log_{10}$ c/mL at 1 week (*Lancet* 2001;358:1760; *J Acquir Immune Defic Syndr* 2002;30:167), a decrease of 1.5-2 $\log_{10}$ to <5,000 c/mL at 4 weeks (*J Acquir Immune Defic Syndr* 2000;25:36; *AIDS* 1999;13:1873; *J Acquir Immune Defic Syndr* 2004;37:1155), <500 c/mL at 8 to 16 weeks (*Ann Intern Med* 2001;135:945; *J Acquir Immune Defic Syndr* 2000;24:433), and <50 c/mL at 24-48 weeks. The 2003 Swiss guidelines define treatment failure by the failure to decrease VL by 1.5 log 10 c/ mL within 4 weeks or to achieve undetectable virus by 4 months (*Scand J Infect Dis* 2003;35:155). The time to viral load nadir is dependent on pretreatment viral load as well as potency of the regimen, adherence, pharmacology, and resistance. Patients with high baseline viral loads take longer to achieve suppression. Failure to reduce viral load by 1 $\log_{10}$ c/mL (90%) at 4 weeks suggests non-adherence, pre-existing resistance, or inadequate drug exposure, and failure to reduce viral load by 1 $\log_{10}$ c/mL at 8 weeks constitutes virologic failure according to the IAS-USA guidelines (*JAMA* 2002;288:228). The target of therapy is a viral load that is

2 Laboratory Tests

■ TABLE 2-5: **Comparison of FDA-approved Assay Methods for Viral Load**

	Roche	Bayer	bioMérieux
Contact	800-526-1247	800-434-2447	800-682-2666
Trade name	*Amplicor* HIV Monitor 1.5	*Versant* HIV-1 RNA 3.0	*NucliSens* HIV-1 QT
Technique	RT-PCR	bDNA	NASBA
Comparison of results	Results with the RT-PCR assay are similar to bDNA (*Versant*) results using version 2.0 or 3.0.	Results with are comparable with RT-PCR (*Amplicor*) assays.	Results appear comparable with RT-PCR and bDNA assays, but supporting data are less robust.
Advantages/ disadvantages	■ Fewer false-positives in patients without HIV infection compared with Bayer.	■ Technician time demands are less. ■ Good dynamic range, but higher threshold for no detectable virus.	■ May be used with tissue or body fluids such as genital secretions. ■ Greatest dynamic range.
Dynamic range	■ Standard: (*Amplicor* 1.5) 400 to 750,000 c/mL ■ Ultrasensitive: (*Ultra-Direct* 1.5) 50 to 100,000 c/mL	bDNA Version 3.0: 75 to 500,000 c/mL*	*NucliSens* HIV-1 QT: 176-3,500,000 c/mL depending on volume
Subtype amplified	■ Version 1.5: A to G	A to G	A to G
Specimen volume	■ *Amplicor*: 0.2 mL ■ Ultrasensitive: 0.5 mL	1 mL	10 μL to 2 mL
Tubes	EDTA (lavender top)	EDTA (lavender top)	EDTA, heparin, whole blood, any body fluid, PBMC, semen, tissue, etc.
Requirement	Separate plasma <6 hours and freeze prior to shipping at -20°C or -70°C.	Separate plasma <4 hours and freeze prior to shipping at -20°C or -70°C.	Separate serum or plasma <4 hours and freeze prior to shipping at -20°C or -70°C.

* The FDA-cleared lower threshold is 50 c/mL. Outside the U.S. the lower threshold is 50 c/mL.

undetectable, although some authorities claim this threshold to be unsupported by clinical trials (*Lancet* 1999;353:863; *JAMA* 2001; 285:777). An analysis of 13 cohorts with 9323 patients receiving initial HAART showed the viral load and CD4 count at 6 months was the most important predictor of clinical outcome (*Lancet* 2003; 362:679). It should be noted that even with "no detectable virus" as defined by viral load <20-50 c/mL, there is still ongoing viral replication in most patients (*JAMA* 1999;282:1627; *Nat Med* 1999;

Laboratory Tests

5:512). Nevertheless, patients who maintain viral loads <20-50 c/mL show no evidence of viral evolution with emergence of drug-resistant strains (*JAMA* 2001;286:196).

- **Interpretation:** Changes of ≥50% (0.3 $\log_{10}$ c/mL) are considered significant.

- **Factors not measured by viral load tests:** Immune function, CD4 regenerative reserve, susceptibility to antivirals, infectivity, syncytial vs nonsyncytial inducing forms, and viral load in compartments other than blood (e.g., lymph nodes, CNS, GI tract, and genital secretions).

- **Factors that increase viral load**
  - □ Switch from non-syncitium virus (RS trophic) to syncitium-inducing virus (x4 trophic).
  - □ Progressive disease
  - □ Failing antiretroviral therapy due to inadequate potency, inadequate drug levels, nonadherence, and resistance.
  - □ Active infections; active TB increases viral load 5- to 160-fold (*J Immunol* 1996;157:1271); pneumococcal pneumonia increases viral load 3- to 5-fold.
  - □ Immunizations such as influenza and *Pneumovax* (*Blood* 1995; 86:1082; *N Engl J Med* 1996;335:817; *N Engl J Med* 1996;334: 1222). Increases are modest and transient (2 to 4 weeks).

- **Falsely low viral loads:** 1) Non-B subtypes using the *Amplicor* (Roche) version 1.0, (*J Clin Microbiol* 2004;73:167), 2) HIV-2 infection, 3) Dual HIV-1 and HIV-2 infection, 4) Use of Amplicor v. 1.0 compared to v. 1.5 (*J Clin Microbiol* 2004;42:2819).

- **Relative merit of tests:** The *Versant* version 3.0 assay has good reproducibility for viral load levels of 75 to 500,000 c/mL. The linear range for *Amplicor* is 50 to 100,000 c/mL for the ultrasensitive test. It should not be used in patients expected to have higher viral loads (*J Clin Microbiol* 2000;38:2837). The *NucliSens* assay has a broad dynamic range (176 to 3,500,000 c/mL) and can be used for HIV quantification on blood or on various body fluids or tissue such as seminal fluid, CSF, breast milk, saliva, and vaginal fluid (*J Clin Microbiol* 2000;38:1414).

CD4 Cell Count

This is a standard test to assess prognosis for progression to AIDS or death, to formulate the differential diagnosis in a symptomatic patient (Table 1-1, p. 2), and to make therapeutic decisions regarding antiviral treatment and prophylaxis for opportunistic pathogens. It is the most reliable indicator of prognosis (*Ann Intern Med* 1997;126:946; *Lancet* 2002;360:119; *Lancet* 2003;362:679). CD8 cell counts have not been found to predict outcome (*N Engl J Med* 1990;322:166); HIV-specific CD8 cells (CD38 cells) are important for controlling HIV levels but

Laboratory Tests

2

cannot be routinely measured (*Science* 1999;283:857; *J Acquir Immune Defic Syndr* 2002;29:346).

Technique: The standard method for determining CD4 count uses flow cytometers and hematology analyzers that are expensive, require fresh blood (<18 hours old), and generally cost $50 to $150. An alternative system that uses EIA technology is the *TRAX* CD4 Test Kit (*J Acquir Immune Defic Syndr* 1995;10:522). This may be attractive in resource-limited areas, although most clinicians who do not have access to CD4 counts will probably use total T-lymphocyte counts (TLC) (*Scaling Up Antiretroviral Therapy in Resource Limited Settings*, WHO, 2002).

Normal Values: Normal values for most laboratories are a mean of 800 to 1050 cells/mm³, with a range representing two standard deviations of approximately 500 to 1400 cells/mm³ (*Ann Intern Med* 1993;119:55).

Frequency of Testing: The CD4 count should be repeated every 3 to 6 months in untreated patients and at 2 to 4 month intervals in patients on antiretroviral therapy (*Clin Infect Dis* 2001;33:1060; *JAMA* 2002;288:222; *Ann Intern Med* 2002;137:381). The test should be repeated when results are inconsistent with prior trends. Frequency will vary with individual circumstances. In the absence of therapy, the average rate of CD4 decline is 4% per year for each log_{10} HIV RNA c/mL (*J Infect Dis* 2002;185:905). With initial therapy or a change in therapy, the recommendation is that CD4 counts (and viral load) be measured at 4, 8 to 12, and 16 to 24 weeks (IAS-USA guidelines, *JAMA* 2002;288:228).

Reproducibility: Both clinicians and patients must be aware of the variability in CD4 test results, especially if they will be used to make clinical decisions, such as initiation of antiretroviral therapy or opportunistic infection prophylaxis. The 95% confidence range for a true count of 200 cells/mm³, for example, is 118-337 cells/mm³ (*J Acquir Immune Defic Syndr* 1993;6:537). Results that are inconsistent with prior trends should be repeated.

Factors that Influence CD4 Cell Counts: Factors include analytical variation, seasonal and diurnal variations, some intercurrent illnesses, and corticosteroids. Substantial analytical variations, which account for the wide range in normal values (usually about 500 to 1400 cells/mm³), reflect the fact that the CD4 cell count is the product of three variables: the white blood cell count, percent lymphocytes, and the percent CD4 cells (cells that bear the CD4 receptor). There are also seasonal changes (*Clin Exp Immunol* 1991;86:349) and diurnal changes, with the lowest levels at 12:30 PM and peak values at 8:30 PM (*J Acquir Immune*

Defic Syndr 1990;3:144); these variations do not clearly correspond to the circadian rhythm of corticosteroids. Modest decreases in the CD4 cell count have been noted with some acute infections and with major surgery. Corticosteroid administration may have a profound effect, with decreases from 900 cells/mm³ to less than 300 cells/mm³ with acute administration; chronic administration has a less pronounced effect (*Clin Immunol Immunopathol* 1983;28:101). Acute changes are probably due to a redistribution of leukocytes between the peripheral circulation and the marrow, spleen, and lymph nodes (*Clin Exp Immunol* 1990;80:460).

Deceptively high CD4 counts may occur with HTLV-1 co-infection or splenectomy. HTLV-1 is closely related to HTLV-2, and most serologic assays do not distinguish between the two, but only HTLV-1 causes deceptively high CD4 cell counts. Serologic studies in the United States show HTLV-1/2 infection rates of 7% to 12% in injection drug users and 2% to 10% in commercial sex workers (*N Engl J Med* 1990;326:375; *JAMA* 1990;263:60); 80% to 90% of these are HTLV-2 in both populations. High rates of concurrent HIV and HTLV-1 have been reported in Brazil (*JAMA* 1994;271:353) and Haiti (*J Clin Microbiol* 1995;33:1735). Analysis of patients with co-infection suggests that CD4 counts are 80% to 180% higher than in controls for comparable levels of immunosuppression (*JAMA* 1994;271:353). Splenectomy results in a prompt, sustained increase in CD4 count. The CD4 percentage more accurately reflects immunocompetence (*Clin Infect Dis* 1995;20:768; *Arch Surg* 1998;133:25).

The following have minimal effect on the CD4 cell count: gender, age in adults, risk category, psychological stress, physical stress, and pregnancy (*Ann Intern Med* 1993;119:55).

CD4 Count Percentage: The CD4 cell percentage is sometimes used in preference to the absolute number because this reduces the variation to a single measurement (*J Acquir Immune Defic Syndr* 1989;2:114). In the AIDS Clinical Trial Group (ACTG) laboratories, the within-subject coefficient of variation for percent CD4 was 18% compared with 25% for the CD4 count (*J Infect Dis* 1994;169:28). Data from a large observational database suggested that the CD4 count is the most useful predictor of the risk for development of opportunistic infections (*J Acquir Immune Defic Syndr* 2004;36:1028). Corresponding CD4 cell counts and percentages are provided in the table below.

■ TABLE 2-6: **Approximate CD4/CD4% Equivalents**

CD4 Cell Count	% CD4
>500/mm³	>29%
200 to 500/mm³	14% to 28%
<200/mm³	<14%

2 Laboratory Tests

21

Response to HAART: The CD4 count typically increases ≥50 cells/mm³ at 4 to 8 weeks after viral suppression with HAART and then increases an additional 50-100 cells/mm³/year thereafter (*JAMA* 2002;288:222; *J Infect Dis* 2002;185:471; *AIDS* 2001;15:735). Factors that correlate with good response include high baseline VL and low baseline CD4 count (*J Infect Dis* 2004;190:1860). Despite good virological response, there may be an initial delay in CD4 response that cannot be explained (*JAMA* 2002;288:222). The CD4 response generally correlates with viral load suppression, but discordant results are common (*J Infect Dis* 2001;183:1328). Nevertheless, population-based studies show the most important factor in CD4 response to HAART is the duration of virologic control (*J Infect Dis* 2004;190:148). The CD4 count usually declines rapidly, up to 100-150 cells/mm³ in 3 to 4 months, when therapy is discontinued (*Clin Infect Dis* 2001;33:344; *Clin Infect Dis* 2001;32:1231; *N Engl J Med* 2003;349:837). This decrease may be seen with or without antecedent viral suppression and is ascribed either to reduced replication capacity due to resistant mutations (*N Engl J Med* 2003;349:837) or to loss of partial antiviral activity despite resistance.

Total Lymphocyte Count (TLC): The TLC is sometimes used as a surrogate for CD4 count in resource limited areas (*JAMA* 1993;269:622; *Am J Med Sci* 1992;304:79). TLC of <1200/mm³ combined with clinical symptoms is recommended as a surrogate for a CD4 count of <200 cells/mm³ as an indication for antiretroviral therapy in the DHHS guidelines (*Scaling Up Antiretroviral Therapy in Resource Limited Settings*, WHO, 2003). The addition of a hemoglobin ≤12 g/dL improves the sensitivity of detecting CD4 counts <200/mm³ when the TLC is 1200-2000/mm³ (*AIDS* 2003;17:1311).

CD4 Repertoire: Progressive immunodeficiency in HIV infection is associated with both quantitative and qualitative changes in CD4 cells. The two major categories of CD4 cells are naïve cells and memory cells. In early life, all cells are naïve and express the isoform of CD45RA⁺. Memory cells (CD45RA⁻) represent the component of the T-cell repertoire that has been activated by exposure to antigens. These are the CD4 cells with specificity for most opportunistic infections, such as *P. carinii*, cytomegalovirus, and *Toxoplasma gondii*. It is the depletion of these cells that accounts for the inability to respond to recall antigens, a defect noted relatively early in the course of HIV infection. Studies of HIV infected patients show a preferential decline in naïve cells. With HAART, there is a three-phase component to the CD4 rebound. The initial increase is due primarily to redistribution of CD4 cells from lymphatic sites. The second phase is characterized by an influx of CD4 memory cells with reduced T-cell activation and improved response to recall antigens. In the third phase there is an increase in naïve cells following at least 12 weeks of HAART (*Nat Med*

Laboratory Tests

1997;5:533; *Science* 1997;277:112). By 6 months the CD4 repertoire is diverse. The competence of these cells is evidenced by favorable control of selected chronic infections such as cryptosporidiosis, microsporidiosis, and molluscum contagiosum, the ability to discontinue maintenance therapy for disseminated MAC and CMV, and the ability to safely discontinue primary prophylaxis for PCP and MAC in responders. Nevertheless, some patients with immune reconstitution have deficits in CTL responses to specific antigens that may result in PCP or relapses in CMV retinitis despite CD4 counts >300 cells/mm^3 (*J Infect Dis* 2001;183:1285).

Idiopathic CD4 Lymphocytopenia (ICL): Idiopathic CD4 lymphocytopenia (ICL) is a syndrome characterized by a low CD4 cell count that is unexplained by HIV infection or other medical conditions. Case definition criteria include: 1) CD4 less than 300 cells/mm^3 or a CD4 percent less than 20% on two or more measurements; 2) lack of laboratory evidence of HIV infection; and 3) absence of alternative explanation for the CD4 cell lymphocytopenia including Sjogrens Syndrome, sarcoid, radiation, atopic dermatitis, collagen vascular disease, steroid therapy, or lymphoma. Transient, unexplained decreases in CD4 cells may occur in healthy persons (*Chest* 1994;105:1335; *Eur J Med* 1993;2:509; *Am J Med Sci* 1996;312:240). One study of 430 HIV negative TB patients showed 62 (14%) had ICL (*J Infect Dis* 2000;41:167). The CDC receives notice of about one ICL case/month (Dr. T.J. Spira, personal communication). Conclusions from the experience with patients having ICL are: 1) They lack risk factors for HIV infection; 2) There is no evidence of an infectious agent based on clustering or contact evaluations; 3) They have fewer OIs than AIDS patients for a given CD4 level; 4) The predominant OIs associated with ICL are cryptococcosis, molluscum, and histoplasmosis – infections with *P. jiroveci*, *Candida*, and HHV-8 [KS] are unusual; 5) Their CD4 counts tend to remain stable, and their prognosis is relatively good; 6) Recommended prophylaxis is TMP-SMX with persistent counts <200/mm^3; and 7) Treatment of ICL has included IL-2 and gamma interferon, but the experience is very limited (*Lancet* 1992;340:273; *N Engl J Med* 1993;328:373; *N Engl J Med* 1993;328:380; *N Engl J Med* 1993;328:386; *N Engl J Med* 1993;328:393; *Clin Exp Immunol* 1999;116:322; *Clin Infect Dis* 2000:3:E20; *Clin Infect Dis* 2001;33:E125). Cases of this syndrome should be reported to local/state health departments rather than reported directly to the CDC as originally advocated.

Resistance Testing (see *N Engl J Med* 2004;350:1023)

The prevalence of ≥1 major resistance mutation in patients receiving antiretroviral therapy is about 50% (*Lancet* 2002;359:49; *Nature Med* 2001;7:1016). The frequency of ≥1 major resistance mutation in treatment-naïve, recently infected patients is 10-25% (*Nat Med* 2001;

Laboratory Tests

2

7:1016; *Br Med J* 2001;322:1087; *AIDS* 2001;15:601; *JAMA* 2002;288: 181; *N Engl J Med* 2002;347:385). These observations have made resistance testing an increasingly important component of HIV care, but many feel that both the technology and the interpretation still need substantial improvement. The limitations include the following:

- Resistance assays measure only dominant species at the time the test is performed; resistant variants that account for <20% of the total viral population in blood and species in "sequestered havens" (CNS, latent CD4 cells, genital tract, etc.) are not detected.

- There must be a sufficient viral load to perform the test, usually ≥500 to 1,000 c/mL.

- Genotypic assays are often difficult to interpret because multiple mutations are required for drug resistance for antiretroviral agents other than 3TC and non-nucleoside reverse transcriptase inhibitors (NNRTIs).

- Phenotypic assays may be difficult to interpret due to the arbitrary thresholds used to define susceptibility, particularly for some RTV-boosted regimens, and they are also less sensitive at detecting emerging resistance.

- Clinical trials with resistance tests compared with "standard care" for selection of salvage regimens have shown variable results (*AIDS* 2002;16:579; *AIDS* 2002;16:209; *Antivir Ther* 2000;5[suppl 3]:78; *AIDS* 2000;14:F83; *J Infect Dis* 2001;183:401).

As a result of these limitations, the following conclusions can be drawn:

- **Resistance testing most reliably identifies drugs that should be avoided** but is less reliable at detecting the drugs that are most likely to be active.

- **Testing is most reliable for indicating activity of drugs being given or recently given,** because discontinuation of therapy eventually results in the reemergence and proliferation of wild-type virus. The time required for reappearance of wild-type virus after discontinuation of antiretrovirals appears to be longer than previously thought. For example, S. Little et al showed persistence of K103N, TAMS, and PI mutations for up to 1 year after acute HIV infection without therapy (11th CROI, San Francisco, Feb. 2004, Abstr 36 LB). Nevertheless, usual recommendation is that resistance testing should be performed while the patient is on therapy or within 2 to 3 weeks of stopping.

- **Interpretation of results in patients who have received prior antiretroviral agents is difficult**, which may account for variations in clinical trials. The problem is failure to detect "archived strains" or "minority species." Thus, prior drug history and outcome are important factors in regimen selection. This was shown in ACTG 398, in which EFV-experienced patients failed EFV therapy. Routine resistance tests at baseline showed EFV was active but single genome sequencing revealed resistance in minority species (*Antivir Ther* 2003;8:S150).

- **A viral load of 500 to 1,000 c/mL is usually required.**
- **There is a general preference** for genotypic resistance, at least for the initial virologic failures. This is based on better clinical trial results and reduced price. The relative merits of the available assays are discussed below ("Test Methods").
- **Expert interpretation improves results.**

Indications for Resistance Testing

DHHS Guidelines (http://www.aidsinfo.nih.gov/guidelines, Oct. 29, 2004; and IAS-USA Guidelines (http://www.iasusa.org; *JAMA* 2004;292:251; *Top HIV Med* 2004;12:119; *Antivir Ther* 2004;9:829)

CHRONICALLY INFECTED PATIENT WITH VIROLOGIC FAILURE
(Recommended by virtually all guidelines – see Table 2-7)

Most guidelines make the following recommendation for resistance testing for chronically infected patients receiving ART who meet one of the following criteria:

- Failure to decrease viral load >0.5 to 0.7 $\log_{10}$ c/mL by 4 weeks.
- Failure to decrease viral load >1 $\log_{10}$ c/mL by 8 weeks.
- Viral load >1000 c/mL after 16 to 24 weeks.

■ TABLE 2-7: **Comparison of Recommendations for Resistance Testing (*J Acquir Immune Defic Syndr* 2001;26:551)**

Category	British HIV Assoc.**	European Assoc.*	IAS-USA[†]	USA-DHHS[‡]
Acute HIV (within 6-12 months of transmission)	Recommend	Recommend	Recommend	Recommend
Chronic HIV				
Rx naïve and chronically infected	Recommend	Consider	If infected <1 yr	Consider
Virologic failure	Recommend	Recommend	Recommend	Recommend
Pregnancy	Recommend	Recommend	Recommend	Only for above indications

* *AIDS* 2001;15:309
** *HIV Med* 2003;4 Suppl:1
[†] *Antivir Ther* 2004;9:829
[‡] http://www.aidsinfo.nih.gov, Oct. 2005

EVALUATION: A meta-analysis of published reports and conference presentations through February 2001 compared virologic results at 3 to 6 months after using resistance testing vs clinician decision or standard

Laboratory Tests

2

of care (SOC) for salvage regimens (*HIV Clin Trials* 2002;3:1). For genotypic analysis, there was a modest but statistically significant benefit with genotypic testing. Results were significantly better with expert interpretation of the resistance assay. There was no significant benefit with phenotypic resistance testing compared with SOC (although the analyses were done prior to currently accepted thresholds to define resistance). Results for viral suppression at 6 months after regimen change based on aggregate data for genotypic analysis vs SOC were genotype 168/432 (39%) vs SOC 115/400 (29%). Many studies showed only short-term benefit (*AIDS* 2002;16:369). An exception is the NARVL analysis with a mean follow-up of 600 days; there was no benefit with either genotypic or phenotypic tests vs no tests in terms of virologic control after failure, but there was a cost benefit in the rescue regimen selected (*Clin Infect Dis* 2004;38:723). Possibly the most important studies of the value of resistance testing with therapeutic failure was TORO 1 and TORO 2 (*N Engl J Med* 2003; 348:2175 and 2293). These studies showed that the optimal regimen in 334 patients with virologic failure resulted in a median viral load decrease of 0.8 $\log_{10}$ c/mL and a median CD4 increase of 32-38/mm^3.

Conclusions of the IAS-USA are: 1) there is at least short term benefit with both phenotypic and genotypic testing; but it is hard to show; 2) evidence of benefit is strongest for genotypic testing; and 3) expert interpretation notably improves results (*Clin Infect Dis* 2003;17:37).

The currently available tests are standardized for clade B strains; utility for the other clades is not known (*Scand J Infect Dis* 2003;35[Suppl 106]:75).

RESISTANCE TESTING IN OTHER SETTINGS

- **Primary HIV infection (advocated in most guidelines):** Studies of HIV resistance with acute HIV infection in untreated patients show substantial variation in results over time and geographic area. In the US the rates of resistance, increased rapidly in the late 1990s, and then stabilized. The largest study is the report by S. Little et al of 377 patients in the U.S. with acute HIV, with samples taken from 1995 to 2000. The rate of resistance by phenotypic analysis (IC50 <10x wild-type) to ≥1 agent was 3.4% for 1995-98 compared to 12.4% for 1999-2000. Genotypic analysis of these strains showed the most common resistance mutations on the RT gene were at codons 103, 118, 184 and 215; for the protease gene it was codons 82 and 90 (*N Engl J Med* 2002;347:385). The greatest increase by class during the 5-year study was NNRTIs, which increased from 1.9% to 7.1%. More recent studies by S. Little et al have shown no substantial increase in resistance with recent HIV infection in the U.S. (*Antivir Ther* 2002;7:S188). Other reports show rates of resistance to at least one class of drug in 10-12% of recently infected persons. This rate has stabilized; similar results are reported from North America and Europe (Table 2-8).

■ TABLE 2-8: **Results of Resistance Tests in Patients with Acute or Recent HIV Infection**

Study	Citation	N	Yr.	Result
10 U.S. cities	N Engl J Med 2002;347:385	377	1995-2000	Phenotypic resistance 1995-98: 3.1%; 1999-00: 8.4%
Swiss cohort	AIDS 2001;15:2287	197	1999-2001	1996: 8.6%; 1997: 14.6%; 1998: 8.8%; 2000: 5%
CATCH (16 European cities)	IAS, Paris, 2003 Abstract LB-1	596	1996-2002	1996-98: 14.5% 2001-02: 9.5%
CDC 10 U.S. cities	Antivir Ther 2002;8:S133	182	1997-2002	12%
Switzerland	11th CROI 2003, Abstract 680	453	1996-2002	11%
France	Antivir Ther 2002;8:S137	296	2001-2002	11%
Montreal	Antivir Ther 2002;8:S136	170	1996-2003	12%
England	Antivir Ther 2002;8:S138	157	1996-2003	17%

■ **Chronically infected treatment-naïve patients:** There is an increasing trend toward routine resistance testing in treatment-naïve, chronically infected patients prior to initiation of HAART. Multiple studies of this practice show the frequency of resistance to at least one drug or class of drug is 5-7%, based on five reports for an aggregate total of 4012 patients studied in 1996-2003 (Antivir Ther 2003;8:S122, S133, S136, S137 and S138). Nevertheless, there is concern about the validity of these tests for initial testing, and guidelines generally recommend them only within 1-2 years of the acute infection. The concern is that the resistant strains are often minority species and consequently undetected in the absence of selective pressure of antiviral agents. Nevertheless, some resistance mutations have been found to persist ≥2 years, especially the K103N mutation conferring NNRTI resistance (N Engl J Med 2002;347:385). IAS-USA guidelines recommend testing within 12 months of transmission if the duration of infection is known (Clin Infect Dis 2003;17:113). Recommendations of the Primary Care Guidelines, IDSA (Clin Infect Dis 2004;39:609) are for testing if the patient is to be treated and has been infected <2 years "and perhaps longer." For patients with a longer duration of infection, an alternative strategy is to test after 4-6 weeks of therapy if virologic goals are not achieved, since this allows sufficient time to select minority species (Topics in HIV Med 2003;11:150). The IAS-USA recommendation is to perform this test at 8-12 weeks of the initial regimen (Clin Infect Dis 2003;17:113).

■ **Pregnancy:** Some guidelines recommend routine resistance tests for pregnant women, although the rationale, beyond the indications cited above, is unclear (Table 2-7).

Laboratory Tests

2

Test Methods: There are two types of tests, genotypic and phenotypic assays. These are compared in Table 2-9, p. 29 (*J Antimicrob Chemother* 2004;53:555).

GENOTYPIC ASSAYS: Genotype analysis identifies mutations associated with phenotypic resistance. Testing may be performed using commercial kits or "home brews." There is 98% concordance when two commercial kits are tested by the same laboratory (*Antivir Therapy* 2000;5 suppl 4:60; *Antivir Therapy* 2000; suppl 3:53). Another study showed 0.3% frequency of false positive results and a 6.4% frequency of false negative results (*Antivir Therapy* 2001;6 suppl 1:1). Assays vary in cost, number of mutations tested, and method of reporting and interpretations of results. The methodology involves: 1) Amplification of the reverse transcriptase (RT) and protease (Pr) gene, by RT PCR. 2) DNA sequencing of amplicons generated for the dominant species (mutations are limited to those present in >20% of plasma virions). 3) Reporting of mutations for each gene using a letter-number-letter standard, in which the first letter indicates the amino acid at the designated codon with wild type virus, the number is the codon position, and the second letter indicates the amino acid substituted in the mutation. Thus, the RT mutation K103N indicates that asparagine (N) has replaced lysine (K) on codon 103. Table 2-9 (p. 29) shows the amino acids and corresponding letter codes used to describe mutations in genotype analyses. Interpretation is based on judgement using lists of drug resistance mutations or computerized rules-based algorithms. Updated information on resistance testing can be obtained at http://www.iasusa.org or http://hivdb.stanford.edu.

PHENOTYPIC ASSAYS: Phenotype analysis measures the ability of HIV to replicate at different concentrations of tested drugs. It is available from three commercial labs, which show generally good concordance when compared (*Antivir Therapy* 2001;6 suppl 1:129; *Antivir Therapy* 2000;5 suppl 3:49). The test involves insertion of the RT and protease genes from the patient's strain into a backbone laboratory clone by cloning or recombination. Replication is monitored at various drug concentrations and compared with a reference wild type virus. This assay is comparable with conventional *in vitro* tests of antimicrobial sensitivity, in which the microbe is grown in serial dilutions of antiviral agents. Results are reported as the IC_{50} for the test strain relative to that of a reference or wild-type strain. The interpretation was previously based on interassay variation of control, but current interpretations use either biologic thresholds based on the normal distribution of wild-type virus from untreated patients or, for some drugs, clinical thresholds based on data from clinical trials.

VIRTUAL PHENOTYPE: This is a prediction of the phenotype of the test strain based on genotypic analysis. The mutational pattern of the test strain is compared with results of phenotypic assay using strains

28

showing similar mutations from a databank of >55,000 HIV isolates. Lack of sufficient paired genotype and phenotype assays in the database preclude results in about 20% (*Antivir Therapy* 2003;8:S103).

RELATIVE MERITS: Genotypic resistance tests are generally preferred for baseline (pretreatment) testing and with first and second failures. The rationale is that clinical trial data show better outcomes in this setting when compared to the standard of care (GART [*AIDS* 2000;14:F83], VIRADAPT [*Lancet* 1999;353:2195]; HAVANA [*AIDS* 2002;16:209]) or when compared to phenotypic testing (REALVIRFEN [*Antivir Ther* 2003;8:577]; NARVAL [*Antivir Ther* 2003;8:427]). Genotypic testing is also less expensive and appears cost-effective when used for first or second regimen failures (*Ann Intern Med* 2001;134:440; *J Acquir Immune Defic Syndr* 2000;24:227). Phenotype resistance may be preferred or may supplement genotypic test results in patients with multiple regimen failures (CERT [*Clin Infect Dis* 2004;38:723] and TORO [*N Engl J Med* 2003;348:2175]).

■ TABLE 2-9: **Comparison of Genotypic and Phenotypic Assays**

Genotypic Assays	
Advantages	**Disadvantages**
■ Less expensive ($300 to $480/test). ■ Short turn-around of 1 to 2 weeks. ■ Well standardized ■ Good reproducibility ■ Possibility of virtual phenotype* ■ More sensitive for detection of emerging resistance (mixtures) ■ Favored in comparative studies with first or second regimens that fail.	■ Detect resistance only in dominant species (>20%). ■ Interpretation requires expertise. ■ Technician experience influences results. ■ All resistance mutations are not known. ■ May show discrepancy with phenotype. ■ Requires viral load >1000 c/mL.
Phenotypic Assays	
■ Interpretation more straightforward and familiar. ■ Assesses total effect, including mutational interactions. ■ Does not require data on genotypic correlates of resistance (advantageous with newer agents). ■ Reproducibility is good. ■ Advantage over genotype when there are multiple mutations. ■ Provides drug levels necessary to treat resistant virus.	■ More expensive (usually $800 to $1000). High cost may affect reimbursement. ■ Report takes longer than genotypic assay. ■ Clinically determined thresholds not available for all drugs and PI thresholds do not always account for ritonavir boosting. ■ Detects resistance only to single drug, not combinations. ■ Detect resistance only in dominant species (>20%). ■ Require viral load >500-1000 c/mL.

Virtual phenotype is rapid, easily done, and less expensive than phenotypic assays; disadvantages are inability to perform when database is inadequate.

Laboratory Tests

2

■ TABLE 2-10: **Letter Designations for Amino Acids***

A	Alanine	I	Isoleucine	R	Arginine
C	Cytosine	K	Lysine	S	Serine
D	Aspartic acid	L	Leucine	T	Threonine
E	Glutamic acid	M	Methionine	V	Valine
F	Phenylalanine	N	Asparagine	W	Tryptophan
G	Glycine	P	Proline	Y	Tyrosine
H	Histidine	Q	Glutamine		

* Amino acids and corresponding single-letter codes used in describing genotypes.

■ TABLE 2-11: **Resistance Mutations Adapted From IAS-USA (*Top HIV Med* 2004:12:251). Updated at http://www.iasusa.org (accessed April 1, 2005). Also see: http://hivdb.stanford.edu/pages/seqAnalysis.html**

Drug	Codon Mutations*	Comment
Nucleosides and Nucleotides		
AZT	41L, 44D, 67N, 70R, 118I, 210W, 215YF, 219QE	Mutations are "TAMs" – reduce susceptibility to AZT, d4T, ABC, ddI, ddC, TDF, 3TC; TAMs infrequently coexist with 65R; most frequent TAMS are 41L, 210W and 215Y.
d4T‡	41L, 44D, 65R, 67N, 70R, 118I, 210W, 215YF, 219QE	The d4T-specific mutation at 75 and confers low level d4T resistance.
3TC	44D, 65R, 118I, 184VI	184 – high level 3TC resistance, increases activity of d4T, AZT, and TDF but clinical significance is unknown and it can be overcome by TAMs. Reduces susceptibility to ddI, ddC, ABC, though not clinically significant with M184V alone. 44D and 118I are not selected by 3TC, but they confer moderate 3TC resistance.
FTC	65R, 184VI	Similar or identical to 3TC
ddC	65R, 69D, 74V, 184V	
ddI	65R, 74V	Presence of 74 or 65 alone or combined with TAMs is associated with resistance to ddI.
ABC‡	65R, 74V, 115F, 184V	Resistance depends on number of TAMs ± M184V; 184 alone does not confer resistance. Presence of M184V plus ≥3-4 TAMs associated with ABC resistance.
TDF	65R	Reduced activity with K65R and resistance with 69 insertion.
Multinucleoside resistance – A-Q151M complex	62V, 75I, 77L, 116Y, 151M	Occurs with or without TAMs. Confers resistance to all NRTIs but not to tenofovir.

Drug	Codon Mutations*	Comment
Nucleosides and Nucleotides		
Multinucleoside resistance – 69 insertion	41L, 62V, 67N, 69 insert, 70R, 210W, 215YF, 219QE	Confers resistance to all NRTIs and TDF but not to DAPD.
Multinucleoside resistance – Multiple TAMs	41L, 44D, 67N, 70R, 118I, 210W, 215YF, 219QE	Confer resistance to all NRTI including TDF. AZT and d4T select for TAMS.
Non-nucleoside Reverse Transcriptase Inhibitors (NNRTIs)		
NVP	100I, 103N, 106AM, 108I, 181CI, 188CLH, 190A	Y181C is favored mutation with NVP, unless combined with AZT, in which case K103N is favored.
DLV	103N, 106M, 181C, 188L, 236L	
EFV	100I, 103N, 106M, 108I, 181CI, 188L, 190SA, 225H	181 CI is not selected, but its presence contributes to low-level cross resistance. Resistance with 188L but not 188C or 188H 108 and 225.
Multi-NNRTI resistance	103N, 106M, 188L	Either mutation substantially reduces activity of all NNRTIs.
Multi-NNRTI resistance accumulation	100I, 106A, 181CI, 190SA, 230L	≥2 of these mutations substantially reduces activity of all NNRTIs. The 106M mutation is found only in clade C HIV.

Drug	Major†	Minor‡	Comment
Protease Inhibitors (PIs)			
IDV	46IL, 82AFT, 84V	10IRV, 20MR, 24I, 32I, 36I, 54VI, 71VI, 73SA, 77I, 90M	At least 3 mutations required for resistance (>4x decrease in susceptibility).
NFV	30N, 90M	10FI, 36I, 46IL, 71VT, 77I, 82AFTS, 84V, 88DS	D30N most common mutation: No PI cross-resistance. L90M occurs in some, leading to greater PI cross-resistance.
RTV	82AFTS, 84V	10FIRV, 20MR, 32I, 33F, 36I, 46IL, 54VL, 71VT, 77I, 90M	Cross resistance with IDV common.
SQV	48V, 90M	10IRV, 54VL, 71VT, 73S, 77I, 82A, 84V	90 develops 1st, then 48; Codon 48 mutation unique, but L90M contributes to PI cross-resistance.
APV and FPV	50V, 82A, 84V	10FIRV, 32I, 46IL, 47V, 54LVM, 73S, 90M	I50V is associated with cross-resistance to LPV.
LPV/r		10FIRV, 20MR, 24I, 32I, 33F, 46IL, 47VA, 50V, 53L, 54VLAMTS, 63P, 71VT, 73S, 82AFTS, 84V, 90M	Major and minor mutations have not been determined. ≥6 mutations cause reduced response; the number may be as low as 4. I50V (selected by APV) decreases LPV susceptibility.

(continued)

Laboratory Tests

2

Drug	Major[†]	Minor[‡]	Comment
Protease Inhibitors (PIs)			
ATV	50L	10IFV, 20RMI, 24I, 32I, 33IF, 36ILV, 46I, 48V, 54V, 71V, 73CSTA, 82A, 84V, 88S, 90M	Selects for 50L and 71 when initial PI; in PI experienced patients selects for 54 and 84
TPV	33IF, 82AFLT, 84V	10IV, 20MLT, 46I, 54V	
Multi-PI resistance	46IL, 82AFTS, 84V, 90M	10FIRV, 32I, 54VML	≥4 usually cause multiple PI resistance.
Fusion Inhibitors			
Enfuvirtide (T20)		36DS, 37V, 39R, 42T, 43D	Resistance in the gp41 envelope gene at positions 36-45.

* The distinction between primary and secondary mutations has been eliminated for NRTIs NNRTIs by the International AIDS Society Expert Committee; this distinction has been retained for PIs, but with the terms "Major" or "Minor."

[†] **Major mutations** develop first or are associated with decreased drug binding or reduced viral activity; these effect phenotype resistance.

[‡] **Minor mutations** appear later and, by themselves, do not significantly change phenotype resistance.

Mutation Category	Mutation	Comment
Thymidine analog mutations (TAMs)	M41L, D67N/G, K70R, L210W, T215F/Y, K219E/Q/N	Selected by thymidine analogs (AZT, d4T) but cause resistance to all NRTIs. 41L/210W/215Y pattern more common and causes higher-level NRTI resistance than 67N/70R/219. T215C/D/E/S/I/V are "revertants" that typically indicate "back mutations" after initial infection with NRTI-resistant virus. Revertants do not cause resistance themselves, but may indicate presence of resistant virus.
Accessory mutations	E44D, VI118I	Contribute to NRTI resistance when accompanied by multiple TAMs.
Non-TAM nucleoside analog mutation	K65R	Selected by TDF, ABC, ddI. Causes variable decrease in susceptibility to those drugs and to 3TC/FTC, but hypersusceptibility to AZT. Rarely occurs in patients on AZT-containing regimens or in setting of TAMs. d4T susceptibility maintained, though selection by d4T can occur.
Non-TAM nucleoside analog mutation	L74V	Selected by ABC, ddI. (L74V more common than K65R with ABC/3TC-containing regimens). Causes variable decrease in susceptibility to ABC and ddI, but hypersusceptibility to AZT, TDF. Rarely occurs in patients on AZT-containing regimens or in setting of TAMs.
3TC/FTC resistance mutation	M184V	Selected by 3TC, FTC. Causes high-level resistance to both drugs and modest decrease in susceptibility to ABC, ddI (not clinically significant when present alone). Increases susceptibility to AZT, d4T, TDF. Delays emergence of TAMs in thymidine analog-containing regimens.
Multi-nucleoside resistance mutations	T69 insertion	Selected by thymidine analogs, but rare in HAART era, especially with 3TC- or FTC-containing regimens. Causes high-level resistance to all NRTIs and TDF.
Multi-nucleoside resistance mutations	Q151M complex	Selected by thymidine analogs, but rare in HAART era, especially with 3TC- or FTC-containing regimens. Causes high-level resistance to all NRTIs when combined V75I, F77L, F116Y. TDF may retain activity.
d4T mutation	V75T/M/A	Selected by d4T *in vitro* and results in decreased d4T susceptibility, but uncommon with clinical use of d4T.
ABC mutation	Y115F	Selected by ABC, resulting in ~3-fold decrease in ABC susceptibility.

Laboratory Tests

2

■ TABLE 2-13: **Non-nucleoside Reverse Transcriptase Inhinitor (NNRTI) Resistance Mutations by Category**

Mutation	Comment
A98G	Selected by NVP (uncommon), resulting in minimal decrease in NVP susceptibility.
L100I	Usually occurs with K103N, resulting in further loss of NNRTI susceptibility.
K101E/P	**K101E:** Selected by NVP and EFV (uncommon), resulting in minimal decrease in NNRTI susceptibility. **K101P:** Usually occurs with K103N, resulting in further loss of NNRTI susceptibility.
K103N/S	**K103N:** Commonly selected by all NNRTIs, resulting in high-level NNRTI resistance. K103S less common, resulting in lower degree of resistance to DLV and EFV, but moderate resistance to NVP. **K103R:** Polymorphism with minimal effect on NNRTI susceptibility.
V106M/A	**V106M:** Selected by NVP (common with subtype C), resulting in NVP/EFV resistance and unknown effect on DLV. **V106A:** Selected by NVP (uncommon), resulting in NVP resistance and minimal effect on DLV/EFV susceptibility. V106I is polymorphism that does not cause NNRTI resistance.
V108I	Selected by NVP and EFV (uncommon), resulting in minimal decrease in NVP/EFV susceptibility.
V179D/E	Selected by NNRTIs (uncommon), resulting in minimal decrease in NNRTI susceptibility.
Y181C/I	Selected by NVP and DLV, causing resistance to both. Causes only low-level resistance to EFV maintained, but clinical response to EFV unlikely, possibly because of presence of viral subpopulations with other resistance mutations. Increases susceptibility to AZT and tenofovir.
Y188L/H/C	**Y188L:** Selected by NVP, DLV, and EFV (uncommon) resulting in resistance to all 3 drugs. **Y188H/C:** Selected by NVP; cause lower-level NVP resistance and minimal EFV resistance. Unknown effects on DLV.
G190S/A/E	**G190A:** Selected by NVP and EFV, causing high-level resistance to both drugs. G190A/S cause hypersusceptibility to DLV. **G190E:** Causes low-level resistance to DLV. Clinical significance of DLV hypersusceptibility unknown; other NNRTI mutations may be present in viral subpopulations.
P225H	Usually occurs with K103N, resulting in further loss of NNRTI susceptibility.
F227L	Sometimes seen in combination with V106A, resulting in further loss of NVP susceptibility.
M230L	Selected by NNRTIs (uncommon), resulting in moderate NNRTI resistance.
P236L	Selected by DLV (uncommon), resulting in DLV resistance.
K238T/N	Selected by NNRTIs (uncommon), usually in combination with K103N or other NNRTI mutations, resulting in further loss of NNRTI susceptibility.
F318L	Selected by NNRTIs (uncommon), resulting in moderate loss of DLV susceptibility.

Laboratory Tests

Mutation	Comment
L10I/V/F/R/V	Accessory mutations that can contribute to reduced susceptibility in the presence of other PI mutations. **L10V:** Contributes to TPV resistance in presence of other TPV mutations.
I13V	Contributes to TPV resistance in presence of other TPV mutations.
K20R/I/M/T/V	Accessory mutations/polymorphisms that may contribute to reduced susceptibility in the presence of other PI mutations. **K20M/R/V:** Contribute to TPV resistance in presence of other TPV mutations.
L23I	Uncommon mutation; low-level NFV resistance.
L24I/F	**L24I:** PI resistance, especially to IDV, when combined with other PI mutations. **L24F:** Rare mutation with unknown effect on PI susceptibility.
D30N	Primary PI mutation selected only by NFV, especially with subtype B virus; intermediate NFV resistance; further loss of susceptibility with N88D/S.
V32I	Accessory mutation that confers low-level resistance to IDV, RTV, APV, LPV.
L33F/I/V	**L33F:** decreases susceptibility to RTV, APV, LPV, ATV, and TPV in presence of other PI mutations. **L33I/V:** Polymorphisms not known to be associated with drug resistance.
E35G	Contributes to TPV resistance in presence of other TPV mutations.
M36I/V/L	**M36I/V:** Accessory mutations that contribute to reduced PI susceptibility in the presence of other PI mutations. **M36I:** Contributes to TPV resistance in presence of other TPV mutations. **M36L:** Unknown effect on PI susceptibility.
K43T	Contributes to TPV resistance in presence of other TPV mutations.
M46I/L/V	**M46I/L:** Accessory mutation that contributes to reduced PI susceptibility in the presence of other PI mutations. **M46L:** Contributes to TPV resistance in presence of other TPV mutations. **M46V:** Uncommon mutation with unknown effect on PI susceptibility.
I47A/V	**I47V:** Reduced susceptibility to APV, IDV, RTV, LPV, TPV in combination with other PI mutations. **I47A:** Moderate to high-level LPV resistance.
G48V/M	**G48V:** selected by SQV; intermediate SQV resistance; low-level resistance to other PIs. **G48M:** Effect on PI susceptibility unknown.
I50V/L	**I50V:** Selected by APV in PI-naïve patients; intermediate APV resistance; low-to-intermediate resistance to RTV, LPV. **I50L:** Selected by ATV in PI-naïve patients; moderate to high-level ATV resistance; susceptibility to other PIs maintained or increased.
F53L	Associated with PI resistance when combined with other PI mutations.
I54V/M/L/T/ S/A	**I54V:** Increases resistance to PIs when combined with other PI mutations. **I54M/L:** Selected by APV or FPV, causing low to intermediate resistance. **I54T/S/A:** Effect on PI susceptibility unknown. **I54A/M/V:** Contribute to TPV resistance in presence of other TPV mutations.

(continued)

2 Laboratory Tests

Mutation	Comment
Q58E	Contributes to TPV resistance in presence of other TPV mutations.
L63A/C/E/H/P/ Q/R/S/T/V/I	**L63P:** Common polymorphism that increases PI resistance when combined with other PI mutations. **Others:** Effect on PI susceptibility unclear.
H69K	Contributes to TPV resistance in presence of other TPV mutations.
A71V/T/I	**A71V/T:** Decreases susceptibility to all PIs when combined with other mutations. **A71I:** Effect on PI susceptibility unknown.
G73S/C/T/A	**G73S/C/T:** Resistance to NFV, IDV, SQV, ATV in combination with other PI mutations. **G73A:** Uncommon variant.
T74P	Contributes to TPV resistance in presence of other TPV mutations.
L76V	Decreases LPV susceptibility to unknown degree.
V77I	Polymorphism associated with slight decrease in NFV susceptibility.
V82A/T/F/S/ I/G/L	**V82A/T/F/S:** Primary PI mutation that reduces susceptibility to LPV, IDV, RTV, and also to NFV, SQV, APV, ATV when combined with other PI mutations. **V82I:** Polymorphism with minimal effect on PI susceptibility. **V82M:** Seen with subtype G infection; reduces IDV susceptibility. **V82L/T:** Contribute to TPV resistance in presence of other TPV mutations.
N83D	Contributes to TPV resistance in presence of other TPV mutations.
I84V/A/C	**I84V:** Decreases susceptibility to all PIs: greatest effect on APV, NFV, SQV, lowest on LPV. Contributes to TPV resistance in presence of other TPV mutations. **I84A/C:** Effects similar to I84V, but rare.
N88S/D	**N88D:** Intermediate resistance to NFV; low-level resistance to SQV, ATV. **N88S:** Intermediate resistance to NFV, ATV; low-level resistance to IDV; hypersusceptibility to APV.
L90M	By itself, causes intermediate resistance to SQV and NFV and low-level resistance to other PIs except TPV.
T91S	Emerges *in vitro* with exposure to LPV; effect on susceptibility unknown.
I93L/M	**I93L:** Common polymorphism that increases PI resistance when combined with other PI mutations. **I93M:** PI mutation with unknown effect on PI susceptibility.

Screening Laboratory Tests

The usual screening battery advocated for patients with established HIV infection is summarized in Table 2-16, pp. 38-39 (Primary Care Guidelines IDSA, *Clin Infect Dis* 2004;39:609).

Complete Blood Count: The CBC is important, because anemia, leukopenia, lymphopenia and thrombocytopenia are common due to HIV per se or to medications (*J Acquir Immune Defic Syndr* 1994;7:1134; *J Acquir Immune Defic Syndr* 2001;28:221). Repeat at 3- to 6-month intervals and more frequently in patients with symptoms

Drug	ViroLogic PhenoSense		Virco Antivirogram	
	Cutoff	Clinical (C) or Biological (B)	Cutoff	Clinical (C) or Biological (B)
NRT/NtRTI				
abacavir	4.5	C	2.1	B
didanosine	1.3 (lower) 2.2 (upper)	C	2.3	B
emtricitabine	3.5	B	3.7	B
lamivudine	3.5	C	2.1	B
stavudine	1.7	C	2.4	B
tenofovir	1.4	C	2.5	B
zidovudine	1.9	B	2.7	B
NNRTI				
delavirdine	2.5	B	—	
efavirenz	2.5	B	3.4	B
nevirapine	2.5	B	5.2	B
PI				
fosamprenavir	2	B	1.8	B
indinavir	2.1	B	2.1	B
indinavir/ritonavir	10	C*	—	
lopinavir/ritonavir	10	C	1.6	B
nelfinavir	2.5	B	2.3	B
ritonavir	2.5	B	—	—
saquinavir	1.7	B	1.7	B
atazanavir	2.2	C	2.0	B
atazanavir/ritonavir	5.2	C	—	—
tipranavir/ritonavir	4.0	C	—	—
FI				
enfuvirtide	—	—	—	—

*Clinical cutoff for IDV/r based on studies using IDV/RTV 800/200 mg bid

(headache, fatigue), those receiving marrow-suppressing drugs such as AZT, and in those with marginal or low counts.

Serum Chemistry Panel: This panel is advocated in the initial evaluation of HIV infection due to high rates of hepatitis (*J Infect Dis* 2002;186:231), to help stage the disease, and to obtain baseline values in patients who are likely to have multisystem disease due to HIV or its treatment. Up to 75% of HIV-infected patients have abnormal transaminases at baseline, 20% have severe abnormalities, and about half have elevated lactic dehydrogenase (LDH) levels (*J Acquir Immune Defic Syndr* 1994;7:1134).

Laboratory Tests

2

■ TABLE 2-16: **Routine Laboratory Tests in Asymptomatic Patients**

Test	Cost*	Frequency and Comment
Serologic Tests		
CMV IgG**	$10 to $15	Advocated for low-risk patients (not MSM or IDU); seroprevalence in U.S. adults is 50% to 60%, and for MSM and IV drug abuse patients it is ≥90%. Rationale is to alert for need for CMV-negative or leukocyte-reduced blood products if needed.
Total anti-HAV antibody**	$20 to $30	Screen for HAV vaccine candidates
anti-HBc or anti-HBs**	$10 to $15	HBV: Screen for vaccine candidates with anti-HBc or anti-HBs. If prior HBV vaccination, then test anti-HBs.
HBsAg**	$20 to $25	Screen for chronic hepatitis B.
anti-HCV**	$25 HCV EIA	Screen with anti-HCV IgG; confirm positives with quantitative HCV RNA at $150. Consider qualitative or quantitative HCV RNA in HCV-seronegatives at high risk and/or with abnormal transaminases.
Hepatitis screen	$60 to $80	Abnormal transaminase levels – "hepatitis screen": anti-HAV IgM, anti-HCV and HBsAg ± anti-HBc IgM
HIV (see p. 6)	$30 to $60	Repeat test for patients with positive test results and inadequate confirmation.
Syphilis – VDRL or RPR**	$5 to $16	Repeat annually in sexually active patients. Confirm positives with FTA-ABS.
anti-*Toxoplasma* IgG**	$12 to $15	Screen all patients at baseline, and repeat in sero-negatives if CD4 cell count is ≤100/mm³ and patient does not take TMP-SMX for *P. carinii* prophylaxis or has symptoms suggestive of toxoplasmis encephalitis. Agglutination assays for IgG are preferred. IgM is not useful.
Varicella IgG*		If negative history for chickenpox to promote protections against exposure, varicella vaccination and/or post-exposure ZIG.
Chemistry		
Chemistry panel**	$10 to $15	Includes LFTs and renal function. Repeat annually or more frequently in patients with abnormal results and with administration of hepatotoxic or nephrotoxic drugs.
G6-PD	$14 to $20	Test: 1) Susceptible hosts: Primarily men (X-linked), with the following ancestry African-American, Italian, Sephardic Jew, Arab, and those from India and South-east Asia; 2) Those with drug-induced hemolipses fol-lowing recovery (see p. 46). Options are testing suscep-tible patients at baseline or before use of oxidant drugs – sulfonamides, dapsone or primaquine.
Lipid profile and blood glucose (fasting) (HAART recipients)**	$20 to $40	Therapeutic monitoring recommended for patients receiving antiretroviral regimens that include a PI or NNRTI; consider at baseline and at 3 to 6 months with subsequent measurements annually or more frequently based on initial results and risks.**

Laboratory Tests

Test	Cost*	Frequency and Comment
Hematology		
Complete blood count (CBC)**	$6 to $8	Repeat at 3 to 6 months, more frequently for low values and with marrow-toxic drugs.
CD4 cell count and %**	$60 to $150	Repeat every 3 to 6 months and repeat for discordant results, including those results with results that are inconsistent with prior trends. Routine testing when counts are <50 cells/mm³ is of minimal use except for monitoring response to antiretroviral therapy.
Other		
Chest x-ray	$40 to $140	May be routine or restricted to those with past pulmonary disease, chronic pulmonary disease or a positive PPD*
PAP smear**	$25 to $40	Repeat at 6 months and then annually if results are normal. Results reported as "inadequate" should be repeated. Refer to a gynecologist for results showing atypia or greater on the Bethesda scale (see pp. 41-43).
PPD skin test**	$1	Test at baseline. Annual testing should be considered in previously PPD-negative patients who have risk for tuberculosis, and repeat testing should be considered if initial test was negative and the CD4 count has subsequently increased to >200 cells/mm³ in response to HAART.
Urine NAAT–*N. gonorrhoeae* & *C. trachomatis* (optional)**	$60 to $100	Recommended by CDC HIV prevention guidelines for "consideration" in sexually active male patients (*MMWR* 2003;52(RR-12):1-24). Advocated as marker of high risk behavior (and need for enhanced counseling) and for treatment + contact tracing. Repeat annually in sexually active patients. and more often in high-risk patients (see p. 30) (NAAT=nucleic acid amplification test).
Wet mount for *Trichomonas* (women)**		Repeat annually.

*Common charges are based on survey of five laboratories.
** Recommendations of Primary Care Guidelines of IDSA (*Clin Infect Dis* 2004;39:609).

Syphilis Serology (*MMWR* 2002;51[RR-6]:19):

Screen with a nontreponemal test (VDRL or RPR) at baseline and annually thereafter due to high rates of co-infection. Up to 6% of patients with HIV infection have biologic false-positive (BFP) screening tests. Risk factors for biologic false-positive results include injection drug use, pregnancy, and HIV infection (*Clin Infect Dis* 1994;19:1040; *J Infect Dis* 1992;165: 1124; *J Acquir Immune Defic Syndr* 1994;7:1134; *Am J Med* 1995;99: 55). Nontreponemal tests give antibody titers that correlate with disease activity. Positive screening tests are confirmed with a fluorescent treponemal antibody adsorbed (FTA-ABS) or *T. pallidum* particle agglutination (TP-PA test). Many patients will have positive treponemal tests for life, but the VDRL and RPR usually become negative or persist at low titer. Some HIV-infected patients have "atypical serology" with unusually high, unusually low, or fluctuating titers, but "for most HIV infected patients, serologic tests are accurate and reliable for the diagnosis of syphilis and for the response to therapy" (*MMWR* 2002;51[RR-6]:19). For management guidelines see pp. 350-351.

Urine Screen for Other Sexually Transmitted Diseases: Infections with *N. gonorrhoeae* and/or *C. trachomatis* are common with HIV infection (*AIDS* 2000;14:297) and are often asymptomatic in both men and women (*Sex Transur Dis* 2001;28:33; *Clin Infect Dis* 2002;35:1010). STDs are of interest because 1) usually indicate ongoing high-risk behavior, 2) many enhance transmission of HIV, and 3) detection can reduce likelihood of transmission (*Sex Transm Infect* 1999;75:3; *Lancet* 1995;346:530). Urine-based nucleic acid amplification tests (NAATs) are now generally available for *N. gonorrhoeae* and *C. trachomatis* with advantages of good specificity and ease of specimen collection. NAAT with endocervical or intraurethral swabs are more sensitive (*MMWR* 2002;51[RR-15]:1). The usual cost is $60-$100. Screening for *N. gonorrhoeae* and *C. trachomatis* is advocated for sexually active patients and those with syptoms, but the language in the CDC guidelines is softened to "consider" because NAAT testing is expensive and has no proven efficacy in preventing HIV transmission (*MMWR* 2003;52(RR-12):6).

Screening for Other Sexually Transmitted Diseases: The 2003 CDC HIV prevention guidelines recommend the following tests on the first visit (*MMWR* 2003;52RR-12:6):
- RPR or VDRL for syphilis
- Consider screen for *N. gonorrhoeae* and *C. trachomatis* with urethral culture (men) or cervical culture (women) or urine (first 10-30 mL) for NAAT testing to detect either or both
- Trichomoniasis screen in women with wet mount or culture of vaginal secretions
- Patients reporting anal sex: consider anal swab for culture for *N. gonorrhoeae* and *C. trachomatis* if available.
- Patients reporting oral sex: Consider pharyngeal culture for *N. gonorrhoeae*.

REPEAT TESTS: Consider repeating these tests annually in sexually active patients and at 3- to 6-month intervals if at high risk. The purpose is to detect high-risk behavior that might not otherwise be apparent (for enhanced counseling), for contact tracing, and for treatment.

Chest X-Ray: The frequency of lung disease with HIV infection is high even in the HAART era (*Am Rev Respir Crit Care Med* 2001;164:21; *Chest* 2001;120:1888). A routine baseline chest X-ray is recommended by the CDC (*MMWR* 1986;35:448), both for detection of asymptomatic tuberculosis and as a baseline for patients who are at high risk for pulmonary disease. Nevertheless, in a longitudinal study of 1,065 patients at various stages of HIV infection, showed routine X-rays performed at 0, 3, 6, and 12 months (*Arch Intern Med* 1996;156:191) detected an abnormality in only 123 (2%) of 5,263 X-rays. None of the asymptomatic PPD negative patients had evidence of active tuberculosis, and only 1 of 82 with a positive PPD had an abnormality on X-ray. The authors concluded that routine chest X-rays in HIV infected patients with negative PPD skin tests are not warranted. DHHS Guidelines recommend an X-ray "when clinically indicated" (*MMWR* 1998;47[RR-1]:38). In resource-limited regions the WHO policy is to obtain a chest X-ray to exclude active TB in patients with a positive PPD, but a study of 563 asymptomatic HIV-infected patients in Botswana showed only one (0.02%) with active disease (*Lancet* 2003;362:1551). The authors argued that in resource-limited areas, X-rays could be limited to those with symptoms.

PPD Skin Testing: The CDC recommends the Mantoux method TST (Tuberculin Skin Test), using 5 TU of PPD, for HIV-infected patients who have not had a prior positive test. TST should be repeated annually if initial test(s) were negative and if the patient belongs to population with a high risk of tuberculosis (eg, residents of prisons or jails, injection drug users, and homeless individuals). The PPD should also be repeated following immune reconstitution when the CD4 count increases to >200 cells/mm^3 (2002 USPHS/IDSA Guidelines for the Prevention of Opportunistic Infections (*MMWR* 2002;51[RR-6]). Induration of ≥5 mm at 48 to 72 hours constitutes a positive test. Anergy testing is not recommended.

Pap Smear: The CDC recommends a gynecological evaluation with pelvic exam and Pap smear be performed at baseline, repeated at 6 months and annually thereafter (*MMWR* 2002;517[RR-6]:59; *JAMA* 1994;271:1866; *MMWR* 1999;48[RR-10]:31), with management according to guidelines in Table 2-17, p. 42. More aggressive testing is recommended because of a several-fold increase in rates of squamous intraepithelial lesion (SIL) (33% to 45% HIV+ vs 7% to 14% HIV-) and a 0 to 9-fold increase in rates of cervical cancer in women with HIV (*Arch Pediatr Adolesc Med* 2000;154:127; *Obstet Gynecol Clin N Am* 1996; 23,861; *J Acquir Immune Defic Syndr* 2003;32:527; *J Acquir Immun Defic Syndr* 2004;36:978)). Severity and frequency of cervical dysplasia increase with progressive immune compromise. There is a strong association between HIV infection and detectable and persistent HPV infection by HPV types associated with cervical cancer (16, 18, 31, 33, and 35); this association increases with progressive immunosuppression (*Clin Infect Dis* 1995;21[suppl 1]:S121; *N Engl J Med* 1997;337:1343; *J Infect Dis* 2001;184:682).

2 Laboratory Tests

■ TABLE 2-17: **Recommendations for Intervention Based on Results of Pap Smear** (*MMWR* 2002;51[RR-6]:58; *JAMA* 1989;262:931; *JAMA* 2002;287:2114)

Results	Management
Severe inflammation	Evaluate for infection; repeat Pap smear, preferably within 2 to 3 months.
Atypia, atypical squamous cells of undetermined significance (ASCUS) ■ ASC-US (undetermined significance) ■ ASC-H (cannot exclude HSIL). ASC-H is intermediate between ASC-US and HSIL	Consider HPV testing: If high risk type (16, 18, 31, 33, or 35) – colposcopy. Alternative without HPV testing is follow-up. Follow-up Pap without colposcopy every 4 to 6 months x 2 years until three are negative; if second report of ASCUS, perform colposcopy.
Low-grade squamous intraepithelial lesion (LSIL)	Colposcopy ± biopsy or follow with Pap smear every 4 to 6 months, as above, with colposcopy and biopsy if repeat smears are abnormal.*
High-grade squamous intraepithelial lesion (HSIL) (carcinoma *in situ*)	Referral for colposcopy ± biopsy.
Invasive carcinoma	Colposcopy with biopsy or conization; treat with surgery or radiation.

* Most gynecologists recommend evaluation with any abnormality due to the high prevalence of underlying SIL.

METHOD: The cervix is scraped circumflexually using an *Ayer* spatula or a curved brush; a sample from the posterior fornix or the "vaginal pool" may also be included. The endocervical sample is taken with a saline-moistened cotton-tipped applicator or straight ectocervical brush that is rolled on a slide and immediately fixed in ethyl ether plus 95% ethyl alcohol or 95% ethyl alcohol alone. The yield is 7-fold higher with the brush specimen. The following are important steps in obtaining an adequate sample:

- Collect Pap prior to bimanual exam.
- Avoid contaminating sample with lubricant.
- Obtain Pap before samples for STD testing.
- Carefully remove large amounts of vaginal discharge (if present) with large swab before obtaining Pap smear.
- Obtain ectocervical sample before endocervical sample.
- Defer Pap smear if patient is bleeding heavily (small amounts of blood will not interfere with cytologic sampling).
- Apply collected material to slide uniformly, with no clumping. Fix rapidly to avoid air drying. If spray fixatives are used, the spray should be held at least 10 inches away from the slide to prevent disruption of cells by propellant.

When performing speculum examination, if an ulcerative or exophytic lesion suspicious for invasive cancer is noted, the patient should be referred for possible biopsy.

Newer methods of cytologic evaluation using liquid-based collection and thin-layer processing increase sensitivity, decrease frequency of inadequate smears, permit HPV testing, and provide better resolution of ASCUS.

Analysis for HPV-DNA: Screening of Pap smears for high-risk HPV DNA types (including 16, 18, 31, 33, and 35) was compared with standard thin layer Paps for detecting intraepithelial neoplasia (CIN grade 3) or cancer (*JAMA* 2002;288:1749). Testing for these high-risk HPV types showed higher sensitivity (91% vs 61%) but less specificity (73% vs 82%).

ANAL PAP SMEAR FOR SIL AND CARCINOMA IN MSM

Anal cancer is similar to cervical cancer in many ways, including the facts that both are caused by HPV infection, several HPV types appear to be oncogenic, low-grade lesions often progress to high-grade lesions, and Pap smear may be an effective screening method (*Am J Med* 2000;108:674). The prevalence of HPV in MSM is 60% to 75% (*J Infect Dis* 1998;177:361), the frequency of anal carcinoma in men with HIV infection is about 80 times that of the general population (*Lancet* 1998;351:1833) and rates increase with CD4 counts <500/mm^3 (*AIDS* 1998;12:495). Some authorities recommend anal Pap smears in MSM at 3-year intervals, which is comparable with cervical Pap smear with regard to cost-effectiveness (*Am J Med* 2000;108:634). More recent studies suggest this risk applies to all men with HIV, leading some to recommend routine anal cytology regardless of a history of receptive anal intercourse, especially those with a low CD4 count (*Ann Intern Med* 2003;183:453). Anal Pap shows sensitivity similar to cervical Pap but less accurately indicates grade of abnormality. Therefore, abnormal anal Paps should lead to referral for anoscopy and biopsy (*Clin Infect Dis* 2004;38:1490). HAART is also important due to its profound impact on survival (*Dis Colon Rectum* 2004;47:1305).

Hepatitis A Serology: HAV serology (total anti-HAV antibody) is performed to identify candidates for HAV vaccine, which is indicated for susceptible persons with chronic HCV infection, injection drug use, MSM, persons with clotting disorders, persons with chronic liver disease, and travelers to HAV-endemic areas (*MMWR* 1996;45[RR-15]:1). Some authorities believe that all HIV-infected persons who are susceptible should be vaccinated. The prevalence of anti-HAV IgG is 62% in injection drug users and 32% in MSM (*Clin Infect Dis* 1997;25:726; *MMWR* 1999;48:[RR-12]:1). To diagnose acute hepatitis the preferred test is anti-HAV IgM. The anti-HAV IgG becomes positive at 8 to 16 weeks.

2 Laboratory Tests

Hepatitis B Serology: All HBV seronegative patients with HIV should receive the standard 3-dose HBV vaccine series. The standard screening test is anti-HBc or anti-HBs (*MMWR* 2002;51RR-6:63). HBV seroprevalence is 35-50% for MSM, 60-80% for hemophilia patients, 5-20% for heterosexuals with multiple partners, and 3-14% for the general population. For patients with prior vaccination the appropriate test is anti-HBs, but the titer wanes with time and many [patients-?] have protection despite negative serology several. years post-vaccination, presumably due to cell-mediated immunity (*Ann Intern Med* 2005;142:333). The CDC now recommends post-vaccination serology with anti-HBs in patients with HIV infection at 1 to 2 months after the third dose of vaccine to confirm an antibody response (*MMWR* 1999;48:33). Response is defined as HBsAb levels ≥10 IU/mL (*MMWR* 2001;50[RR-1]). Patients who fail to respond should be considered for revaccination using the standard 3 dose regimen (*Ann Intern Med* 1982;97:362; *MMWR* 2002;51[RR-6]:64). Additional doses with non-response to the second series are not advocated. Rates of non-response increase with age >30 years (*Clin Infect Dis* 2002;35:1368) and with HIV infection, especially when associated with low CD4 counts (*Addiction* 2002;97:985; *Scand J Infect Dis* 2004;36:131).

Patients with chronic HBV infection: Patients with unexplained liver disease and negative HBV serology should be evaluated for chronic HBV infection with serology for HBsAg. Prevalence of chronic HBV is 0.2-1.0% in the general population and 6-7% for MSM, IDUs and hemophilia patients.

Chronic carriers of HBsAg should be evaluated with LFTs, HBeAg and HBV DNA to determine the replicative status and possible indication for liver biopsy and therapy. HBV co-infection is complicated in patients with HIV due to the frequent use of antivirals with anti-HBV activity including 3TC, FTC, and TDF (see p. 99).

HCV Testing (*MMWR* 2004;53,[RR-15]:1): The seroprevalence of HCV is 1.8% in the general population, 4%-6% in MSM, and 70%-90% in IDUs and hemophilia patients. All HIV infected persons be tested for HCV infection using the third generation EIA screening assay for anti-HCV antibodies. The third generation EIAs have a sensitivity and specificity of >99% in immunocompetent patients, but there may be false-negatives with severe immunosuppression as with CD4 count <100 cells/mm^3 (*J Acquir Immune Defic Syndr* 2002;31:154). The qualitative HCV RNA assay could help with suspected false-negatives (*J Infect Dis* 1994;170:433; *Blood* 1993;82:1010). For patients with a positive EIA screening test, qualitative HCV RNA assay is commonly recommended for confirmation but generally unnecessary with risk factors for HCV infection and an abnormal ALT. Qualitative HCV RNA assays have a threshold of detection of 50-100 IU/mL and may be used to confirm the diagnosis of HCV infection in persons with positive serology. A negative test doesn't exclude HCV because HCV RNA levels may periodically decline below limits of detection; repeat testing is required to confirm chronic HCV infection. Quantitative HCV assays (bDNA or RNA PCR) are viral load assays that have a threshold of detection of 500 IU/ mL and may be used in place of the qualitative RNA test to establish the diagnosis. The principal use is to monitor response to therapy. Patients with chronic HCV infection should have hepatic function tests. Those who are considered candidates for HCV therapy should be evaluated as indicated on p. 407.

■ TABLE 2-18: **Tests for HCV**

Test	Cost	Comment
Anti-HCV EIA	$25 to $45	Indicates past or present HCV infection. Sensitivity of the third generation tests is >99%. EIA lacks specificity in low-prevalence populations – supplemental assay required for confirmation. RIBA – of little utility in HIV infected patients.
Qualitative HCV RNA (HCV RT-PCR)	$160 to $200	RT-PCR technology to detect HCV RNA; may have false-positives and negatives. Threshold for detection is 50 IU/mL. Usual use is to confirm serology results.
Quantitative HCV PCR or bDNA	$160 to $225	Determines concentration using RT-PCR or bDNA technology. Less sensitive than qualitative RT-PCR. Threshold of detection is 500 IU/mL; most patients with chronic HCV infection have 10^5 to 10^7 c/mL. HCV RNA level is not useful for determining prognosis; it is used to monitor response to therapy. Magnitude of HCV RNA level may predict response. It has largely supplanted qualitative HCV RNA tests due to adequate sensitivity and comparable cost.
Genotype	$200 to $250	6 genotypes – genotype 1 predominates in United States (70%) and shows poorest response to therapy.

Toxoplasmosis Serology:

Toxoplasma serology (anti-*Toxoplasma* IgG) is recommended to assist in the differential diagnosis of complications involving the CNS, to identify candidates for toxoplasmosis prophylaxis (*Ann Intern Med* 1992;117:163), and to counsel patients on preventive measures if seronegative. The preferred method is an agglutination assay for IgG; IgM assays are not useful, and the Sabin-Feldman dye test is less accurate than the agglutination assay. Toxoplasmosis seroprevalence among adults in the United States is 10% to 30%, and the seroconversion rate is up to 1%/year. The sensitivity of the test is 95% to 97%. Most infections in AIDS patients represent relapse of latent infection, which is noted in 20% to 47% with CD4 counts <100 cells/mm^3, positive toxoplasmosis serology, and no prophylaxis (*Clin Infect Dis* 1992;15:211; *Clin Infect Dis* 2002;34:103).

2 Laboratory Tests

A negative *Toxoplasma* serology should be repeated after the CD4 cell count is ≤100 cells/mm^3 if the patient does not take atovaquone or TMP-SMX phophylaxis for PCP (2002 USPHS/IDSA Guidelines for the Prevention of Opportunistic Infections, *MMWR* 2002;51:[RR-6]) or whenever the diagnosis toxoplasmosis encephalitis is being considered and when prior tests were negative.

CMV Serology: This is advocated by the USPHS/IDSA Guidelines for HIV infected persons who have low risk for CMV infection, specifically those who are not MSM or injection drug users (*MMWR* 2002;51[RR-8]:17). This information has the following possible applications: 1) Identification of seronegative patients for counseling on CMV prevention (although the message is not different from the "safe sex message" for preventing HIV transmission); 2) Assessment of the likelihood of CMV disease in late-stage HIV infection; 3) Identification of seronegative individuals who should receive CMV-antibody-negative blood or leukocyte-reduced blood products for nonemergent transfusions (*JAMA* 2001;285:1592). Seroprevalence for adults in the United States is about 50%; in MSM and injection drug users it is >90% (*J Infect Dis* 1985;152:243; *Am J Med* 1987;82:593). It should be noted there are multiple methods to detect CMV, including p65 antigen assays, CMV DNA PCR assays, NASBA early antigen assays, and culture of blood and urinary tests using culture and urinary CMV DNA PCR. None of the recommended strategies has proven effective in predicting CMV disease in HIV-infected persons (*J Clin Microbiol* 2000;38:563).

Glucose-6-Phosphate Dehydrogenase Levels (G6-PD): G6-PD deficiency is a genetic disease that predisposes to hemolytic anemia following exposure to oxidant drugs commonly such as dapsone, primaquin and TMP-SMX. Over 150 G6-PD variants are inherited on the X chromosome, but the most frequent are Gd^{A-}, which is found in 10% of black men and in 1% to 2% of black women, and Gd^{med}, found predominantly in men from the Mediterranean area (Italians, Greeks, Sephardic Jews, Arabs), India, and Southeast Asia. With most defects, the hemolysis is mild and self-limited because only the older red cells are involved, and the bone marrow can compensate even with continued administration of the implicated drug. The important exception is Gd^{med}, which may cause life-threatening hemolysis. The limited hemolysis in patients with Gd^{A-} may be significant in patients with HIV infection, who often have anemia from other causes. The severity of anemia also depends on the concentration of the drug in red cells and the oxidant potential of the inducing agent: The most likely offending agents are dapsone and primaquine. Sulfonamides cause hemolysis less commonly. G6-PD deficiency may be partial, in which case the contraindication for oxidant drugs is relative. Options for screening include: 1) test at baseline in all patients; 2) restricting testing to those most likely to have a defect; and 3) reserving testing for the occasional case of hemolytic anemia following exposure to typical inducing agents. Typical findings with this hemolysis include elevated indirect bilirubin, elevated LDH, decreased haptoglobin, methemoglobinemia, reticulocytosis, and a peripheral smear showing the characteristic "bite cells." During hemolysis, G6-PD levels are usually normal because the susceptible red cells are destroyed; testing must consequently be delayed until about 30 days after discontinuation of the offending agent. Some laboratories report results as units/g Hgb, with fewer than three indicating severe deficiency, in men and homozygous women; other labs report qualitative results.

Adverse Drug Reaction Monitoring

Adverse drug reactions attributed to antiretroviral agents include diabetes mellitus, blood lipid changes associated with risks for coronary artery disease and stroke, lactic acidosis/steatosis attributed to nucleoside analogs, periperal neuropathy, and hepatic toxicity (see p. 110 and Table 4-30).

Laboratory Tests

3 | Disease Prevention: Prophylactic Antimicrobial Agents and Vaccines

Recommendations of the 2002 USPHS/IDSA Guidelines for the Prevention of Opportunistic Infections in Persons Infected with Human Immunodeficiency Virus (*MMWR* 2002;51[RR-8]:1; www.aidsinfo.nih.gov)

■ TABLE 3-1: **Categories Reflecting Strength and Quality of Evidence**

Rating System for Strength of Recommendation and Quality of Evidence Supporting the Recommendation	
Category	Definition
Categories Reflecting the Strength of Each Recommendation	
A	Both strong evidence for efficacy and substantial clinical benefit support recommendation for use. Should always be offered.
B	Moderate evidence for efficacy, or strong evidence for efficacy, but only limited clinical benefit, supports recommendation for use. Should generally be offered.
C	Evidence for efficacy is insufficient to support a recommendation for or against use, or evidence for efficacy may not outweigh adverse consequences (eg, toxicity, drug interactions, or cost of the chemoprophylaxis or alternative approaches). Optional.
D	Moderate evidence for lack of efficacy or for adverse outcome supports a recommendation against use. Should generally not be offered.
E	Good evidence for lack of efficacy or for adverse outcome supports a recommendation against use. Should never be offered.
Categories Reflecting Quality of Evidence Supporting the Recommendation	
I	Evidence from at least one properly randomized, controlled trial
II	Evidence from at least one well-designed clinical trial without randomization, from cohort or case-controlled analytic studies (preferably from more than one center), or from multiple time-series studies or dramatic results from uncontrolled experiments.
III	Evidence from opinions of respected authorities based on clinical experience, descriptive studies, or reports of expert committees.

Strongly Recommended as Standard of Care
Pneumocystis jiroveci (P. carinii)

NOTE: The new name from Stringer et al is *P. jiroveci* (*Emerg Infect Dis* 2002;8:891), but the term PCP (*Pneumocystis jiroveci* Pneumonia) continues to be used.

RISK: CD4 count <200/mm³, prior PCP or HIV-associated thrush, or unexplained fever x 2 weeks (Category AII from Table 3-1)

PREFERRED REGIMEN: TMP-SMX 1 DS/day or 1 SS/day (AI)

ALTERNATIVE REGIMENS

- TMP-SMX 1 DS 3x/week (BI)
- Dapsone 100 mg/day or 50 mg PO bid (BI)
- Dapsone 50 mg/day plus pyrimethamine 50 mg/week plus leucovorin 25 mg/week (BI)
- Dapsone 200 mg/week plus pyrimethamine 75 mg/week plus leucovorin 25 mg/week (BI)
- Aerosolized pentamidine 300 mg/month by *Respirgard II* nebulizer using 6 mL diluent delivered at 6L/min from a 50 psi compressed air source until reservoir is dry (usually 45 min), with or without albuterol (2 whiffs) to reduce cough and bronchospasm (BI)
- Atovaquone 1500 mg PO qd with meals (*N Engl J Med* 1998;339: 1889) (BI)

RISK: The risk of PCP without prophylaxis is 60% to 70% per year in those with prior PCP and 40% to 50% per year for those with a CD4 count <100/mm^3. The mortality for patients hospitalized and treated for PCP is 15% to 20%. PCP prophylaxis reduces the risk of PCP 9-fold, and patients who get PCP despite prophylaxis have a lower mortality rate (*Am J Respir Crit Care Med* 1997;155:60). The major reasons for PCP prophylaxis failure are CD4 count <50/mm^3 and non-compliance (*JAMA* 1995;273:1197; *Arch Intern Med* 1996;156:177). TMP-SMX has established efficacy for reducing the incidence of bacterial infections and toxoplasmosis. This drug is active against *Nocardia*, *Legionella*, most *Salmonella*, most methicillin-sensitive *S. aureus*, community-acquired MRSA (USA 300 strains), many gram-negative bacilli, most *H. influenzae*, and about 70% of *S. pneumoniae*. No other PCP prophylaxis regimen has this spectrum of activity.

ADVERSE REACTIONS: Adverse reactions sufficiently severe to require discontinuation of the drug are noted in 25% to 50% with TMP-SMX, 25% to 40% with dapsone, and 2% to 4% with aerosolized pentamidine (*N Engl J Med* 1995:332:693). Patients who have a non-life-threatening reaction to TMP-SMX should continue this drug if it can be tolerated. Those who have had such a reaction in the past should be rechallenged, possibly using desensitization (see pp. 317-318). Gradual initiation of TMP-SMX prophylaxis reduces the rate of rash and/or fever by about 50% (*J Acquir Immune Defic Syndr* 2000;24:337). This suggests that most reactions are not allergic or IgE mediated. Patients given dapsone should be tested for G6-PD deficiency if at risk. Fansidar is rarely used due to possible severe hypersensitivity reactions.

IMMUNE RECONSTITUTION: Patients who have increases in CD4 count to >200/mm^3 x ≥3 months may safely discontinue primary PCP prophylaxis (AI) (*N Engl J Med* 1999;340:1301; *Lancet* 1999;353:1293; *Lancet* 1999;353:201; *J Infect Dis* 2000;181:1635) and secondary

Disease Prevention: Prophylactic Antimicrobial Agents and Vaccines prophylaxis (BII) (*N Engl J Med* 2001;344:159; *N Engl J Med* 2001; 344:168). Prophylaxis should be restarted when the CD4 count falls to <200/mm³ (AIII). A meta-analysis of 14 controlled trials involving discontinuation of PCP prophylaxis found (*Clin Infect Dis* 2001;33:1901) no difference in risk for PCP between those who continued prophylaxis and those who discontinued for a CD4 count >200/mm³. The rates were 19.1 vs 18.2 PCP episodes per 1000 patient-years for primary prophylaxis and 43.5 vs 41.9 PCP cases per 1000 patient-years for secondary prophylaxis. The rate of adverse reactions was 34.5 vs 8.6 cases per 1000 patient-years favoring discontinuation. A more recent review with follow-up averaging 40 months in 78 patients showed no cases of PCP (*AIDS* 2004;18:2047).

TRANSMISSION RISK: Some authorities recommend avoidance of "high-intensity exposure," meaning that a patient with PCP should not room with a vulnerable patient (*N Engl J Med* 2000;342:1416; *Am J Respir Crit Care Med* 2000;162:167; *Emerg Infect Dis* 2004;10:1713). Recent reports do not support this recommendation (*JAMA* 2001;286:2450).

M. tuberculosis

RISK (*MMWR* 1998;47:[RR-20]): Positive PPD (≥5 mm induration) without prior prophylaxis or treatment (AI), recent TB contact (AII), or history of inadequately treated TB that healed (AII) (*MMWR* 2000;49[RR-6]). The rate of active TB in those with a positive PPD is magnified 7- to 80-fold by HIV co-infection (*Lancet* 2000;356:470; *MMWR* 2000;49[RR-6]). It also appears that active TB accelerates the rate of HIV progression (*J Acquir Immune Defic Syndr* 1998;19:361; *BMJ* 1995;311:1468; *J Infect Dis* 2004;190:869). HIV-positive persons who are close contacts of active TB cases should be evaluated to exclude active disease and should receive treatment for latent TB infection regardless of PPD results.

PREFERRED REGIMEN FOR COMPLIANT PATIENT LIKELY TO COMPLETE 9-MONTH COURSE (*MMWR* 2000;49[RR-6]; *MMWR* 2001;50:773)

- INH 300 mg + pyridoxine 50 mg PO qd x 9 months (AII); or
- INH 900 mg + pyridoxine 100 mg PO 2x/week x 9 months (BII).

PREFERRED REGIMEN FOR PATIENT UNLIKELY TO COMPLETE 9-MONTH INH COURSE WITHOUT CONCURRENT PI OR NNRTI

- Rifampin 600 mg qd + PZA 15-20 mg/kg qd x 2 months (AI) For use of rifamycins with HAART, see p. 367. Note that the rifampin/ ritabutin + PZA combination has been associated with high rates of hepatotoxicity and requires frequent monitoring (see below).
- **Alternative regimen:** Rifampin 600 mg/day x 4 months (BII). There is no experience in HIV-infected patients, and there is concern for rifampin resistance.

Disease Prevention: Prophylactic Antimicrobial Agents and Vaccines

3

CONTACT WITH INH-RESISTANT STRAIN: Rifampin plus PZA x 2 months (above doses) (AI). Alternative: Rifabutin/PZA (above doses x 2 months) (BIII); rifabutin 300 mg/day PO x 4 months (CIII). See caution with requirement for frequent monitoring for hepatotoxicity (below) and recommendations for rifamycins with HAART (p. 367).

CONTACT WITH STRAIN RESISTANT TO INH AND A RIFAMYCIN: Use two agents with anticipated activity – ethambutol (EMB)/PZA or levofloxacin/PZA. Levofloxacin dose – 500 mg bid (*Arch Chest Dis* 2002;57:39); moxifloxacin also has good activity (*Antimicrob Agents Chemother* 1999;43:85).

PREGNANCY: INH regimens

MONITORING: Recipients of PZA + rifampin/rifabutin: There have been 40 cases of severe hepatotoxicity, including 7 deaths reported with the PZA + rifampin 2-month regimen (*MMWR* 2001;50:733; *MMWR* 2002;51:998; *Am Rev Respir Crit Care Med* 2001;164:1319). None of these patients was known to have HIV infection or concurrent active viral hepatitis; 3 had prior INH-associated hepatotoxicity. A subsequent analysis of this study showed only 15 of 721 HIV-infected patients who received RIF/PZA had ALT levels >250 U/L. This rate was similar for INH recipients (12/745). The conclusion was that hepatotoxicity is rare in HIV-infected patients given RIF/PZA (*Clin Infect Dis* 2004;39:561). Consequently, this regimen is still preferred for HIV infected patients who are considered unlikely to complete the 9-month INH regimen, providing there is no prior INH-associated hepatotoxicity. Monitoring should include patient visits at 0, 2, 4, 6, and 8 weeks with bilirubin + ALT measurements at 0, 2, 4, and 6 weeks. Prophylaxis should be discontinued with ALT elevations of 5x ULN in asymptomatic patients and with any elevation of ALT when accompanied by hepatitis symptoms (*MMWR* 2002;51:998). Cases of severe liver injury with this regimen should be reported to the CDC: 404-639-8116.

RECIPIENTS OF INH: Clinical monitoring at monthly intervals. Bilirubin ALT, AST, and CBC measurements at baseline, 3 months, and prn. Patient should report any symptoms of hepatitis – jaundice, dark urine, nausea, vomiting, abdominal pain, and/or fever >3 days. INH should be discontinued with ALT elevation to >5x ULN without symptoms or ALT >3x ULN with symptoms.

Toxoplasmà gondii

RISK: CD4 count <100/mm³ plus positive IgG serology for *T. gondii*. The risk of toxoplasmosis encephalitis in the pre-HAART era in patients with low CD4 counts and no prophylaxis was 33%/year (*J Infect Dis* 1996;173:91; *Clin Infect Dis* 2001;33:1747).

PREFERRED: TMP-SMX 1 DS/day (AII)

ALTERNATIVES

- TMP-SMX 1 SS/day (BIII)
- Dapsone 50 mg/day PO + pyrimethamine 50 mg/week + leucovorin 25 mg/week (BI)
- Dapsone 200 mg/week PO + pyrimethamine 75 mg/week PO + leucovorin 25 mg/week PO
- Atovaquone 1500 mg/day ± pyrimethamine 25 mg/day + leucovorin 10 mg/day (CIII)

IMMUNE RECONSTITUTION: Studies confirm the safety of discontinuing primary and secondary prophylaxis for toxoplasmosis (*Lancet* 2000;355:2217; *J Infect Dis* 2000;181:1635; *AIDS* 1999;13:1647; *AIDS* 2000;14:383; *Ann Intern Med* 2002;137:239).

- **Primary prophylaxis:** Discontinue prophylaxis with CD4 count >200/mm³ for >3 months (AI); restart when CD4 count is <100-200/mm³ (AIII).
- **Maintenance therapy:** Discontinue prophylaxis with CD4 count >200/mm³ for ≥6 months providing initial therapy for ≥6 wks has been completed and the patient is asymptomatic for toxoplasmosis (CIII). Some authorities would include MRI evaluation in this decision. Restart prophylaxis when CD4 count is <200/mm³ (AIII).

M. avium complex

RISK: CD4 count <50/mm³. The incidence of MAC with a CD4 <50/mm³ and no HAART or prophylaxis is 20-40% (*J Infect Dis* 1997;176:126; *Clin Infect Dis* 1993;17:7).

PREFERRED: Clarithromycin 500 mg PO bid (AI) or azithromycin 1200 mg PO weekly (AI). Note: Physician compliance with MAC prophylaxis recommendations is only about 50%, compared with 80% for PCP prophylaxis (*N Engl J Med* 2000;342:1416).

ALTERNATIVE: Rifabutin 300 mg/day PO (BI) or azithromycin 1200 mg/week plus rifabutin 300 mg/day (CI) (see rifabutin dose adjustment for use with PIs or NNRTIs, p. 291). Use caution when rifabutin is combined with clarithromycin due to drug interactions resulting in reduced levels of clarithromycin (*J Infect Dis* 2000;181:1289).

IMMUNE RECONSTITUTION: It is safe to discontinue primary and secondary MAC prophylaxis with immune reconstitution (CII) (*N Engl J Med* 1998;338:853; *N Engl J Med* 2000;342:1085; *Ann Intern Med* 2000;133:493; *J Infect Dis* 1998;178:1446; *HIV Med* 2004;5:278).

- **Primary prophylaxis:** Discontinue prophylaxis with CD4 count >100/mm³ for >3 months (AI); restart when CD4 count is <100/mm³ (AIII).

3 Disease Prevention: Prophylactic Antimicrobial Agents and Vaccines

- **Maintenance therapy:** Discontinue when CD4 cell count is >100/mm³ for >6 months, 12 months of therapy have been completed, and the patient is asymptomatic for MAC (CIII). Some authorities recommend blood cultures for MAC even in asymptomatic patients before discontinuing therapy. Restart when CD4 count is <100/mm³ (AIII).

Varicella zoster virus (VZV)

RISK (PRIMARY INFECTION): Significant exposure to chickenpox or shingles in individuals who are either seronegative for VZV or have no history of primary or secondary VZV.

PREFERRED: VZIG 625 U for patients >40 kg and 500 U for those <40 kg IM within 96 hours of exposure, preferably within 48 hours (AIII).

ALTERNATIVE: Prophylactic acyclovir was included in the 1995 USPHS/IDSA Guidelines, but was deleted from the 1999 version due to lack of supporting clinical evidence of efficacy.

Vaccines

S. pneumoniae

RISK: All patients with HIV infection. Risk for invasive pneumococcal infection is 50- to 100-fold greater than in the general population (*Ann Intern Med* 2000;132:182; *J Infect Dis* 1996;173:857; *J Acquir Immune Defic Syndr* 2001;27:35; *AM J Respir Crit Care Med* 2000;162:2063).

PREFERRED: *Pneumovax* 0.5 mL IM x 1 (CD4 count >200/mm³ – BII; CD4 count <200/mm³ – CIII).

REVACCINATE: When CD4 count increases to >200/mm³ if initial immunization was given with CD4 count <200/mm³ (CIII) (*MMWR* 1999;[RR-10]:16). Revaccination is recommended at 3- to 5-year intervals (*N Engl J Med* 2000;342:1416), though there is no evidence of efficacy for revaccination.

ALTERNATIVE: The 7 valent protein-conjugated pneumococcal vaccine approved by the FDA in March 2000 is recommended only for children. Use of this vaccine in adults shows no advantage over Pneumovax in terms of antibody levels (*Vaccine* 2001;20:545).

NOTE: Studies of pneumococcal vaccine in HIV infected persons have shown variable results. A CDC report indicated 49% efficacy (*Arch Intern Med* 2000;160:2633), but others found poor efficacy in immunosuppressed hosts (*N Engl J Med* 1986;315:1318; *JAMA* 1993;270:1826), and a controlled study in Uganda showed increased rates of pneumococcal disease in vaccine recipients (*Lancet* 2000;355:2106). Long-term follow-up continued to show a 1.6-fold increase in pneumonia from all causes in the Pneumovax recipients, but there was

Disease Prevention: Prophylactic Antimicrobial Agents and Vaccines

also a paradoxical increase in survival in this group (*AIDS* 2004;18:1210). Another report from Uganda showed a poor antigenic response to this vaccine (*J Infect Dis* 2004;190:707). Based on the controversial data regarding efficacy and virtually no vaccine-associated risks, the OI Guidelines Panel continues to recommend *Pneumovax*, but with low priority (CIII) and does not endorse its use as a recommended performance indicator (*Clin Infect Dis* 2000;30:51).

Hepatitis B

RISK: Negative anti-HBc or anti-HBs screening test.

PREFERRED: *Recombivax HB* 10 ug IM x 3 (at 0, 1, and 6 mos) (BII) or *Engerix-B* 20 µg IM x 3 (BII).

Influenza

RISK: All patients annually.

PREFERRED: Influenza vaccine 0.5 mL IM each year, preferably October to November (BIII).

ALTERNATIVE: The OI Panel recommends amantadine 100 mg PO bid (CIII) or rimantadine 100 mg PO bid (CIII). Zanamivir (*Relenza*, 10 mg inhaled/day) and oseltamivir (*Tamiflu*, 75 mg/day) are active against most strains of influenza B as well as influenza A, but are more expensive. Oseltamivir, rimantadine, and amantadine are FDA-approved for prophylaxis. The AWP price/month for standard dose in 2005 is $36/month for amantadine, $132/month for rimantadine, and $210/month for oseltamivir.

Hepatitis A

RISK: 1) MSM, 2) illegal drug users (injection and non-injection), and 3) persons with chronic liver disease, including chronic HBV and HCV (*MMWR* 2002;51[RR-6]:61). Susceptibility is defined by negative total anti-HAV antibody which is present in 33% of American adults. Some authorities recommend HAV for all susceptible patients as defined by negative HAV serology (total anti-HAV antibody).

PREFERRED: HAV vaccine 0.5 mL IM x 2 separated by 6 months (BIII).

Not Recommended for Most Patients; Consider for Selected Patients

Histoplasmosis

RISK: CD4 count <100/mm³ plus residence in endemic area. The risk is 2-5% for AIDS patients not receiving HAART in the Midwest and Puerto Rico (*Clin Infect Dis* 2000; 30:S5).

RECOMMENDATION: Consider primary prophylaxis if CD4 <100/mm³, residence in endemic area and occupational or other special risk.

Disease Prevention: Prophylactic Antimicrobial Agents and Vaccines

3

PREFERRED: Itraconazole 200 mg/day PO, AI Alternative is amphotericin B 1 mg/kg q week (AI)

Coccidioidomycosis

RISK: CD4 count <250/mm^3 (*J Infect Dis* 2000;181:1428) plus exposure in an endemic area (Southeast U.S.). The frequency in the endemic area is about 4% per year in untreated AIDS patients, 0.2% per year for HIV without AIDS, and 0.015% per year in the general population (*J Infect Dis* 2000;181:1428).

RECOMMENDATION: Primary prophylaxis is not recommended.

4 | Antiretroviral Therapy

Recommendations for Therapy

Based on the recommendations of DHHS as of April 7, 2005: http://www.aidsinfo.nih.gov and International AIDS Society-USA (*JAMA* 2004;292:251).

Goals of Therapy

CLINICAL GOALS: Prolongation of life and improvement in quality of life.

VIROLOGIC GOALS: Greatest possible reduction in viral load (preferably to <20-50 c/mL) for as long as possible to halt disease progression and prevent or delay progression.

IMMUNOLOGIC GOALS: Immune reconstitution that is both quantitative (CD4 cell count in normal range) and qualitative (pathogen-specific immune response).

THERAPEUTIC GOALS: Rational sequencing of drugs in a fashion that achieves clinical, virologic, and immunologic goals while maintaining treatment options, limit drug toxicity and facilitate adherence.

EPIDEMIOLOGIC GOALS: Reduce HIV transmission

Indications for Therapy (see Tables 4-3 (DHHS guidelines), 4-4 (IAS-USA guidelines), 4-5 (European guidelines), and 4-6 (WHO guidelines)

Recommendations are based on CD4 cell count, symptoms, and viral load. It is assumed that the patient is ready and willing to start therapy and understands the critical importance of adherence.

The CD4 count is the most important indicator for initiating treatment according to guidelines, and all agree that treatment is indicated for all patients with a CD4 count <200 cells/mm³. Whether to initiate therapy in the CD4 stratum between 200-350 cells/mm³ is more controversial. Some studies show no clear benefit with initiation at this stage (*JAMA* 2001;286:2560; *JAMA* 2001;286:2568; *AIDS* 2002;16:1371; *Ann Intern Med* 2003;138:620; *AIDS* 2001;15:2551; *J Infect Dis* 2004;190:1043), and others demonstrate only modest or no benefit (*Lancet* 2002;360:119; *Lancet* 2003;362:679; *AIDS* 2002;16:2455; *JAMA* 2001;286:2568). Factors that influence prognosis are the viral load, CD4 trajectory, age, patient readiness (meaning likelihood of adherence), and risk (IDU vs. other). (See risk calculator based on analysis of >9,000 patients receiving initial HAART in 13 cohorts.

Antiretroviral Therapy

4

www.art-cohort-collaboration.org). An argument by Phillips and colleagues is that short-term studies (≤3 years) will show treatment benefit even at high CD4 counts if the sample size is large enough. The problem is the inability to determine long-term benefit, since the period of response may be limited, and new developments in the field are unpredictable (*AIDS* 2003;17:1863). The probability of AIDS or death within 3 years in the pre-HAART era is summarized in Table 4-1.

■ TABLE 4-1: **Probability of Developing an AIDS-Defining OI Within 3 Years in the Absence of ART, Based on Baseline CD4 Count and Viral Load. Data from Multicenter AIDS Cohort Study (MACS) (*Ann Intern Med* 1997;126:946; updated June, 2002 per A. Munoz)**

VL (RT-PCR)* c/mL	% AIDS-Defining Complication			
CD4 <200 cells/mm³	**N**	**3 yrs.**	**6 yrs.**	**9 yrs.**
7,000-20,000	7	14	29	64
20,000-55,000	20	50	75	90
>55,000	70	84	98	100
CD4 201-350 cells/mm³	**N**	**3 yrs.**	**6 yrs.**	**9 yrs.**
1,500-7,000	27	0	20	37
7,000-20,000	44	7	44	66
20,000-55,000	53	36	72	85
>55,000	104	64	89	93
CD4 >350 cells/mm³	**N**	**3 yrs.**	**6 yrs.**	**9 yrs.**
<1,500	119	2	6	13
1,500-7,000	227	2	16	30
7,000-20,000	342	7	30	54
20,000-55,000	323	15	51	74
>55,000	262	40	72	85

* Plasma HIV RNA levels in c/mL using RT-PCR.

■ TABLE 4-2: **Risk of AIDS-defining OI or Death in 3 Years According to Baseline CD4 and VL in Patients Given HAART***

CD4	VL ≤100,000	VL >100,000
<50	19%	24%
50-99	15%	19%
100-199	12%	15%
200-349	6%	9%
>350	4%	5%

*Calculations are made for age <50 yrs., CDC stage A or B, and risk category other than IDU. For CD4 <50 and VL >100,000 c/ mL, age of >50 years increases the 24% to 36%; IDU increased it to 31% (www.art-cohort-collaboration.org).

When to Start Antiretroviral Therapy

DHHS GUIDELINES

■ TABLE 4-3: **Indications to Initiate Antiretroviral Therapy – DHHS Guidelines,)Oct. 10, 2005 (http://www.aidsinfo.nih.gov)**

Clinical Category	CD4 Cell Count	Plasma HIV RNA	Recommendation
Symptomatic (AIDS or severe symptoms)*	Any value	Any value	Treat
Asymptomatic	<200/mm³	Any value	Treat
Asymptomatic	200 to 350/mm³	Any value	Treatment should be offered; controversy exists for patients with viral load <20,000 c/mL due to low probability of AIDS-defining diagnosis within 3 years.
Asymptomatic	>350/mm³	≥100,000 c/mL	Most clinicians would defer therapy.

* Unexplained fever or diarrhea >2-4 wks, thrush or unexplained weight loss of >10% baseline weight

IAS-USA GUIDELINES:

■ TABLE 4-4: **When to Start Antiretroviral Therapy: IAS-USA Guidelines — 2004 (*JAMA* 2004;292;251)**

Disease Stage	Recommendations
Symptomatic HIV	ART recommended
Asymptomatic	
• CD4 <200/mm³	ART recommended
• CD4 200-350/mm³	ART considered. Defer if viral load low, CD4 slope <50/mm³/yr, patient reluctance. Treat if VL >100/mm³/yr, CD4 slope >100/mm³/yr
CD4 >350/mm³	Usually defer. Consider if high viral load or rapid CD4 slope

■ Table 4-5: **When to Start Treatment: British HIV Association 2005 Draft Guidelines (www.bhiva.org/guidelines/2005/BHIVA-guidelines/index.html, accessed June 25, 2005)**

Disease Stage	Recommendation
Acute HIV infection	Limited trials show no evidence of long term benefit; recommend participation in clinical trial.
Chronic HIV infection 1. Symptomatic or AIDS	ART recommended; active TB possible exception.
2. Asymptomatic	
• CD4 <200/mm³	ART recommended
• CD4 200-350/mm³	ART should start within this range depending on symptoms, viral load, CD4 slope, patient preference and co-morbidities such as hepatitis C
• CD4 >350/mm³	Defer ART

Antiretroviral Therapy

4

WHO GUIDELINES

Scaling up antiretroviral therapy in resource-limited settings.
WHO, December 2003 (draft version, http://www.who.int/hiv/pub/prev_care/en/WHO_ARV_Guidelines_Update.pdf)

Indications for initiating antiretroviral therapy are divided into two categories, depending on whether CD4 cell counts are available or not. The total lymphocyte count (TLC) is used as a "less useful" substitute for the CD4 count. The threshold for initiation of therapy using the CD4 count is 200 /mm³ with or without symptoms.

Table 4-6: **When to Start Antiretroviral Therapy – WHO Guidelines (March 2004)**

CD4 count available
WHO stage IV* (AIDS-defining diagnosis)
WHO Stage III (including HIV wasting, chronic enigmatic diarrhea, chronic enigmatic FUO, active pulmonary tuberculosis, recurrent invasive bacterial infections or recurrent/persistent mucosal candidiasis) with consideration of using CD4 counts <350/mm³ to assist decision making
WHO stage I-II* plus CD4 <200 /mm³
CD4 count not available
WHO stage IV*
WHO Stage III (including HIV wasting, chronic enigmatic diarrhea, chronic enigmatic FUO, active pulmonary tuberculosis, recurrent invasive bacterial infections or recurrent/persistent mucosal candidiasis regardless of TLC)
WHO stage II* plus TLC <1200 cells/mm³

*Clinical stages
- Clinical stage I: Asymptomatic or PGL, and/or normal activity
- Clinical stage II: Weight loss <10%, minor mucocutaneous conditions, zoster <5 years, recurrent URIs, and/or symptomatic plus normal activity
- Clinical stage III: Weight loss >10%, unexplained diarrhea >1 month, unexplained fever >1 month, thrush, oral hairy leukoplakia, pulmonary TB in past year, or severe bacterial infection, and/or bedridden <50% of days in the past month
- Clinical stage IV: CDC-defined AIDS and/or bedridden >50% of days in the past month

The Initial Regimen (see *Lancet* 2004;363:1248)

REGIMEN SELECTION: Preferred regimens for initial therapy are summarized according to guidelines for DHHS (Table 4-7), IAS-USA (Table 4-8), WHO (Table 4-9) pp. 61-62. It is becoming common practice to obtain pretreatment resistance tests in patients who are chronically infected. These results should be included in the choice of initial therapy, but it is emphasized that while these results are useful in identifying drugs to avoid, the lack of detectable resistance to a drug does not guarantee susceptibility, since resistant strains that are minority species (accounting for <20%) will not be detected with standard genotypic resistance tests. Technology to detect resistance in minority species exists, but is not yet commercially available (*J Infect Dis* 2005;192:24). There are also host factors that influence regimen selection, such as pregnancy (p. 114), tuberculosis (p. 361), hepatitis B or C coinfection, and HIV-2 infection.

■ TABLE 4-7: **Initial Regimen: DHHS Guidelines (October 6, 2005)**

Preferred
efavirenz + (lamivudine or emtricitabine) + (zidovudine or tenofovir DF) – except for pregnant women or women with pregnancy potential**
lopinavir/ritonavir (co-formulated as Kaletra®) + (lamivudine or emtricitabine) + zidovudine
Alternatives (may be preferred in some patients)
efavirenz + (lamivudine or emtricitabine) + (didanosine or abacavir or stavudine) except for pregnant women or women with pregnancy potential**
nevirapine + (lamivudine or emtricitabine) + (zidovudine or stavudine* or tenofovir or didanosine or abacavir) (Avoid for initial therapy in women with CD4 counts >250/mm³ and men with CD4 counts >400/mm³ due to high rates of hepatotoxicity.)
fosamprenavir + (lamivudine or emtricitabine) + (zidovudine or stavudine* or abacavir or tenofovir or didanosine)
fosamprenavir/ritonavir[†] + (lamivudine or emtricitabine) + (zidovudine or stavudine* or abacavir or tenofovir or didanosine)
atazanavir + (lamivudine or emtricitabine) + (zidovudine or stavudine* or abacavir or didanosine) or (tenofovir + ritonavir 100 mg/d)
indinavir/ritonavir[†] + (lamivudine or emtricitabine) + (zidovudine or stavudine* or abacavir or tenofovir or didanosine)
lopinavir/ritonavir (co-formulated as Kaletra®) + (lamivudine or emtricitabine) + (zidovudine or stavudine* or tenofovir or didanosine)
nelfinavir + (lamivudine or emtricitabine) + (zidovudine or stavudine* or abacavir or tenofovir or didanosine)
saquinavir (Invirase) /ritonavir[†] + (lamivudine or emtricitabine) + (zidovudine or stavudine* or abacavir or tenofovir or didanosine)
abacavir + lamivudine + zidovudine – only when an NNRTI- or a PI-based regimen cannot or should not be used

*Higher incidence of lipoatrophy, hyperlipidemia, and mitochondrial toxicities reported with stavudine than with other NRTIs

**"Women with child-bearing potential" includes women who want to conceive or who are not using effective contraception

[†] Low-dose (100-400 mg) ritonavir

4 Antiretroviral Therapy

■ TABLE 4-8: **Initial Regimen: IAS-USA (_JAMA_ 2004;292:251)**

Class	Preferred	Alternatives
2 NRTIs _plus_ NNRTI or boosted PI		
PI	Atazanavir/ritonavir Lopinavir/ritonavir Saquinavir/ritonavir Indinavir/ritonavir	Fosamprenavir//ritonavir Atazanavir Nelfinavir
NNRTI	Efavirenz	Nevirapine
NRTI pairs	(Zidovudine or tenofovir) + (lamivudine or emtricibine) Didanosine + emtricitabine	Abacavir + lamivudine Didanosine + tenofovir Didanoside + lamivudine Zidovudine + abacavir Stavudine + lamivudine
Regimen for special circumstances: zidovudine + lamivudine + abacavir		

■ TABLE 4-9: **Preferred Initial Regimens – British HIV Association, June, 2005 (draft)**

	A	B	C
Choose one from each column (A, B, and C)			
Preferred	EFV LPV/r	AZT, ABC, TDF, ddl	3TC FTC
Alternative	FPV/r SQV/r		
Special groups*	NVP* ATV[†] ATV/r[†]		
Not recommended	ABC[§] Unboosted PI[‡]	d4T	

* NVP restricted to women with baseline CD4 <250/mm³ and men with baseline CD4 <400/mm³.

[†] ATV was not licensed in the UK at the time these guidelines were developed.

[‡] ATV and NFV in pregnancy are exceptions.

[§] Use as "third drug" only if PI and NNRTI cannot be given.

Antiretroviral Therapy

Initial Regimen for Resource-Poor Settings: WHO Guidelines (March, 2004)

Regimen	Toxicity*	Pregnancy issue	Concurrent TB Rx	Fixed dose
NVP/d4T/3TC	d4T, NVP	Yes	Alternative	Yes
NVP/AZT/3TC	AZT, NVP	Yes	Alternative	Yes
EFV/d4T/3TC	EFV, d4T	Alternative	OK	No
EFV/AZT/3TC	EFV, AZT	Alternative	OK	No

*Toxicity
   d4T: peripheral neuropathy, lipoatrophy
   ZDV: anemia, neutropenia, GI intolerance
   NFV: hepatotoxicity, skin rash
   EFV: CNS toxicity, teratogenicity

■ TABLE 4-11: **Advantages and Disadvantages of Antiretroviral Agents and Combinations for Initial Therapy**

Agents	Advantages	Disadvantages
2 NRTIs + 1 PI or RTV-boosted PI*		
Atazanavir + ritonavir	■ Low pill burden ■ Once daily dosing ■ No effect on lipids or insulin resistance ■ Fewer GI side effects	■ Food requirement ■ Hyperbilirubinemia/jaundice ■ Drug interactions including TDF and EFV (use ATV/r 300/100 qd) ■ Potential for QTc prolongation ■ Absorption dependent on acidic pH (PPI contraindicated) ■ No resistance data in PI-naïve patients
Fosamprenavir + ritonavir	■ Once daily regimen available (FDA-approved without prior PI failure) ■ No food effect ■ No PI resistance with failure	■ Limited experience ■ Cross resistance with LPV (I50V) ■ Rash, nausea ■ PI class toxicity
Indinavir + ritonavir*	■ Long term experience documenting sustained benefit ■ RTV boosting eliminates food effect	■ Nephrolithiasis, skin/hair side effects ■ IDV/RTV 400/400 bid – Poor GI tolerance 800/100 bid – Increased nephrolithiasis
Lopinavir + ritonavir	■ Co-formulation ■ High potency documented ■ Comparable potency with viral load >100,000 c/mL ■ No PI resistance with initial failure ■ Durable potency established ■ Once daily therapy FDA approved	■ Nausea, diarrhea ■ Limited experience in pregnancy ■ Food requirement ■ After initial therapy

4 Antiretroviral Therapy

Agents	Advantages	Disadvantages
Nelfinavir	■ Generally well tolerated ■ No PI cross-resistance with D30N ■ Extensive experience establishing favorable pharmokinetics and safety in pregnancy	■ Diarrhea ■ PI class toxicity ■ Reduced potency compared with boosted PIs ■ Decreased efficacy with viral load >100,000 c/mL and/or low CD4 count ■ Fatty food requirement ■ PI cross-resistance with L90M ■ Poor boosting with RTV
Saquinavir (Invirase) + ritonavir*	■ Extensive experience	■ Poor GI tolerability ■ PI class toxicity

2 NRTI + NNRTI

Agents	Advantages	Disadvantages
Delavirdine	■ Increases PI levels	■ Minimal efficacy data ■ tid dosing ■ Rash ■ Single mutation confers class resistance
Efavirenz	■ High potency documented ■ Comparable potency with viral load >100,000 c/mL ■ One tab per day ■ May use with rifampin ■ Durable potency established	■ Neuropsychiatric toxicity and rash ■ Contraindicated in pregnancy and with pregnancy potential ■ Single mutation confers class resistance ■ Methadone interaction ■ Reduces PI levels
Nevirapine	■ Fewer drug interactions ■ Low pill burden ■ No food effect ■ Minimal lipid changes	■ Hepatotoxicity including lethal hepatic necrosis especially with pre-treatment CD4 counts >250 (F) or >400 (M) ■ High rate of rash, including life-threatening hypersensitivity ■ Single mutation confers class resistance ■ Methadone interaction ■ Reduces PI levels ■ Less clinical trial data than with EFV

3 NRTIs

Agents	Advantages	Disadvantages
AZT/3TC/ABC	■ Extensive experience ■ Low pill burden ■ Preserves PI and NNRTI options ■ Minimal drug interactions ■ Co-formulated	■ Reduced potency at all VL levels compared to EFV-based HAART ■ ABC hypersensitivity reactions ■ AZT effects (see below)

Antiretroviral Therapy

Agents	Advantages	Disadvantages
2 NRTIs (as component of HAART regimen)		
AZT/3TC or AZT/FTC	■ Extensive experience ■ Low pill burden ■ Co-formulated (AZT/3TC) ■ No food effect ■ M184V slows AZT resistance ■ Gradual accumulation of TAMs with failure	■ AZT toxicity: Anemia, neutropenia, GI intolerance ■ TAMs and NRTI cross-resistance with prolonged failure ■ Mitochondrial toxicity (AZT) including lipoatrophy and lactic acidosis
TDF/3TC or TDF/FTC	■ Once daily regimen ■ Both effective against HBV ■ Well tolerated ■ Low pill burden ■ Avoids TAMs ■ Coformulated (TDF/FTC) ■ Low potential for mitochondrial toxicity	■ Risk of ABC and ddI cross-resistance after failure (K65R) ■ TDF interaction to decrease levels of ATV (use ATV/r)
ddI/3TC or ddI/FTC	■ Once daily regimen ■ Low pill burden ■ Avoid TAMs	■ Minimal data ■ ddI toxicity: Pancreatitis, neuropathy, GI intolerance, mitochondrial toxicity ■ Food effect (ddI) ■ Risk of K65R with ABC and TDF cross-resistance
d4T/3TC or d4T/FTC	■ Good short-term tolerability ■ No food effect ■ Low pill burden ■ M184V (3TC) slows d4T resistance	■ d4T toxicity: Neuropathy, lipoatrophy, hyperlipemia, ascending paralysis (rare), lactic acidosis ■ TAMs and cross-resistance with prolonged failure
ABC/3TC or ABC/FTC	■ No food effect ■ Once daily regimen ■ Low pill burden ■ Well tolerated ■ Avoids TAMs	■ ABC hypersensitivity reaction ■ Risk of ddI cross-resistance (L74V) or TDF and ddI cross-resistance (K65R)
ddI/d4T (not commonly used)	■ Extensive prior experience ■ Low pill burden	■ Contraindicated in pregnancy ■ ddI/d4T toxicity: Lactic acidosis, peripheral neuropathy, pancreatitis, lipoatrophy, and hyperlipidemia ■ Food effect (ddI) ■ May increase risk of TAMs and multi-nucleoside resistance mutations

continued on next page

Antiretroviral Therapy

4

■ TABLE 4-11: **Advantages and Disadvantages of Antiretroviral Agents and Combinations** *(Continued)*

Agents	Advantages	Disadvantages
AZT/ddl (not commonly used)	■ Extensive prior experience ■ Low pill burden	■ Side effects of AZT + ddl ■ May increase risk of TAMs and multi-nucleoside resistance mutations ■ Complex dosing (AZT tolerability improved with food, ddl taken on empty stomach) ■ Mitochondrial toxicity (AZT and ddl) including lipoatrophy and lactic acidosis
TDF/ddl (not recommended)	■ Once daily regimen	■ High rates of viral failure with 3rd NRTI or with NNRTI ■ Possible reduced CD4 response ■ Drug interaction requiring reduced dose of ddl ■ Possible increased risk of pancreatitis and lactic acidosis

*All PIs except ATV are associated with class adverse reactions (hyperlipidemia, insulin resistance, fat redistribution).

All PIs preserve the NNRTI option.

All PIs are boosted to give better pharmacokinetics, except nelfinavir.

■ TABLE 4-12: **Once-Daily Drugs**

Class	FDA-approved	Possibly Effective Based on Pharmacology
NRTI	■ ddl 400 mg ■ ABC 600 mg ■ TDF 300 mg ■ 3TC 300 mg ■ FTC 200 mg	
NNRTI	EFV 600 mg	NVP 400 mg (higher incidence of hepatotoxicity)
PI	■ ATV 400 mg ■ ATV + RTV 300/100 mg ■ FPV + RTV 1400/200 mg* ■ LPV/r 800/200 mg	■ SQV/RTV (*Invirase*) 2000/100 mg

*Treatment naïve patients only

Antiretroviral Therapy

- **HIV-2 treatment** (*Clin Infect Dis* 2004;38:1771)
  - □ This strain should be suspected in patients with an epidemiologic link to West Africa (see p. 5).
  - □ There is no commercially available test for HIV-2 viral load, although some labs have "home brews."
  - □ Experience with treatment is limited
    - NRTIs are as effective as with HIV-1
    - NNRTIs are largely ineffective
    - PIs appear variable. IND may be less active vs. HIV-2 compared to HIV-1. SQV, RTV and NFV appear to have comparable activity.

Factors That Influence Probability of Prolonged Viral Suppression

REGIMEN POTENCY: A review was provided for trials of treatment using 3 or 4 antiretroviral agents in publications or presentations from 1994 until March 2004. Criteria for inclusion were ≥30 previously treatment-naïve patients in each arm of the study, study duration ≥24 wks, and results for virologic control defined as proportion of subjects <50 c/mL by intent-to-treat analysis (12th CROI, Boston, Feb. 2005, Abstr. 586). There were 49 trials, 85 treatment arms and 15,147 patients. NNRTI- and boosted PI-based HAART regimens were comparable and that both were superior to unboosted PI-based HAART regimens (p <0.01). Of the top 20 regimens, EFV-based HAART accounted for 13, LPV/r for 4 and NVP for 3. The proportion of patients achieving suppression to <50 c/mL by ITT analysis for 19 of these top 20 regimens was 65%-82%.

ADHERENCE: Obvious but critical, as shown in a study that demonstrated a strong correlation between virologic response and adherence (*Ann Intern Med* 2000;133:21). Most important was the demonstrated need for >95% adherence to achieve viral suppression in 80%. The virologic failure rate with <95% adherence is reported at >50% (Table 4-11). Multiple other studies have shown similar results (*AIDS* 2001;15:2109; *Clin Infect Dis* 2001;33:386; *AIDS* 2000;14:357; *Clin Infect Dis* 2002;34:115; *J Gen Intern Med* 2002;17:377; *AIDS* 2004;35:S35). However, many of the studies involved unboosted PI-based regimens, and there is reason to believe that requirements for adherence are less stringent for NNRTI- and boosted PI-based regimens.

Antiretroviral Therapy

4

■ TABLE 4-13: Correlation Between Adherence and Virologic Response to HAART (*Ann Intern Med* 2000;133:21)

Adherence to HAART*	Viral Load <400 c/mL at 6 Months
>95% adherence	78%
90 to 95% adherence	45%
80 to 90% adherence	33%
70 to 80% adherence	29%
<70% adherence	18%

* Number of doses prescribed/number taken

ADHERENCE AND RESISTANCE: Poor adherence predicts virologic failure but not necessarily resistance. The highest risk of resistance to a PI-based regimen is with virologic failure in the face of good adherence (*J Acquir Immune Defic Syndr* 2002;30:278; *AIDS* 2000;14:357; *AIDS* 2001;15:1701). In one study, 23% of patients with virologic failure ascribed to resistance had 92% to 100% adherence based on unannounced pill counts (*AIDS* 2003;17:1925). In another study, 88% of patients with resistance mutations were in patients who consumed >70% of prescribed doses (*Clin Infect Dis* 2003;37:1112). Both reports showed virologic failure but virtually no resistance mutations with consumption of <60% of prescribed doses. More recent data suggest this association between adherence and resistance may be drug class-related, with high rates of resistance correlates better with good adherence to unboosted PIs, but to low adherence to NNRTI-based regimens (XV Intl AIDS Conference 2004, Abstr. WePeB5820).

GUIDANCE FOR IMPROVED ADHERENCE

ADHERENCE ISSUES

- Common strategies
  - □ Establish patient readiness before initiating treatment
  - □ Use a standardized approach to assess adherence
  - □ Use the entire health care team to reinforce adherence messages
  - □ Understand that health care professionals are poor predictors of who will adhere
  - □ Understand that patients will usually over-report their adherence
  - □ Understand that adherence usually decreases with time, becoming significantly worse at 6-12 mos than it is initially (*Topics HIV Med* 2003;11:185)
  - □ Adherence is more effective in a medical setting than in a social service setting (HRSA)

Antiretroviral Therapy

- Patients need to understand that the regimen most likely to succeed is the first one
- Address obvious issues of convenience; adherence is sometimes related to pill burden, frequency of daily administrations, food or fasting requirements, tolerance and/or pill size

- **Factors that correlated with reduced adherence:** Intolerance, mental illness, active substance abuse, comorbidities such as TB and diabetes, asymptomatic status of patient when treatment begins, poverty issues (homelessness, transportation problems), poor understanding of regimen, inadequate pharmacy service (*Topics HIV Med* 2003;11:185; American Public Health Association, "Recommendations for Best Practices," www.apha.org/ppp/hiv).

- **Adherence review and recommendations of the British HIV Association, http://www.bhiva.org/guidelines/2004/adherence/index.html**
  - Treatment simplification: Once-daily therapy has not proven better with treatment of hypertension (*Am J Hyperten* 2000;13:184). A review of the HIV literature on this point found only one study demonstrating a better outcome with once-daily HAART (*JAMA* 2002;288:2868); however, it is generally preferred by patients.
  - Improvement in knowledge: Two reports show benefit with educational sessions (*J Acquir Immune Defic Syndr* 2003;34:191; *Patient Educ Couns* 2003;50:187). Other reports show no benefit with individual counseling by a trained counselor or group support (*J Acquir Immune Defic Syndr* 2003;34:174; *J Assoc Nurses AIDS Care* 2003;14:52).
  - Pagers, alarms, phones: One large randomized study showed significantly more virologic failure in patients using a dose time alarm vs. controls (XV Int'l AIDS Conf 2004, Abstr. LbOrB15).
  - Practice with placebo: One controlled trial with a 2-mo training period showed no benefit (12th CROI, 2005, Abstr. 614).
  - Directly observed therapy: Two studies show improved virologic outcomes using DOT with methadone maintenance (*Clin Infect Dis* 2004;38[suppl 5]:S409; *Clin Infect Dis* 2004;38[suppl 5]:S414).
  - Clinical trial with enfuvirtide injections: Compliance to >95% of doses was achieved by patient report in 84% of participants (XV Int'l AIDS Conf., 2004, Abstr. WePeB5822).

RECOMMENDATIONS

- Data do not support frequent, intensive or prolonged contact with adherence specialists; use the entire HIV medicine team of health care providers rather than an adherence specialist.
- Brief individualized interventions may be beneficial.

Antiretroviral Therapy

4

- Regimens should not be simplified if it reduces potency.
- Medication alarms may reduce adherence.

BASELINE VIRAL LOAD: Some studies show a correlation between baseline viral load and probability of achieving viral suppression to <50 c/mL or <500 c/mL (*AIDS* 1999;13:187; *Clin Infect Dis* 1999;29:75; *Arch Intern Med* 2000;160:1323; *AIDS* 2001;15:1793; *JAMA* 2001;286:2560; *N Engl J Med* 2004;350:1850) and the durability of the response (*Clin Infect Dis* 2003;37:702). This does seem to apply to highly potent regimens such as EFV- or LPV/r-based HAART (*N Engl J Med* 1999;341: 1865; *N Engl J Med* 2002;346:2039; *N Engl J Med* 2003;349:2293).

PRIOR EXPOSURE TO ANTIRETROVIRAL AGENTS: Multiple studies demonstrate an inverse correlation between response and the extent of prior antiretroviral therapy as determined by number of agents, number of classes, and duration of treatment. In the Swiss Cohort study for example, the probability of achieving a viral load <500 c/mL with HAART therapy was 91% in treatment-naïve patients compared with 75% in treatment-experienced patients (*Lancet* 1999;353:863). Among patients who achieved undetectable viral loads, the probability of maintaining a viral load <500 c/mL at 2 years was 80% for treatment-naïve patients compared with 62% for treatment-experienced patients. The conclusion of many authorities is that the initial regimen is the most important regimen because it is associated with the greatest probability of achieving prolonged viral suppression (*J Acquir Immune Defic Syndr* 2000;24:115).

VIRAL LOAD NADIR: Multiple studies demonstrate that the viral load nadir predicts the durability of response (*AIDS* 2002;16:1521; *JAMA* 1998;279:930; *Lancet* 2001;358:1760; *J Acquir Immune Defic Syndr* 2002;30:167; *AIDS* 1998;12:F9). An analysis of 22 cohorts with 9323 patients started on an initial HAART regimen, the most important predictor of mortality or development of an AIDS-defining event was the VL and CD4 count 6 months after starting (*Lancet* 2003;362:92).

RAPIDITY OF VIRAL LOAD RESPONSE: The trajectory of the viral load response predicts the nadir plasma HIV RNA level and consequently the durability of HIV response. To achieve an optimal and durable virologic response, treatment-naïve patients treated with HAART should respond as follows:

- Decrease 0.7-1.0 $\log_{10}$ c/mL at 1 week (*Lancet* 2001;358:1760; *J Acquir Immune Defic Syndr* 2002;30:167)
- Decrease 1.5-2.0 $\log_{10}$ c/mL to <5,000 c/mL at 4 weeks (*AIDS* 1999;13:1873; *J Acquir Immune Defic Syndr* 2000;25:36). One review of 656 treatment-naïve patients given HAART showed a VL reduction to <1000 c/mL by week 4 predicted with an 82%-95%

Antiretroviral Therapy

probability of VL <50 c/mL at week 24 (*J Acquir Immune Defic Syndr* 2004;37:1155).

- Decrease to <500 c/mL at 8 to 16 weeks and <50 c/mL at 16 to 24 weeks (*Ann Intern Med* 2001;135:954; *J Acquir Immune Defic Syndr* 2000;24:433)

Failure to achieve these goals suggests lack of antiretroviral potency, non-adherence, resistance or inadequate drug levels due to drug interactions, poor absorption, etc.

FACTORS THAT PREDICT CLINICAL PROGRESSION (AIDS-DEFINING DIAGNOSIS OR DEATH) AFTER INITIATING HAART: Based on an analysis of 9323 patients from 13 cohorts given initial regimen of HAART, the following factors correlate with clinical outcomes defined by mortality or an AIDS-defining event (see www.art.cohort-collaboration.org for Risk Calculator):

- **Baseline VL:** High VLs arbitrarily defined at 100,000 c/mL correlate with probability of virologic control (<50 c/mL by 24-48 wks) with some HAART regimens but not others (*J Infect Dis* 2004;190:280). This depends on the potency of the regimen. The most important predictors of long-term success are CD4 count and VL at 6 months post-treatment.
- CD4 count represents a continuum in the risk stratification.
- Age >50 years decreases the probability of long-term success.
- Injection drug use is the only HIV risk category with increased risk of progression or death (*J Acquir Immune Defic Syndr* 2004;35:46). Multiple studies show that HCV coinfection is a risk factor for HIV progression, but this appears to reflect HCV as a surrogate for IDU (*J Acquir Immune Defic Syndr* 2003;33:365; Lancet 2003;362:877). However, one study found that rehabilitated IDUs had outcomes comparable to those who never used injection drugs (*AIDS* 2001;27:251).
- Therapy with a PI or NNRTI reduced risk of progression by 60% and were comparable.
- The most important predictor was VL and CD4 count at 6 months of therapy.

When to Modify Therapy

DEFINING TREATMENT FAILURE

- **Virologic Failure:** The goal of therapy is a sustained VL level <50 c/mL, according to 2004-05 guidelines of IAS-USA (*JAMA* 2004;292:26), the U.S. DHHS (http://AIDSinfo.nih.gov) and the British HIV Association (http://www.bhiva.org/guidelines/2005/BHIVA-guidelines/index.html).

Antiretroviral Therapy

- Rapidity of response: Response in treatment-naïve patients should be a decrease of 0.7-1.0 log c/mL at 1 wk, 1.5-2.0 log c/mL decrease at 4 wks and <50 c/mL at 16-24 wks (see p. 16).

- Blips: Blips are defined as a transient VL >50 c/mL preceded and followed by measurements <50 c/mL without a change in treatment. One study that measured VL every 2-3 days for 3-4 mos found that blips were common (9/10 patients), low-level (median of 79 c/mL), transient (<3 days), unrelated to clinical events (illness, vaccination, etc.) and appeared to represent a statistical variation around the mean HIV level below 50 c/mL (*JAMA* 2005;293:817). Levels >200 c/mL or sustained VL >50 c/mL usually indicate virologic failure.

- Frequency of virologic failure: Analysis of 12 reports with 1,197 patients in the U.S. showed 62% failed to achieve the goal of VL <50 c/mL by 24 wks (*Clin Infect Dis* 2004;38:614).

- Rationale for the 50 c/mL threshold: Sequence analysis of HIV clones from patients with sustained VL <50 c/mL show no sequence evolution with emergence of resistance mutations (*J Infect Dis* 2004;189:1444; *J Infect Dis* 2004;189:1452). A similar analysis in patients with persistent low-level viremia (50-400 c/mL) showed acquisition of resistance mutations in 9/21 patients at a median follow-up of 11 mos (*Clin Infect Dis* 2004;39:1030).

- **Immunologic failure:** This is arbitrarily defined as failure of the CD4 count to increase 25-50/mm^3 in the first year of HAART (DHHS, http://AIDSinfo.nih.gov, April 7, 2005). The CD4 response correlates with viral suppression; the increase averages 50/mm^3 at 4-8 wks with good viral suppression and then increases 100-150/ mm^3/year thereafter (*JAMA* 2002;288:222; *J Infect Dis* 2002;185:471; *JAMA* 2004;292:1911). As expected, the response correlates with the duration of HIV suppression. Using virologic failure as the reference, a review of 596 patients followed for a median of 2.5 yrs showed annual increase of 5.2 cells/mm^3/yr for each 10% cumulative time spent with viral suppression to <400/ mm^3 (*J Infect Dis* 2004;190:1860).

  Although this correlation is consistent in population-based studies, individual variation is great and discordant changes in both directions are relatively common (*J Infect Dis* 2001;183:1328; *Clin Infect Dis* 2002;35:1005). The problem is that there are no strategies with established merit to deal with the discordance; e.g., the patient with viral suppression and a blunted CD4 response.

- **Clinical failure:** This is defined as the occurrence or re-occurrence of an AIDS-defining opportunistic complication after 3 mos of HAART. Immune reconstitution syndrome (p. 419) does not qualify as a clinical failure and should be excluded.

Antiretroviral Therapy

■ TABLE 4-14: **Monitoring Response to Therapy Adapted from Primary Care Guidelines (*Clin Infect Dis* 2004;39:609)**

Rx	Test	Time	Comment
New Rx	VL	1-4 wks	• Optional; purpose is to determine response. assess adherence and resistance. • Expect VL decrease 0.7-1.0 $\log_{10}$ c/mL
New Rx	VL	3-4 mo	• Standard practice. • If VL does not suppress to <400 c/mL or if persistently >400 c/mL after good viral suppression or failure to achieve this level at 24-48 wks, review adherence and test resistance if VL >1000 c/mL.
	CD4	3-4 mo	• Standard practice. • Expected increase with viral suppression of 30-70/mm³ in the first 4 mo, then 100-150/mm³/year.
D/C ART	VL CD4	1, 2 & 3 mo	• Expected response is CD4 decrease by 30-50/mm³/mo; VL increase to pretreatment levels. • Usually, restart HAART at predetermined values for CD4 count.

■ TABLE 4-15: **Therapeutic Drug Monitoring – Target Trough Levels for Wild-type Virus (Adapted from DHHS Guidelines, March 23, 2004)**

Drug	Concentration (ng/mL)
Amprenavir*	400
Atazanavir†	≥150-850
Fosamprenavir	400
Efavirenz	3400
Indinavir	100 (max. 10,000)
Lopinavir‡	1000
Nelfinavir	800
Nevirapine	3400
Ritonavir	2100 (as single PI)
Saquinavir	100-250

* APV trough of 1200 ng/mL suggested for PI-experienced patients

† Added by author based on 12th CROI, Boston, Abstr. 645

‡ LPV trough of 4000 ng/mL suggested for PI-experienced patients

4 Antiretroviral Therapy

Adverse Reactions		
Toxicity	**Routine Tests**	**Comment**
Lactic acidosis; d4T AZT, ddl	None	■ Serum lactate only with symptoms and with high risk groups receiving NRTIs: pregnancy, history of lactic acidosis. ■ See p. 103
Hyperlipidemia (*Clin Infect Dis* 2002;34:838); d4T, PIs (except ATV)	Fasting total, LDL, HDL cholesterol and triglycerides at baseline, then at 3-6 months, then at least annually	■ Treat according to Framingham risks and National Cholesterol Education Program (NCEP) guidelines ■ Associated with PIs, especially RTV (dose dependent). Also more associated with d4T among NRTIs and EFV among NNRTIs. ■ Consider switch to non-PI-based regimen or ATV. ■ See p. 106
Insulin Resistance: Most PIs	FBS at baseline + every 3 to 6 months (IAS-USA) or at 1-3 mo, then q 3-4 mo (DHHS)	■ Associated with most PIs (not ATV). ■ Treat hyperglycemia, preferably with insulin sensitizing agents, or switch to non-PI-containing or ATV-containing regimen. ■ See p. 105
Fat accumulation and lipoatrophy d4T, AZT (lipoatrophy), PIs, EFV (fat accumulation)	No screening test	■ Glucose tolerance test at baseline is not indicated. ■ Cosmetic issue; patient perception is usually most important. ■ Best monitoring: Waist or waist/hip and breast measurement. ■ No established treatment, but drug switches (PI- to non-PI-based regimens for fat accumulation, d4T or AZT to TDF or ABC switches for lipoatrophy) may be helpful. ■ See p. 100
Hepatitis NVP (hepatic necrosis), EFV, NVP, all PIs (transaminitis) d4T, AZT, ddl (steatosis)	■ Regular monitoring of ALT/AST q 3-4 mo (all PI and NNRTI regimens) ■ NVP: Monitor more closely for hepatotoxicity (see comments)	■ NVP: DHHS: ALT/AST at baseline, 2, 4, 8, 12, 16 wks, than q 3 mo. ■ TPV/r monitoring in patients at risk for hepatitis. ■ See p. 110

Antiretroviral Therapy

- The standard goal is viral suppression with the specific targets to decrease VL ≥1 $\log_{10}$ c/mL (90%) within 4 weeks and viral load <20-50 c/mL by 16 to 24 weeks. Studies show that <5% of all AIDS-defining complications occur in patients with a viral load of <5,000 c/mL, suggesting that thresholds that define virologic failure and clinical failure may be different (*AIDS* 1999;13:1035; *AIDS* 1999;13:341; *J Acquir Immune Defic Syndr* 2001;27:44; *J Acquir Immune Defic Syndr* 2002;30:154). However, long-term studies show that virologic failure will eventually lead to clinical and immunologic failure (*J Infect Dis* 2004;190:280), and studies of HIV show no sequence evolution with new resistance mutations over a 1-yr period when the VL is maintained at <50 c/mL (*J Infect Dis* 2004;189:1444; *J Infect Dis* 2004;189:1452). Unfortunately, reviews of large cohorts show this level of viral suppression is hard to achieve and sustain (*Ann Intern Med* 1999;131:18; AIDS 1999;13: F35). The HIV Cost and Services Utilization Study Consortium (HCSUS) study suggests that only about 28% of persons in the United States who were receiving HIV care in the U.S. in 1996-98 had a viral load <500 c/mL (*J Acquir Immune Defic Syndr* 2000;25:115). Based on these observations, most authorities consider a reduction to <50 c/mL to be the ultimate goal of therapy but acknowledge that this may be unrealistic in some patients. More importantly, the attempt to achieve unrealistic virologic responses may severely limit future therapeutic options due to the evolution of resistance.

CD4 RESPONSE: The CD4 response is generally a mirror image of the HIV RNA decay curve, with increases that average 50-60 cells/mm^3 in the first 4 months with subsequent increases at a rate of 8-10 cells/mm^3/month or 100-150 cells/mm^3/year with good viral suppression (*J Infect Dis* 2002;185:471; *Ann Intern Med* 2001;135:954; *AIDS* 2001;15:1793; *AIDS* 2001;15:983). However, many patients (up to 20%-30%) have discordant results, either with minimal CD4 response despite good viral suppression or with a CD4 increase despite a poor virologic response (*J Infect Dis* 2001;183:1328; *JAMA* 2001;285:777). Therapeutic decisions are usually made based on viral load data. One exception is the combination of TDF/ddI, which has been associated with a blunted CD4 response even with ddI dose adjustment and viral suppression (*Clin Infect Dis* 2005;41:901).

CAUSE OF VIROLOGIC FAILURE: Inadequate virologic response is ascribed to (1) resistance or (2) failure of the drugs to reach the virus (inadequate adherence, altered metabolism, drug interaction).

GUIDELINES FOR CHANGING ANTIRETROVIRAL REGIMEN
(Modified from DHHS Guidelines, April 2005 and IAS-USA Guidelines, 2004)

- **Assessing failure:**
  - *Adherence:* Address issues of access, depression, tolerability, convenience (food effect, pill burden, multiple dosing regimens), substance abuse, patient comprehension, dementia (see p. 71)
  - *Convenience*

    Once-daily regimen (see Table 4-11, p. 63)

4 Antiretroviral Therapy

Low pill burden: 2 to 4 pills/day, EFV, NVP, ATV, FPV-based HAART. Coformulation of EFV, TDF and FTC will permit 1 pill/day and is expected in 2006.

Food effect: see below

□ *Tolerability*

GI intolerance is most common. Treatment may be symptomatic with anti-emetic, antidiarrheal agent, or fiber supplement; administration with food often improves tolerability, but this is not possible with ddI or unboosted IDV

Single-drug substitutions

□ *Pharmacokinetic issues*

Food effect: fasting requirements – ddI, unboosted IDV, and EFV (first 2-3 wks); Food requirement – ATV, TPV/r, LPV/r, NFV, and SQV

□ *Drug interactions* (see Table 4-22, pp. 92-95) – Avoid TDF and unboosted ATV, d4T/AZT, TDF/ddI (unless ddI is dose reduced)

□ *Resistance:* resistance testing requires expertise for reliable interpretation. These tests are most reliable for evaluating only drugs being taken at the time the test is performed or within 4 wks of the test. They do not reliably detect minority species (<20%) and consequently are more useful in determining which agents are unlikely to be effective than to determine which drugs are likely to be effective. To assess minority strains, consider prior resistance test results, treatment history, including duration of therapy in presence of virologic failure and agent-specific genetic barriers to resistance (high barrier with most boosted PIs and thymidine analogs; low barrier with 3TC and NNRTIs).

The validity of testing after ART is discontinued depends on the time off treatment and the drug evaluated (*Antimicrob Agents Chemother* 2004;48:644). Wild-type virus may become dominant in ≥4 wks after treatment is discontinued, so this represents the anticipated minimal duration of resistance test validity. Nevertheless, some mutations such as K103N may persist 9 to 12 months or longer (*J Clin Lab Anal* 2002;16:76), possibly because this mutation does not alter replication capacity (*J Med Virol* 2003;69:1). The M184V mutation more strongly influences replication capacity (*AAC* 2003;47:3377) and usually cannot be detected 5-20 wks after discontinuation for 5 to 20 weeks (*AAC* 2002;46:2255; *Antimicrob Agents Chemother* 2004;48:644).

- **Guidance for changes based on intolerance**

□ Changes based on ADRs or intolerance can be made with single agent substitution, provided the patient has an appropriate virologic response to the original regimen.

□ Changes for class adverse reactions (see pp. 100-113)

STRATEGIES FOR VIROLOGIC FAILURE

In general, the probability of success with a second regimen is nearly as great as with the first, but with subsequent regimens it becomes increasingly difficult to achieve viral suppression.

- **First regimen failure:** In most cases the usual regimen change after virologic failure to the initial regimen is to switch classes (NNRTI-based HAART to PI-based HAART or vice versa), each combined with NRTI changes selected by sensitivity tests (*Clin Infect Dis* 2004;38:613).

- **Virologic failure and no resistance mutations:** If the test was performed on therapy, the anticipated cause is failure of the drug to reach the target, usually due to inadequate adherence but sometimes due to drug interactions, noncompliance with food requirements, etc.

  □ *Limited prior exposure but VL up to 1000 c/mL:* Consider intensification or new regimen. With intensification, should reach virologic goals within 2 to 3 weeks (*AAC* 2002;46:3907) (with VL >1000 decision should be made based on resistance test results).

  □ *Limited prior exposure with resistance to one drug:* Consider single drug substitution based on resistance test results.

- **PI-based regimen with virologic failure**

  □ Patients failing boosted PI-based regimens frequently have no resistance mutations in which case the cause of failure is often due to non-adherence. Options are: (1) continue this regimen with stress on adherence and repeat VL test after 2-4 wks of re-treatment; (2) use of alternative PIs; (3) change to NNRTI-based HAART, or (4) intensify the NRTI backbone if there is reason to suspect NRTI resistance.

  □ With PI resistance mutations, the options are dictated largely by specific mutations, combined with any historic data on drug exposures and prior resistance tests. Options are:

    1. NNRTI-based HAART

    2. Double-boosted PI, such as LPV/r/SQV or LPV/r/ATV, for which pharmacokinetic data indicate effective plasma levels of both PIs (*AIDS* 2004;18:503), although there are sparse clinical data indicating efficacy

    3. Combinations of a PI and NNRTI, especially in patients with few or no NRTI options and no prior exposure to NNRTIs. It is emphasized that EFV and NVP reduce exposure to all PIs studied except NFV. The best-studied combinations are LPV/r using 533/133 (4 tabs) bid + EFV in standard doses (*Antimicrob Agents Chemother* 2003;47:350; *Antiviral Ther* 2002;17:165) and IDV/r/EFV in standard doses (*N Engl J Med* 1999;341: 1865). However, EFV-based HAART with 2 active NRTIs is

Antiretroviral Therapy

4

superior to LPV/r/EFV for both viral suppression and tolerability (12th CROI, 2005, Abstr. 162).

4. The favored PIs for salvage have been LPV/r, ATV and TPV. LPV/r and ATV/r appear comparable in patients who have failed one prior PI-based regimen (*Clin Infect Dis* 2004;38:1599). TPV is used in this setting and is most effective if the TPV mutation score is low (see TPV section in Chapter 5). Analysis of the RESIST-1 study showed superior viral and CD4 response in TPV/r recipients compared to the subset in the control group that received LPV/r (12th CROI, 2005, Abstr. 560).

5. Enfuvirtide is an important component of therapy in patients with limited options (*N Engl J Med* 2003;348:2175; *N Engl J Med* 2003;348:2186). It must be combined with at least one additional active agent.

- **NNRTI-based regimen with failure:** Resistance to EFV or NVP results in cross-resistance to all currently available members of the class; resistance is high-level, meaning it cannot be overcome with pharmacologic modification; and there is no apparent benefit to maintaining resistant strains with respect to either reducing replication capacity or providing partial virologic suppression (*J Med Virol* 2003;69:1). Furthermore, continuation of NNRTIs in a failing regimen leads to accumulation of additional resistance mutations that may lead to cross-resistance to second-generation NNRTIs currently in development. For these reasons, NNRTIs should be used only in fully suppressive regimens.

- **NRTI resistance with virologic failure:** The dual-NRTI component of HAART is standard and appears superior to various combinations of PIs and NNRTIs tested to date (*N Engl J Med* 1999;341:1865; *N Engl J Med* 2003;349:2293). In general, 3TC or FTC are included in most regimens even with the 184V mutation due to good tolerability and documented antiviral effect attributed to reduction in replication capacity and/or partial antiviral effect (3rd IAS Conf, 2005, Abstr. WeFo0204).

- **Rescue Therapy: Treatment following three class failures:** The definition of rescue has changed during the HAART era. This discussion applies to patients with virologic failure with exposure to all three classes of antiretrovirals, sometimes referred to as rescue or salvage therapy.

  □ ***Criteria for success:*** In some patients the standard goal of viral suppression to <50 c/mL is simply unrealistic. The goal of therapy in these cases may be redirected to maintaining or increasing the CD4 count and preventing opportunistic infections. Studies indicate that stable or even rising viral loads may be associated with stable or increasing CD4 count in patients on HAART.

- **Discontinuation of HAART:** Discontinuation of HAART after virologic failure is usually not recommended. Prior reports showed that discontinuation resulted in a median increase in VL of 0.8-1.0 $\log_{10}$ c/mL and a decrease in CD4 of 85-100/mm³ within 3 months (*N Engl J Med* 2003;349:837; *J Infect Dis* 2000;181:946). Nevertheless, the decision to continue a failing regimen must be considered carefully, because it will allow further accumulation of resistance mutations, with the possible consequence of loss of future treatment options (*J Infect Dis* 2003;188:1001). Discontinuation must also be regarded as a temporizing tactic, in that immunologic failure with HIV-associated complications is still expected, even if delayed (*AIDS* 2002;16:201). Considerations must include current options, future drugs and disease stage. Aggressive treatment becomes critical with a CD4 count of 20/mm³ and far less compelling with a CD4 count of 200/mm³. An important goal of current research is to identify key components of the failing regimen that could achieve the temporizing goal without the unnecessary consequence of side effects or resistance mutations. Most experts recommend continuation of 3TC or FTC (3rd IAS Conf, 2005, Abstr. WeFo0204) and discontinuation of NNRTIs in this setting. Beyond that, there are few clear directions.

- **Rescue regimens:** Two agents have been FDA-approved exclusively for salvage therapy: enfuvirtide (T20, ENF) and tipranavir (TPV). Clinical trials tested ENF combined with an optimized ART background vs. the optimized background alone in 995 patients with virologic failure and three-class exposure. ENF recipients had a significantly better virologic response, but required combination with at least one additional antiretroviral agent that was active in vitro. TPV was subsequently tested in RESIST-1 and -2 in patients with three-class exposure and resistance, with the option to add ENF. Virologic response was superior in TPV recipients; the outcome was most successful in patients who received TPV + ENF. The following chart summarizes the 24-wk data:

Study	Regimen	N	VL <50	VL <400
TORO 1 & 2	ENF/optomized regimen	826	16%*	30%*
	Optomized regimen only[†]		6%	15%
RESIST 1 & 2	TPV/r/2 NRTIs/ENF	577	33%*	47%*
	CPI/r/2 NRTIs/ENF[†]		14%	22%

- Significantly better than comparator (*p* <0.05)

[†] Control group (CPI = comparator PI)

4 Antiretroviral Therapy

- □ ***New agents:*** Another option is participation in a clinical trial that gives access to an investigational drug, which includes both new drugs in existing classes as well as drugs in novel classes, such as integrase inhibitors and coreceptor antagonists (CCR5 or CXCR4 inhibitors). Among drugs that will target resistant strains, the furthest along in development are TMC-114 (a new PI), TMC-125 (a new NNRTI) and D-d4FC (a new NRTI).

- □ ***Mega-HAART:*** This term refers to the use of 6 or 7 antiretroviral agents with the usual inclusion of 3 PIs, 1 or 2 NNRTIs and ≥2 NRTIs. Trial outcomes have been variable and toxicity rates are high (*AIDS* 2001;15:61; *J Acquir Immune Defic Syndr* 2002;29:58).

TREATMENT INTERRUPTION STRATEGIES

- ■ **Virologic failure:** The strategy is to suspend antiretroviral therapy in patients with virologic failure and multiple resistance mutations. The rationale is that the resistance mutants are associated with reduced fitness and therefore will be replaced by drug-susceptible wild-type HIV when antiviral pressure is eliminated. The largest controlled trial was CPCRA 064, in which 270 patients with VL >5000 c/mL and three-class exposure and resistance were randomized to treatment interruption (TI) for 16 wks vs continued HAART (*N Engl J Med* 2003;349:837). The TI group had a significant decrease in CD4 count (mean decrease 85/mm^3 at 4 mos) and a significant increase in AIDS-defining events (17 vs. 5). Similarly poor results were reported in a study from Spain (*Clin Infect Dis* 2004;39:569). Others have had better success with shorter periods of TI (8 wks) and salvage with "mega-HAART" using 6-8 drugs (*AIDS* 2004;18:217). Nevertheless, the theoretical concept in this trial was flawed because the new regimen was introduced when resistance mutations were still present. This strategy cannot be recommended as a way to manage treatment failure (DHHS Guidelines, April 7, 2005).

- ■ **Autovaccination for chronic infection with virologic control:** The rationale is that TI in patients with good virologic control would permit viral rebound, which would augment HIV-specific CD4 and CD8 cell responses, thereby improving immunologic control. The largest trial was the Swiss-Spanish Intermittent Treatment Trial (SSITT), in which patients with VL <50 c/mL for ≥6 mos stopped HAART for 2 wks, then restarted for 8 wks. After four cycles, a sustained virologic response with VL <5000 c/mL was achieved in <20% of 133 participants (*AIDS* 2002;16:S5157). This treatment strategy is not recommended.

- ■ **Autovaccination for acute HIV infection:** The rationale is the same as above, but with the assumption, based in part on success in primate studies (*Science* 2000;290:1591; *Nat Med* 2000;6:1140),

Antiretroviral Therapy

that there would be a more robust immune response in patients treated during primary infection. Clinical studies demonstrated preservation of HIV-specific CD4 and CD8 cells when HAART is initiated during primary HIV infection (*Nature* 2000;407:523). Initial results with this treatment were promising, but long-term follow-up showed lack of virologic control in 11/14 (11th CROI, 2003, Abstr. 24). This approach is not recommended except in properly designed clinical trials (*PLoS Med* 2004;1:e36).

- **Intermittent treatment interruption (ITI):** The rationale for ITI is to reduce drug cost, toxicity and inconvenience while maintaining viral suppression. Two small NIH studies used ITI with EFV or IDV-based HAART given every other week after achieving good viral suppression with standard therapy (*Proc Natl Acad Sci* 2001;98:15161; *J Infect Dis* 2004;189:174). Results at 48 wks showed persistent viral suppression with no resistance. However, other ITI trials have been far less successful. The STACCATO trial attempted the alternate-weeks strategy with various regimens; the rate of virologic failure was 53% in the experimental treatment group compared to 5% in controls given continuous HAART (*Clin Infect Dis* 2005;37:1541). A more rational approach is "5 days on, 2 days off," (Five On Two Off, or FOTO) with NNRTI-based HAART. (The NNRTI maintains antiviral activity over the weekend.) The initial experience with 17 participants in the FOTO trial has shown continued viral suppression (XV Int'l AIDS Conference, 2004, Abstr. TuPeB4575). These strategies should be reserved for patients in clinical trials until more experience is achieved.

- **CD4-guided treatment interruption:** The rationale is that antiretroviral therapy is not recommended with a CD4 count >350/mm^3, but many patients have immune reconstitution to much higher levels, suggesting it may be safe to suspend therapy when there is a good response. There are at least 12 reports, including 2 prospective analyses (*AIDS* 2005;19:287; *AIDS* 2004;18:439), 6 retrospective reviews (*J Infect Dis* 2002;186:851; *Clin Infect Dis* 2003;37:1541; *J Acquir Immune Defic Syndr* 2004;37:1351; *Clin Infect Dis* 2005;40:728; *HIV Med* 2005;6:12; *AIDS* 2004;18:2381) and 5 presentations at the 12th CROI in 2005 (Abstrs. 100, 584, 585, 679, 682).

Nearly all trials use similar criteria: patients who achieve virologic control and a CD4 count >500/mm^3 discontinue treatment until the CD4 declines to <350/mm^3, when treatment is restarted, usually with the same regimen. Results based on an aggregate total of 770 cases are excellent, with an average of 8-12 months off treatment. There have been no intercurrent OIs and essentially uniform response to re-administration of HAART. The best predictor of the duration off therapy is the nadir (pretreatment) CD4 count; the lower the nadir CD4 count, the shorter the time off treatment.

Antiretroviral Therapy

4

Recommendations for using this strategy

☐ It should be elective, since the large formal study with proper controls (SMART study) is being done and should provide a scientific basis and specific guidelines.

☐ Patients should be warned that they will have rapid return of VL to pretreatment levels, which will have potential consequences for HIV transmission. The CD4 count usually decreases abruptly for 3 mos, then decreases at a lower rate.

☐ About 3% of patients have a clinical syndrome comparable to the acute retroviral syndrome. Excluding patients with high pre-treatment viral loads may decrease this risk.

☐ The time off therapy correlates best with the nadir pretreatment CD4 count. This strategy works best in patients who initiated HAART at a CD4 level that is no longer an indication for treatment.

☐ The greatest risk associated with CD4-guided TI is the consequence of simultaneous discontinuation of all antiretrovirals, especially with NNRTI-based HAART. This risks effective NNRTI monotherapy and resistance.

☐ It should be noted that as HAART becomes simpler, better tolerated, and less toxic, there may be a stronger rationale for earlier initiation of therapy, in which case the rationale for treatment intervention may become weaker.

STOPPING HAART: There are many reasons to discontinue HAART, including severe drug toxicity, intercurrent severe illness or major procedure, CD4-guided interruption (described above), lack of drug supply or discontinuation when ART is given only to prevent perinatal transmission. The standard recommendation is to stop all drugs together, but there is concern about the long half-life and low genetic barrier to resistance of EFV and NVP. Discontinuation of NNRTI-based regimens results in monotherapy, which can lead to NNRTI resistance. The concern is based largely on the experience with single-dose NVP to prevent perinatal transmission, which has resulted in class resistance due to K103N mutations in up to 60-80% of women (*J Infect Dis* 2005;192:24). The issue has not been studied adequately to give precise recommendations, but these are suggested options:

■ Discontinue EFV or NVP and continue the NRTIs for 1 additional week (British HIV Association guidelines, 2005)

■ Discontinue EFV or NVP and substitute a PI for 1 wk, then stop all drugs together (British HIV Association guidelines, 2005). The Moore Clinic policy is to substitute PIs for 3-4 wks due to prolonged half-life of EFV (36-100 h) and NVP (25-30 h).

Antiretroviral Therapy

Antiretroviral Agents

Antiretroviral Agents Approved by the FDA

■ TABLE 4-17: **Antiretroviral Drugs Approved by the FDA for Treatment of HIV Infection**

Generic Name (Abbreviation)	Brand Name	Manufacturer	FDA Approval Date
Zidovudine (AZT, ZDV)	*Retrovir*	GlaxoSmithKline	March 1987
Didanosine (ddl)	*Videx*	Bristol-Myers Squibb	October 1991
Zalcitabine (ddC)	*Hivid*	Hoffman-La Roche	June 1992
Stavudine (d4T)	*Zerit*	Bristol-Myers Squibb	June 1994
Lamivudine (3TC)	*Epivir*	GlaxoSmithKline	November 1995
Saquinavir (SQVhgc)	*Invirase*	Hoffman-La Roche	December 1995
Ritonavir (RTV)	*Norvir*	Abbott Laboratories	March 1996
Indinavir (IDV)	*Crixivan*	Merck & Co., Inc.	March 1996
Nevirapine (NVP)	*Viramune*	Boehringer Ingelheim	June 1996
Nelfinavir (NFV)	*Viracept*	Agouron Pharmaceuticals	March 1997
Delavirdine (DLV)	*Rescriptor*	Pfizer	April 1997
Zidovudine/Lamivudine (AZT/3TC)	*Combivir*	GlaxoSmithKline	September 1997
Saquinavir (SQVsgc)	*Fortovase*	Hoffman-La Roche	November 1997
Efavirenz (EFV)	*Sustiva*	DuPont Pharmaceuticals	September 1998
Abacavir (ABC)	*Ziagen*	GlaxoSmithKline	February 1999
Amprenavir (APV)	*Agenerase*	GlaxoSmithKline	April 1999
Lopinavir/Ritonavir (LPV/r)	*Kaletra*	Abbott	September 2000
Zidovudine/lamivudine/ abacavir (AZT/3TC/ABC)	*Trizivir*	GlaxoSmithKline	November 2000
Tenofovir DF (TDF)	*Viread*	Gilead Sciences	October 2001
Enfuvirtide (ENF)	*Fuzeon*	Roche	March 2003
Atazanavir (ATV)	*Reyataz*	Bristol-Myers Squibb	June 2003
Emtricitabine (FTC)	*Emtriva*	Gilead Sciences	July 2003
Fosamprenavir (FPV)	*Lexiva*	GlaxoSmithKline	November 2003
Tipranavir (TPV)	*Aptivus*	Boehringer Ingelheim	June 2005

4 Antiretroviral Therapy

Non-Nucleoside Reverse Transcriptase Inhibitors (NNRTIs)

■ TABLE 4-18: **Nucleoside Analogs**

Generic/Trade name	AZT, ZDV	ddI	ddC	d4T	3TC	ABC	TDF	FTC
	Zidovudine/*Retrovir*	Didanosine/*Videx* and *Videx EC*	Zelcitabine/*Hivid*	Stavudine/*Zerit*	Lamivudine/*Epvir*	Abacavir/*Ziagen*	Tenofovir DF/*Viread*	Emtricitabine/*Emtriva*
How supplied	■ 100 mg caps and 300 mg tabs ■ 300 mg + 3TC 150 mg as *Combivir* caps ■ 300 mg + 3TC 150 mg + ABC 300 mg as *Trizivir* tabs ■ 10 mg/mL IV solution ■ 10 mg/mL po solution	■ 125, 200, 250, and 400 mg enteric coated cap (*Videx EC*) ■ 25, 50, 100, 150, and 200 mg buffered tabs ■ 125, 200, 250 & 400 EC	■ 0.375 and 0.75 mg tabs	■ 15, 20, 30, and 40 mg caps ■ 1 mg/mL oral solution	■ 150 and 300 mg tabs ■ 150 mg with AZT 300 mg as *Combivir* caps ■ 150 mg with AZT 300 mg and ABC 300 mg as *Trizivir* tabs ■ 300 mg + 600 mg ABC as *Epzicom* ■ 10 mg/mL oral solution	■ 300 mg tabs ■ 300 mg + AZT 300 mg + 3TC 150 mg as *Trizivir* tabs ■ 600 mg + 3TC 300 mg as *Epzicom* ■ 20 mg/mL solution	■ 300 mg tabs ■ 300 mg + 200 mg FTC as *Truvada*	■ 200 mg caps ■ 200 mg + 300 mg TNF as *Truvada*
Dosing recommendations	■ 300 mg bid (or 200 mg tid) *Combivir* – 1 bid *Trizivir* – 1 bid)	■ >60 kg *Videx EC*: 400 mg qd *Videx* tabs: 200 mg bid or 400 mg qd ■ <60 kg *Videx EC*: 250 mg qd *Videx* tabs: 250 mg qd or 125 mg bid with TDF: 200 mg/d	■ 0.75 mg tid	■ >60 kg: 40 mg bid ■ <60 kg: 30 mg bid	■ 150 mg bid ■ *Combivir* – 1 bid ■ *Trizivir* – 1 bid ■ *Epzicom* – 1 qd	■ 300 mg bid or 600 mg qd ■ *Trizivir* – 1 bid ■ *Epzicom* – 1 qd	■ 300 mg qd ■ *Truvada* – 1 qd	■ 200 mg qd ■ *Truvada* – 1 qd
Oral bioavailability	■ 60%	■ 30% to 40%	■ 85%	■ 86%	■ 86%	■ 83%	■ 25% to 39%	■ 90%
Food effect	■ None; may be better tolerated with food.	■ Levels ↓55% with food – Take 1hr before and 2 hrs after meal	■ None	■ None	■ None	■ None ■ Alcohol ↑ ABC levels 41%	■ None	■ None

Generic/Trade name	AZT, ZDV	ddI	ddC	d4T	3TC	ABC	TDF	FTC
	Zidovudine/Retrovir	Didanosine/Videx and Videx EC	Zalcitabine/Hivid	Stavudine/Zerit	Lamivudine/Epivir	Abacavir/Ziagen	Tenofovir/Viread	Emtricitabine/Emtriva
Serum half-life	■ 1.1 hour	■ 1.6 hours	■ 1.2 hour	■ 1.0 hour	■ 5 to 7 hours	■ 1.5 hours	■ 12 to 26 hours	■ 10 hours
Intracellular half-life	■ 7 hours	■ 25 to 40 hours	■ 3 hours	■ 7.5 hours	■ 18 to 22 hours	■ >3.3 hours	■ >60 hours	■ >20 hours
CNS penetration (% serum levels)	■ 60%	■ 20%	■ 20%	■ 30 to 40%	■ 10%	■ 30%	■ ?	■ ?
Elimination	■ Metabolized to AZT Glucuronide (GAZT) ■ Renal excretion of GAZT	■ Renal excretion 50%	■ Renal excretion 70%	■ Renal excretion 50%	■ Renal excretion unchanged	■ Metabolized ■ Renal excretion of metabolites 82%	■ Renal excretion	■ Renal excretion
Major toxicity Class toxicity	■ Bone marrow suppression: Anemia and/or neutropenia ■ Subjective complaints: GI intolerance, headache, insomnia, asthenia, fatigue ■ Lactic acidosis ■ Lipoatrophy	■ Pancreatitis ■ Peripheral neuropathy ■ Lactic acidosis ■ GI intolerance – nausea, diarrhea. ■ Avoid combination with d4T especially with pregnancy‡	■ Peripheral neuropathy ■ Lactic acidosis ■ Lipo-atrophy ■ Stomatitis	■ Peripheral neuropathy ■ Lactic acidosis ■ Lipoatrophy ■ Avoid combination with ddI especially pregnancy‡	■ Minimal toxicity	■ Hypersensitivity (5%), with fever, GIs, cough, dyspnea, malaise, morbilliform rash, usually first 6 wks ■ Re-challenge may be life-threatening	■ Minimal toxicity ■ Occasional GI intolerance ■ Nephrotoxicity	■ Minimal toxicity ■ Occasional hyperpigmentation (palms, sides)
Drug interactions (Antiretroviral drugs & methadone)	■ Antagonism with d4T – avoid	■ Methadone ↓ ddI levels 41%; consider ddI dose increase ; ddI EC not affected (prefered) ■ Tenofovir increases ddI AUC 44%. Use 250 mg/d (>60 kg) or 200 mg/d (<60 kg) ■ Ribavirin – avoid combo ■ ATV and IDV – avoid buffered ddI	■ None	■ Methadone ↓ d4T levels 27%. No dose adjustment. ■ Antagonism with AZT – avoid ■ ddI AUC increased use ddI 250 mg/d (>60 kg) or 200 mg/d (<60 kg)	■ None	■ None	■ Increases ddI AUC 44%; 250 mg/d (>60 kg) or 200 mg/d (<60 kg) ■ Decreases ATV AUC 25% – use ATV/r 300/100 qd ■ LPV/r increases TDF AUC 34%; no dose adjustment	■ None

* For adults, ddI pediatric oral solution can be mixed by the pharmacist with liquid antacids. See package insert for instructions.

4 Antiretroviral Therapy

■ TABLE 4-19: **Non-Nucleoside Reverse Transcriptase Inhibitors**

	NVP	DLV	EFV
Generic/ Trade Name	Nevirapine/ *Viramune*	Delavirdine/ *Rescriptor*	Efavirenz/ *Sustiva*
Form	■ 200 mg tabs ■ 50 mg/5 mL oral solution	■ 100 mg and 200 mg tabs	■ 50, 100, 200 mg caps ■ 600 mg tabs
Dosing recommendations	■ 200 mg PO qd x 14 days, then 200 mg PO bid	■ 400 mg PO tid	■ 600 mg PO qd hs
Oral bioavailability	■ >90%	■ 85%	■ Not known
Food effect	■ No effect	■ No effect	■ High fat meal increases C_{max} 29% with caps and 79% with tabs; take on empty stomach
Serum half-life	■ 25 to 30 hours	■ 5.8 hours	■ 40 to 55 hours
Elimination	■ Metabolized by cytochrome P450 (CYP3A4 inducer); ■ 80% excreted in urine (glucuronidase metabolites, <5% unchanged), 10% in feces	■ Metabolized by cytochrome P450 (CYP3A4 inhibitor); ■ 51% excreted in urine (<5% unchanged), 44% in feces	■ Metabolized by cytochrome P450 enzymes (CYP3A4 mixed inhibitor/inducer); ■ 14% to 34% excreted in urine (<1% unchanged), 16% to 61% in feces
Major toxicity Class toxicity	■ Rash (15% to 30%); discontinuation required in 7%; rare cases of Stevens-Johnson syndrome usually in first 6-12 wks ■ Hepatitis with hepatic necrosis ■ Risks: Baseline CD4 >250/mm³ in women, >400/mm³ in men ■ Elevated ALT/AST ■ Class ADRs See p. 100	■ Rash (10% to 15%); discontinuation required in 4% ■ Elevated ALT/AST ■ Headache ■ Class ADRs See p. 100	■ CNS: Dizziness, "disconnectedness," somnolence, insomnia, abnormal dreams, confusion, amnesia, agitation, hallucinations, poor concentration – 40% to 50%, usually resolves within 2 to 3 weeks; discontinuation in 2-6% ■ Rash (5% to 10%); discontinuation required in 1% to 7%; rare reports of Stevens-Johnson syndrome ■ Teratogenic in monkeys; avoid in first trimester and with pregnancy potential. ■ False-positive drug screening test for cannabinoids – marijuana ■ Elevated ALT/AST ■ Class ADRs. See p. 100

Antiretroviral Therapy

■ TABLE 4-20: **Drugs That Should Not Be Used With Protease Inhibitors or NNRTIs***

Category	Drugs	PIs or NNRTIs contraindicated
Cardiac	■ Flecainide ■ Propafenone ■ Amiodavone ■ Quinidine	■ LPV/r, RTV, DLV, FPV, RTV, SQV, TPV ■ RTV, LPV/r, FPV, SQV, TPV ■ RTV, LPV/r, SQV, TPV ■ RTV, SQV, TPV
Lipids	■ Simvastatin* ■ Lovastatin*	■ All PIs and DLV ■ All PIs and DLV
Antimycob.	■ Rifampin ■ Rifabutin	■ All PIs and NNRTIs except EFV ■ DLV
Ca++ channel blocker	■ Bepridil	■ RTV, APV, TPV
Antihistamine	■ Astemizole* ■ Terfenadine*	■ All PIs, all NNRTIs but NVP ■ All PIs and NNRTIs but NVP
Neuroleptic	■ Pimozide	■ All PIs and DLV
Psychotrophic	■ Midazolam* ■ Triazolam* ■ Alprozalam	■ All PIs and NNRTIs but NVP ■ All PIs and NNRTIs but NVP ■ DLV
Ergot alkaloids	■ Ergots	■ All PIs and NNRTIs except NVP
Herbs	■ St. John's wort	■ All PIs and NNRTIs
GI	■ Proton pump inhib ■ Cisapride	■ ATV, DLV ■ All PIs and NNRIs except NVP
Antifungal	■ Voriconazole	■ RTV (including low-dose RTV), EFV

*Alternatives: Antihistamines – Loratadine, fexofenadine, cetirizine; Psychotropics – temazepam, lorazepam; Lipid lowering – atorvastatin, pravastatin, possibly rosuvastatin.

Antiretroviral Therapy

4

Protease Inhibitors (PIs)

■ TABLE 4-21: **Protease Inhibitors**

	Indinavir (IDV)	Ritonavir (RTV)	Saquinavir (SQV)
	Crixivan	*Norvir*	*Invirase*
Form	■ 200, 333, 400 mg caps	■ 100 mg caps ■ 600 mg/7.5 mL PO sol'n	■ 200, 500 mg caps
Usual unboosted dose	■ 800 mg q8h ■ Separate buffered ddI dose by 1 hour	■ 600 mg bid* (rarely used) ■ Separate buffered ddI dose by 2 hrs	■ Should not be prescribed without RTV boosting
RTV boosted dose (mg)	IDV/RTV ■ 800/100-200 bid ■ 400/400 bid	NA	SQV/RTV ■ 1000/100 bid ■ 2000/100 qd ■ 400/400 bid
Food effect	■ Levels ↓ 77% ■ Take 1 hr before or 2 hrs after meals or take with low-fat snack or skim milk ■ No food effect when taken with RTV	■ Levels ↑ 15% ■ Take with food if possible to improve tolerability	■ Take with RTV and within 2 hrs of meal
Bioavailability	■ 65% (on empty stomach)	■ Not determined	■ 4% (unboosted)
Storage	■ Room temp 59-86°F	■ Room temp or refrigerate if stored >30 days	■ Room temp
Serum half-life	■ 1.5 to 2 hours	■ 3 to 5 hours	■ 1 to 2 hours
CNS penetration	■ Moderate	■ Poor	■ Poor

Nelfinavir (NFV)	Tipranavir (TPV)	Lopinavir/ritonavir (LPV/r)	Atazanavir (ATV)	Fosamprenavir (FPV)
Viracept	*Aptivus*	*Kaletra*	*Reyataz*	*Lexiva*
■ 625 mg tabs ■ 250 mg caps ■ 50 mg/g oral powder	■ 250 mg caps	■ 133 mg LPV + 33 mg RTV caps bid ■ 80 mg LPV + 20 mg RTV/mL oral soln bid	■ 100, 150, 200 mg caps	■ 700 mg tabs
■ 1250 mg bid or 750 mg tid	■ Requires boosting	■ 400/100 mg (3 caps or 5 mL) bid ■ 800/200 mg (4 caps or 10 mL) qd	■ 400 mg qd (with TDF or EFV use ATV/RTV 300/100 mg qd)	■ 1400 mg bid
NFV/RTV ■ 500-750/400 bid (not recommended)	TPV/RTV ■ 500/200 bid	■ co-formulated	ATV/RTV ■ 300/100 qd	FAPV/RTV ■ 700/100 bid ■ 1400/200 qd
■ Levels ↑ 2x to 2- to 5- fold (high fat) ■ Take with meal or snack; high fat meal preferred	■ AUC ↑ 2x ■ Take with meal	■ Fat ↑ AUC 50% to 80% ■ Take with food	■ ↑ bioavail 70% Take with food	■ No food effect
■ 20% to 80%	■ Not determined	■ Not determined	■ Not determined	■ Not determined
■ Room temp 59-86° F	■ Room temp	■ Up to 77° F for 2 mo	■ Up to 77° F	■ Up to 77° F
■ 3.5 to 5 hours	■ 2.5-3.9 hours	■ 5 to 6 hours	■ 7 hours	■ 7.7 hours
■ Moderate	■ Not known	■ Not known	■ Not known	■ Moderate

continued on next page

Antiretroviral Therapy 4

	Indinavir (IDV)	Ritonavir (RTV)	Saquinavir (SQV)
	Crixivan	*Norvir*	*Invirase*
Elimination	■ Cytochrome P450, CYP3A4 inhibitor	■ Cytochrome P450, CYP3A4>2D6; most potent 3A4 inhibitor; mild inducer	■ Cytochrome P450, CYP3A4 inhibitor (weak)
Side effects*	■ GI intolerance (10% to 15%) ■ Nephrolithiasis or nephrotoxicity (10% to 20%) take >1.5 L/day; ■ Increased transaminases ■ Miscellaneous: Headache, blurred vision, thrombocytopenia, hepatitis, asthenia, dizziness, rash, metallic taste, ITP, alopecia, dry skin, chapped lips, paronychia ■ Lab: Increase indirect bilirubinemia (inconsequential) ■ Class ADRs, p. 100	■ GI intolerance (20% to 40%): Diarrhea ■ Circumoral and extremities extremitis paresthias (10%) ■ Taste perversion (10%) ■ Lab: Increased transaminase, CPK and/or uric acid levels ■ Miscellaneous: Asthenia, hepatitis, alcohol content of oral solution contains EtOH, possible disulfiram reaction ■ Class ADRs, p. 100	■ GI intolerance (10% to 20%) ■ Headache ■ Increased transaminases ■ Class ADRs, but little or no lipid effect, p. 100

* Dose escalation for boosted RTV: days 1 and 2, 300 mg bid; days 3 to 5, 400 mg bid; days 6 to 13, 500 mg bid; day 14, 600 mg bid.

Antiretroviral Therapy

Nelfinavir (NFV)	Tipranavir (TPV)	Lopinavir/ritonavir (LPV/r)	Atazanavir (ATV)	Fosamprenavir (FPV)
Viracept	Aptivus	Kaletra	Reyataz	Lexiva
■ Cytochrome P450, CYP3A4 inhibitor	■ Cytochrome P450, CYP3A inducer; TPV/r produces net inhibition ■ Excreted primarily in stool	■ Cytochrome P450, CYP3A4 inhibitor and inducer	■ Cytochrome P450, CYP3A4 inhibitor	■ Cytochrome P450, CYP3A4 inhibitor
■ Diarrhea (10% to 30%) ■ Increased transaminase levels ■ Class ADRs, p. 100	■ GI intolerance: Nausea, vomiting, diarrhea ■ Increased transaminases Gr 3/4-8% ■ Rash: women 13%; men 4% ■ Class ADRs, p. 100	■ GI intolerance: Nausea, vomiting, diarrhea ■ Asthenia ■ Increased transaminases ■ Oral solution is 42% EtOH – possible disulfiram reaction ■ Class ADRs, p. 100 ■ ↑ lipid	■ GI Intolerance ■ Lab: Increased indirect bili (inconsequential) ■ Jaundice or scleral icterus ■ Prolonged PR interval ■ Increased transaminases ■ Class ADRs but not dyslipidemia p. 100	■ GI intolerance ■ Skin rash (19%) ■ Increased transaminase ■ Class ADRs p. 100

4 Antiretroviral Therapy

Drug Interactions

■ TABLE 4-22: **Drug Interactions Requiring Dose Modifications or Cautious Use**

Drugs Affected	IDV	RTV	SQV	NFV	FPV
Antifungals					
Ketoconazole	■ Levels: IDV ↑68% ■ IDV 600 mg tid	■ Ketoconazole ↑3x ■ Use ≤200 mg/d	■ Levels: SQV ↑3x ■ Dose: Standard	■ No dose adjustment necessary	■ Ketoconazole ↑44% APV ↑31% ■ Keto dose ≤400 mg/d; or ≤200 with FPV/r
Voriconazole	■ Standard doses ■ No interaction ■ With IDV/r: See RTV	■ Vori AUC 82% ■ RTV in therapeutic dose: Contraindicated ■ Low dose RTV (100-400 mg/d): No data; some advise avoidance	■ No data ■ Potential for bidirectional inhibition; monitor toxicity ■ See RTV	■ No data ■ Potential for bidirectional inhibition; monitor toxicity	■ No data ■ Potential for bidirectional inhibition; monitor toxicity ■ FPV/r: See RTV
Antimycobacterials					
Rifampin	■ IDV ↓89% ■ Contraindicated	■ RTV ↓35% ■ Consider RBT	■ SQV ↓84% ■ Contraindicated	■ NFV ↓82% ■ Contraindicated	■ APV ↓82% ■ Contraindicated
Rifabutin	■ IDV ↓32% ■ Rifabutin ↑2x ■ ↓ Rifabutin to 150 mg qd or 300 mg 3x/wk IDV 1,000 mg tid ■ IDV/RTV: See RTV	■ Rifabutin ↑4x ■ ↓ Rifabutin to 150 mg qod or dose 3x/wk ■ With boosted PIs: Standard dose for PI and RTV + RBT 150 mg qod or 150 mg 3x/wk	■ SQV ↓40% ■ SQV + RTV: See RTV	■ NFV: No change with 1250 mg bid ■ Rifabutin ↑2x ■ ↓ Rifabutin to 150 mg qd or 300 mg 3x/wk ■ NFV: 1250 mg bid	■ APV ↓15% ■ Rifabutin ↑193% ■ ↓ Rifabutin to 150 mg qod or 300 mg 3x/wk ■ FPV dose standard ■ FPV/r: See RTV
Clarithromycin	■ Clarithromycin ↑53% ■ No dose adjustment	■ Clarithromycin ↑77% ■ Dose adjust for renal insufficiency	■ Clarithromycin ↑45% ■ SQV ↑177% ■ No dose adjustment	■ No data	■ APV ↑18% ■ No dose adjustment
Oral contraceptives	■ No dose adjustment	■ Use alternative method	■ No data	■ Use alternative method	■ Use alternative method

LPV/r	ATV	TPV	NVP	EFV
Antifungals				
■ Ketoconazole ↑3x ■ LPV ↑13% ■ Do not exceed 200 mg/d of ketoconazole	■ Unboosted – no dose change ■ No dose change ■ ATV/r: See RTV	■ Ketoconazole levels ↑ ■ Do not exceed 200 mg/d	■ Ketoconazole ↓63% ■ NVP ↑15% to 30% ■ Not recommended	■ No data
■ Bidirectional inhibition; see RTV		■ Potential for bidirectional inhibition: monitor for toxicities	■ No data NVP ↑ and Vori ↓	■ ↓ Vori AUC 77% ↑ EFV 44% ■ Contra-indicated
Antimycobacterials				
■ LPV AUC ↓75% ■ Avoid	■ Avoid	■ Contra-indicated	■ NVP 20-58% ■ Not recom-mended due to potential hepatotoxicity; if used – moni-tor LFTs	■ EFV ↓25% ■ EFV dose 800 mg/d
■ LPV ↓17% ■ Rifabutin: ↑3x, ↓ Rifabutin dose to 150 mg qod or 150 mg 3x/wk ■ LPV/r standard	■ Rifabutin ↑2.5x ■ Rifabutin 150 mg qod or 150 mg 3x/wk ■ ATV standard ■ ATV/r: See RTV	■ RBT ↑3x ■ RBT dose 150 mg qod or 3x/wk	■ NVP ↓16% Rifabutin: No change ■ NFV: No dose change ■ Rifabutin: standard dose	■ EFV unchanged ■ Rifabutin ↓35% ■ Dose ↑ Rifabutin to 450 mg/day or 600 mg 3x/wk ■ EFV dose: Standard
■ Clarithromycin AUC ↑ 77%,; adjust dose with renal failure	■ Clarithromycin ↑94%, risk ↑ QTc ■ Clarithromycin ↓ dose 50%; consider azithro.	■ TPV ↑ 66% ■ No dose change except with renal fail-ure: ↓ clari dose 50% for CrCl 30-60 mL/min + 75% of CrCl <30	■ NVP ↑26% ■ Clarithromycin ↓30% ■ Dose: Stan-dard; consider azithro	■ Clarithromycin ↓39% but 14-OH metabolite ↑34% ■ High rate of rash ■ Monitor for efficacy or use azithromycin
■ Use alterna-tive method	■ Use alterna-tive method	■ Use alterna-tive method	■ Use alterna-tive method	■ Use alterna-tive method

continued on next page

4 Antiretroviral Therapy

Drugs Affected	IDV	RTV	SQV*	NFV	FPV
Lipids					
Atorvastatin	■ Caution – start 10 mg/d ■ No data	■ Statin SQV/RTV ↑450% ■ Start 10 mg dose	■ SQV/RTV – statin ↑450% ■ Start 10 mg/d	■ Statin ↑74% ■ Start 10 mg dose	■ Statin ↑ 150% ■ Start 10 mg dose
Pravastatin	■ No data	■ SQV/RTV-statin ↓50% ■ Standard dose	■ SQV/RTV-statin ↓50% ■ Standard dose	■ Pravastatin↓ ■ No data	■ No data
Anticonvulsants					
Phenobarbital Phenytoin Carbamazepine	■ Carbamazepine ↓IDV levels substantially ■ Use alternative ART or RTV + IDV or IDV TDM ■ Consider valproic acid or levetivacetaur	■ Use with caution ■ Monitor anticonvulsant levels ■ Consider valproic acid or levetivacetaur	■ Unknown, but may ↓ SQV levels substantially ■ Monitor anticonvulsant levels ■ Consider valproic acid or levetivacetaur	■ Phenytoin AUC ↓ 20-40% ■ May ↓ NFV: Consider NFV TDM ■ Monitor anticonvulsant levels ■ Consider valproic acid or levetivacetaur	■ May ↓ APV levels substantially ■ Consider FPV TDM ■ Monitor anticonvulsant levels ■ Consider valproic acid or levetivacetaur
Methadone (see p. 253)	■ No change in methadone levels ■ No change in IDV	■ Methadone ↓37% ■ Slight ↓ in active R isomer ■ May require ↑ methadone	■ Slight ↓ in active R isomer	■ NFV decrease methadone ■ No change in active R isomer ■ APV C$_{min}$ ↓25%	■ No data ■ Methadone levels ↓35% ■ No change in active R isomer
Miscellaneous	■ Grapefruit juice ↓IDV levels by 26% ■ Sildenafil: Do not exceed 25 mg/48 hours ■ Vardenafil: ≤2.5/72 hrs with RTV ■ Tadalafil: ≤10 mg/72 hrs ■ Amlodipine: AUC amlodipine ↑90% with IDV/r: Monitor	■ Desipramine ↑145% ■ Theophylline ↓47%, monitor levels ■ Trazodone: AUC ↑2.4x – monitor for toxicity ■ Sildenafil: Do not exceed 25 mg/48 hours ■ Vardenafil: ≤2.5 mg 72 hrs ■ Tadalafil: ≤10 mg/72 hr	■ Grapefruit juice ↑SQV levels ■ Dexamethasone ↓SQV levels ■ Sildenafil: Do not exceed 25 mg/48 hours ■ Vardenafil: ≤2.5/72 hrs with RTV ■ Tadalafil: ≤10 mg/72 hr	■ Sildenafil: Do not exceed 25 mg/48 hours ■ Vardenafil: ≤2.5/72 hrs with RTV ■ Tadalafil: ≤10 mg/72 hr	

LPV/r	ATV	TPV	NVP	EFV
Lipids				
■ Statin ↑5.9x ■ Start 10 mg dose	■ No data, anticipate ↑↑ statin AUC ■ Caution – start 10 mg/d	■ Statin ↑9x ■ Start 10 mg/d	■ No data	■ Atorvastatin AUC ↓43% ■ Do not exceed maximum dose
■ Statin ↑33% ■ Standard dose	■ No data	■ No data	■ No data	■ No data
Anticonvulsants				
■ Phenytoin: ↓levels LPV, RTV and phenytoin – Avid or LPV TDM ■ Carbamazepine ↑ with RTV ■ Monitor anticonvulsant levels ■ Consider valproic acid, levetivacetaur or lamotuigine	■ May ↓ ATV substantially ■ Monitor anticonvulsant ■ Consider valproic acid, levetivacetaur or lamotuigine ■ Consider TDM ATV	■ Decrease TPV levels ■ Effect on anti-convulsants variable – monitor or use valproic acid levetiracetam or lamotuigine	■ Unknown ■ Monitor anticonvulsant level	■ Unknown ■ Use with caution ■ Monitor anticonvulsant levels
■ Methadone ↓53% ■ Monitor; may need to ↑ methadone dose	■ No interaction	■ Methadone: May need methadone dose increase	■ NVP unchanged ■ Methadone ↓60% ■ Titrate metha-done dose	■ Methadone levels ↓52% ■ Titrate methadone dose; withdrawal reported
■ Sildenafil: Do not exceed 25 mg/48 hours ■ Vardenafil: ≤2.5/72 hrs with RTV ■ Tadalafil: ≤10 mg/72 hr	■ H₂ receptor antagonist – separate dose 12 hrs ■ Antacids give – ATV 2 hrs before or 1 hr after ■ Proton pump inhibitors: Avoid ■ Vardenafil: ≤2.5 mg/d; ≤2.5/72 hrs with RTV ■ Sildenafil: Do not exceed 2.5 mg in 48 hours ■ Tadalafil: Do not exceed 10 mg/72 hr ■ Ca⁺⁺ channel blockers: Titrate dose, monitor EKG	■ Sildenafil: Do not exceed 25 mg/48 hours ■ Vardenafil: Do not exceed 2.5 mg/72 h ■ Antacids: Separate co-administration by ≥2 hrs ■ AZT: AUC ↓31-42% dose adjustment ? ■ ddI: Separate dosing ddI EC by ≥2 hrs	■ Fluconazole: NVP levels ↑ 100% – possible hepatotoxicity	■ Monitor warfarin when used concomitantly

■ TABLE 4-23: **Drug Interactions: PIs and NNRTIs Effect of Drug on Levels (AUCs)/Dose**

Drugs Affected	RTV	SQV	NFV	LPV/r	ATV
IDV	■ IDV ↑2 to 5x ■ Dose: IDV 400 mg bid + RTV 400 mg bid, or IDV 800 mg bid + RTV 100-200 bid – ↑ risk renal stones	■ IDV no effect ■ SQV ↑4-7x[†] ■ Dose: Insufficient data	■ IDV ↑50% NFV ↑80% ■ Dose: Limited data for IDV 1200 mg bid + NFV 1250 mg bid	■ IDV ↑ C_{min} 240% ■ Dose: IDV 600 or 666 mg bid + LPV/r standard (3 caps bid)	■ Not recommended
RTV	—	■ RTV no effect ■ SQV ↑20x*[†] ■ Dose: *Invirase*/r 1000/100 bid or 2000/100 qd	■ RTV no effect ■ NFV ↑1.5x ■ Dose: RTV 400 mg bid + NFV 500 to 750 mg bid (insufficient data)	■ Co-formulated	■ ATV ↑2.4x ■ ATV 300 mg + RTV 100 mg qd
SQV	—	—	■ SQV ↑3 to 5x ■ NFV ↑20%[†] ■ Dose: NFV 1250 mg bid	■ SQV ↑ AUC ■ Dose: *Invirase* 1000 mg bid + LPV/r standard	■ SQV: 1200 qd + ATV 400 mg qd
NFV	—	—	—	■ LPV ↓27% ■ NFV ↑27% ■ Dose: LPV 4 caps bid, NFV 1000 mg bid	■ NFV: No data
LPV/r	—	—	—	—	■ No data
ATV	—	—	—	—	—
FPV	—	—	—	—	—

Antiretroviral Therapy

NVP	FPV	TPV	EFV
■ IDV ↓28% ■ NVP no effect ■ Dose: IDV 999 mg q8h; standard NVP or IDV 1000 + RTV 100 bid + NVP standard	■ Inadequate data	■ No data	■ Levels: IDV ↓31% ■ Dose: IDV 999 mg q8h; EFV 600 mg hs ■ Consider IDV 800 mg bid + RTV 200 mg bid + EFV 600 mg hs
■ RTV ↓11% ■ NVP no effect ■ Dose: Standard for both drugs	■ APV ↑2x ■ PI-experienced: FPV 700 mg + RTV 100 mg bid. ■ PI-naïve: FPV 700 mg + RTV 100 mg bid or FPV 1400 mg qd + RTV 200 mg qd	■ Co-admin required (TPV 500 mg bid + RTV 200 mg bid)	■ Levels: RTV ↑18% ■ EFV ↑21% ■ Dose: Standard for both drugs
■ SQV ↓25% ■ NVP no effect ■ Dose: NVP standard + *Invirase* 1000 mg bid + RTV 100 mg bid	■ SQV ↓32% ■ APV ↓39% ■ No recommendation	■ Contraindicated	■ Levels: SQV ↓62% ■ EFV ↓12% ■ Co-administration not recommended without RTV ■ Consider SQV 400 mg + RTV 400 mg bid + EFV 600 mg hs
■ NFV ↑10% ■ NVP no effect ■ Dose: Standard for both drugs	■ No recommendation	■ Contraindicated	■ Levels: NFV ↑20% ■ Dose: Standard for both drugs
■ LPV ↓55% ■ LPV/r 533/133 mg bid + NVR standard	■ C_{min} LPV ↓64% ■ LPV/r 533/133 bid + FPV 1400 mg bid (minimal data)	■ Contraindicated	■ Levels: LPV ↓40% ■ EFV – no change ■ LPV/r – 533/133 mg bid + EFV SD
■ ATV ↓ ■ Not recommended	■ No data	■ Contraindicated	■ ATV AUC ↓74% ■ ATV 300 + RTV 100 mg + EFV SD
■ No data ■ Consider FPV 700/RTV 100 bid; NVP standard dose	—	■ No data	■ APV C_{min} ↓36% ■ Dose: FPV 700/RTV 100 mg bid + EFV SD or FPV 1400 + RTV 300 qd

4 Antiretroviral Therapy

■ TABLE 4-24: **Dosing of ART Agents in Renal and Hepatic Failure**

Drug	Standard Dose	Dose for Renal Insufficiency CrCl = mL/min			Dosing in Hemodialysis	Hepatic Dysfunction
AZT	300 mg bid	CrCl <15: 100 mg tid or 300 mg qd			100 mg tid or 300 mg qd[†]	Consider decreased dose
ddl	>60 kg 400 mg qd <60 kg 250 mg qd	CrCl*	>60 kg	<60 kg	As with CrCl <10 mL/min[†]	Usual dose
		30-59	200 mg/d	125 mg/d		
		10-29	125 mg/d	100 mg/d		
		<10	125 mg/d	75 mg/d		
d4T	>60 kg 40 mg bid <60 kg 30 mg bid	CrCl*	>60 kg	<60 kg	As with CrCl 10-25 mL/min[†]. Dose after HD	Not defined; use caution
		26-50	20 mg bid	15 mg bid		
		10-25	20 mg qd	15 mg qd		
ddC	0.75 mg tid	CrCl 10-40: 0.75 mg bid CrCl <10: 0.75 mg qd			No data	Usual dose
TDF	300 mg qd	CrCl 30-49: 300 mg q 48h 10-29: 300 mg 2x/wk <10: no recommendation			300 mg/wk after HD	Usual dose
3TC	300 mg qd or 150 mg bid	CrCl 30-49: 150 mg qd 15-29: 150 mg, then 100 mg qd 5-14: 150 mg, then 50 mg qd <5: 50 mg, then 25 mg qd			No data	Usual dose
FTC	200 mg qd	CrCl 30-49: 200 mg q 48h 15-29: 200 mg q 72h <15: 200 mg q 96h			200 mg q96h	Not defined
ABC	300 mg bid	Usual dose	Usual dose	Usual dose	Usual dose	200 mg bid CPC class A contra-indicated class B & C

Drug	Usual Adult Dose	Dosing for GFR >50 mL/min	Dosing for GFR 10-50 mL/min	Dosing for GFR <10 mL/min	Dosing in Hemodialysis	Hepatic Failure
EFV	600 mg qd	Usual dose likely	Usual dose	Usual dose likely	Usual dose	Use with caution
NVP	200 mg qd x 14 days then 200 mg bid	Usual dose	Usual dose	Usual dose	Usual dose	Avoid use with severe liver disease
NFV	1250 mg bid	Usual dose	Usual dose	Usual dose	Usual dose Must give post dialysis	Use with caution
IDV	800 mg tid[§]	Usual dose	Usual dose	Usual dose	Usual dose	600 mg q8h
RTV	600 mg bid[§]	Usual dose	Usual dose	Usual dose	Usual dose	Use with caution
TPV/r	500/200 mg bid	Usual dose	Usual dose	Usual dose	Usual dose	Usual dose for mild hepatic disease

*Lactic acidosis syndrome should be ruled out before treating for hepatic failure.

(For other notes, see p. 99)

■ TABLE 4-24: **Dosing of ART Agents in Renal and Hepatic Failure** *(Continued)*

Drug	Usual Adult Dose	Dosing for GFR >50 mL/min	Dosing for GFR 10-50 mL/min	Dosing for GFR <10 mL/min	Dosing in Hemodialysis	Hepatic Failure
SQV	Boosted (see p. 291)	Usual dose	Usual dose	Usual dose	Usual dose	Use with caution
LPV/r	400/100 mg bid	Usual dose	Usual dose	Usual dose	Usual dose	Use with caution
ATV	400 mg qd§	Usual dose	Usual dose	Usual dose	Usual dose	*CP Score*** C: 300 mg qd >9: Avoid
FPV	1400 mg bid§	Usual dose	Usual dose	Usual dose	Usual dose	*CP Score*** C: 700 mg bid 9-12: Avoid Avoid RTV boosing with hepatic failure
ENF	90 mg SC bid	Usual dose	Usual dose	Usual dose	Usual dose	Usual dose

* CrCl = creatinine clearance in mL/min (Cockcroft-Gault equation). For men it is

$$\frac{(140 - \text{age in yrs}) \times \text{wt (kg)}}{72 \times \text{serum creatinine}}$$; for women it is this value x 0.85.

† Administer post-dialysis on dialysis days. Hemodialysis removes significant amounts of ddI (*Clin Pharm Ther* 1996;60:535); d4T (*Antimicrob Agents Chemother* 2000;44:2149); ddC; 3TC; TDF; and NFV (*AIDS* 2000;14:89). Hemodialysis little or none of the following: AZT (*J Acquir Immune Defic Syndr* 1992;5:242); ABC; EFV (*AIDS* 2000;14:618); NVP (*Nephrol Dial Transplant* 2001;16:192); IDV (*Nephrol Dial Transplant* 2000;15:1102); RTV (*Nephron* 2001;87:186); SQV (*Nephron* 2001;87:186); and LPV/r (*AIDS* 2001;15:662). There are sparse data for most antiretroviral agents for dose adjustments based on removal with peritoneal dialysis. Removal is anticipated or established with d4T, and ddC, which should be dosed post dialysis. TDF is not recommended with peritoneal dialysis. Others are not removed or are not expected to be removed.

‡ Avoid APV liquid due to its propylene glycol content.

§ Dose modified when combined with second PI – see Table 4-21, p. 88.

**CP Score=Child-Pugh Score

Antiretroviral Therapy

- **Impact of hepatic dysfunction** (*J Infect Dis* 2005;40:174)
  - □ NRTIs: Minimal effect because these drugs have limited first-pass metabolism and low protein binding and are eliminated primarily by renal excretion. No dose adjustments with liver disease except ABC use 200 mg bid for Child-Pugh Class A; avoid for Class B and C.
  - □ NNRTIs: Liver dysfunction has minimal effect on trough levels of EFV and NVP.
  - □ PIs: These are extensively metabolized by CYP enzymes; recommendations are:
    - □ NFV: Increased levels, but inconsequential
    - □ IDV: Recommended dose is 600 mg q 8h; for boosting: IDV/r 200/100 mg bid
    - □ SQV: Standard
    - □ LPV/r: No data; consider therapeutic drug monitoring
    - □ ATV: Child-Pugh B – 300 mg qd; C – avoid. 300-400 mg qd; RTV boosting not recommended

Adverse Drug Reactions (ADRs) to Antiretroviral Agents

Sources: DHHS Guidelines (April 7, 2005), IAS-USA (*J Acquir Immune Defic Syndr* 2002;31:257), federal nutrition guidelines (*Clin Infect Dis* 2003;31:Suppl 2)

For reviews from authoritative sources, see *J Acquir Immune Defic Syndr* 2002;31:257 (IAS-USA guidelines); *Clin Infect Dis* 2003;31:Suppl 2 (nutrition guidelines); *Clin Infect Dis* 2003;31:216 (dyslipidemia guidelines); *N Engl J Med* 2005;352:48 (review of cardiovascular risk and body fat abnormalities).

Lipodystrophy
(*N Engl J Med* 2005;352:48)

Lipodystrophy consists of two components, that may be seen together or independently: fat accumulation and fat atrophy. Fat accumulation is seen within the abdominal cavity ("Crix-belly" or "protease paunch"), the upper back (dorsocervical fat pad or "buffalo hump"), the breasts (gynecomastia), and in subcutaneous tissue (peripheral lipomatosis). Some patients show the combination of abdominal obesity, hypertension, dyslipidemia and insulin resistance that simulates the metabolic syndrome, or "syndrome X" (*J Intern Med* 1994;764:13). Lipoatrophy includes loss of subcutaneous fat in the face, extremities, and buttocks. Lipoatrophy is ascribed to NRTIs, especially d4T, and to

Antiretroviral Therapy

a lesser extent to AZT and ddI (*Sex Trans Infect* 2001;77:158). The cause of fat accumulation is less clear.

- **Frequency:** Lipodystrophy is reported in 20% to 80% of patients receiving antiretroviral therapy, a wide range reflecting a heterogeneous population and the lack of a standard case definition (*AIDS* 1999;13:1287; *AIDS* 1999;13:2493; *Lancet* 2000;356:1423; *Clin Infect Dis* 2002;34:248; *Clin Infect Dis* 2003;36[suppl 2]:S84; *J Acquir Immune Defic Syndr* 2005;38:18). The incidence based on perceived changes in body fat sufficiently severe to be detected by both the patient and physician in patients receiving 2 NRTIs plus a PI was 17%, with a median follow-up of 18 months (*Lancet* 2001;357:592). The frequency of abdominal fat accumulation was 9.2/100 pt-yrs, and 7.7/100 pt-yrs for lipoatrophy. A meta-analysis of 5 series with 5435 HAART recipients showed fat accumulation was reported in 17% to 67% of studies and fat atrophy in 20% to 75% of studies (*Clin Infect Dis* 2003;36:S84).

- **Antiretroviral Agents**

  □ Fat accumulation is often associated with PI-based HAART (*AIDS* 2001;15:231; *AIDS* 1999;13:2493) with an odds-ratio in controlled trials of 2.6 to 3.4 (*Clin Infect Dis* 2003;36[suppl 2]:S84). Nevertheless, it may be seen with HIV infection in the absence of PI exposure. The changes may occur without hyperlipidemia (*J Acquir Immune Defic Syndr* 2000;23:351; *Arch Intern Med* 2000;150:2050).

  □ Lipoatrophy is more closely linked with NRTIs, especially d4T and less frequently AZT (*AIDS* 2000;14:F25; *AIDS* 1999;13:1659), although some data are conflicting (*Lancet* 2001;15:231; *Antiviral Ther* 2000;5:S55). The presumed mechanism is inhibition of DNA polymerase gamma resulting in depletion of mitochondrial DNA (*N Engl J Med* 2002;346:81).

- **Evaluation** (*Lancet* 2000;356:1412; *Lancet* 2001;357:592; *AIDS* 1999;13:2493; *Clin Infect Dis* 2003;36[suppl 2]:S63)

  □ Patient perception

  □ Physical examination, serial photography

  □ Waist-hip ratio (>0.85 for women, >0.95 for men): Safe, portable and inexpensive*

  □ Dual energy X-ray absorptiometry (DEXA): Good for measuring limb fat but not visceral fat*

  □ Ultrasound: Limited published experience*

  □ Computed tomography and MRI: Gold standards*

  □ Bioelectric impedence: not validated, not recommended*

---

*Evaluation by IAS-USA review (*J Acquir Immune Defic Syndr* 2002;31:2570)

Antiretroviral Therapy

4

- **Treatment**
  - □ **Low fat diet and aerobic exercise** can be partly effective in treating fat accumulation (*AIDS* 1999;13:231; *Cochrane Database Syst Rev* 2005;18:CD001796), although they may exacerbate lipoatrophy.

  - □ **Growth hormone** (up to 6 mg/kg/day) may reduce fat accumulation (*Ann Intern Med* 1996;125:873; *AIDS* 1999;13:2099; *J Clin Endocrinol Metab* 1997;82:727), but the benefits disappear after treatment is stopped (*J Acquir Immune Defic Syndr* 2002;35:249). Disadvantages include high price and side effects, including hyperglycemia, fluid retention, hypertension, carpal tunnel syndrome, further loss of subcutaneous fat, and the need for maintenance treatment. Current studies are exploring the utility of lower doses of growth hormone (*J Acquir Immune Defic Syndr* 2002;30:379; *J Acquir Immune Defic Syndr* 2004;35:367).

  - □ Growth hormone-releasing hormone (GHRH): Initial results of a trial (1 mg SC bid x12 wks) showed significant decrease in visceral fat and increase in extremity fat with no change in blood lipids or insulin resistance (*JAMA* 2004;292:210). Problems with this treatment are bid SC injection requirement and monthly cost of about $1800.

  - □ **Thiazolidinediones:** There was preliminary evidence of efficacy for lipoatrophy (*Ann Intern Med* 2000;133:263), but a placebo-controlled trial showed no benefit of rosiglitazone (4 mg bid x48 wks) in 108 patients with lipoatrophy (*Lancet* 2004;363:429).

  - □ **Metformin** (500 mg bid) improves insulin sensitivity and results in weight loss and decreased intra-abdominal fat in patients with fat accumulation and insulin resistance (*JAMA* 2000;284:472; *AIDS* 1999;13:1000). It may also improve some markers of cardio-vascular risk (*J Clin Endocrinol Metab* 2002;87:4611). These initial studies are considered preliminary and inconclusive (*Clin Infect Dis* 2003;36[suppl 2]:S96).

  - □ **Restorative surgery** for fat accumulation includes removal of lipomas, breast/fat tissue or dorso-cervical fat pad by either surgery or liposuction. A number of methods with implants and injections are being investigated for facial fat atrophy. Injectable poly-L-lactic acid (*Sculptra*) has gained favor for facial atrophy and is FDA-approved for this indication. Injections of fat or collagen are associated with rapid resorption, so the changes are short-lived.

  - □ **Regimen changes** with a switch from PIs to an NNRTI are sometimes partially successful in reversing fat accumulation, although data are conflicting and changes are slow (*J Infect Dis* 2001;184:914; *Clin Infect Dis* 2000;31:1266). Switches from d4T or AZT to ABC or TDF may lead to gradual improvements in lipoatrophy (*JAMA* 2002;288:207; 3rd IAS, 2005, Abstr.

Antiretroviral Therapy

TuPe2.2B12; 12th CROI, Boston, 2005, Abstr. 44LB; 12th CROI, Boston, 2005, Abstr. 45LB; *Clin Infect Dis* 2004;38,263; *AIDS* 2005;19:15). The TARHEEL study showed that the switch from d4T to ABC or AZT was associated with significant increases in arm, leg and trunk fat at 48 wks, but improvement was noted in <40% and was greater with DEXA than by self-report (*Clin Infect Dis* 2004;38:263).

Lactic Acidosis/Hepatic Steatosis

Hyperlactatemia is defined as a venous lactate level >2 mM. It can be asymptomatic or can be associated with overt, sometimes fatal lactic acidosis. It appears to be a complication of NRTI therapy. Although it was originally described as a rare but potentially fatal complication of AZT therapy in the early 1990s, it is now seen primarily as a complication of d4T, ddI or both; AZT is a less frequent cause (*Clin Infect Dis* 2002;34:838). Initial reports focused on critically ill patients, with a mortality rate of 55% (*Clin Infect Dis* 2002;34:838). Mild asymptomatic elevations of lactic acid are now seen more frequently, and treatment strategies are evolving. The mechanism is nucleoside analog-mediated inhibition of DNA polymerase gamma, leading to depletion of mitochondrial DNA (*N Engl J Med* 2002;346:811; *Nat Med* 1995;1:417; *J Clin Invest* 1995;96:126).

- **Frequency:** This depends on the definition, duration of NRTI exposure, specific agents used, and demographics of the population studied and adequacy of lactic acid measurements, which often show falsely high levels unless testing is done very carefully. Lactic acidemia without symptoms or with mild symptoms is noted in 8% to 20% of patients given prolonged courses of nucleosides (*Clin Infect Dis* 2003;36[suppl 2]:S96; *Arch Intern Med* 2000;160:2050). This does not predict serious lactic acidosis, however, and may not require treatment. In fact, in an ACTG trial only 1 of 83 asymptomatic NRTI recipients had elevated LA levels, which were normal when repeated (*J Acquir Immune Defic Syndr* 2004;35:274). The conclusion was that most such elevations in asymptomatic patients reflect faulty collection methods. Most reports show a rate of symptomatic hyperlactatemia of 0.5-1/100 patient-years of NRTI exposure (*AIDS* 2001;15:717; *Clin Infect Dis* 2001;33:1931; *AIDS* 2000;14:2723; *Lancet* 2000;356:1423). Using *in vitro* assays of mitochondrial toxicity due to inhibition of DNA polymerase γ, the frequency in rank order is d4T/ddI, d4T, ddI and AZT; other NRTIs (3TC, FTC, TDF and ABC) are infrequent or only theoretical causes (*Clin Infect Dis* 2002;34:838; *N Engl J Med* 2002;346:811; *Clin Infect Dis* 2000;31:162; *Clin Infect Dis* 2001;33:2072; *AIDS* 2001;15:717). Duration of treatment is inconsistently correlated (*Clin Infect Dis* 2002;34:558; *J Acquir Immune Defic Syndr* 2002;31:257). Risk factors include female sex, pregnancy, obesity, and use of ddI

4 Antiretroviral Therapy

combined with d4T, ribavarin or hydroxyurea. This risk accounts for the contraindication for giving ribavarin and ddI and for combining d4T + ddI in pregnancy.

- **Diagnosis:** Patients with elevated serum lactate levels may be asymptomatic, critically ill, or may have non-specific symptoms, such as fatigue, myalgia, nausea, vomiting, diarrhea, abdominal distention, weight loss, or dyspnea (*Ann Intern Med* 2000;133:192; *Clin Infect Dis* 2002;34:838). Diagnosis is established with an elevated lactic acid level, which requires the use of a pre-chilled fluoride-oxalate tube and blood sampling without a tourniquet, with blood delivered rapidly to the lab on ice for processing within 4 hours. The patient should not exercise for 24 hours prior to sampling and should be well hydrated. Errors in quality control and over-diagnosis are common. ACTG A5129 showed elevated lactic acid levels in only 1/83 patients with clinical or laboratory evidence of hyperlactemia associated with NRTI therapy (*J Acquir Immune Defic Syndr* 2004;35:274). In general, lactic acid levels correlate with prognosis: 0-2 mM is normal; 5-10 mM is associated with a 7% mortality; 10-15 mM with a >30% mortality, and >15 mM with a >60% mortality (*Clin Infect Dis* 2002;34:838). Other common lab test abnormalities that suggest this diagnosis are elevated CPK, LDH, amylase or AST, increased anion gap (Na - [Cl + CO_2] >16); low serum albumin, pH or bicarbonate, and CT scan, ultrasound, or biopsy of liver showing hepatic steatosis.

- **Indications for lactic acid levels** (federal nutrition guidelines, *Clin Infect Dis* 2003;36[suppl 2]:596): (1) Symptoms suggesting this diagnosis in NRTI recipients, including otherwise unexplained dyspnea, nausea, abdominal pain, wasting and/or liver failure. (2) Unexplained lab abnormalities: anion gap, increased transaminase levels, and increased amylase. (3) Selected patients: Pregnant women getting NRTIs and patients with prior lactic acidosis who are now retreated.

- **Treatment:** Lactic acid levels <5 mM may not require treatment or may be managed with modification of NRTI therapy. Symptomatic patients usually have levels >5 mM and typically require discontinuation of NRTIs. In some cases, a switch from d4T, ddI, or AZT to ABC, 3TC, FTC, or TDF may be reasonable, provided the patient is not seriously ill and can be carefully observed. Lactic acid levels >10 mM, if properly obtained, should be viewed as a medical emergency because of the high mortality. Seriously ill patients require supportive care, which may include intravenous hydration, mechanical ventilation, and/or dialysis. Recovery is protracted. The half-life of mitochondrial DNA ranges from 4.5 to 8 weeks, and the time required for clinical recovery is 4 to 28 weeks (*AIDS* 2000;14:F25); *N Engl J Med* 2002;346:811). Anecdotal case reports show possible benefit of thiamine, riboflavin, L-carnitine, vitamin C, and antioxidants (*Clin Infect Dis* 2002;34:838). The experience with riboflavin (50 mg/day) appears to be the most extensive and favorable. NRTI therapy with agents less likely to cause lactic acidosis should be delayed until the lactate level measured monthly for at least 3 months is normal. The alternative is to use NRTI-sparing regimens.

Insulin Resistance

Insulin resistance (impaired uptake of glucose by muscle and inhibition of hepatic glucogenesis) is common with PI-based HAART, but diabetes (fasting blood sugar >126 mg/dL) is infrequent and rarely requires insulin, except in patients who are prone to diabetes (first-degree relative).

- **Frequency:** Insulin resistance is noted in 30% to 90% of patients treated with protease inhibitors, and overt diabetes occurs in 1% to 11%, with a mean of approximately 7% at 5 years (*AIDS* 1999;13:F63; *Lancet* 1999;353:2093; *Arch Intern Med* 2000;160: 2050). In an analysis of the MACS database, the incidence of diabetes mellitus (fasting blood glucose >126 mg/dL) was 4.7/100 person-years for HAART recipients, a 4.1-fold risk compared to untreated controls (*Arch Intern Med* 2005;165:1179). Insulin resistance has been demonstrated with administration of LPV/r, IDV, and RTV to uninfected individuals. No changes are seen with ATV (*J Infect Dis* 2004;182:209). No data are available for SQV, FPV or NFV. The changes in blood glucose are usually apparent within 2 to 3 months and can be detected with a fasting blood glucose (*Lancet* 1999;353:2093). With indinavir, insulin resistance can be detected after a single dose (*AIDS* 2002;16:F1).

SCREENING

- Random blood glucose, fasting blood glucose, and HgA1c measurements are insensitive methods to measure insulin resistance, due to compensatory increases in insulin. PI-treated patients with normal fasting blood glucose levels may have severe insulin resistance demonstrated by glucose clamp techniques (*AIDS* 2000;25:312).

- The 2004-05 DHHS and IAS-USA guidelines recommend fasting blood glucose levels at baseline and at 3- to 6-month intervals in PI-treated patients, with more measurements when indicated by initial results and diabetes risk. More aggressive testing may include fasting insulin levels, C-peptide, and oral glucose tolerance testing for those with borderline fasting glucose levels (110-126 mg/dL).

RISK: A practical importance of insulin resistance is its role as a risk factor for atherosclerosis (*N Engl J Med* 1996;334:952; *Am J Med*

Antiretroviral Therapy

4

1997;103:152), especially when accompanied by dyslipidemia, hypertension, and visceral fat accumulation, e.g., the components of metabolic syndrome or "syndrome X" (*J Intern Med* 1994;736:13). Risk assessment should include assessment of risk factors for diabetes and atherosclerosis, including family history, smoking, hypertension, obesity, and dyslipidemia.

TREATMENT: Standard guidelines are recommended for management of diabetes (*Diabetes Care* 2000;23[suppl 1]:S32). Most cases are type 2 and can be managed with diet and exercise. The daily diet should consist of 50% to 60% carbohydrates, 10% to 20% protein, and <30% fat, with <100 mg cholesterol per day and <10% of total calories from saturated fat. When drug therapy is necessary, the two major classes of agents are insulin secretagogues (sulfonylureas) and insulin-sensitizing agents (metformin and thiazolidinediones). Metformin or a thiazolidinedione have the potential advantage of improving insulin resistance and decreasing visceral fat accumulation (*AIDS* 1999;13: 100; *JAMA* 2000;284:472), with a possible reduction in cardiovascular risk. LFTs need to be monitored (ALT q 2 months x 12 months) with thiazolinediones; a baseline ALT >2.5 ULN contraindicates use. A baseline elevation of creatinine or lactic acid to ≥2 x ULN contraindicates metformin. An alternative strategy is to change the HAART regimen to a non-PI-based regimen or ATV-based HAART (*AIDS* 1999;13:805; *J Acquir Immune Defic Syndr* 2001;27:229; *Clin Infect Dis* 2000;31:1266).

Hyperlipidemia

Changes in blood lipids have emerged as an important concern with HAART, due to the potential for premature atherosclerosis and coronary artery disease. The risk of this complication with relatively short-term follow-up appears to be modest but real (*N Engl J Med* 2003;349:1993). Studies in the pre-HAART era showed that HIV progression was associated with elevated triglyceride levels and decreased cholesterol levels (*Am J Med* 1991;90:154; *JAMA* 2003; 289:2978). With PI-based HAART there is usually an increase in triglycerides, cholesterol and LDL cholestrol (*J Infect Dis* 2004;189: 1056). Most cholesterol is carried in low-density lipoprotein (LDL-C); high concentrations of LDL-C are associated with increased risk of atherosclerosis, especially coronary artery disease. High triglyceride levels also increase this risk. Triglyceride levels may increase to >1000 mg/dL, levels associated with an increased risk of both pancreatitis and atherosclerosis. Total and LDL cholesterol levels increase an average of about 30 mg/dL, but there is substantial individual patient variation, which is poorly understood (*J Acquir Immune Def Syndr* 2000;23:35; *Arch Intern Med* 2000;160:2050; *J Aquir Immune Defic Syndr* 2000;23:261; *Lancet* 1998;352:1031; *AIDS* 1998;12:F51; *Circulation*

1999;100:700; *J Infect Dis* 2004;189:1056). With regard to agents, the analysis of 23,000 HIV-infected patients in D:A:D showed the highest risk was with RTV and boosted PIs (*J Infect Dis* 2004;189:1056). Lipid changes with ATV are nil (*J Acquir Immune Defic Syndr* 2004;36:1011). D4T is also associated with elevated triglyceride levels (*JAMA* 2004;292:191). Effects are less with NNRTIs in general and less with NVP compared to EFV (*AIDS* 2003;17:1195). HAART-associated changes are usually apparent within 2 to 3 months of initiating therapy.

- **Risk:** An increased risk of cardiovascular disease associated with HAART was initially assumed based on serum lipid changes. The most comprehensive study of serum lipid changes is D:A:D (Data Collection on Adverse Events of anti-HIV Drugs), an observational study of 11 HIV cohorts with data on >20,000 HIV-infected patients in 188 clinics. The initial results showed 126 MIs among 23,468 patients. The relative rate for HAART recipients was 1.25; and for smoking it was 2.2 (*N Engl J Med* 2003;349:1993). Other studies also show a modest increased risk of coronary events with use of HAART (*JAMA* 2003;289:2978; *AIDS* 2003;17:1179). Assessment needs to include a review of other cardiovascular risk factors as defined by NCEP, as summarized in Table 4-25 (*JAMA* 2001;285:2486).

- **Management:** Based on recommendations of ACTG and IDSA (*Clin Infect Dis* 2003;37:613) and the National Cholesterol Education Program guidelines III (*JAMA* 2001;285:2486). Note that LDL-C guidelines were modified based on more recent data to target LDL-C at 70 and 100 mg/dL in the two highest risk groups (*J Am Coll Cardiol* 2004;44:720).

- **Baseline assessment:** Lipid profile, including cholesterol, LDL + HDL cholesterol, and triglycerides after fasting at least 8 (preferably 12) hours. Fasting is necessary for accurate measurement of triglycerides and the calculation of LDL cholesterol but has minimal effect on total cholesterol. LDL cholesterol measurements are unreliable with triglyceride levels >400 mg/dL.

- **Monitoring:** The lipid profile should be repeated at 3 to 4 months, and then with a frequency depending on the 3- to 4-month values and risk assessment. It should be repeated at least once per year.

- **Therapeutic life changes:** Diet, exercise, smoking cessation, treatment of HBP and diabetes, and weight loss for obesity should be recommended for triglycerides >400 mg/dL, cholesterol >240 mg/dL, and HDL <35 mg/dL.

- **Statin regimens to treat elevated LDL-C:** Pravastatin 20-80 mg/day, atorvastatin 10-40 mg/day, fluvastatin 20-40 mg/day or rosuvastatin 10-40 mg/day

4 Antiretroviral Therapy

- **Sequencing:** Initiate non-drug therapy unless there are extreme elevations; e.g. LDL-C >220 mg/dL or triglyceride >1000 mg/dL + history of pancreatitis

- **Switch therapy:** PI → NNRTI or ATV

- **Triglyceride levels >1000 mg/dL (ACTG guidelines) or >500 mg/dL (NCEP guidelines):** Therapeutic life changes + drug therapy, usually gemfibrozil 600 mg bid or fenofibrate 48-145 mg qd.

- TABLE 4-25: **National Cholesterol Education Program Guidelines** (*Circulation* 2004;110:227)

Risk category	LDL goal (m/dL)	Lifestyle change*	Drug therapy
Atherosclerosis, diabetes or multiple risk factors	<70	>100	>130 optional – 100-130
≥2 risk factors: smoking, HBP, HDL, >40, hereditary factors*			
10 yr risk 10-20%	<100	<130	>130
10 yr risk <10%	<130	<130	>160
0-1 risk factors*	<160	<190	optional 160-190 >190

* Age: male >45 yrs, female >55 yrs; HDL-C <40 mg/dL; BP >140/90 or antihypertension drugs; smoking; coronary artery disease in a first-degree male relative <55 yrs or female relative <65 yrs

TREATMENT OF HYPERLIPIDEMIA

- **Lifestyle changes**
  - □ Diet – Reduce saturated fat to <7%; reduce cholesterol to <200 mg/d; increase fiber to 20-30 gm/d; LDL-lowering plant stanols/sterols 2 gm/d; protein, 15% of calories; carbohydrates, predominantly complex and 50-60% of calories
  - □ Exercise
  - □ Weight reduction
  - □ Smoking cessation
  - □ Control of hypertension, diabetes

DRUG THERAPY

- **LDL-C elevation: statins**
  - □ ***Basics:*** Statins are the most effective drugs to reduce LDL-C; they also decrease triglycerides. Statins may produce a modest increase in HDL-C and decrease CRP (*N Engl J Med* 2005;352:73). The clinical benefit correlates with the LDL-C decrease. Meta-

analysis of 58 placebo-controlled trials showed coronary artery events decreased by 20%, 31% and 51% with decreases of 20 mg/dL, 40 mg/dL and 62 mg/dL, respectively. Once started, statins are usually continued for a lifetime. If stopped, lipid levels return to baseline within 2-3 wks.

- □ **PI interactions:** Most statins are metabolized using cytochrome P3A4; all PIs inhibit CYP3A4. the greatest effect is with lovastatin and simvastatin; atorvastatin is only partially metabolized by CYP3A4; fluvastatin is metabolized mainly by CYP2C9; pravastatin and rosuvastatin are not metabolized by this mechanism.

- □ **Adverse effects:** Myalgias and muscle weakness, with or without elevated CPK, is common (*JAMA* 2003;289:1681). Rhabdomyolysis and myoglobinemia with renal failure are rare. These risks are dose-related and increased with PIs. Obtain baseline CPK levels and repeat the test if myalgias develop; some recommend discontinuing statins or lowering the dose if the level is 3-5x ULN (*Treatment Guidelines, Med Letter* 2003;3:15). Other ADRs include increased transaminase levels in 1-2%, which is often corrected by use of an alternative statin. A rare polyneuropathy has been reported (Neurology 2002;58:1333).

■ TABLE 4-26: **Statins**

Agent	Form	Dose (FDA)		Decrease LDL
		Initial mg/day	Max mg/day	
Atorvastatin (*Lipitor*)	Tabs – 10, 20, 40, 80 mg	10	80	35-60%
Fluvastatin (*Lescol*)	caps – 20, 40 mg; 80 mg XL	20	80	20-40%
Pravastatin (*Pravachol*)	tabs – 10, 20, 40, 80 mg	20-40	80	30-40%
Rosuvastatin (*Crestor*)	tabs – 5, 10, 20, 40 mg	10	40	45-60%

Lovastatin (*Mevacor*) and simvastatin (*Zocor*) are not included due to major drug interactions with all PIs and EFV.

■ TABLE 4-27: **Drug Interactions**

Statin*	ATV	FPV	IDV	LPV	NFV	RTV	SQV	EFV
Atorvastatin	ND	1.5x	↑	↑5.9x	↑74%	↑	↑4.5%	↓0.4x
Pravastatin	ND	ND	ND	↑33x	ND	↓	↓50%	ND

ND = no data;   ↑ = anticipated increase in AUC of statin;   ↑0.7x = statin AUC increased 70%; ↑4.5x = statin AUC increased 450%

* Data are not provided for simvastatin or lovastatin because all are contraindicated for concurrent use with all PIs; EFV decreases AUC of simvastatin 58% and there are no data for NVP.

Antiretroviral Therapy

4

Agent	Form	Regimen
Gemfibrozil (*Lopid*)	Tabs – 600 mg	600 mg bid before meals
Fenofibrate (*TriCor*) Generic	Tabs – 48, 145 mg Caps – 67, 100, 200 mg	145 mg qd 200 mg qd

Hepatotoxicity (see *Clin Liver Dis* 2003;7:475)

Most antiretroviral agents have been implicated as potential causes of hepatotoxicity, but frequency, severity, and mechanism are highly variable (Table 4-29). Many cases are confounded by the concurrent presence of pre-existing liver disease ascribed to HBV, HCV or alcoholism. The most common manifestation is an asymptomatic increase in transaminase levels, which often resolves without discontinuation of the implicated agent.

■ TABLE 4-29: **Grading of Hepatotoxicty (ACTG)**

Grade	ALT/AST (x ULN)	AlkPhos x ULN	Bili x ULN
1	1-2.5x	1-2.5x	1.0-1.5x
2	2.5-5x	2.5-5x	1.5-2.5x
3	5-10x	5-10x	2.5-5x
4	>10x	>10x	>5x

Antiretroviral Therapy

■ TABLE 4-30: **Hepatotoxicity of Antiretrovirals***

Class & Agent	Frequency Grade 3-4	Mechanism
NRTI		
d4T, AZT, ddI	6-13%	Mitochondrial toxicity with hepatic steatosis; d4T most common
FTC, TDF, 3TC; withdrawal or development of HBV resistance with chronic HBV	6% (?)	HBV hepatitis flare Resistance most likely with 3TC and FTC
ABC	5%	Hypersensitivity; genetic component
Protease inhibitors		
All agents	3-10%	Mechanism unknown; consequences unknown; transaminase levels may return to normal while continuing PI. Greatest risk with HCV or HBV coninfection.
IDV and ATV	Most	Elevated indirect bilirubin; jaudice; 3-5%; not associated with hepatotoxicity.
NNRTI		
NVP	1-11%	Symptomatic hepatitis (usually with nausea, vomiting, rash and/or fever in the first 12-16 wks of treatment; *J Infect Dis* 2005;191:825). Risks: baseline CD4 count >250/mm^3 in women, >400/mm^3 in men; rate is 11% in women initally treated with CD4 >250/mm^3 and <2% with CD4 <250/mm^3. Delayed hepatotoxicity can also occur. Mechanism is unknown. Analogous to hepatitis with PIs. Greatest risk with HBC or HCV co-infection.
EFV, DLV	8-15%	Mechanism unknown Analogous to hepatitis with PIs. Greatest risk with HBV or HCV co-infection.

* Adapted from Olgledigbe, A, and Sulkowski, M. *Clin Liver Dis* 2003;7:475 and Sanne I, *J Infect Dis* 2005;191:825)

- **HBV or HCV co-infection:** Both are associated with increased mortality with HIV co-infection, although the mechanisms are unclear. HCV often represents a marker of injection drug use, which may account for the difference (*J Acquir Immune Defic Syndr* 2003;33:365; *Clin Infect Dis* 2003;36:363). HBV is immune-mediated, so immune restoration with HAART may account for an increase in HBV progression.

Antiretroviral Therapy

4

- **NRTIs:** Three mechanisms of liver injury are described: hepatic steatosis that accompanies lactic acidosis, abacavir hypersensitivity, and flares of chronic hepatitis due to HBV that accompany either withdrawal of drugs active against HBV or the development of HBV resistance to those drugs (*J Infect Dis* 2002;186:23). Antiretroviral agents that are active against HBV include 3TC, FTC, and TDF. The frequency of resistance to 3TC and presumably FTC is 30% to 50% after 1 year of exposure; it is <2% with TDF (*AIDS* 2003;17:1649). The abacavir hypersensitivity reaction is a serious multisystem reaction that is seen in 4% to 5% of abacavir recipients with >90% occurring in the first 6 weeks of treatment. This requires immediate withdrawal of the drug without rechallenge, which could be fatal (*Clin Infect Dis* 2002;34:1137). Lactic acidosis usually occurs after months of treatment with NTRIs, primarily with regimens that include d4T, ddI and/or AZT (*Clin Infect Dis* 2003;36[suppl 2]:S96) (see pp. 103-105).

- **NNRTIs:** All three NNRTIs may cause hepatotoxicity with elevated transaminases. Reported rates of grade 3-4 hepatotoxicity are 8% to 15%, and highest with NVP (*HIV Clin Trials* 2003;4:115; *AIDS* 2003;17:2191; *J Hepatol* 2002;36:283). NVP appears to cause liver disease by two possibly distinct mechanisms. The serious form is symptomatic, sometimes associated with hepatic necrosis, usually occurs in the first 6 weeks of treatment, is accompanied by a systemic response (fever, rash, GI symptoms) and resembles a hypersensitivity reaction (*AIDS* 2003;17:2209). This reaction is reported in 11% in women who start NVP as initial treatment with a CD4 count >250/mm^3; the risk is also increased in previously untreated men who initiate NVP with a CD4 count >400/mm^3. This reaction may not be reversible even when detected early. Frequent monitoring of transaminase levels is commonly advocated, but there is no evidence that this predicts the event. See p. 263 for management guidelines. The second type of hepatotoxicity usually occurs later in the course and is seen with PIs, NVP, DLV, and EFV, especially in patients with HBV or HCV co-infection. Most are asymptomatic. Current recommendations are to discontinue the NNRTI only when there are symptoms or the transaminase levels reach an arbitrary threshold of 5 or 10x ULN, plateau. Many will spontaneously resolve even when treatment is continued with ALT levels >10x ULN (*Clin Liver Dis* 2003;7:475; *AIDS* 2003;17:2209).

- **PIs:** Hepatotoxicity with PIs is usually characterized by asymptomatic elevations in transaminase levels caused by unknown mechanisms. Liver biopsies in such cases are usually nonspecific and do not show drug-induced injury. Most have resolution of the abnormal tests despite continuation of the implicated drug. Grade 3-4 toxicity (ALT to 5-10x ULN) is most common in patients with HBV or HCV co-infection; it appears to be most frequent with RTV (*JAMA*

2000;283:74) and is dose-related (>300 mg RTV bid) The recommended intervention is to alter therapy if hepatitis is symptomatic or if the ALT increases above an arbitrary threshold of 5x-10x ULN in the absence of symptoms.

Increased Bleeding in Patients With Hemophilia

Increased spontaneous bleeding epsodes in patients with hemophilia A and B have been observed with the use of PIs. Most of the reported episodes involved joints and soft tissues. However, more serious bleeding episodes, including intracranial and GI bleeding, have also been reported. The bleeding episodes occurred a median of 22 days after initiation of PI therapy. Some patients received additional coagulation factor while continuing PI therapy (*Hemophilia* 2000; 6:487).

Osteopenia/Osteoporosis and Osteonecrosis/Avascular Necrosis

Osteonecrosis with avascular necrosis is another possible late complication that may be due to HAART. By 2002 there had been 67 reported cases of osteonecrosis in HIV-infected patients (*Clin Infect Dis* 2000;31:1488; *Ann Intern Med* 2002;137:17). Reported prevalence based on routine MRI scans is 1.3% to 4.4%. The most common site is the femoral head; many patients have other risk factors, including alcohol abuse, hyperlipidemia, lipid lowering agents, testosterone therapy, corticosteroid use, and hypercoagulability. X-rays are not sensitive for detecting avascular necrosis. Screening of asymptomatic patients is not recommended. CT scan or MRI should be considered in patients with symptoms and risk.

Bone density studies using dual energy X-ray absorptiometry (DEXA) scanning show that osteopenia and osteoporosis are relatively common, although there is no clear association with specific agents, drug classes, or lipodystrophy (*AIDS* 2000;14:F63).

Antiretroviral Therapy

4

Recommendations For Antiretroviral Therapy In Pregnancy

(Based on Revised DHHS Guidelines of November 2004;
http://www.aidsinfo.nih.gov)

■ TABLE 4-31: **Recommended Antiretroviral Therapy in Pregnancy (based on DHHS Guidelines, April, 7, 2005. www.aidsinfo.nih.gov)**

Nucleosides and nucleotides	
Recommended	AZT and 3TC (standard doses)
Alternatives	ddI, FTC, d4T, ABC (standard doses)
Insufficient data	TDF
Not recommended	ddC
Non-nucleoside RT inhibitors	
Recommended	NVP (should not be used as initial therapy in women with baseline CD4 count >250 mm³) (standard doses)
Not recommended	EFV, DLV
Protease inhibitors	
Recommended	NFV (1250 mg bid),* SQV/r (800/100 mg bid)*
Alternatives	IDV (800/100 ng bid)*, LPV/r (400/100 mg bid)
Insufficient data	APV, FPV, ATV
Fusion inhibitors	
Insufficient data	ENF

*Doses of PIs (*N Engl J Med* 2002;346:1879; *AIDS* 2003;17:1195)

- NVP: PACTG 353 9th CROI, Seattle, 2002, Abstr. 795W
- SQV/r: AAC 2004;48:430
- IDV: *AIDS* 2000;14:1061
- IDV and LPV/r: may need therapeutic drug monitoring

Principles (*N Engl J Med* 2002;346:1879)

■ **HIV progression:** Pregnancy has no clear effect on HIV progression.

■ **Pregnancy complications:** Data from developing countries show HIV infection is associated with increased rates of preterm delivery, low birth weight, and stillbirth. This has not been observed in industrialized countries.

■ **Viral load:** Probability of perinatal transmission is directly related to viral load at the time of delivery. Other risks include substance abuse, premature rupture of membranes, HCV coinfection, and preterm gestation.

■ **When to treat:** All pregnant women should be offered antiretroviral agents to reduce perinatal transmission and improve maternal health. HAART is recommended for treatment of HIV in the pregnant woman based on guidelines that apply to the general population, with few exceptions for agent selection (see next bullet). HAART is also recommended to prevent perinatal transmission in any woman with a viral load >1000 c/mL. With viral load <1000 c/mL (without treatment), some authorities accept AZT monotherapy.

- **Drugs to use:** Avoid hydroxyurea, EFV, TDF, and d4T + ddI. When possible, include AZT (but not AZT + d4T). Preferred regimens in DHHS guidelines: AZT/3TC + either NFV 1250 mg bid or SQV/r 1000/100 mg bid; in WHO guidelines: 2 NRTIs + either NVP, or NFV.

- **NVP:** New data suggest NVP should be avoided in women who initiate treatment with a CD4 count >250/mm³ (*J Infect Dis* 2005;19:825). (This does not pertain to the single dose of NVP given intrapartum to prevent perinatal transmission.)

- **C-section:** Elective cesarean section reduces risk of perinatal transmission and should be offered at 38 weeks to pregnant women with viral loads likely to be >1,000 c/mL at delivery. There is no evidence of benefit after onset of labor, after rupture of membranes, or with viral load <1000 c/mL. See p. 117 for more on this subject.

Interventions for Preventing Perinatal Transmission

The largest U.S. report is the Women and Infants Transmission Study (WITS) Group (*J Acquir Immune Defic Syndr* 2002;29:484).

- Antiretroviral agents: Results for perinatal transmission for 1542 patients from 1990 to 2000 showed the following: No antiretrovirals – 20.0%, AZT monotherapy – 10.4%, dual NRTIs – 3.8%, and HAART – 1.2% (*J Acquir Immune Defic Syndr* 2002;29:484). The rate was 18.1% for 1990-92 and decreased to 1.6% in 1999-2000 (*J Acquir Immune Defic Syndr* 2005;38:87). The rate in the European Collaborative Study for 2001-02 was 1% (*Clin Infect Dis* 2005;40:458).

HIV Testing and Counseling

HIV TESTING: Standard serologic test with counseling is recommended for all pregnant women. Testing should be repeated at 28 weeks. The rapid test (see p. 10) is recommended for previously untested women presenting in labor and some high-risk women. Women with symptoms suggesting acute HIV infection in the third trimester should have HIV RNA tests.

COUNSELING (*MMWR* 2001;50[RR-19]:1): Minimum information to be conveyed includes the following:

- HIV is the virus that causes AIDS and is spread by sex and drugs.
- Women may be infected and not know it.

- There are effective interventions that protect the infant and reduce morbidity and mortality in adults.
- HIV serology is recommended for all pregnant women.
- Services are available to help pregnant women prevent HIV transmission.
- Women who refuse the test will receive the usual care for themselves and their infants.

LEGAL ISSUES (UNITED STATES): Testing and counseling pregnant women has been endorsed by most professional societies and implemented by most states, but with substantial variations in strategy. No states mandate testing pregnant women without informed consent, but CDC guidelines issued in 2003 recommend routine testing of newborns from women who did not have prenatal screening. Obstetricians in some states simply show a list of tests that includes HIV serology and ask if any tests are refused ("opt-out testing").

Factors that Reduce Perinatal Transmission

For women who do not breastfeed, intrauterine transmission previously accounted for 25% to 40% and delivery for 60% to 75% (*MMWR* 2001;50[RR-19]:63). More recent data from the WITS study in the U.S. shows *in utero* transmission now accounts for more than half of MTCT in the US (*J Acquir Immune Defic Syndr* 2005;38:87). A study of 315 twin births in Malawi showed equal risks for the first- and second-born (*J Infect Dis* 2003;188:850). This has been interpreted to suggest exposure occurs due to microtransfusion at the time of placental disruption rather than exposure with passage through the birth canal. It should be emphasized that all three components of the AZT regimen (pre-natal, perinatal, and post-natal) have merit.

VIRAL LOAD: There is a direct correlation between maternal viral load and probability of perinatal transmission varying from 41% with a VL >100,000 c/mL to 0% with a VL <1000 c/mL (*N Engl J Med* 1999;13: 407; *J Infect Dis* 2001;183:206; *J Acquir Immune Defic Syndr* 2002;29: 484). Despite these findings, it should be emphasized that there is no viral load that can be regarded as safe because other factors also play a role (*AIDS* 1999;13:1377; *AIDS* 1999;13:407; *J Infect Dis* 1999;179: 590). In an analysis of seven prospective studies, there were 44 cases of HIV in babies born to 1,202 women with viral loads <1,000 c/mL (*J Infect Dis* 2001;183:539).

AZT: This drug should be included when possible because it has the largest experience for safety and efficacy. This includes significant reduction in perinatal transmission that is independent of viral load (*N Engl J Med* 1996;335:1621; *Lancet* 1999;354:156) and possibly independent of AZT resistance (*J Infect Dis* 1998;177:557). Analysis of ACTG 076 showed that AZT significantly reduces perinatal transmission even when the baseline viral load is <1,000 c/mL (*J Infect Dis* 2001;183:539). This provides the rationale for AZT monotherapy in untreated pregnant women with a baseline viral load <1,000 c/mL, although some authorities would recommend this treatment only if a standard HAART regimen was refused.

NVP: NVP is the best studied drug other than AZT. It is generally well tolerated and the preferred "third drug" in the 2003 WHO guidelines for HIV-infected patients who are pregnant or have pregnancy potential. Two concerns are HIV resistance even with a single dose at delivery (*N Engl J Med* 2004;351:229) and the high rate of hepatotoxicity of NVP in women with a CD4 count >250/mm³ (*J Acquir Immune Defic Syndr* 2004;36:772; see Nevirapine, p. 260). Efficacy in preventing perinatal transmission has been shown in multiple studies, most performed in resource limited areas with a single maternal dose of 200 mg PO at delivery and one infant dose of 2 mg/kg. A study from Thailand compared AZT (076 protocol) with a single intrapartum dose to the mother and to the infant. This reduced the rate of perinatal transmission to 2% (*N Engl J Med* 2004;351:229). However, an analysis of 229 participants given NVP at 6 to 8 weeks postpartum showed NVP resistance mutations in 66 (32%), including the K103N mutation in 48 (21%). These mutations were often undetectable at 13 to 18 months, but the probability that they were archived is supported by a lower rate of response to subsequent treated with NVP-based HAART (*N Engl J Med* 2004;351:229). More recent reports using more sensitive methods to detect genotypic resistance show that K103N or other NNRTI resistance mutations are present in 60%-80% of patients after single-dose NVP (*J Infect Dis* 2005;192:24). The clinical significance of this is being vigorously pursued. Safety concerns (rash, hepatotoxicity) do not apply to single-dose NVP.

CESAREAN SECTION: C-section has established efficacy in reducing perinatal transmission when maternal viral load exceeds 1,000 c/mL. A meta-analysis of 15 studies with 8,533 mother-infant pairs showed a 2-fold reduction in perinatal transmission in women given AZT vs no antiretroviral and a 4-fold reduction when AZT was combined with cesarean section (Table 4-32, p. 118). A study of the European Mode of Delivery Collaboration randomly assigned patients to vaginal delivery vs C-section. The C-section group had a perinatal transmission rate of 3/170 (1.8%) compared with 21/200 (10.5%) in the vaginal delivery group. However, C-section confers far less benefit for pregnant women given HAART due to the substantial reduction in perinatal transmission rates with effective viral suppression (*Br Med J* 2001;322:511). The C-section decision is based on the risk/benefit ratio. There appears to be a slightly increased risk of this surgery to

4 Antiretroviral Therapy

both mother and infant (*Am J Obstet Gynecol* 2002;186:784; *J Acquir Immune Defic Syndr* 2001;26:236; *Am J Obstet Gynecol* 2000;183:100; *Am J Obstet Gynecol* 2001;184:1108). The rate of reduction in perinatal transmission varies with antiretroviral therapy and maternal VL at delivery (*AIDS* 2000;14:263; *Clin Infect Dis* 2001;33:3). Current DHHS guidelines (2005) recommend offering C-section to HIV-infected women with a VL >1000 c/mL at 36 weeks pregnancy. Table 4-32 shows the relative rates of perinatal transmission with and without C-section in the HAART era, as well as an unexplained large difference in the frequency of C-sections in Europe compared to the US. C-section performed at the time of labor or in a patient with ruptured membranes incurs a 5- to 7-fold increased risk of infectious complications and no benefit for reducing perinatal transmission. Other risks for adverse outcome(s) are non-elective C-section, malnutrition, obesity, smoking, genital infection, low socioeconomic status, prolonged labor, and membrane rupture. The major complications noted in these patients are wound infections, pneumonia, and endometritis. In the largest U.S. study (WITS), there were 2 deaths among 207 HIV-infected women who underwent C-section, both had PCP (*J Acquir Immune Defic Syndr* 2001;26:218).

■ TABLE 4-32: **Rates and Results of Cesarean Section to Prevent HIV infection in Europe and the U.S.**

	Europe* n = 1579	U.S.[†] n = 1398
Mode of Delivery		
Vaginal	369 (23%)	1098 (79%)
Elective C-section	971 (61%)	108 (8%)
HIV transmission		
Vaginal	24/369 (6.5%)	38/1398 (3.5%)
C-section	16/971 (1.7%)	1/108 (1%)

Elective cesarean section performed to prevent perinatal transmission should be done at 38 weeks instead of the usual 39 weeks.

BREASTFEEDING: The risk of HIV transmission with breastfeeding is 10%-16% (*J Infect Dis* 1996;174:722; *JAMA* 2000;283:1167; *Lancet* 1992;340:385; *JAMA* 2000;283:1175). The risk appears to be greatest in the first 4 to 6 months (*JAMA* 1999;282:744). The risk is increased 2-fold with mastitis and 50-fold with a breast abscess. Other risk factors include cracked nipples, infant with thrush, primary HIV infection during pregnancy, and prolonged breastfeeding. Breast-feeding is consequently discouraged for HIV-infected women in the developed world; the issue is more complex in developing countries,

Antiretroviral Therapy

where breastfeeding is critical for infant nutrition and survival (*JAMA* 2000;238:1167). It is estimated, for example, that 1.7 million babies develop HIV each year due to breastfeeding but that 1.5 million babies would die each year if not breastfed (*Br Med J* 2001;322:511).

Issues with Antiretroviral Agents

SAFETY OF ANTIRETROVIRAL THERAPY (see Table 4-34, P. 124): To date the data support the safety of all commonly used antiretroviral agents in pregnancy except for ddI + d4T, EFV, and hydroxyurea (*J Acquir Immune Defic Syndr* 2000;25:306; *MMWR* 2002;51[RR-7]:1; *N Engl J Med* 2002;346:1879). The combination of **ddI + d4T** should be avoided or used cautiously due to reports of three maternal deaths ascribed to lactic acidosis and/or hepatotoxicity. **EFV** should be avoided in the first trimester due to neural tube defects in 3 of 20 monkeys and neural tube defects in 5/206 infants born to women exposed in the first trimester of pregnancy (EFV package insert). EFV now has a class D pregnancy rating. Safety in the second and third trimesters is not established. EFV exposures should be reported to the Pregnancy Registry (contact information on next page). **NVP** appears safe when given at delivery (*J Acquir Immune Defic Syndr* 1999;354:795) but shows high rates of hepatotoxicity, including fatal hepatic necrosis and death when given to pregnant women with a CD4 count >250/mm³ (see Nevirapine, p. 240). **TDF** given in high doses to gravid monkeys caused a reduction in body length and reduction in insulin-like growth factor (*J Acquir Immune Defic Syndr* 2002;29:207). Implications for humans are unclear. **Hydroxyurea** is unsafe in pregnancy and carries a class D FDA rating. A report from France suggested mitochondrial toxicity with neurologic sequelae in 8 of 1754 infants exposed to **AZT** alone or AZT/3TC *in utero* (*Lancet* 1999;354:1084). Evaluation of over 16,000 infants exposed to AZT *in utero* has not confirmed the report and showed no evidence of immunologic, cardiac, oncogenic, or neurologic consequences (*N Engl J Med* 2000;3:805). The conclusion is that AZT exposure *in utero* causes mitochondrial toxicity in ≤0.3% (*N Engl J Med* 2002;346:1879). Rodent studies show an increase in vaginal tumors but only at 30 times the size-adjusted dose in humans (*J Nat Cancer Inst* 1997;89:1602). There are no supporting data in humans (*J Acquir Immune Defic Syndr* 1999;20:43). Liquid **APV** contains large quantities of propylene glycol and should be avoided in pregnancy.

THE ANTIRETROVIRAL PREGNANCY REGISTRY [Antiretroviral Pregnancy Registry, Research Park, 1011 Ashes Drive, Wilmington, NC 28405; toll-free (from US and Canada (800) 258-4263, fax (800) 800-1052; from other countries (910) 256-0238; Web www.apregistry.com]: The purpose of the registry is to detect major teratogenic effects of antiretroviral agents. The summary from January 1, 1989 to July 31, 2004 showed 110 outcomes with birth defects among 4391 live births

Antiretroviral Therapy

4

(2.5/100). This prevalence is not significantly different from the CDC population-base birth defects surveillance system, which reported 3.1/100 live births. First trimester exposures compared to second- and third-trimester exposures showed no significant difference (3.1/100 vs. 2.2/100 live births). The largest experience is with AZT (2.8%) and 3TC (3.0%). The sample size was large enough to have detected a twofold increase in birth defects, but none was noted (www.apregistry.com, accessed June 5, 2005).

PHARMACOLOGY: All NRTIs and NVP cross the placenta; PIs cross poorly (*AIDS* 2002;16:889). Passage of antiretrovirals into breast milk is assumed; it is established for AZT, 3TC, and NVP. NFV shows good pharmacokinetics with 1250 mg bid. SQV/RTV also shows good pharmacokinetic results in pregnancy (*HIV Clin Trials* 2001;2:460). These studies were done with *Fortovase* in the regimen of 800/100 mg bid. It assumed that *Invirase* will be similar, but this is not established. Other PIs either show low serum levels during pregnancy (IDV, LPV, RTV) or have not been adequately studied (ATV, APV, FPV) (*AIDS* 2003;17:1195; *N Engl J Med* 2002;346:1879).

RESISTANCE TESTING: The frequency of AZT resistance in pregnant women who participated in the 076 trial was about 10% in both those who received AZT and those in the placebo group (*J Acquir Immune Defic Syndr* 2003;32:170). When transmission occurred it was usually wild-type virus rather than resistant strains. Single-dose NVP has been associated with high rates of NNRTI resistance mutations, especially K103N, as discussed above at p. 117. The prevalence of resistance to antiretrovirals in treatment-naïve patients is relatively low at 10-20% for any resistance mutation in treatment-naïve patients (*J Infect Dis* 2004;189:2174). The International AIDS Society-USA and Euro Guidelines Group for HIV Resistance recommend routine resistance testing for all pregnant women (*JAMA* 2000;283:2417; *AIDS* 2001;15:309). The DHHS HIV Guidelines Panel (June 23, 2004) and DH Watts (*N Engl J Med* 2002;346:1879) recommend testing only for the same indications used for non-pregnant patients.

- **Regimen discontinuation:** Discontinuation of EFV- or NPV-based HAART is complicated by the long half-lives of these drugs, giving a prolonged period of monotherapy with the risk of resistance if all drugs are stopped together; see p. 82.

ISSUES FOR DEVELOPING COUNTRIES (*Lancet* 2002;359:992): The rate of perinatal transmission without intervention is 19% to 36% (*AIDS* 2001;15:379). The prevalence of HIV in pregnant women in some locations is as high as 25%. Antiretroviral drugs, including AZT, AZT + 3TC and NVP ± AZT/3TC, have established merit in preventing perinatal transmission and are cost-effective (*Br Med J* 1999;318:1650). These regimens include short course AZT, short-course AZT + 3TC, single-dose nevirapine regimens and combinations of NPV with AZT ± 3TC (*JAMA* 1999;281:151; *N Engl J Med* 1999;340:1042; *Lancet* 1999;354:795; *N Engl J Med* 2000;343:982). Nevertheless, there is concern about these regimens. For AZT, resistance requires 4 to 6 months, and AZT-resistant strains are infrequently transmitted (*Clin Infect Dis* 1995;20:1321; *J Infect Dis* 2001;183:1688; *AIDS* 1998;12:2281). By contrast, 3TC and NVP may develop high-level resistance rapidly and with a single mutation. In trials of single-dose NVP, 15% to 24% had NVP-resistant virus at 6 weeks postpartum that was no longer detected at 12 months (*J Infect Dis* 2002;186:181; *AIDS* 2001;15:1951). The obvious concern is the archiving of resistant strains that could cause limitations to subsequent HAART response both in individual patients and on a population basis (*J Acquir Immune Defic Syndr* 2003;34:308). The high rate of virologic failure in women exposed to NVP during delivery compared to those who did not supports this concern (*N Engl J Med* 2004;351:229). Using a more sensitive method to detect resistance mutations (*Nat Methods* 2004;1:141), the frequency of NVP resistance with single-dose exposure is 60-70% and is higher with clade C than with clades A or B (*J Infect Dis* 2005;192:24).

Adverse Effects of Antiretroviral Agents

GI INTOLERANCE: Nausea and vomiting associated with early pregnancy may complicate drug administration or exacerbate the GI side effects of HAART regimens. Possible solutions are delay in initiation of antiretroviral therapy or temporary suspension of treatment.

HYPERGLYCEMIA: All PIs are associated with insulin resistance, and gestational diabetes is a concern with pregnancy. Some authorities advocate a glucose tolerance test with a 50-gm glucose load in early pregnancy and at 24 to 28 weeks' gestation.

MITOCHONDRIAL TOXICITY: Pregnancy is associated with increased susceptibility to mitochondrial toxicity with lactic acidosis (*N Engl J Med* 1999;340:1723; *Semin Perinatol* 1999;23:100), so caution is advised when using d4T, ddI and, to a lesser extent, AZT with respect to this complication. The combination of ddI/d4T should be avoided if possible; 3 deaths attributed to lactic acidosis in pregnant women who received this combination have been reported by the FDA. This combination may be confused with the acute fatty liver of pregnancy or the HELLP (hemolysis, elevated liver enzymes and low platelets) syndrome of pregnancy.

NEVIRAPINE: This drug has been widely advocated for pregnant women based on extensive experience, but most of this is single-dose treatment to prevent perinatal transmission at delivery. NVP is associated with severe rashes and symptomatic hepatitis including death in at least 6 pregnant women (*J Acquir Immune Defic Syndr* 2004;36:772). Most severe rash reactions and liver toxicity occur in the first 6-18 wks. The risk of symptomatic hepatitis is up to 11% in women who initiate NVP with a CD4 count >250/mm^3, so the drug should be avoided in this group. With lower CD4 counts the drug may be given with careful monitoring in the first 18 wks to detect hypertoxicity (transaminase levels), rash, fever and GI symptoms. Women already receiving NVP should simply continue it.

ACTG 076 Protocol (*MMWR* 2002;51[RR-7]:1)

ANTEPARTUM: AZT 300 mg bid or 200 mg tid from week 14 to delivery*

INTRAPARTUM: AZT IV 2 mg/kg 1st hour, then 1 mg/kg/hour until delivery

POSTPARTUM: AZT syrup, 2 mg/kg q6h (or 1.5 mg/kg q6h IV) x 6 weeks for the infant

---

* Even when AZT resistance or AZT intolerance requires use of alternative drugs, the mother should receive IV AZT intrapartum, and oral AZT should be given to the infant (DHHS Guidelines, April 7, 2005).

SCENARIOS

- **No prior HIV therapy**
  - Standard clinical, immunologic and virologic testing
  - VL >1000 c/mL: HAART including the 3-part AZT regimen of PACTG 076 (usually AZT/3TC + NFV or SQV/r)
  - VL >1000 c/mL: May give HAART or AZT only using the PACTG protocol
  - May delay initiation of therapy to 10-12 weeks gestation

- **HIV-infected women receiving antiretroviral therapy**
  - First trimester: counsel on benefits and risks of antiretroviral therapy. If therapy is stopped in the first trimester, discontinue all drugs simultaneously; note precautions with NNRTIs at p. 82.
  - Include AZT in the regimen according to the PACTG 076 protocol after the first trimester when feasible.

- **Presents postpartum**
  - Infant should receive 6-wk course of AZT per ACTG 076 protocol, starting ASAP.
  - Mother should have standard evaluation for HIV.
  - Infant should have HIV testing.

Regimen	Maternal	Infant
AZT	AZT 2 mg/kg IV 1st hr, then 1 mg/kg IV until delivery	AZT syrup 2 mg/kg q 6 h x 6 wks*
AZT/3TC	AZT: 600 mg po onset labor, then 300 mg q 3h 3TC: 150 mg po onset labor, then 150 mg po q 12 h	AZT – 4 mg/kg q 12 h + 3TC – 2 mg/kg q 12 h x 7 days
NVP/AZT	AZT: 2 mg/kg IV bolus, then 1 mg/kg/hr NVP: 200 mg at onset of labor	AZT – 2 mg/kg po q 6 h x 6 wks + NVP – 2 mg/kg po at 48-72 h (single dose)[†]

* AZT for infants <35 wks gestation: give 1.5 mg/kg IV or 2 mg/kg PO q 12 h, then q 8 h and 2-4 wks

† If NVP <1 h prior to delivery, first infant dose should be given ASAP after birth and second infant dose at 48-72 h.

MONITORING DURING PREGNANCY: CD4 counts, viral load, and resistance tests should be performed according to standards for non-pregnant patients.

Postexposure Prophylaxis (PEP)

Occupational Exposure

RISK OF TRANSMISSION (*MMWR* 2005;54:RR-9)

- A total of 23 studies of needle sticks among health care workers (HCWs) demonstrate HIV transmission in 20 of 6,135 (0.33%) exposed to an HIV-infected source (*Ann Intern Med* 1990;113:740). With mucosal surface exposure, there was one transmission among 1,143 exposures (0.09%), and there were no transmissions among 2,712 skin exposures. As of June 2004, there were a total of 57 HCWs in the United States who had occupationally acquired HIV-infection as indicated by seroconversion in the context of an exposure to an HIV infected source. This group includes six HCWs who received PEP using recommended regimens initiated within 2 h after exposure. There are an additional 136 HCWs who had possible occupationally acquired HIV; these latter HCWs did not have documented seroconversion in the context of an exposure (*N Engl J Med* 2003;348:826). Occupations among 56 confirmed cases: Nurses (23), laboratory technicians (20), and physicians (6). All transmissions involved blood or bloody body fluid except for three involving laboratory workers exposed to HIV viral cultures. Exposures were percutaneous in 48, mucocutaneous in 5, and both in 2 cases.

Antiretroviral Therapy

4

■ TABLE 4-34: **Safety of Antiretroviral Agents in Pregnancy (Adapted from *Guidelines for Use of Antiretroviral Drugs in Pregnant HIV-1 Infected Women for Maternal Health and Interventions to Reduce Perinatal HIV-1 Transmission in the U.S. [MMWR 2002;51(RR-7):1]*)**

Anti-retroviral Drug	FDA Cate-gory*	Placental Passage Newborn:Maternal Drug Ratio	Long-term Animal Carcinogenicity Studies	Rodent Teratogen
AZT	C	Yes (human) [0.85]	Positive (rodent, vaginal tumors)	Positive (near lethal dose)
ddC	C	Yes (rhesus) [0.3-0.50]	Positive (rodent, thymic lymphomas)	Positive (hydrocephalus at high dose)
ddI	B	Yes (human) [0.5]	Negative (no tumors, lifetime rodent study)	Negative
d4T	C	Yes (rhesus) [0.76]	Not completed	Negative (but sternal bone calcium decreases)
3TC	C	Yes (human) [~1.0]	Negative (no tumors, lifetime rodent study)	Negative
FTC	B	Unknown	Not completed	Negative
ABC	C	Yes (rats)	Not completed	Positive (anasarca and skeletal malformations at 1,000 mg/kg, 35 x human exposure, during organogenesis)
TDF	B	Yes (rats and monkeys)	Not completed	Negative
SQV	B	Minimal (human)	Not completed	Negative
IDV	C	Minimal (human)	Not completed	Negative (but extra ribs in rats)
RTV	B	Minimal (human)	Positive (rodent liver adenomas and carcinomas in male mice)	Negative (but cryptorchidism in rats at maternally toxic doses)
NFV	B	Minimal (human)	Not completed	Negative
APV and FPV	C	Unknown	Not completed	Positive (thymic elongation; incomplete ossification of bones; low body weight)
NVP	C	Yes (human) [~1.0]	Not completed	Negative
DLV	C	Unknown	Not completed	Ventricular septal defect
EFV	D	Yes (cynomolgus monkeys, rats, rabbits) [~1.0]	Not completed	Anencephaly; anophthalmia; microphthalmia (cynomolgus monkeys)
LPV/r	C	Unknown	Not completed	Negative (but delayed ossification and increase in skeletal variations in rats at maternally toxic doses)
ATV	B	Unknown	Not completed	Negative

* See p. 136 for pregnancy categories.

Antiretroviral Therapy

To date, there are no confirmed seroconversions in surgeons and no seroconversions with exposures to a suture needle.

- A retrospective case-control study of needle-stick injuries from an HIV-infected source by the CDC included 33 cases who seroconverted and 739 controls (*MMWR* 1996;45:468; *N Engl J Med* 1997;337:1485). The risks for seroconversion included: 1) deep injury; 2) visible blood on the device; 3) needle placement in a vein or artery; and 4) a source with late-stage HIV infection (presumably reflecting high viral load). There was also evidence that AZT prophylaxis was associated with a 79% reduction in transmission rates. Nevertheless, there are at least 21 cases of failures with PEP prophylaxis (*N Engl J Med* 2003;348:826).

■ TABLE 4-35: **Risk of Viral Transmission with Sharps Injury from Infected Source**

Source		Prevalence (U.S.-general population)	Risk/exposure with sharps injury
HIV		0.3%	0.3%
HBV	HBsAg	0.1-0.3%	1-6%*
	HBeAg	0.05-0.1%	22-31%*
HCV		1.8%	1.9%

* Unvaccinated HCW

PEP RECOMMENDATIONS AND CHOICE OF REGIMEN: Recommendations are based on the type of exposure, HIV status of the source, or, if the status is unknown, the risk status of the source.

MANAGEMENT RESOURCES

- National Clinicians' Postexposure Prophylaxis Hotline (HRSA, AETC, CDC) (available at all times): 888-448-4911 or http://www.ucsf.edu/hivcntr/
- Hepatitis hotline: 888-443-7232 or http://www.cdc.gov/hepatitis
- CDC Reporting (occupationally acquired HIV and PEP failure): 800-893-0485
- FDA: Unusual or severe toxicity of antiretrovirals: 800-332-1088 or http://www.fda.gov/medwatch
- HIV/AIDS Treatment Information: http://www.aidsinfo.nih.gov

Antiretroviral Therapy

4

■ TABLE 4-36: **HIV Postexposure Prophylaxis for Percutaneous Injuries**

Exposure	Status of Source		
	Source HIV+ and Low Risk*	Source HIV + and High Risk*	HIV Status of Source is Unknown
Not severe: Solid needle, superficial	2-drug PEP[†]	3-drug PEP[†]	Usually none; consider 2-drug PEP[‡]
Severe: Large bore, deep injury, visible blood in device, needle in patient artery/vein	3-drug PEP[†]	3-drug PEP[†]	Usually none; consider 2-drug PEP[‡]

* Low risk: Asymptomatic HIV or viral load <1,500 c/mL. High risk: Symptomatic HIV, AIDS, acute seroconversion, and/or high viral load.

[†] Concern for drug resistance: Initiate prophylaxis without delay and consult an expert.

[‡] Consider 2-drug PEP if source is high risk for HIV or exposure is from an unknown source with HIV infection likely.

■ TABLE 4-37: **HIV Post Exposure Prophylaxis for Mucous Membranes and Non-intact Skin Exposures***

Exposure	Status of Source		
	HIV+ and Low Risk[†]	HIV + and High Risk[†]	Unknown
Small volume (drops)	Consider 2-drug PEP	2-drug PEP	Usually no PEP; consider 2-drug PEP[‡]
Large volume (major blood splash)	2-drug PEP	3-drug PEP	Usually no PEP; consider 2-drug PEP[‡]

* Non-intact skin: Dermatitis, abrasion, wound

[†] Low risk: Asymptomatic or viral load <1500 c/mL; high risk: Acute seroconversion or high viral load

[‡] Consider if source has HIV risk factors or exposure from unknown source where HIV infected source is likely.

- **Two-drug regimens:** AZT/3TC, AZT/FTC, d4T/3TC, d4T/FTC, TDF/3TC, TDF/FTC

- **Three-drug regimens:** Two NRTIs (above) plus LPV/r; **Alternatives:** SQV/r, ATV/r, ATV, IDV/r, or EFV

- **Drugs not recommended:** NVP, ABC, DLV, ddC

■ TABLE 4-38: **Drugs for PEP**

Agent	Comment
Nucleoside Analogs	
AZT	Only drug with established efficacy; note high rates of GI intolerance, fatigue and headache; monitor CBC
3TC	In most regimens due to good tolerability, potency, and qd dosing; may need to check for 184V/I resistance in source
d4T	Potent; good short-term tolerability; avoid combining with AZT
ABC	Concern for hypersensitivity reaction (reported in 5-9%)
ddI	Concerns are fasting requirement and GI intolerance
TDF	Well tolerated, effective for PEP in primate model, benefit of qd dosing
FTC	Similar to 3TC
Non-nucleoside RTIs	
EFV	Potent, but concern for short-term CNS toxicity in HCW
NVP	Avoid: FDA has reports of 22 PEP recipients with serious reactions to NVP, including 12 hepatotoxicity cases (one requiring a liver transplant) and 14 skin reactions, including 3 with Stevens Johnson syndrome
Protease Inhibitors	
LPV/r	Potent and favored among PIs; note food requirement and probable diarrhea
ATV ± RTV	Potent, well tolerated, qd dosing, boosted well with RTV; note food requirement, risk of jaundice, boosting requirement for TDF, multiple drug interactions
NFV	Well tolerated except for diarrhea that usually responds to Imodium; note fatty food requirements and diarrhea
FPV ± RTV	Potent, reliatively low pill burden, option of once-daily therapy; no food effect
IDV/r	Note need for q 8 h dosing unless boosted with RTV; note need for food, ≥1.5 L fluid/day, risk of nephrolithiasis
SQV/r	Potent, option for once daily therapy
Entry Inhibitors	
ENF	Some theoretical advantage with blocking entry, but no experience in PEP and requirement for injections

4 Antiretroviral Therapy

TESTING IN THE SOURCE PATIENT: If there is no recent positive or negative serology, a rapid test (see p. 10) is preferred. Results should be available in <1 h. Rapid tests are as reliable as standard serology for excluding HIV infection (false negatives in "window" period), and testing is highly cost effective in preventing unnecessary empiric short-term courses of antiretroviral agents (*Infect Control Hosp Epidemiol* 2001;22:289). Standard serologic tests may take 3 to 7 days, but a negative EIA screening assay is usually available in 24 to 48 hours and is adequate for the decision to discontinue PEP if the rapid test is not available. Most states permit testing the source of a health care worker exposure without informed consent. If the source has had an illness compatible with acute HIV syndrome, testing should include plasma HIV RNA levels.

MONITORING AND COUNSELING THE HCW

- **Testing the HCW:** HIV serology should be performed at the time of injury, and repeated at 6 weeks, 3 months, and 6 months. It should be repeated at 12 months in HCW who acquired HCV with the injury, since this may delay HIV seroconversion (*N Engl J Med* 2003;348: 826; *Am J Infect Control* 2003;31:168).

- **Viral load:** VL testing is sometimes done since HIV viremia precedes positive serology. This is not recommended due to high rates of false positives (*J Infect Dis* 2004;190:598). Confine VL testing to patients with a febrile illness consistent with the acute retroviral syndrome.

- **Precautions to prevent sexual transmission:** The HCW should be advised to practice safe sex or abstain until serology is negative at 6 months postexposure. The greatest risk is the first 6 to 12 weeks, and many authorities recommend these precautions only to the 3-month test.

- **Time:** PEP should be initiated as quickly as possible, preferably within 1 to 2 hours of exposure and up to 36 hours postexposure. The median time from exposure to treatment in 432 HCWs with HIV exposure from October 1996 to December 1998 was 1.8 hours (*Infect Control Hosp Epidemiol* 2000;21:780).

- **Side effects:** For HCWs who receive PEP, about 74% experience side effects, primarily nausea (58%), fatigue (37%), headache (16%), vomiting (16%), or diarrhea (14%). About 50% discontinue treatment before completion of the 4-week course due to multiple factors including side effects of drugs (*Infect Control Hosp Epidemiol* 2000;21:780). A similar experience with PEP was reported from France, where ADRs occurred in 85%, most commonly with GI intolerance (*Clin Infect Dis* 2001; 32:1494)

Antiretroviral Therapy

- **Pregnancy:** EFV, TDF, and the combination of ddI + d4T should be avoided in pregnancy. The favored agents for HCWs who are pregnant are summarized on Table 4-31, p. 114. Note that some authorities delay initiating ART in pregnant women with established HIV infection due to concerns about toxicity of these drugs. In each case there needs to be a risk-benefit assessment, preferably by an HIV expert. CDC guidelines state that pregnancy should not preclude ART. Counseling non-pregnant HCWs with childbearing capacity should include a discussion of these risks and the limited data regarding safety of many antiretroviral agents, especially during the first trimester. Drugs with the most extensive data from the Pregnancy Registry to establish safety in pregnancy are AZT, 3TC, and d4T (see p. 114).

- **Breastfeeding:** Consider temporary discontinuation of breastfeeding during antiretroviral therapy.

- **Resistance testing:** Guidance for drug selection based on anticipated resistance mutations may be available from prior resistance tests in the source. This testing may also be done in the source at the time of injury if there is an adequate VL, although the time required for test results mandates rapid institution on the basis of empiricism or anticipated resistance according to prior test results or drug history and virologic response. Most authorities recommend that decisions be based on the drug history and viral load of the source. In a review of 52 patients who were the source of occupational exposures, 39% involved stains with major mutations conferring resistance (*N Engl J Med* 2003;348:826). This is another issue for which assistance from an HIV expert is appropriate.

HEALTH CARE WORKER TO PATIENT TRANSMISSION

- **Health care worker to patient transmission:** This became a topical issue in 1990 with the case of a Florida dentist, who was identified as the source of HIV infection for 6 dental patients (*Ann Intern Med* 1992;116:798; *Ann Intern Med* 1994;121:886). The source of the virus was established by genetic sequencing (*J Virol* 1998;72:4537), but the mechanism of transmission was never established. This disclosure led to a series of "look backs," in which serologic tests were performed on >22,000 patients who received care from 59 health providers with known HIV infection. No transmissions were identified (*Ann Intern Med* 1995;122:653). Since this time, there have been 2 additional cases in France, one traced to a total hip procedure and the other to a C-section (*Ann Intern Med* 1999;130:1). The totals for known transmissions from infected surgeon to patient are 375 for HBV and 7 for HCV as of 2002 (*Hosp Infect Control* 2003;7:88).

Antiretroviral Therapy

4

- **Management of HIV-infected HCW**
  - Concern about the incident with the Florida dentist led to a federal law in 1991 requiring states to establish guidelines for HIV-positive HCWs. Most states adopted CDC recommendations that required persons who perform "exposure-prone invasive procedures" (surgery in a blind body cavity) to: 1) advise the patient of the HCW's serostatus and 2) obtain written informed consent from the patient. This applies to surgeons, nurses, and other members of the operating team.
  - A review by Julie Gerberding, an expert in this topic and Director of the CDC, did not mention these recommendations in her review of management of HIV infected health care workers (*Ann Intern Med* 1999;130:64) but she did emphasize the following: Patients who have exposures analogous to what would be defined as a potentially high-risk occupational exposure from a health care worker should be managed by standard guidelines with respect to counseling, serologic testing, and antiretroviral therapy. Concerns are that such disclosure is illegal and unethical for the HCW regarding patient confidentiality issues, but the reverse is not true; the result may be a truncated career despite a risk that is virtually nonexistent. Few hospitals currently actively endorse these guidelines and many are unaware they exist (*Hosp Infect Control* 2003;7:88).

OCCUPATIONAL EXPOSURE TO HEPATITIS B VIRUS (HBV)

- **Efficiency of transmission:** Highly dependent on vaccine status of HCW and the HBeAg status of the source.

- **HBV postexposure prophylaxis:** Recommendations are based on the vaccine status of the healthcare worker, evidence of serologic response, (anti-HBs levels >10 mIU/mL), and the HBsAg status of the source. Responder status of the HCW is best assessed with serology at 1-6 months after completion of the 3-dose series. Response is age-related; 95% for persons 20 to 30 years of age, 86% at 40 to 50 years of age, and 45% at ≥65 years of age. Titers decrease an average of 10%/year, but prior responders with antibody titers >10 mIU/mL are probably protective. Non-responders have a 55% probability of response to re-vaccination.

- Vaccine efficacy: 80% to 95% when considering all vaccine recipients; 99% for responders.

Antiretroviral Therapy

■ TABLE 4-39: **HBV Postexposure Prophylaxis**

Vaccination Status of HCW	Features of Source	
	HBsAg Positive	**Source Unknown**
Unvaccinated	HBIG* + vaccine series (3 doses)	HBV vaccine (3 doses)
Vaccinated		
Responder[†]	No Rx	No Rx
Non responder	HBIG x 1 + vaccine series or HBIG x 2[‡]	Rx as source positive if high risk
Antibody status unknown	Test for anti-HBs ■ Anti-HBs >10 mIU/mL – no Rx ■ Anti-HBs <10 mIU/mL – HBIG x 1 + vaccine booster	Test for anti-HBs ■ Anti-HBs >10 mIU/mL – no Rx ■ Anti-HBs <10 mIU/mL – HBV vaccine series with titer at 1-2 mo

* HBIG = Hepatitis B immune globulin; dose is 0.06 mL/kg IM. Should be given as soon as possible and within 7 days.

† Responder defined by antibody to HBsAg of >10 mIU/mL.

‡ HBIG + the vaccine series is preferred for non-responders who did not complete the 3 dose series; HBIG x 2 doses is preferred if there were 2 vaccine series and no response.

OCCUPATIONAL EXPOSURE TO HEPATITIS C VIRUS (HCV)

■ Efficiency of transmission: A review of 25 studies published from 1991 to 2002 found that the rate of HCV transmission following a sharps injury from an HCV-infected source was 44/2357 (1.9%) (*Clin Microbiol Rev* 2003;16:546). Cutaneous exposure to contaminated blood with intact skin does not appear to confer risk.

■ **Seroprevalence of HCV (U.S.):** General population, – 1.8%; HCW – 0.5% to 2%; gay men – 2% to 6%; hemophilia patients – 60% to 90%; injection drug users – 60% to 90%.

■ **HCV postexposure management**

  □ Source testing: Anti-HCV; confirm positives with qualitative PCR

  □ HCW: Anti-HCV and ALT at baseline and at 3 to 6 months. Confirm positive serology with qualitative PCR.

  □ HCV RNA may be tested at 4 to 6 weeks to detect acute HCV prior to seroconversion. Persons with documented acute HCV infection should have positive quantitative HCV PCR at 2-4 weeks, usually accompanied by asymptomatic elevation of ALT. This precedes anti-HCV seroconversion.

  □ No prophylaxis with immune globulin (*Clin Infect Dis* 1993;16:335) or with antiviral agents (interferon + ribavirin) is recommended (*Clin Infect Dis* 1993;16:335; *J Infect Dis* 1996;173:822; *Clin Microbiol Rev* 2003;16:546).

Antiretroviral Therapy

4

- **Management of patients with occupationally acquired HCV:**
Postexposure monitoring with HCV PCR will detect early seroconversion. A controversial issue at this juncture is the utility of treatment with peginterferon + ribavarin. One report from Germany showed a high rate of HCV cure with treatment of acute HCV (*N Engl J Med* 2001;345:1452) and others have had a similar experience in 5/6 HCWs with occupationally acquired HIV (*Infection* 2005;33:30). Nevertheless, this tactic has received varying degrees of endorsement (*Infect Control Hosp Epidemiol* 2001;22:53). The major concerns are the drug-associated toxicity for an infection that has a 20% to 40% probability of spontaneous clearance (*Hepatology* 2001;34:341; *Hepatology* 2002;S195; *Hepatology* 2001;34:341; *Hepatology* 2002;36:1020), the relatively benign long-term prognosis in persons without additional risk factors (*Hepatology* 1999;29:908) and the lack of data to show treatment at this stage is superior in any way to standard guidelines for management of chronic infection (*Clin Microbiol Rev* 2003;16:546). Treatment in the acute phase should therefore be considered experimental.

Non-Occupational HIV Exposure (Sexual Contact or Needle Sharing)
RISK OF TRANSMISSION

- TABLE 4-40: **Risk of HIV Transmission with Single Exposure from an HIV-Infected Source**

Exposure	Source	Risk/10,000 exposures
Blood transfusion	Donegan E, *Ann Int Med* 1990;113:733	9,000
Needle sharing IDU	*J Acquir Immun Defic Syndr* 1995;10:175	67
Receptive anal intercourse	*Br Med J* 1992;304:809	50
Needlestick injury	*Am J Med* 1997;102:9	30
Receptive vaginal intercourse	*Br Med J* 1992;304:809 *Sex Transm Dis* 2002;29:38 *Am J Epid* 1998;148:88	10
Insertive anal intercourse	*Br Med J* 1992;304:809 *Sex Transm Dis* 2002;29:38	6-7
Insertive vaginal intercourse	*Br Med J* 1992;304:809 *Sex Transm Dis* 2002;29:38	5

Risk of HIV Transmission in 415 Untreated Discordant Couples (*N Engl J Med* 2000;342:921)

Viral Load	Transmissions/100 Person-years
<400 c/mL	0
400-3,500 c/mL	4.8
3,500-50,000 c/mL	14.0
>50,000 c/mL	23.0

- **Follow-up:** A more recent report indicated the risk was greatest with acute HIV infection when the VL was highest (0.008/coital act in 5 months after conversion compared to 0.0007/coital act in 8 year with chronic infection; *J Infect Dis* 2005;191:1403).

CDC RECOMMENDATIONS (*MMWR* 2004;54[RR-2:1])

Recommendations are based to a large extent on probability of HIV infection in the source, the ability to deliver PEP within 72 hours of exposure and the type of exposure. The recommendations are summarized in the following table.

■ TABLE 4-42: **CDC Recommendations for HIV Prophylaxis After Non-occupational Exposure (nPEP)**

nPEP is recommended if there is substantial risk of exposure within 72 hours and: 1. Eposure of vagina, rectum, eye, mouth, other mucosal surface, nonintact skin or subcutaneous **and** 2. Exposure with: Blood, semen, vaginal secretions, rectal secretions, breast milk, bloody fluid **and** 3. From: Source likely to be infected **and** 4. Time from exposure: <72 hours
nPEP is not recommended if there is: 1. Delay >72 hours from time of exposure **or** 2. Negligible risk based on exposure with: urine, nasal secretions, saliva, sweat or tears if not visibly contaminated with blood (regardless of HIV status of source)
nPEP recommended on case-by-case basis if: 1. Substantial risk exposure (defined above) 2. Within 72 hours of exposure **and** 3. Source patient HIV status unknown
Recommended regimens: The recommendations follow the 10/29/04 recommendations of DHHS guidelines for the initial treatment of HIV infection with the exception that nevirapine has been removed from the list
Preferred regimens ■ EFV* + (3TC or FTC) + (AZT or TDF) ■ LPV/r + (3TC or FTC) + AZT

(continued)

4 Antiretroviral Therapy

■ TABLE 4-42: **CDC Recommendations for HIV Prophylaxis After Non-occupational Exposure (nPEP) (*Continued*)**

Alternative regimens
■ EFV* + (3TC or FTC) + (ABC, ddI, or d4T)
■ ATV + (3TC or FTC) + (AZT d4T, ABC, or ddI) or (RTV 100 mg/d + TDF)
■ FPV + (3TC or FTC) + (AZT or d4T) or (ABC, TDF, or ddI)
■ FPV/r + (3TC or FTC) + (AZT d4T, ABC,TDF, or ddI)
■ IDV/r + (3TC or FTC) + (AZT d4T, ABC,TDF, or ddI)
■ LPV/r + (3TC or FTC) + (d4T, ABC, TDF, or ddI)
■ NFV + (3TC or FTC) + (AZT or d4T, ABC, TDF, or ddI)
■ SQV/r + (INV or TFV) + (3TC or FTC) + (AZT, d4T, ABC, TDF, or ddI)
■ ABC + AZT + 3TC (*Trivizir*)

──────

*Avoid in pregnancy

■ TABLE 4-43: **Recommended Tests on Exposed Person and Source**

Exposed Person	Baseline	During PEP	4-6 wks	3 mo	6 mo
HIV serology	+		+	+	+
CBC/LFT/BUN or creatinine	+	+			
STD (GC, CT, syphilis)	+	+*	+*	−	−
HBV	+	−	+*	+*	−
HCV	+	−	−	+	+
Pregnancy	+	+*	+*		
If HIV seroconversion					
HIV viral load			+	+	+
Resistance test			+	+	+
CD4 count			+	+	+

* As clinically indicated

Source: tests at baseline: HIV serology, STD screen (GC, *C. trachomatis*, and syphilis), HBVsAg, HCV Ab

Antiretroviral Therapy

5 | Drug Information

DRUG PROFILES are listed alphabetically by generic drug names.

TRADE NAME and pharmaceutical company source are provided unless there are multiple providers. Trade names are for United States brands.

COST is based on average wholesale price (AWP) according to Price Alert, First DataBank, San Bruno, California, January 2004. Prices are generally given for generic products when generics are available.

PHARMACOLOGY, SIDE EFFECTS, AND DRUG INTERACTIONS: Data are from Drug Information 2004, American Hospital Formulary Service, Bethesda, MD; *PDR* 2004.

CREATININE CLEARANCE

- **Males:** $\dfrac{\text{Weight (kg)} \times (140 - \text{age})}{72 \times \text{serum creatinine (mg/dL)}}$

- **Females:** Determination for males x 0.85

- **Obese patients:** Use lean body weight.

- **Formula assumes stable renal function.** Assume creatinine clearance (CrCl) of 5-8 mL/min for patients with anuria or oliguria.

- **Pregnancy and volume expansion:** GFR may be increased in third trimester of pregnancy and with massive parenteral fluids.

PATIENT ASSISTANCE PROGRAMS: Most pharmaceutical companies that provide this service require all of the following:

- Income eligibility criteria such as an annual income <$12,000 for an individual or <$15,000 for a family.

- Non-availability of prescription drug payment from public or private third party sources.

- A prescription and a letter of verification.

Note: Most will provide a 3-month supply subject to re-review after that time (see http://www.needymeds.com).

CLASSIFICATION FOR DRUG USE IN PREGNANCY BASED ON FDA CATEGORIES: Ratings range from "A" for drugs that have been tested for teratogenicity under controlled conditions without showing evidence of damage to the fetus to "D" and "X" for drugs that are definitely teratogenic. The "D" rating is generally reserved for drugs with no safer alternatives. The "X" rating means there is absolutely no reason to risk using the drug in pregnancy.

Category	Interpretation
A	**Controlled studies show no risk.** Adequate, well-controlled studies in pregnant women have failed to demonstrate risk to the fetus.
B	**No evidence of risk in humans.** Either animal findings show risk, but human findings do not, or, if no adequate human studies have been performed, animal findings are negative.
C	**Risk cannot be ruled out.** Human studies are lacking, and animal studies are either positive for fetal risk, or lacking as well. However, potential benefits may justify the potential risk.
D	**Positive evidence of risk.** Investigational or postmarketing data show risk to the fetus. Nevertheless, potential benefits may outweigh the potential risk.
X	**Contraindicated in pregnancy.** Studies in animals or humans, or investigational or postmarketing reports, have shown fetal risk that clearly outweighs any possible benefit to the patient.

PREGNANCY REGISTRY FOR ANTIRETROVIRAL DRUGS: This is a joint project sponsored by staff from pharmaceutical companies with an advisory panel with representatives from the CDC, NIH obstetrical practitioners, and pediatricians. The registry allows anonymity of patients and birth outcome follow-up is obtained by registry staff. Healthcare professionals should report prenatal exposures to antiretroviral agents to: Antiretroviral Pregnancy Registry, 155 N. Third Street, Suite 306, Wilmington, NC 28401; 800-258-4263; fax 800-800-1052 (www.apregistry.com).

CLASSIFICATION OF CONTROLLED SUBSTANCES

Category	Interpretation
I	**High potential for abuse and no current accepted medical use.** Examples are heroin and LSD.
II	**High potential for abuse.** Use may lead to severe physical or psychological dependence. Examples are opioids, amphetamines, short-acting barbiturates, and preparations containing codeine. Prescriptions must be written in ink or typewritten and signed by the practitioner. Verbal prescriptions must be confirmed in writing within 72 hours and may be given only in a genuine emergency. No renewals are permitted.
III	**Some potential for abuse.** Use may lead to low-to-moderate physical dependence or high psychological dependence. Examples are barbiturates and preparations containing small quantities of codeine. Prescriptions may be oral or written. Up to five renewals are permitted within 6 months.
IV	**Low potential for abuse.** Examples include chloral hydrate, phenobarbital, and benzodiazepines. Use may lead to limited physical or psychological dependence. Prescriptions may be oral or written. Up to five renewals are permitted within 6 months.
V	**Subject to state and local regulation.** Abuse potential is low; a prescription may not be required. Examples are antitussive and antidiarrheal medications containing limited quantities of opioids.

ABACAVIR (ABC)

TRADE NAME: *Ziagen* (GlaxoSmithKline)

CLASS: Nucleoside analog

FORMULATIONS, REGIMEN AND PRICE

- **ABC**
  - □ Formulations: 300 mg tab
  - □ Regimen: 300 mg bid or 600 mg qd
  - □ AWP: $400/month
- ***Trivizir:*** AZT/ABC/3TC (300/300/150 mg tab)
  - □ Regimen: 1 bid
  - □ AWP: $1,020/month
- ***Epzicom:*** ABC/3TC (600/300 mg tab)
  - □ Regimen: 1 qd
  - □ AWP: $760/month

FOOD: Take without regard for meals

RENAL FAILURE: ABC – no dose adjustment; *Trizivir* and *Epzicom* – not recommended with CrCl <50 mL/min; use separate component with dose adjustment

HEPATIC FAILURE: Standard dose for ABC, *Trizivir* and *Epzicom*

ADVANTAGES: Well tolerated, potent antiviral activity, once-daily therapy, no food effect

DISADVANTAGES: Hypersensitivity reaction in 5%-8%% of patients

CLINICAL TRIALS: With monotherapy, ABC reduced viral load 1.5-2.0 logs – significantly more than AZT, ddI, d4T; not more than TDF, 3TC, FTC.

5 Drugs: Abacavir

■ TABLE 5-1: **Clinical Trials of ABC in Initial Therapy**

Study	Regimen	N	Dur (wks)	VL <50	VL <400
CNA 3014 *Curr Med Res Opin* 2004;20:1103	AZT/3TC/ABC	164	48	60*	66%*
	AZT/3TC/IDV	165		50*	50%
CNA 3005 *JAMA* 2001;285:1155	AZT/3TC/ABC	262	48	31%	51%
	AZT/3TC/IDV	265		45%*	51%
ABCDE 12th CROI, #587	AZT/3TC/EFV	237	96	61%*	
	d4T/3TC/EFV			48%	
ACTG 5095 *N Engl J Med* 2004;350:1850	AZT/3TC/ABC	382	48	61%*	74%†
	AZT/3TC/EFV±ABC	765		83%	89%†
CNA 30024 *Clin Infect Dis* 2004;39:1038	ABC/3TC/EFV	324	48	70%	
	AZT/3TC/EFV	325		69%	
CNA 30021 (ZODIAC) *J Acquir Immun Defic Syndr* 2005;38:417	ABC (qd)/3TC/EFV	384	48	66%	—
	ABC (bid)/3TC/EFV	386		68%	—
EES 30009 3rd IAS, #WePe12.2C23	ABC/TDF/3TC	102	12**		51%**
	ABC/3TC/EFV	169	48	71%	75%*
EES 30008 12th CROI, #572	ABC/3TC (qd) + 3rd agent	130	48	82%	
	ABC/3TC (bid) + 3rd agent	130		81%	

* Superior to comparitor (*P*<0.05)
** Study terminated due to high failure rate
† VL <200 c.mL

SWITCH STUDIES

- **The RAVE Study:** Patients with lipoatrophy attributed to AZT or d4T were switched to TDF or ABC; results with 105 patients at 48 weeks showed significant and comparable increases in limb fat with continued viral suppression (12th CROI, Boston, Feb. 2005 Abstr. 44).

- **EES 40003:** 104 patients on PI-based HAART complicated by hyperlipidemia were switched to ABC (*n* = 52) or continued PI-based HAART (*n* = 52). Analysis at 28 weeks showed improved cholesterol levels in the ABC group and no changes in viral suppression, insulin resistance or waist-hip ratio (*BMC Infect Dis* 2005;5:2).

Comparison of AZT/3TC vs. ABC/3TC

- **CNA 30024** compared these two regimens, each with EFV, in 699 treatment-naïve patients. At 48 weeks VL was <50 c/mL in 69% and 70%, respectively, by ITT analysis (*Clin Infect Dis* 2004;39:1038). ABC/3TC was associated with less anemia, nausea, and vomiting, but more hypersensitivity, than AZT/3TC. This paved the way to coformulation with *Epzicom*.

Drugs: Abacavir

Comparison of ABC/3TC qd vs. bid

- **ESS 30008** compared twice-daily vs. once-daily regimens in patients with viral suppression with ABC/3TC twice-daily, combined with a PI or NNRTI. Viral suppression was sustained at 48 weeks in 81% in the once-daily ABC/3TC group vs. 82% in the twice-daily group. Toxicity and CD4 responses were similar, and there were no ABC hypersensitivity reactions. Adherence was better in the once-daily group. (12th CROI, Boston, Feb. 2005, Abstr. 572).

- **Summary:** ABC is a potent NRTI. The ATC/3TC/ABC (*Trizivir*) regimen was previously used as a preferred regimen throughout much of the world. However, ACTG 5095 demonstrated the superiority of EFV-based HAART compared to *Trizivir*. The study was stopped prematurely by the data safety and monitoring board, and *Trizivir*, along with all other "triple nucleoside" regimens, was rapidly deleted from all guidelines in the world. Nevertheless, *Trizivir* has the advantages of preserving NNRTI and PI treatment options, convenient dosing regimen and potency that is comparable to at least some of the currently recommended HAART regimens. It is clearly superior to all other triple nucleoside regimens and may be particularly useful in selected patients, including some with active tuberculosis or pregnancy. Disadvantages include the potential for the ABC hypersensitivity reaction, reduced potency, twice-daily dosing, the potential for broad NRTI cross-resistance with persistent failure, and AZT-associated side effects including anemia and mitochondral toxicity. ABC does not appear to be effective as a component of salvage therapy in patients with extensive NRTI experience. The combination of ABC and 3TC as a dual NRTI component of HAART is attractive due to convenience (1 pill daily) good tolerability, low potential for mitochondrial toxicity, and no thymidine analog mutations after failure; the disadvantages are the ABC hypersensitivity reaction, including the potential for confusion between this reaction and NNRTI hypersensitivity, as well as the potential for development of the K65R or L74V mutation, with resulting cross-resistance to ddl and TDF in the case of K65R.

RESISTANCE: ABC selects primarily for 74V, and to a lesser extent K65R (ICAAC 2003; Chicago abstr H-1722b). The 184V mutation leads to complete cross-resistance to 3TC, but by itself does not significantly decrease ABC susceptibility unless there are TAMs. Mutations at RT codons 65R and 74V lead to cross-resistance to ddl and ddC, and K65R leads to variable loss of susceptibility to TDF, especially when not accompanied by M184V. Each of these mutations results in a 2- to 4-fold decrease in susceptibility to ABC. Significant resistance requires multiple mutations, usually in addition to the 184V mutation. Clinical trials indicate that the presence of the 184V mutation plus at least three thymidine analog mutations (TAMs) predicts ABC failure (*Antivirol Ther* 2004;9:37). In combination with TDF there is selection for 65R

Drugs: Abacavir

5

(*Antimicrob Agents Chemother* 2004;48:1413). TAMs that accumulate via the 41/210/215 pathway cause higher-level ABC resistance than those in the 67/70/219 pathway.

PHARMACOLOGY

- **Bioavailability:** 83%; alcohol increases ABC levels by 41% (clinical significance unknown).

- **T½:** 1.5 hours (serum); intracellular T½ : >12 hours. The active metabolite, carbovir triphosphate, has an intracellular half-life of >20 hours (ICAAC 2003; Chicago, Abstr. A-1797). CSF levels: 27% to 33% of serum levels.

- **Elimination:** 81% metabolized by alcohol dehydrogenase and glucuronyl transferase with renal excretion of metabolites; 16% recovered in stool, and 1% unchanged in urine. Metabolism does not involve the cytochrome P450 pathway. Plasma clearance correlates with body weight, suggesting the possibility of suboptimal levels in patients with greater body weight (*Br J Clin Pharmacol* 2005;59:183).

- **Dose modification in renal failure:** None (*Nephron* 2000;87:186)

SIDE EFFECTS

- **Hypersensitivity reaction (Black box FDA warning):** In an analysis of 30,595 participants in clinical trials and expanded access programs, 1302 (4.2%) had definite or probable hypersensitivity reactions, and 19 were lethal, for a mortality rate of 0.03% (3/10,000) (*Clin Ther* 2001;23:1603). Of the 19 deaths, 6 occurred with re-challenge. The median time of onset is a 9 days; 90% occur in the first 6 weeks. Clinical features include fever (usually 39°C to 40°C), skin rash (maculopapular or urticarial), fatigue, malaise, GI symptoms (nausea, vomiting, diarrhea, abdominal pain), arthralgias, cough, and/or dyspnea. The rash occurs in 70% (*Clin Infect Dis* 2002;34:1137). Laboratory changes may include increased CPK, elevated liver function tests, and lymphopenia. Nearly all true hypersensitivity reactions have symptoms involving ≥2 organs (12th CROI, Boston, Feb. 2005, Abstr. 836). A more recent FDA review of 2670 ABC recipients in clinical trials indicated an incidence of 8% for investigator-defined H5R (12th CROI, Boston, Feb. 2005, Abstr. 835); none was fatal.

Susceptibility to this reaction appears to be genetic and has been associated with the HLA-DR7 and HLA-DQ3 haplotypes. This 57-1 ancestral haplotype was found in 78% of Caucasians from western Australia with typical ABC hypersensitivity reactions and 3% of controls in one report (*Lancet* 2002;359:727). Subsequent studies showed a susceptibility locus within the 57.1 haplotype that was present in 94% of patients with ABC hypersensitivity vs 1.7% controls (OR 960; *P* <0.00001). Patients with hypersensitivity show increased TNF expression by monocytes with ABC exposure *ex vivo* (*PNAS* 2004;101:4180). HLA typing is available in many laboratories

Drugs: Abacavir

at a cost of $500-$800, but there is concern about the generalizability of the Australian data, and the fact that negative results do not eliminate the risk (*Lancet* 2002;359:722). Re-challenge results in a reaction within hours and may resemble anaphylaxis in 20% with hypotension, bronchoconstriction, and/or renal failure (*AIDS* 1999:13:999). Treatment is supportive with IV fluids, ventilator support, dialysis, etc. Steroids and antihistamines are not effective. Re-challenge has been associated with death, but this is rare. Hypersensitivity reactions should be reported to the Abacavir Hypersensitivity Registry at 800-270-0425. For more information call 800-334-0089.

Patients should be warned to consult their provider immediately if they note fever plus skin rash, typical GI symptoms, cough, dyspnea, or constitutional symptoms, especially during the first month of therapy. A warning sheet is usually provided to the patient by pharmacists. An obvious concern is that common intercurrent illnesses, especially during flu season, or other drug reactions may be erroneously attributed to this reaction, preventing the subsequent use of the drug. A possible solution in unclear cases is administration under observation, because patients experiencing true ABC hypersensitivity will experience worsening symptoms with each dose.

- **Other side effects** include nausea, vomiting, malaise, headache, diarrhea, or anorexia.
- **Lactic acidosis**. Patients taking ABC can presumably develop lactic acidosis with or without hepatic steatosis, although this is rare and may not occur with ABC at all.

DRUG INTERACTIONS: Alcohol increases ABC levels by 41%; ABC has no effect on alcohol levels (*Antimicrob Agents Chemother* 2000;283:1811). ABC AUC ↓40% with TPV/r co-administration; clinical significance unknown.

PREGNANCY: Category C. Rodent teratogen test showed skeletal malformations and anasarca at 35x the comparable human dose. Placental passage positive in rats. There are no studies of ABC in pregnant women. It is considered an alternative NRTI in the DHHS Guidelines (Apr. 7, 2005) for antiretroviral drugs in pregnant women.

ACYCLOVIR (also includes famciclovir and valacyclovir)

TRADE NAME: *Zovirax, Valtrex* (valacyclovir) (GlaxoSmithKline), *Famvir* (famciclovir) (Novartis), or generic

FORMS AND PRICES

- **Acyclovir:** Caps: 200 mg at $1.12. Tabs: 400 mg at $2.16, 800 mg at $4.21. Suspension: 200 mg/5 cc at $118/480 mL. IV vials: 1 gm at $35.00. 5% ointment: 15 g at $78.01 (utility limited)

- **Famciclovir (*Famvir*):** Tabs: 125, 250, 500 mg; 250 mg at $4.37; 500 mg at $8.80

- **Valacyclovir:** Tabs: 500 mg at $4.90, 1000 mg at $8.62

CLASS: Synthetic nucleoside analogs derived from guanine

PATIENT ASSISTANCE PROGRAM: 800-722-9294 (acyclovir and valacyclovir)

INDICATIONS AND DOSES: For oral therapy, valacyclovir and famciclovir are generally preferred for the immunosuppressed host (*Lancet* 2001;353:1513). Acyclovir is also available in an IV formulation in this class. The following acyclovir doses are based on recommendations primarily for immunocompetent patients (*N Engl J Med* 1999;340:1255; *N Engl J Med* 2002;347:340; *Lancet* 2001;357:1513; *MMWR* 2002;51[RR-6]:14; *Lancet* 2001;357:1513). For doses of valacyclovir and famciclovir, see Table 5-2, p. 143.

- **HSV and HIV:** HSV genital infection increases the risk of both HIV transmission and HIV acquisition, presumably because of the risk associated with genital ulcer disease. Also, whether symptomatic or asymptomatic, these ulcers are associated with high concentrations of activated CD4 cells, which represent the target of HIV (*J Clin Invest* 1985;75:226; *J Infect Dis* 1994;169:956). This observation presumably explains the significant reduction in risk of HIV seroconversion in discordant partners receiving HSV suppressive therapy (*J Infect Dis* 2003;187:19) and the 4-fold increase in risk of HIV associated with recent HSV seroconversion (*J Infect Dis* 2003;187:1513). Another observation concerns the possible impact of HSV co-infection on the rate of HIV progression. HSV suppression with acyclovir is associated with a significant reduction in HIV VL (*J Infect Dis* 2002;186:1718), possibly due to HSV suppression.

- **HSV herpes labialis:** See Table 5-1. *Medical Letter* preference is valacyclovir (*Med Letter* 2002;44:95). Topical penciclovir cream is an alternative to acyclovir in mild cases but requires q2h application (*Arch Dermatol* 2001;37:1153). Patients with severe disease and/or advanced HIV should be treated according to guidelines for genital and progressive mucocutaneous HSV.

- **HSV genital and perirectal** (see Table 5-2, p. 143):
  - Progressive mucocutaneous: Acyclovir, 5-10 mg/kg IV q8h x 7 to 14 days
  - Prophylaxis: Standard doses for immunocompetent hosts are summarized in Table 5-2; doubling the dose may be required for AIDS patients. Prophylaxis is contraindicated in pregnancy.
  - Acyclovir-resistant: May try high-dose acyclovir (800 mg PO 5x/day or 10 mg/kg IV q8h) or valacyclovir (2-3g/day PO); more predictable is foscarnet, 40 mg/kg IV q8h and cidofovir systemic or topical (*J Infect Dis* 1997;176:892). Probability of failure with acyclovir-resistant strains using standard dose of acyclovir is 95% (*Antimicrob Agents Chemother* 1994;38:1246).

Drugs: Acyclovir

142

- Encephalitis: 10-15 mg/kg IV q8h x 14 to 21 days.
- **VZV treatment:** Should be started within 4 days or while new lesions are still forming (*N Engl J Med* 2002;347:340).
  - Primary (chickenpox): Acyclovir, 800 mg PO 5x/day x 7 to 10 days
  - Dermatomal zoster (shingles): Famciclovir or valacyclovir are preferred for oral therapy due to easier adherence, better efficacy, or improved drug levels (see Table 5-1, p. 138).
  - Disseminated zoster: 10 mg/kg IV q8h x 7 days; with pneumonia, consider corticosteroids (*Int J Infect Dis* 2002;6:6; *J Chemother* 2002;14:220). Treatment should be started as long as new lesions are forming (*Med Letter* 2002;44:95). Rare strains are acyclovir-resistant and should be treated with foscarnet 60 mg/kg IV 2-3x/day (*N Engl J Med* 1993;308:1448).
  - Note: Varicella vaccine is a live virus vaccine and is contra-indicated in persons with HIV.

- TABLE 5-2: **Comparison of Drugs for Infections Caused by Herpes Simplex and Varicella Zoster** (see *N Engl J Med* 1999;340:1255; *Lancet* 2001;357:1513; *MMWR* 2002;51[RR-2]; *N Eng J Med* 2002;347:340)

Herpes simplex
Orolabial or genital initial or recurrent
■ Acyclovir 400 mg po tid x 7d ■ Famciclovir 500 mg po bid x 7d ■ Valacyclovir 1 gm po bid x 7d
Moderate to severe mucocutaneous
■ Acyclovir 5 mg/kg q 8h IV until lesions begin to regress, then oral agent until lesions are completely healed with daily regimens noted above.
Acyclovir-resistant HSV
■ Foscarnet 120-200 mg/kg/d in 2-3 doses until responding ■ Cidofovir 5 mg/kg qo wk ■ Alternatives – topical trifluridine or cidofovir
Encephalitis
■ Acyclovir 10 mg/kg q 8h x 14-21 d
Varicella-zoster
Chickenpox
■ Acyclovir 10 mg/kg IV q 8h x 7-10 days; may switch to oral agent when afebrile if no visceral involvement ■ Acyclovir 800 mg qid or famciclovir 500 mg tid or valacyclovir 1 gm tid
Dermatomal zoster
■ Famciclovir 500 mg po tid x 7-10 d ■ Valacyclovir 1 gm po tid x 7-10 d
Extensive cutaneous or viscera involved
■ Acyclovir 10 mg/kg IV q 8h until lesions resolved
Retinal necrosis
■ Acyclovir 10 mg/kg IV q 8h + foscarnet 60 mg/kg IV q 8h

5 Drugs: Acyclovir

- **EBV, Oral hairy leukoplakia:** Indications to treat are unclear, but treatment is requested by some patients, usually for cosmetic reasons. One study of 18 patients given valacyclovir 1 gm q 8h x 28 days showed clinical response in 16 (89%) and virologic response in 16 (89%). Recurrence after 1 month off treatment occurred in 2 of 12 patients (18%) (*J Infect Dis* 2003;188:883).

■ TABLE 5-3: **Activity of Antivirals Against Herpesviruses**

	HSV	VZV	EBV	CMV	HHV 6-8
Acyclovir	++	+	+	—	—
Famciclovir	++	+	+	—	—
Valacyclovir	++	+	+	—	—
Ganciclovir	++	+	++	++	+
Foscarnet	+	+	++	+	+
Cidofovir	+	+	++	+	++

PHARMACOLOGY

- **Bioavailability:** 15% to 20% with oral administration
- **T½:** 2.5 to 3.3 hours, CSF levels: 50% serum levels
- **Elimination:** Renal

■ TABLE 5-4: **Acyclovir Dose Modification in Renal Failure**

Usual Dose	Creatinine Clearance	Adjusted Dose
200 mg 5x/day	>10 mL/min	200 mg 5x/day
	≤10 mL/min	200 mg q12h
800 mg 5x/day	10-50 mL/min	800 mg q8h
	<10 mL/min	800 mg q12h
5-10 mg/kg IV q8h	10-50 mL/min	10-20 mg/kg/day
	<10 mL/min	5 mg/kg q24h

- **Famciclovir:** CrCl 40-59 = 500 q12h; 20-39 = 500 q24h; <20 = 250 mg q24h (soon after HD on HD days)
- **Valacyclovir:** CrCl 30-49 = 1 gm q12h; 10-29 = 1 gm q24h; <10 = 500 mg q24h (post-HD on HD days)

SIDE EFFECTS ACYCLOVIR/VALACYCLOVIR (infrequent)

- **IV Acyclovir:** Irritation and phlebitis at infusion site, rash, nausea and vomiting, diarrhea, renal toxicity and crystalluria (especially with rapid IV infusion, prior renal disease, and concurrent nephrotoxic drugs), dizziness, abnormal liver function tests, itching, and headache
- **High doses especially with renal failure:** CNS toxicity-agitation, confusion, hallucination, seizure, coma
- **Others:** Nausea, vomiting, anemia, neutropenia, thrombocytopenia, and hypotension

DRUG INTERACTIONS

- Increased meperidine and theophylline levels
- Probenecid prolongs half-life of acyclovir. No dose adjustment.

PREGNANCY: Acyclovir, famciclovir, and valacyclovir are category B. Acyclovir is not teratogenic, but has potential to cause chromosomal damage at high doses. The CDC Registry shows no increased incidence of fetal abnormalities among 601 women for whom pregnancy outcome data were available (*MMWR* 1993;42:806). The CDC Registry contact number is 800-258-4263. The CDC recommends use of acyclovir during pregnancy for severe HSV outbreaks and varicella. Use for prophylaxis in pregnancy is being investigated.

ALBENDAZOLE

TRADE NAME: *Albenza* (GlaxoSmithKline)

FORM AND PRICE: 200 mg tablets at $1.49

INDICATION AND DOSE: Microsporidiosis; 400 mg PO bid until CD4 count >200/mm^3.

CLINICAL TRIALS: Albendazole (400 mg bid until CD4 >200/mm^3) is highly effective with microsporidiosis involving *Encephalitozoon (Septata) intestinalis* (*Parasitol Res* 2003;90 Suppl 1:S14) but is not effective for *Enterocytozoon bieneusi*, which accounts for about 80% of cases of microsporidiosis in AIDS patients. These species can be distinguished by EM or PCR. It is also used for disseminated microsporidiosis and intraocular infection with *E. cuniculi* (*Int J Med Microbiol* 2005;294:529).

Drugs: Albendazole

5

PHARMACOLOGY

- **Bioavailability:** Low (<5%), but absorption is increased 5-fold if taken with a fatty meal vs in a fasting state. Should be taken with fatty meal.
- **T½:** 8 hours
- **Elimination:** Metabolized in liver to albendazole sulfoxide, then excreted by enterohepatic circulation
- **Dose modification in renal failure:** None

SIDE EFFECTS: Adverse reactions are infrequent and include reversible hepatotoxicity, GI intolerance (abdominal pain, diarrhea, nausea, vomiting), reversible hair loss, hypersensitivity reactions (rash, pruritus, fever), reversible neutropenia, and CNS toxicity (dizziness, headache). Some recommend monitoring and liver function tests every 2 weeks. Fatal pancytopenia has been reported (*Am J Trop Med Hyg* 2005;72:291).

PREGNANCY: Category C. Albendazole is teratogenic and embryotoxic in rodents at doses of 30 mg/kg. Not recommended for use in first trimester of pregnancy.

ALPRAZOLAM

TRADE NAME: *Xanax* (Pharmacia) or generic

FORMS AND PRICES (generic): Tabs: 0.25 mg at $0.62, 0.5 mg at $0.74, 1 mg at $0.94, 2 mg at $1.69

CLASS: Benzodiazepine, controlled substance category IV

INDICATIONS AND DOSES

- **Anxiety:** 0.25-0.5 mg tid; increase if necessary at intervals of 3 to 4 days to maximum of 4 mg/day.
- **Dose reduction or withdrawal:** Decrease by ≥0.5 mg every 3 days; some suggest decrease by 0.25 mg at 3- to 7-day intervals.

PHARMACOLOGY

- **Bioavailability:** >90%
- **T½:** 11 hours, prolonged with obesity and hepatic dysfunction
- **Elimination:** Metabolized and renally excreted

SIDE EFFECTS: See Benzodiazepines (Table 5-9, p. 162). Seizures, delirium, and withdrawal symptoms with rapid dose reduction or abrupt discontinuation. Possible amnesia during drug action. Withdrawal symptoms at 18 hours to 3 days after abrupt discontinuation. Seizures usually occur at 24 to 72 hours after abrupt withdrawal.

DRUG INTERACTIONS: Additive CNS depression with other CNS depressants including alcohol. Disulfiram and cimetidine prolong the half-life of alprazolam. Levels of alprazolam are increased by some PIs, but concurrent use is not contraindicated, but should be used with caution.

RELATIVE CONTRAINDICATIONS: History of serious mental illness, drug abuse, alcoholism, open-angle glaucoma, seizure disorder, severe liver disease.

PREGNANCY: Category D. Fetal harm. Contraindicated. Possible role in cleft lip and heart abnormalities.

AMPHOTERICIN B

TRADE NAME: Parenteral form, generic; oral form is no longer available from commercial sources but can be prepared by a pharmacy.

FORMS AND PRICE: 50 mg vials at $20.45/50 mg vial; *Abelcet* $240/100 mg; *Amphotec* $186/100 mg; *AmBisome* $392/100 mg

CLASS: Amphoteric polyene macrolide with activity against nearly all pathogenic and opportunistic fungi.

INDICATION: Sharply reduced general usage in past year due to concerns about nephrotoxicity and availability of alternatives: Voriconazole, caspofungin, and lipid amphotericin formulations. The main indications for IV amphotericin B is for patients who have normal renal function, will receive short courses (≤2 weeks), and have conditions that cannot be easily treated with azoles. Conventional amphotericin B is still the first line therapy for cryptococcal meningitis.

ADMINISTRATION – ORAL: Oral suspension for thrush is no longer available commercially, but it can be prepared by a pharmacist to a strength of 10 mg/mL of amphotericin B. Dose: 1-5 mL qid; swish as long as possible, then swallow.

ADMINISTRATION – IV: Usual dose is 0.3-1.5 mg/kg/day given by slow IV infusion over ≥2-4 hours (*Br Med J* 2000;332:579). Some authorities advocate a test dose (1 mg in 50 mL DSW given over 30 minutes with cardiovascular monitoring for 4 hours as a test for hypersensitivity.

Drugs: Amphotericin B

5

■ TABLE 5-5: **Systemic (Intravenous) Amphotericin B (*Clin Infect Dis* 2000;30:652)**

Condition	Daily Dose	Total Dose	Comment
Aspergillus	1 mg/kg	30-40 mg/kg	■ Voriconazole is preferred for invasive asperillosis (*N Engl J Med* 2003;347:408). ■ Lipid formulations of ampho B are as effective as ampho B 5 mg/kg/day.
Candida Stomatitis Esophagitis Line sepsis Disseminated	0.3 mg/kg 0.3-0.7 mg/kg 0.3-0.5 mg/kg 0.3-0.8 mg/kg	200-500 mg 2 to 3 weeks 200-500 mg 20-40 mg/kg	■ Reserved for refractory cases ■ Fluconazole is preferred for systemic treatment of most *Candida* infections. ■ Voriconazole and caspofungin are preferred for most fluconazole-resistant *Candida* infections (*N Engl J Med* 2002;347:2020; *Clin Infect Dis* 2003;37:415), but cross-resistance is reported with high level azole resistance.
Coccidioidomycosis Non-meningeal diffuse or disseminated	0.5-1.0 mg/kg	Until clinically stable (usually after total dose of 500-1000 mg)	■ Meningeal disease: Fluconazole. ■ Lipid amphotericin B: Experience is limited. ■ Maintenance: With fluconazole or itraconazole.
Cryptococcal meningitis (+5FC)	0.7 mg/kg	2 weeks	■ Maintenance with fluconazole (preferred), itraconazole, or amphotericin B 1 mg/wk (inferior) ■ *AmBisone* 4 mg/kg/day + 5 FC is at least as effective as ampho B with less nephrotoxicity (*AIDS* 1997;11:1463)
Histoplasmosis	0.7 mg/kg	3 to 10 days	■ IV amphotericin until clinical response ■ Alternative is *Ambisome* 3 mg/kg/day. ■ Maintenance with itraconazole or amphotericin B 1 mg/kg weekly. ■ Meningitis: Ampho B or *AmBisone* x 12-16 weeks
Penicilliosis (severely ill)	0.7 mg/kg	2 weeks	■ Maintenance with itraconazole

PHARMACOLOGY

■ **Bioavailability:** Peak serum levels with standard IV doses are 0.5-2 µg/mL. There is no significant absorption with oral administration – serum levels of 0.05 µg/mL with 400-600 mg/day PO; CSF levels – 3% of serum concentrations.

■ **T½:** 24 hours with IV administration, detected in blood and urine up to 4 weeks after discontinuation.

■ **Elimination:** Serum levels in urine; metabolic pathways are unknown.

Drugs: Amphotericin B

- **Dose adjustment in renal failure:** None

SIDE EFFECTS: Oral form: Rash, GI intolerance, and allergic reactions. Toxicity with IV form is dose-related and less severe with slow administration.

- Chills, usually 1 to 3 hours post infusion and lasting for up to 4 hours post infusion. Reduce with hydrocortisone (10-50 mg added to infusion, but only if necessary due to immunosuppression); alternatives that are now often preferred are meperidine, ibuprofen, or napofam prior to infusion.

- Hypotension, nausea, vomiting, usually 1 to 3 hours post infusion; may be reduced with compazine.

- Nephrotoxicity in up to 80% ± nephrocalcinosis, potassium wasting, renal tubular acidosis. Reduce with gradual increase in dose, adequate hydration, avoidance of concurrent nephrotoxic drugs, and possibly sodium loading. Discontinue or reduce dose with BUN >40 mg/dL and creatinine >3 mg/dL. Lipid amphotericin preparations are less nephrotoxic and could be substituted.

- Hypokalemia, hypomagnesemia, and hypocalcemia corrected with supplemental potassium, magnesium, and calcium.

- Normocytic normochromic anemia with average decrease of 9% in hematocrit.

- Phlebitis and pain at infusion sites: add 1200-1600 units of heparin to infusate.

DRUG INTERACTIONS: Increased nephrotoxicity with concurrent use of nephrotoxic drugs – aminoglycosides, cisplatin, cyclosporine, foscarnet, cidofovir, methoxyflurane, vancomycin; increased hypokalemia with corticosteroids and diuretics. Potential for digoxin toxicity secondary to hypokalemia.

PREGNANCY: Category B. Harmless in experimental animal studies, but no data for humans.

Alternative Preparations

Lipid preparations of amphotericin B include:

- *Abelcet* **(ABLC) (Elan Biopharmaceuticals):** Amphotericin B complexed with 2 phospholipids – DMPC and DMPG

- *Amphotec* **(ABCD) (InterMune, Inc.):** Amphotericin B colloidal dispersion with cholesterol sulfate

- *AmBisome* **(LAmB) (Fugisawa/Gilead Sciences):** Liposomal amphotericin B is a true liposomal delivery system

ADVANTAGES: Compared with amphotericin B in D5W, the newer formulations are advocated primarily to reduce nephrotoxicity and infusion-related reactions (*N Engl J Med* 1999;340:764). Other

5 Drugs: Amphotericin B

potential advantages are increased daily dose and high concentrations in reticulo-endothelial tissue (lungs, liver, spleen). Comparative trials vs amphotericin B consistently show that the lipid preparations are therapeutically equivalent and sometimes superior, especially *AmBisome*. The only reason these drugs are not generally preferred over amphotericin B is cost, which is $11/day vs $400-$1300/day (AWP) for standard doses. With many infections the lipid formulations are more cost-effective due to reduced rates of renal failure and dialysis (*Clin Infect Dis* 2001;32:686; *Clin Infect Dis* 2003;37:415). Relative merits are summarized in Table 5-6.

■ TABLE 5-6: **Relative Merits of Amphotericin B Formulations** (*Clin Infect Dis* 2003;37:415; *N Engl J Med* 1999;340:764; *Clin Infect Dis* 2002;35:359)

Preparation	Amphotericin B	Amphotec ABCD	Abelcet (ABLC)	AmBisome (LAmB)
Dose	0.5-1.2 mg/kg/d	3-4 mg/kg/d	5 mg/kg/d	3-5 mg/kg/d
Cmax (ug/mL)	0.5-2	3.1	1.7	83
Usual cost (AWP)	$11/d	$400-$500/d	$800-$850	$950-$1300
Adverse reactions*				
Chills	30%	53%	15-20%	18%
Fever >38⁵⁰C	16%	27%	10-20%	7%
Creatinine >2x base	30-50%	10-25%	15-20%	19%

*Comparison of ADR is based on *AmBisome* vs. Ampho, *Amphotec* vs. Ampho.

AMPRENAVIR (APV)

TRADE NAME: *Agenerase* (GlaxoSmithKline)

CLASS: Protease inhibitor

FORMS AND PRICE: The only APV formulations now available are pediatric caps (50 mg) and oral solution (15 mg/mL). Fosamprenavir is preferred.

PATIENT ASSISTANCE PROGRAM: 800-722-9294

RECOMMENDED DOSES: 1400 mg PO bid. With RTV boosting, doses are 1400/200 mg qd or 600/100 mg bid.

RESISTANCE: See Fosamprenavir, p. 212.

PHARMACOLOGY

- **Bioavailability:** Estimated at 89%; high-fat meal decreases AUC 21% – can be taken with or without meal, but avoid a high-fat meal.
- **T½:** 7.1 to 10.6 hours

- **Elimination:** Hepatic metabolism – most found in stool; 14% in urine. CYP3A4 inhibition is RTV>IDV=NFV=APV>SQV.
- **Renal disease:** Standard dose.
- **Hepatic disease:** AUC increases 2.5x with liver disease, 4.5x with severe cirrhosis; dose recommendation is based on pharmacokinetic data 450 mg bid with liver disease and 300 mg bid with severe cirrhosis (39th ICAAC, San Francisco, California, 1999, Abstract 326).

SIDE EFFECTS: See Fosamprenavir, p. 212.

The oral solution of APV contains 55% propylene glycol, compared with 5% for the capsules (see black box FDA warning for contraindications). The oral solution is contraindicated in patients with renal failure, hepatic failure, in pregnant women, or in patients receiving disulfiram, metronidazole, or liquid ritonavir. Patients treated with the oral solution should be monitored for adverse effects of propylene glycol, which include seizures, stupor, tachycardia, hyperosmolarity, lactic acidosis, renal failure, and hemolysis. Patients taking the oral solution should change to FPV tab when able to do so, and they should avoid alcoholic beverages when taking the oral solution.

DRUG INTERACTIONS: See Fosamprenavir, p. 212.

PREGNANCY: Category C. There are inadequate data on safety and pharmacokinetics for a recommendation in pregnancy. The oral solution with propylene glycol is contraindicated in pregnancy.

ANADROL – see Oxymetholone (p. 268)

ANCOBON – see Flucytosine (p. 209)

ANDROGEL – see Testosterone (p. 303)

ATIVAN – see Lorazepam (p. 251)

ATAZANAVIR (ATV)

TRADE NAME: *Reyataz* (Bristol-Myers Squibb)

CLASS: Azapeptide protease inhibitor (*Clin Infect Dis* 2004;38:1599)

FORMULATIONS, REGIMEN AND PRICE
- **Forms:** ATV – caps, 100, 150 and 200 mg
- **Regimen:** ATV – 400 mg qd (PI-naïve only); ATV/r – 300/100 mg qd (preferred)

151

5 Drugs: Atazanavir

- **AWP:** $750/month
- **Food:** Take with food
- **Interactions:** Requires gastric acidity; avoid protein-pump inhibitors (omeprazole, etc.), concurrent antacids, etc.; see warnings.
- **Concurrent TDF, EFV, and possibly NVP:** Must use ATV/r.
- **Renal failure:** Standard doses
- **Hepatic failure:** With Child-Pugh score 7-9, dose is 300 mg qd; with Child-Pugh score >9, avoid ATV.
- **Storage:** Room temperature, 15-30°C

PATIENT ASSISTANCE PROGRAM: 800-272-4878

WARNINGS

- Avoid unboosted ATV with TDF, EFV, and NVP (*J Antimicrob Chemother* 2005;56:380); avoid buffered ddI (use ddI-EC)
- Caution with drugs that prolong QTc; with clarithromycin, use half-dose clarithromycin or alternative such as azithromycin.
- Proton pump inhibitors: avoid use
- H_2 receptor antagonists: take H_2 blocker 2 h after ATV, or use ATV/r 400/100 mg qd if concurrent
- Antacids: give ATV 2 hours before or 1 hour after
- Food requirement ↑ ATV AUC 70%. Normal diet.
- Hepatic disease: see dose modification below (Pharmacology)

ADVANTAGES: (1) Potency, esp. with RTV boosting; (2) Convenience of low pill burden and once-daily regimen; (3) Negligible effect on insulin resistance and blood lipids, even with RTV boosting; (4) Unique major resistance mutation (I50L) that does not cause PI cross-resistance; (5) Generally well tolerated (few GI side effects).

DISADVANTAGES: (1) Indirect hyperbilirubinemia – medically inconsequential but may cause jaundice or scleral icterus (<10%); (2) Drug interactions – see warnings; (3) Requirement for food and gastric acid; (4) Need for RTV boosting when combined with TDF, EFV, and NVP.

Drugs: Atazanavir

■ TABLE 5-7: **Clinical Trials with ATV**

Trial	Regimen	No	Dur (wks)	VL <50	VL <200- 400
BMS 034: Treatment naive (*JAIDS* 2004;36:1011)	ATV 400 mg/d AZT/3TC	286	48	32%*	70%
	EFV/AZT/3TC	280		37%*	64%
BMS 043 Failed one PI regimen (*Clin Infect* *Dis* 2004;38:1599)	ATV 400 mg/d/2 NRTI	144	24	59%	—
	LPV/r/2NRTIs	146		77%**	—
BMS 045[†] Failed one PI regimen (*Clin Infect* *Dis* 2004;38:1599)	ATV/r 300/100 mg qd/ 2 NRTIs	120	48[‡]	56%	—
	LPV/r/2 NRTIs	123		58%	—
	SQV 1200 qd/ATV 400 mg qd/2 NRTIs	115		38%**	—
AI 424-009 Failed therapy (*AIDS* 2003;17:1339)	ATV/SQV 400/1200 qd/ 2 NRTIs	34	48	—	41%
	ATV/SQV 600/1200 qd/ 2 NRTIs	28		—	29%
	SQV/RTV 400/400 bid/ 2 NRTIs	23		—	35%

* Low frequency of VL <50 c/mL is attributed to use of inappropriate preservativefor viral load testing.

** Difference is statistically significant vs comparator(s).

[†] Results for >1 $\log_{10}$ c/mL decrease or <400 c/mL.

[‡] VL at 96 wks <50 c/mL in 33% of LPV/r recipients and 30% of ATV/r recipients (7th Internat Congress Drug Therapy 2004; Glasgow, Abstr. PL14.4).

MAJOR TRIALS:

■ **Switch studies:** Two reports with a total of 288 patients switched from PI-based regimens associated with hyperlipidemia showed significant reduction in cholesterol and triglycerides levels at 3-6 months (12th CROI, Boston, Feb. 2005, Abstr. 850 and 858).

■ **Multiple PI failure**

□ **BMS 045:** Patients with multiple PI failures were randomized to TDF/NRTI plus one of three PI regimens (12th CROI, Boston, Feb. 2005, Abstr. 711). Efficacy results are shown below:

Regimen	N	VL (96 wks)	VL with >4 PI mutations
ATV/RTV 300/100 qd	120	-2.3	-1.7
ATV/SQV 400/1200 qd	115	-2.0*	-0.9*
LPV/RTV 400/100 bid	123	-2.1	-1.8

* Significantly less effective.

Drugs: Atazanavir

5

RESISTANCE: The signature mutation is 150L in treatment-naïve patients treated with unboosted ATV, which does not cause cross-resistance with other PIs, including FPV, which has the signature mutation 150V. The 150L mutation reduces ATV activity by a median of 10-fold, reduces replication capacity to 0.3-42%, and increases susceptibility to other PIs (although the significance of this is unknown). Among 78 virologic failures in clinical trials, 23 had both phenotypic resistance and the 150L mutation (*J Infect Dis* 2004;189: 1802). The 150L mutation is often associated with 71V, which increases susceptibility to other PIs (12th CROI, Boston, Feb. 2005, Abstr. 695). 80% of strains with 2 PI resistance-associate mutations (PRAMs) are susceptible to ATV, and 30% are sensitive with 3 PRAMs (*Clin Infect Dis* 2004;38:1599; *Antimicrob Agents Chemother* 2003;47: 1324). ATV given to treatment-experienced patients does not select for 150L but results in emergence of 184V, 90M, 71V/T, 88S/D, and 46I, which causes resistance to ATV and cross-resistance to other PIs (www.reyataz.com). There are no clinical trials in which PI-naïve patients have been treated with ATV/r, so resistance data are not available.

PHARMACOLOGY

- **Absorption:** Requires food and gastric acid for optimal absorption. Food increases AUC 70%. ATV trough levels >150 ng/mL correlate with virologic response (12th CROI, Boston, Feb. 2005, Abstr. 645).

- **Distribution:** Protein-binding 86%, CSF/plasma levels ratio is 0.002-0.02, comparable to IDV and better than other PIs.

- **Serum half-life:** 7 hours

- **Elimination:** Inhibitor and substrate for P450 3A4. Metabolized by the liver, and metabolites are excreted by the biliary tract; only 13% of unmetabolized drug is excreted in urine.

- **Dose adjustment with renal failure:** None

- **Dose adjustment with hepatic failure:** Child-Pugh score 7-9, use 300 mg qd; Child-Pugh score >9, avoid ATV.

SIDE EFFECTS: Generally well tolerated with only 2% discontinuation rate for adverse events in one large trial (BMS 008).

- **Common:** Reversible increase in indirect bilirubinemia due to UGT 1A1 inhibition in 22-47%; this is medically inconsequential but may cause jaundice (reported in 7%). The levels of unconjugated bilirubin correlate with ATV trough levels (12th CROI, Boston, Feb. 2005, Abstr. 645). An increase in bilirubin of ≥0.3 serves as a surrogate marker for ATV adherence (12th CROI, Boston, Feb. 2005, Abstr. 745).

- **Occasional:** GI intolerance with nausea, vomiting, abdominal pain; rash; increase in transaminase.

- **Prolongation of QTc and PR interval**, including asymptomatic first-degree AV block. Use with caution or avoid in patients with

Drugs: Atazanavir

conduction defects and concurrent use with other drugs that alter cardiac conduction, e.g., diltiazem, verapamil, clarithromycin (use half dose of clarithromycin and diltiazem with slow titration). Consider alternatives: azithromycin, quinidine, amiodarone, lidocaine).

- **Rare:** A single case of interstitial nephritis has been reported (*Am J Kidney Dis* 2004;44:e81).

DRUG INTERACTIONS

- **Avoid concurrent use:** Astemizole, bepridil, cisapride, ergotamine, indinavir, irinotecan, lovastatin, midazolam, pimozide, proton pump inhibitors, rifampin, simvastatin, triazolam, St. John's wort, terfenadine, and voriconazole

- **Dose modification:** (ATV standard unless specified)

- **Rifabutin:** 150 mg qod or 3x/week

- **Clarithromycin:** ↑ AUC 94%; use half dose

- **Oral contraceptive:** Estradiol ↑ AUC 48% and norethindrone ↑ AUC 110%; use lowest dose or alternative

- **Statins:** Pravastatin preferred; atorvastatin - use lowest doses

- **Anticonvulsants:** Carbamapezine, phenobarbitol and phenytoin may ↓ ATV levels substantially; avoid or use with caution.

- **Sildenafil:** Maximum of 25 mg q48h

- **Vardenafil:** No data; use ≤2.5 mg/24 hours, and ≤2.5 mg/72 hours with ATV/r.

- **Diltiazem:** ↑ AUC 125%; use half dose and monitor EKG.

- **Calcium channel blocker:** Monitor EKG.

- **H_2 receptor antagonists** (e.g., *Pepcid, Tagomet, Zantac*): Separate doses by as much time as possible, preferably; give ATV 2 h before or 10 h after H_2 blockers.

- **Antacids and buffered medications:** Give 2 h before or 1 h after ATV; use ddI-EC instead of buffered ddI.

- **Proton pump inhibitors** such as omeprazole should be avoided. Co-administration of 40 mg omeprazole with ATV/r 300/100 mg resulted in a 75% reduction in ATV AUC. Attempts to reduce gastric pH with cola were unsuccessful. The restriction includes both the OTC dose of 20 mg and the prescription dose of 40 mg (Bristol-Myers Squibb letter to providers, Jan. 12, 2005) and other PPIs (6th Int Workshop on Clin Pharmacol of HIV, Abstr. 11). This admonition does not apply to other PIs.

- **Methadone:** Unknown.

- **Tenofovir:** ↓ AUC 25% and ↑ TDF AUC 24% (*Antimicrob Agents Chemother* 2004;48:2091); use TDF 300 mg qd + ATV/r 300/100 mg qd.

5 Drugs: Atazanavir

- **PIs:** IDV: avoid (hyperbilirubinemia)
  RTV: ATV/r: 300/100 mg qd
  SQV: ATV/SQV: 400/1200 mg qd (*AIDS* 2004;18:1291) or
  ATV/SQV/RTV: 300/1600/100 mg qd (*AIDS*
  2003;17:1339)
  NFV, APV, FPV, LPV/r: inadequate data
- **NNRTIs:** EFV: Use EFV 600 mg + ATV/r 300/100 mg qd
  NVP: No data. Consider NVP 200 mg bid + ATV/r
  300/100 mg qd based on observational data.
  DLV: No data.
- **Pregnancy:** Category B; there have been no studies of safety or pharmacokinetics in pregnant women. It is not known if the increased indirect bilirubin will increase rates of hyperbilirubinemia in the neonate.

ATORVASTATIN

TRADE NAME: *Lipitor* (Pfizer)

FORMS AND PRICES: Tabs: 10 mg at $2.58, 20 mg at $3.74, 40 mg at $3.47, and 80 mg at $3.47

CLASS: Statin (HMG-CoA reductase inhibitor)

INDICATIONS AND DOSES: Elevated total and LDL cholesterol and/or triglycerides. Recommended statin for hyperlipidemia with PI-based HAART by IAS-USA (*J Acquir Immune Defic Syndr* 2002;31:257) and HIVMA/ACTG (*Clin Infect Dis* 2003;37:613) Other options are fluvastatin, pravastatin, or rosuvastatin. With atorvastatin, the initial dose is 10 mg/day with increases at 2 to 4 week intervals to maintenance doses of 10-80 mg/day in one daily dose. Take with or without food, preferably in the evening.

MONITORING: Blood lipids at ≤4-week intervals until desired results are achieved, then periodically. Obtain transaminase levels at baseline, at 12 weeks, and then at 6-month intervals. Patients should be warned to report muscle pain, tenderness, or weakness promptly, especially if accompanied by fever or malaise. Obtain CPK for suspected myopathy.

PRECAUTIONS: Atorvastatin (and other statins) are contraindicated with pregnancy, breastfeeding, concurrent conditions that predispose to renal failure (e.g., sepsis, hypotension), and active hepatic disease. Alcoholism is a relative contraindication.

PHARMACOLOGY

- **Bioavailability:** 14%
- **T½:** 14 hours
- **Elimination:** Fecal (biliary and unabsorbed) – 98%; renal – <2%

Drugs: Atazanavir

- **Renal failure:** No dose adjustment
- **Hepatic failure:** Levels of atorvastatin are markedly elevated.

SIDE EFFECTS

- **Musculoskeletal:** Myopathy with elevated CPK plus muscle pain, weakness or tenderness ± fever and malaise. Rhabdomyolysis with renal failure reported.
- **Hepatic:** Elevated transaminases in 1% to 2%; discontinue if ALT and/or AST shows unexplained increase >3x upper limit of normal (ULN) x 2.
- **Miscellaneous:** Diarrhea, constipation, nausea, heartburn, stomach pain, dizziness, headache, skin rash, impotence (rare), insomnia

DRUG INTERACTIONS

- **PIs:** Potential for large increase in statin AUC with all PIs (increase with NFV, 74%; LPV/r, 5.8x; SQV/RTV, 4.5x; TPV/r, 9x. Start with 10 mg/day and monitor clinically for myopathy or consider pravastatin; avoid doses >40 mg/d with PIs. EFV ↓ atorvastatin AUC 43%.
- **Grapefruit juice** increases atorvastatin levels up to 24%; avoid large amounts before or after administration.
- **Erythromycin:** Atorvastatin levels increased by 40%.
- **Antacids:** Atorvastatin levels decreased by 35%.
- **Other interactions with increased risk of myopathy:** Azoles (ketoconazole, itraconazole), cyclosporine, fibric acid derivatives, niacin, macrolide antibiotics, nefazodone
- **Niacin and gemfibrozil:** Increased risk of myopathy; rhabdomyolysis reported only with lovastatin + niacin, but could occur with other statins.

PREGNANCY: Category X – contraindicated

ATOVAQUONE

TRADE NAME: *Mepron* (GlaxoSmithKline)

FORM AND PRICE: 750 mg/5 mL: $775 per 210-mL bottle (21-day supply)

PATIENT ASSISTANCE PROGRAM: 800-722-9294

INDICATIONS AND DOSE: PCP: Oral treatment of mild to moderate PCP (A-a O_2 gradient <45 mm Hg and P_AO_2 >60 mm Hg) and PCP prophylaxis in patients who are intolerant of TMP-SMX and dapsone; toxoplasmosis treatment (third line) and prophylaxis (third line).

- **PCP treatment:** 750 mg (5 mL) twice daily with meals x 21 days
- **PCP prophylaxis:** 1500 mg qd or 750 mg bid with meals

5 Drugs: Atorvastatin

- **Toxoplasmosis treatment (alternative):** 1500 mg PO bid with meals alone or combined with either pyrimethamine 200 mg x 1, then 50-75 mg/day or sulfadiazine 1.5 g qid (*Clin Infect Dis* 2002; 34:1243).

PHARMACOLOGY

- **Bioavailability:** Absorption of suspension averages 47% in fed state (with meals) vs 23% with the tablet form. Concurrent administration of fatty food increases absorption by 2-fold. There is significant individual variation in absorption. Administration with fatty food needs emphasis.
- **T½:** 2.2 to 2.9 days
- **Elimination:** Enterohepatic circulation with fecal elimination; <1% in urine
- **CSF/plasma ratio:** <1%
- **Effect of hepatic or renal disease:** No data

SIDE EFFECTS: Rash (20%), GI intolerance (20%), diarrhea (20%). Possibly related headache, fever, insomnia. Life-threatening side effects: none. Percent requiring discontinuation due to side effects: 7% to 9% (rash, 4%).

DRUG INTERACTIONS

- Rifampin: ↓ atovaquone by 54%, ↑ rifampin by 30%; avoid co-administration
- Rifabutin: ↓ atovaquone by 34%, ↑ rifabutin by 19%
- Tetracycline: ↓ atovaquone by 40%; avoid co-administration
- Avoid combination (*MMWR* 1999;48[RR-10]:47). AZT AUC increased 31% due to atovaquone inhibition of AZT gluconuridation (clinical significance unknown).

PREGNANCY: Category C. Not teratogenic in animals; limited experience in humans.

AVENTYL – see Nortriptyline (p. 266)

AZITHROMYCIN

TRADE NAME: *Zithromax* (Pfizer)

FORMS AND PRICES: Tabs: 250 mg tab at $7.83; 600 mg at $19.77; 1 g packet at $22.30. *Z-Pak* with 6 tabs (500 mg, then 250 mg/day x 4 days) at $49.33; *Tri-Pak* with 3 tabs (500 mg x 3 days) for exacerbations of bronchitis at $49.33; IV formulation as 500 mg vial at $29.22

PATIENT ASSISTANCE PROGRAM: 800-207-8990

CLASS: Macrolide

INDICATIONS AND DOSES: see Table 5-8 below.

ACTIVITY: *S. pneumoniae* (about 20% to 30% of *S. pneumoniae* strains are resistant to azithromycin and other macrolides in the U.S.), streptococci (not *Enterococcus*), erythromycin-sensitive *S. aureus, H. influenzae, Legionella, C. pneumoniae, M. pneumoniae, C. trachomatis, M. avium, N. gonorrhea, T. pallidum,* and *T. gondii.* There is concern about high and increasing macrolide resistance by *S. pneumoniae* in the United States and even higher rates in Spain and Asia (*Antimicrob Agents Chemother* 2002;297:1016; *J Infect Dis* 2000;182:1417; *Antimicrob Agents Chemother* 2002;46:265; *Antimicrob Agents Chemother* 2001;45:2147). However, multiple clinical trials show that *in vivo* activity with pneumococcal pneumonia is much better than *in vitro* results. Nevertheless, several cases of breakthrough pneumococcal bacteremia have been reported (*Clin Infect Dis* 2002;35:556). Azithromycn appears to reduce risk of *P. carinii* pneumonia beyond that achieved with standard PCP prophylaxis (*Lancet* 1999;354:891). For MAC bacteremia, one study showed that azithromycin 600 mg/day was equivalent to clarithromycin 500 mg/day (*Clin Infect Dis* 2000;31:1245). The VA trial showed clarithromycin to be superior (*Clin Infect Dis* 31;1245). For syphilis, preliminary studies in patients without HIV infection showed that azithromycin (2 g PO x 1) was equivalent to benzathine penicillin (2.4 mil units IM x 1) for treatment of early syphilis (*Sex Transm Dis* 2002;29:486).

■ TABLE 5-8: **Azithromycin Regimens by Condition**

Indication	Dose[†]
M. avium prophylaxis*	500-600 mg qd + ethambutol (EMB) (*MMWR* 2002;51[RR-8]:1)
M. avium treatment*	500-600 mg qd + EMB ± rifabutin (*Clin Infect Dis* 2000;31:1245)
Pneumonia*	500 mg IV qd x ≥2 days (hospitalized patients), then 500 mg PO qd x 7 to 10 days
Sinusitis*	500 mg x 1, then 250 mg PO/day x 4 (Z-pak) or 500 mg/d x 3 days (Tri-pak)
*C. trachomatis** (nongonococcal urethritis or cervicitis)	1 g or 1.2 g (two 600 mg tablets) PO x 1
Gonococcal urethritis or cervicitis	2 g PO x 1 (poor GI tolerance)
Toxoplasmosis	900-1200 mg PO qd + pyrimethamine 200 mg PO x1, then 50-75 mg/day + leukovorin 10-20 mg qd x ≥6 wks, then half dose of each
Syphilis (primary, secondary, early latent)	2 g PO or 2 g PO x2 separated by 1 week. (*Sex Trans Dis* 2002;29:486; these are considered preliminary results)

* FDA-approved indications.

[†] Caps must be taken ≥1 hour before or >2 hours after a meal; food facilitates absorption and tolerance of tabs and powder.

5 Drugs: Azithromycin

PHARMACOLOGY

- **Bioavailability:** Absorption is ~30% to 40%. The 600 mg tabs and the 1 g powder packet may be taken without regard to food, but food improves tolerability.
- **T½:** 68 hours; detectable levels in urine at 7 to 14 days; with the 1200 mg weekly dose, the azithromycin levels in peripheral leukocytes remain above 32 μg/mL for 60 hours.
- **Distribution:** High tissue levels; low CSF levels (<0.01 μg/mL)
- **Excretion:** Primarily biliary; 6% in urine
- **Dose modification in renal or hepatic failure:** Use with caution.

SIDE EFFECTS: GI intolerance (nausea, vomiting, pain); diarrhea – 14%. With 1200 mg dose weekly, major side effects are diarrhea, abdominal pain, and/or nausea in 10% to 15%; reversible dose-dependent hearing loss is reported in 5% at mean day of onset at 96 days and mean exposure of 59,000 mg (package insert). Frequency of discontinuation in AIDS patients receiving high doses – 6%, primarily GI intolerance and reversible ototoxicity – 2%; rare – erythema multiforme, increased transaminases.

CONTRAINDICATIONS: Hypersensitivity to erythromycin

DRUG INTERACTIONS: Azithromycin increases levels of theophylline and coumadin. Concurrent use with antiretroviral agents, rifampin, and rifabutin is safe. Concurrent use with pimozide may cause fatal arrythmias and must be avoided.

PREGNANCY: Category B (safe in animal studies; no data in humans). Preferred macrolide for MAC prophylaxis and treatment in pregnancy.

AZT – see Zidovudine (p. 323)

BACTRIM – see Trimethoprim-Sulfamethoxazole (p. 315)

BENZODIAZEPINES

Benzodiazepines are commonly used for anxiety and insomnia. They are also commonly misused and abused, with some studies showing that up to 25% of AIDS patients take these drugs. The decision to use these drugs requires careful consideration of side effects along with a discussion of the following issues with the patient:

- **Dependency:** Larger than usual doses or prolonged daily use of therapeutic doses.
- **Abuse potential:** Most common in those with abuse of alcohol and other psychiatric drugs.

Drugs: Azithromycin

- **Tolerance:** Primarily to sedation and ataxia; minimal to antianxiety effects.
- **Withdrawal symptoms:** Related to duration of use, dose, rate of tapering, and drug half-life. Features include: 1) Recurrence of pretreatment symptoms developing over days or weeks; 2) Rebound with symptoms that are similar to but more severe than pretreatment symptoms occurring within hours or days (self-limited); and 3) The benzodiazepine withdrawal syndrome with autonomic symptoms, disturbances in equilibrium, sensory disturbances, etc.
- **Daytime sedation, dizziness, incoordination, ataxia, and hangover:** Use small doses initially and gradually increase. Patient must be warned that activities requiring mental alertness, judgment, and coordination require special caution; concomitant use with alcohol or other sedating drugs is hazardous. Patients often experience amnesia for events during the drug's time of action.
- **Drug interactions:** Sedative effects are antagonized by caffeine and theophylline. Erythromycin, clarithromycin, fluoroquinolones, all PIs cimetidine, omeprazole, and INH may reduce hepatic metabolism and prolong half-life. Midazolam and triazolam are thus contraindicated with co-administration of these drugs. Lovazepam, temazepam, and oxazepam are safer alternatives. Rifampin and oral contraceptives increase hepatic clearance and reduce half-life.
- **Miscellaneous side effects:** Blurred vision, diplopia, confusion, memory disturbance, amnesia, fatigue, incontinence, constipation, hypotension, disinhibition, bizarre behavior
- **Antiretroviral agents:** Concurrent use of triazolam and midazolam with PIs and DLV is contraindicated.

SELECTION OF AGENT AND REGIMEN: Drug selection is based largely on indication and pharmacokinetic properties (see Table 5-9, p. 162). Drugs with rapid onset are desired when temporary relief of anxiety is needed. The smallest dose for the shortest time is recommended, and patients need frequent re-evaluation for continued use. Long-term use should be avoided, especially in patients with a history of abuse of alcohol or other sedative-hypnotic drugs. Dose adjustments are usually required to achieve the desired effect with acceptable side effects. Long-term use (more than several weeks) may require an extended tapering schedule over 6 to 8 weeks (20% to 30% dose reduction weekly) adjusted by symptoms and sometimes facilitated by antidepressants or hypnotics.

5 Drugs: Benzodiazepines

■ TABLE 5-9: **Comparison of Benzodiazepines**

Agent	Trade Name	Anxiety	Insomnia	Tmax (hrs)	Mean Half-life (hrs)	Dose Forms	Regimens
Chlordiazepoxide	Librium	+	−	0.5-4.0	10	5, 10, 25 mg tabs	15-100 mg/day hs or 3 to 4 doses
Clorazepate	Tranxene	+	−	1-2	73	3.75, 7.5, 15, 11.25, 22.5 mg tabs	15-60 mg/day hs or 2 to 4 doses
Diazepam	Valium	+	+	1.5-2.0	73	2, 4, 5, 10 mg tabs	15-60 mg/day hs or 2 to 4 doses
Flurazepam	Dalmane	−	+	0.5-2.0	74	15, 30 mg caps	15-30 mg/day, hs
Quazepam	Doral	−	+	2	74	7.5, 15 mg tabs	7.5-30 mg hs
Alprazolam	Xanax	+	−	1-2	11	0.25, 0.5, 1, 2 mg tabs	0.75-1.5 mg/day in 3 divided doses
Lorazepam	Ativan	+	+	2	14	0.5, 1, 2 mg tabs	0.25-0.5 mg tid up to 4 mg/day
Oxazepam	Serax	+	+	1-4	7	10, 15, 30 mg caps	15-30 mg tid-qid
Temazepam	Restoril	−	+	1.0-1.5	13	15, 30 mg caps	15-30 mg qhs
Triazolam*	Halcion	−	+	1-2	3	0.125, 0.25 mg tabs	0.25 mg hs
Midazolam*	Versed	+	+	2 min	1-5	IV vial	0.03-0.06 mg/kg

* Concurrent use with PIs or DLV is contraindicated.

BIAXIN – see Clarithromycin (p. 169)

BUPROPION

TRADE NAME: *Wellbutrin, Wellbutrin SR, Wellbutrin XL*, and *Zyban* (GlaxoSmithKline)

FORMS AND PRICES: Tabs: 75 mg at $0.72, 100 mg at $0.96, 150 mg sustained-release at $1.69. Wellbutrin comes in 75 and 100 mg tabs; Wellbutrin SR comes in 100, 150, and 200 mg tabs; and Wellbutrin XL comes in 150 and 300 mg tabs.

CLASS: Atypical antidepressant

INDICATIONS AND DOSES: Depression: 150 mg qd x 4 days, then 300 mg qd (XL formulation) or 150 mg bid (SR formulation); antidepressant effect may require 4 weeks. *Zyban* for smoking cessation. Dose same as SR formulation x 7 to 12 weeks.

Drugs: Benzodiazepines

- **Bioavailability:** 5% to 20%
- **T½:** 8 to 24 hours
- **Elimination:** Extensive hepatic metabolism to ≥6 metabolites including two with antidepressant activity; metabolites excreted in urine.
- **Dose modification in renal or hepatic failure:** Not known, but dose reduction may be required.

SIDE EFFECTS: Seizures, which are dose dependent and minimized by gradual increase in dose; dose not to exceed 450 mg/day. Use with caution in seizure-prone patients and with concurrent use of alcohol and other antidepressants.

OTHER SIDE EFFECTS: Agitation, insomnia, restlessness; GI – anorexia, nausea, vomiting; weight loss – noted in up to 25%; rare cases of psychosis, paranoia, depersonalization

BUSPAR – see Buspirone (below)

BUSPIRONE

TRADE NAME: *BuSpar* (Bristol-Myers Squibb)

FORMS AND PRICES: Tabs: 5 mg tab at $0.91, 10 mg tab at $1.34, 15 mg tab at $2.35, 30 mg tab at $4.25

CLASS: Nonbenzodiazepine-nonbarbiturate antianxiety agent; not a controlled substance

INDICATIONS AND DOSES: Anxiety: 5 mg PO tid; increase by 5 mg/day every 2 to 4 days. Usual effective dose is 15-30 mg/day in 2 to 3 divided doses. Onset of response requires 1 week, and full effect requires 4 weeks. Total daily dose should not exceed 60 mg/day.

PHARMACOLOGY

- **Bioavailability:** >90% absorbed when taken with food.
- **T½:** 2.5 hours
- **Elimination:** Rapid hepatic metabolism to partially active metabolites; <0.1% of parent compound excreted in urine
- **Dose adjustment in renal disease:** Dose reduction of 25% to 50% in patients with anuria
- **Hepatic disease:** May decrease clearance and must use with caution.

SIDE EFFECTS: Sleep disturbance, nervousness, headache, nausea, diarrhea, paresthesias, depression, increased or decreased libido, dizziness, and excitement. Compared with benzodiazepines, there is no

5 Drugs: Buspirone

risk of dependency, it does not potentiate CNS depressants including alcohol, it is usually well tolerated by elderly, and there is no hypnotic effect, no muscle relaxant effect, less fatigue, less confusion, and less decreased libido but nearly comparable efficacy for anxiety. Nevertheless, the CNS effects are somewhat unpredictable, and there is substantial individual variation; patients should be warned that buspirone may impair ability to perform activities requiring mental alertness and physical coordination such as driving.

PREGNANCY: Category B

CASPOFUNGIN

TRADE NAME: *Cancidas* (Merck)

FORMS AND PRICE: 50 mg vial $388; 70 mg vial $500

CLASS: Polypeptide antifungal

INDICATIONS: (1) Invasive aspergillosis, in patients intolerant of voriconazole or ampho B; (2) Candidemia and other serious candida infections, including *Candida* esophagitis refractory to azoles

DOSE: 70 mg IV on day 1, then 50 mg/day

- Dose with renal failure: standard
- Dose with hepatic failure: With Child-Pugh score of 7-9, give standard loading dose of 70 mg, then 35 mg qd

PHARMACOLOGY
- **Absorption:** IV only
- **T½:** 9-11 hrs
- **Elimination:** Metabolized by hydrolysis and acetylating; <2% excreted unchanged in urine

ADVERSE REACTIONS: Generally well tolerated. Infrequent or rare side effects are rash, facial swelling, nausea, vomiting, headache, fever, phlebitis, hypokalemia, increased alkaline phosphatase. Rare patients have histamine release symptoms with rash, fever, pruritis and sensation of warmth.

DRUG INTERACTIONS: Cyclosporin increases caspofungin AUC 35%; coadministration is not recommended. Tacrolimus levels reduced 20% with caspofungin; monitor tacrolimus levels. Phenytoin, carbamezapine, and phenobarbitol may decrease caspofungin. Rifampin decreases caspofungin by 30%; increase dose to 70 mg/d.

PREGNANCY: Class C

CHLORAL HYDRATE

TRADE NAME: *Aquachloral Supprettes* suppositories (Polymedica), *Somnote* (Breckenridge Pharmaceutical), or generic

FORMS AND PRICES: Caps: 325 mg, 500 mg at $0.17, and 650 mg; 500 mg at $0.17/cap. Suppositories at $0.19/325 mg. Syrup with 250 and 500 mg, 5 mL syrup at $0.32/500 mg

CLASS: Nonbenzodiazepine-nonbarbiturate hypnotic; controlled substance category IV

INDICATIONS AND DOSES

- **Insomnia:** 500 mg to 1 g PO hs; usually produces sleep within 30 minutes, which lasts 4 to 8 hours.
- **Sedation:** 250 mg PO tid
- **Note:** Tolerance develops within 5 weeks.

PHARMACOLOGY

- **Bioavailability:** >90%
- **T½:** Hepatic metabolism to achieve metabolite (trichloroethanol) with a half-life of 4.0 to 9.5 hours
- **Elimination:** Renal excretion of trichloroethanol
- **Hepatic or renal disease:** Contraindicated

SIDE EFFECTS: Gastric intolerance; dependence and tolerance with long-term use

DRUG INTERACTIONS: Potentiates action of oral anticoagulants

PREGNANCY: Category C

CIDOFOVIR

TRADE NAME: *Vistide* (Gilead Sciences)

FORM AND PRICE: 375 mg in 5 mL vial at $888

PATIENT ASSISTANCE PROGRAM AND REIMBURSEMENT HOTLINE: 800-226-2056

ACTIVITY: Active *in vitro* against CMV, VZV, EBV, HHV-6, pox viruses (molluscum, vaccinia, smallpox), and HHV-8; less active against HSV (*Exp Med Biol* 1996;394:105). CMV strains resistant to ganciclovir are usually sensitive to cidofovir; cidofovir-resistant strains are usually resistant to ganciclovir and sensitive to foscarnet. HSV resistant to acyclovir is often sensitive to cidofovir.

INDICATIONS AND DOSE: CMV retinitis; efficacy in other forms of CMV disease has not been established but is expected (*Arch Intern Med* 1998;158:957).

- **Induction dose:** 5 mg/kg IV over 1 hour* weekly x 2
- **Maintenance dose:** 5 mg/kg IV over 1 hour every 2 weeks*

---

* Probenecid 2 g given 3 hours prior to cidofovir and 1 g given at 2 and 8 hours after infusion (total of 4 g). Patients must receive >1 L 0.95 N (normal) saline infused over 1 to 2 hours immediately before cidofovir infusion.

CLINICAL TRIALS: A Studies of the Ocular Complications of AIDS (SOCA) trial comparing cidofovir vs deferred treatment of patients with CMV retinitis demonstrated a median time to progression of 120 days in the treated group compared with 22 days in the deferred group (*Ann Intern Med* 1997;126:257). Dose-limiting nephrotoxicity was noted in 24%, and dose-limiting toxicity to probenecid was noted in 7%. Another SOCA study showed that cidofovir was comparable with the ganciclovir implant plus oral ganciclovir in 61 patients with CMV retinitis.

NOTES ON ADMINISTRATION

- Cidofovir is diluted in 100 mL 0.9% saline.
- Renal failure: Cidofovir is contraindicated in patients with preexisting renal failure (serum creatinine >1.5 mg/dL, creatinine clearance ≤55 mL/min or urine protein >100 mg/dL or 2+ proteinuria).
- Co-administration of nephrotoxic drugs is contraindicated, including non-steroidal anti-inflammatory agents, amphotericin B, aminoglycosides, and IV pentamidine; there should be a 7-day "washout" following use of these drugs.
- Dose adjustment for renal failure during cidofovir treatment:
  - Serum creatinine increase 0.3-0.4 mg/dL: Reduce dose to 3 mg/kg.
  - Serum creatinine increase ≥0.5 mg/dL or ≥3 + proteinuria: Discontinue therapy.
- Gastrointestinal tolerability of probenecid may be improved with ingestion of food or an antiemetic prior to administration. Antihistamines or acetaminophen may be used for probenecid hypersensitivity reactions.
- Cases of nephrotoxicity should be reported to Gilead Sciences, Inc. 800-GILEAD-5, or to the FDA's Medwatch 800-FDA-1088.

PHARMACOLOGY

- **Bioavailability:** Requires IV administration; probenecid increases AUC by 40% to 60%, presumably by blocking tubular secretion. CSF levels are undetectable.
- **T½:** The elimination half-life of the active intracellular metabolite is 17 to 65 hours permitting long intervals between doses.
- **Excretion:** 70% to 85% excreted in urine.

SIDE EFFECTS: The major side effect is dose-dependent nephrotoxicity. Proteinuria is an early indicator. IV saline and probenecid must be used to reduce nephrotoxicity. Monitor renal function with serum creatinine

Drugs: Cidofovir

and urine protein within 48 hours prior to each dose. About 25% will develop ≥2 + proteinuria or a serum creatinine >2-3 mg/dL, and these changes are reversible if treatment is discontinued (*Ann Intern Med* 1997;126:257,264). Cases of nephrotoxicity should be reported to 800-GILEAD-5.

OTHER SIDE EFFECTS: Neutropenia in about 15% (monitor neutrophil count) and metabolic acidosis with Fanconi's syndrome with proteinuria, normoglycemic glycosuria, hypophosphatemia, hypo-uracemia and decreased serum bicarbonate indicating renal tubule damage. Other side effects include ocular hypotony, anterior uveitis or iritis, and aesthenia. Probenecid causes side effects in about 50% of patients including fever, chills, headache, rash, or nausea, usually after 3 to 4 treatments. Side effects usually resolve within 12 hours. Dose-limiting side effect is usually GI intolerance. Side effects may be reduced with antiemetics, antipyretics, antihistamines, or by eating before taking probenecid (*Ann Intern Med* 1997;126:257).

DRUG INTERACTIONS: Avoid concurrent nephrotoxic drugs including aminoglycosides, amphotericin B, foscarnet, IV pentamidine and NSAIDs. Patients receiving these drugs should have a ≥7 day "washout" prior to treatment with cidofovir. Probenecid prolongs the half-life of acetaminophen, acyclovir, aminosalicylic acid, barbiturates, beta-lactam antibiotics, benzodiazepines, bumetadine, clofibrate, methotrexate, famotidine, furosemide, NSAIDs, theophylline, and AZT.

PREGNANCY: Category C. Use only if potential benefit justifies the risk.

CIPROFLOXACIN –
(see "Fluoroquinolones," see Table 5-21, p. 210, for comparisons)

TRADE NAME: *Cipro* (Bayer); available as generic

FORMS AND PRICES: Tabs: 250 mg, 500 mg at $5.80, 750 mg at $6.28; 500 mg XR at $8.66; 1000 mg XR at $9.86. Vials for IV use: 200 mg at $14.41.

PATIENT ASSISTANCE PROGRAM: 800-998-9180

CLASS: Fluoroquinolone

INDICATIONS AND DOSES

- **Respiratory infections:** 500-750 mg PO bid x 7-14 days (*P. aeruginosa*); use 750 mg PO bid or 400 mg IV q8h.
- **Gonorrhea:** 500 mg x 1 (First line)
- **M. avium:** 500-750 mg PO bid (alternative or 3rd or 4th drug with serious disease)

Drugs: Ciprofloxacin

5

- **Tuberculosis:** 500-750 mg PO bid multidrug-resistant *M. tuberculosis* or liver disease)
- **Salmonellosis:** 500-750 mg PO or IV bid x 7-14 days for mild disease or 4-6 wks for CD4 <200 and/or bacteremia (preferred)
- **UTI:** 250-500 mg PO bid x 3 to 7 days (First line)
- **Traveler's diarrhea:** 500 mg PO bid x 3 days (First line)

ACTIVITY: Active against most strains of *Enterobacteriaceae, P. aeruginosa, H. influenzae, Legionella, C. pneumoniae, M. pneumoniae, M. tuberculosis, M. avium,* most bacterial enteric pathogens other than *C. jejuni* and *C. difficile.* Somewhat less active against *S. pneumoniae* than levofloxacin, gatifloxacin, and moxifloxacin; the clinical significance of this difference is debated when using full doses of ciprofloxacin (750 mg PO bid), and some authorities now feel that levofloxacin should also be used in full dose (750 mg/day) for pneumococcal infections. There is increasing and substantial resistance by *S. aureus* (primarily MRSA) (*Clin Infect Dis* 2000;32: S114), *P. aeruginosa* (*Clin Infect Dis* 2000;32:S146), and *C. jejuni* (*Clin Infect Dis* 2001;32:1201). There is escalating concern about fluoroquinolone-resistant *S. pneumoniae, N. gonorrhea, C. jejuni, S. aureus,* and *P. aeruginosa.* Rates for *S. pneumonia* vary greatly by geographic areas (*Emerg Infect Dis* 2002;8:594), although overall rates in the U.S. remained <1% through 2002 (*Antimicrob Agents Chemother* 2002;46:680; *Antimicrob Agents Chemother* 2002;46:265; *Clin Infect Dis* 2003;36:783).

PHARMACOLOGY

- **Bioavailability:** 60% to 70%
- **T½:** 3.3 hours
- **Excretion:** Metabolized and excreted (parent compound and metabolites) in urine
- **Dose reduction in renal failure:** CrCl>50 mL/min – 250-750 mg q12h; CrCl 10-50 mL/min – 250-500 mg q12h; CrCl<10 mL/min – 250-500 mg q18h or 500 mg q24h

SIDE EFFECTS: Usually well tolerated; most common include:

- **GI intolerance** with nausea – 1.2%; diarrhea – 1.2%
- **CNS toxicity:** Malaise, drowsiness, insomnia, headache, dizziness, agitation, psychosis (rare), seizures (rare), hallucinations (rare)
- **Tendon rupture:** About 100 cases reported involving fluoro-quinolones, with ciprofloxacin accounting for 25% (*Clin Infect Dis* 2003;36:1404). The incidence in a review of 46,776 courses was 0.1% with increased age and steroids as confounding risks (*Brit Med J* 2002;324:1306).

Drugs: Ciprofloxacin

- **Torsades de pointes:** Rates/10 million are: Moxifloxacin – 0, cipro-floxacin – 0.3, levofloxacin – 5.4, gatifloxacin – 27 (*Pharmacother* 2001;21:1468).
- ***Candida* vaginitis**

PREGNANCY: Fluoroquinolones are contraindicated in persons <18 years due to concern for arthropathy, which has been seen in beagle dogs, but application to human disease is debated, and the FDA is reviewing application for pediatric use (*Pediatr Infect Dis J* 2002; 21:345; *Pediatr Infect Dis J* 2002;21:525). Some fluoroquinolones may cause false positive urine screening tests for opiates (*JAMA* 2001;286:3115).

DRUG INTERACTIONS: Increased levels of theophylline, methotrexate, and caffeine; reduced absorption with cations (Al, Mg, Ca) in antacids, sucralfate, milk and dairy products, buffered ddl; gastric achlorhydria does not influence absorption. Take fluoroquinolone 2 h before cations.

PREGNANCY: Category C. Arthropathy in immature animals with erosions in joint cartilages; relevance to patients is not known, but fluoroquinolones are not FDA-approved for use in pregnancy or in children <18 years. Review of >200 first trimester exposures showed no anomalies. Use may be justified in severe MAC or multi-drug-resistant tuberculosis.

CLARITHROMYCIN

TRADE NAME: *Biaxin* (Abbott Laboratories)

FORMS AND PRICES: Tabs: 250 mg at $4.64, 500 mg at $4.64, 500 mg XL at $4.71 (for qd dosing). Suspension: 250 mg/5 mL at $71.61 per 100 mL.

PATIENT ASSISTANCE PROGRAM: 800-659-9050

CLASS: Macrolide

■ TABLE 5-10: **Clarithromycin Indications and Doses**

Indication	Dose Regimen*
Pharyngitis, sinusitis, otitis, pneumonitis, skin and soft tissue infection[†]	250-500 mg PO bid or 1 g 2XL tabs qd
M. avium prophylaxis[†]	500 mg PO bid (*MMWR* 1995;44[RR-8]:1)
M. avium treatment[†] (plus EMB ± ciprofloxacin or rifabutin)	500 mg PO bid
Bartonella	500 mg po bid x ≥3 mo

* Doses of ≥2 g/day are associated with excessive mortality (*Clin Infect Dis* 1999;29:125).

[†] FDA-approved for this indication.

Drugs: Clarithromycin

5

CLINICAL TRIALS: Clarithromycin is highly effective in the treatment and prevention of MAC disease (*N Engl J Med* 1996;335:385; *Clin Infect Dis* 1998;27:1278). Clarithromycin was superior to azithromycin in the treatment of MAC bacteremia in terms of median time to negative blood cultures 4.4 weeks vs >16 weeks (*Clin Infect Dis* 1998;27:1278). However, this point is debated and may be a dose issue (*Clin Infect Dis* 2000;31:1254). There is no evidence that it is superior to azithromycin for MAC prophylaxis. Clarithromycin should be given with caution with rifabutin due to decreased levels of clarithromycin (*N Engl J Med* 1996;335:428). This is the presumed explanation for the lack of superior outcome with rifabutin plus clarithromycin vs clarithromycin alone for prevention of MAC (*J Infect Dis* 2000;181:1289).

ACTIVITY: *S. pneumoniae* (20% to 30% of strains and 40% of penicillin-resistant strains are resistant in most areas of the United States), erythromycin-sensitive *S. aureus, S. pyogenes, M. catarrhalis, H. influenzae, M. pneumoniae, C. pneumoniae, Legionella, M. avium, T. gondii, C. trachomatis,* and *U. urealyticum.* Activity against *H. influenzae* is often debated, although a metabolite shows better *in vitro* activity than the parent compound, and the FDA has approved clarithromycin for pneumonia caused by *H. influenzae.* There is concern about increasing rates of macrolide resistance by *S. pneumoniae* (*J Infect Dis* 2000;182:1417; *Antimicrob Agents Chemother* 2001;45:2147; *Antimicrob Agents Chemother* 2002;46:265), although clinical trials show *in vivo* results that are superior to *in vitro* activity. Nevertheless, excessive rates of breakthrough pneumococcal bacteremia has been reported (*Clin Infect Dis* 2002;35:556).

PHARMACOLOGY

- **Bioavailability:** 50% to 55%
- **T½:** 4 to 7 hours
- **Elimination:** Rapid first-pass hepatic metabolism plus renal clearance to 14 – hydroxyclarithromycin
- **Dose modification in renal failure:** CrCl <30 mL/min half usual dose or double interval.

SIDE EFFECTS: GI intolerance – 4% (vs 17% with erythromycin); transaminase elevation – 1%, headache – 2%, PMC – rare.

DRUG INTERACTIONS: Clarithromycin is a substrate and inhibitor of CYP3A4. It increases levels of rifabutin 56%, and levels of clarithromycin are decreased 50%. May need to decrease rifabutin dose and increase clarithomycin dose or use azithromycin. Clarithromycin should not be combined with rifampin, trimetrexate, ergot alkaloid, carbamazepine (*Tegretol*), cisapride (*Propulsid*), pimozide (*Orap*), and *Seldane*; increased levels of *Seldane*, pimozide, and *Propulsid* may cause fatal arrhythmias. The same concern for arrhythmias applies to concurrent use with atazanavir. (Azithromycin has no substantial interaction with these drugs.) May increase serum level CYP3A4 substrates. See Table 5-11 for interactions and dose adjustments for clarithromycin use with NNRTIs and PIs.

■ TABLE 5-11: **Clarithromycin Interactions with PIs and NNRTIs**

Agent	Clarithromycin	PI/NNRTI	Regimen
IDV	↑53%	↑29%	Standard
RTV	↑77%	↓14 OH clarithro	Reduce clarithromycin dose by 50% if CrCl 30-60 mL/min, and by 75% if CrCl <30 mL/min
SQV	↑45%	↑177%	Standard
NFV	No data	No data	No data
APV	No change	↑18%	Standard
LPV/r	↑77%	—	Reduce clarithromycin dose by 50% if CrCl 30-60 mL/min, and by 75% if CrCl <30 mL/min
NVP	↓30%	↑26%	Standard; monitor for efficacy or use azithro
EFV	↓39%	↑14 OH clarithro 34%	Avoid if possible; consider azithromycin
DLV	↑100%	↑44%	Dose reduction for renal failure; monitor QTc
ATV	↑94%	—	Use half dose clarithromycin and monitor for arrhythmia (QTc prolongation) or use azithromycin

PREGNANCY: Category C; teratogenic in animal studies and no adequate studies in humans.

CLINDAMYCIN

TRADE NAME: *Cleocin* (Pharmacia) or generic

FORMS AND PRICES

- **Clindamycin HCl caps:** 75 mg, 150 mg, 300 mg at $5.00
- **Clindamycin PO$_4$ with 150 mg/mL in 2, 4, and 6 mL vials:** 600 mg/mL vial at $10.41; 900 mg at $12.75

PATIENT ASSISTANT PROGRAM: 800-242-7014

INDICATIONS AND DOSES

- **PCP:** Clindamycin 600-900 mg q6h-q8h IV or 300-450 mg q6-8h PO + primaquine 15-30 mg (base)
- **Toxoplasmosis:** Clindamycin 600 mg IV or PO q6h + pyrimethamine 200 loading dose, then 50-75 mg/day PO/leucovorin, 10-20 mg day

5 Drugs: Clindamycin

- **Other infections:** 600 mg q8h IV or 300 mg PO q6h-q8h

ACTIVITY: Most Gram-positive cocci are susceptible except *Enterococcus* and some *Staphylococci*. Nosocomial MRSA are usually resistant; community-acquired MRSA are usually sensitive. Most anaerobic bacteria are susceptible, but new IDSA guidelines for intra-abdominal sepsis do not include clindamycin, due to increasing resistance by *B. fragilis*.

PHARMACOLOGY

- **Bioavailability:** 90%
- **T½:** 2 to 3 hours
- **CNS penetration:** Poor
- **Elimination:** Metabolized; 10% in urine
- **Dose modification in renal failure:** None

SIDE EFFECTS: GI – diarrhea in 10% to 30%. Six percent of patients develop *C. difficile*-associated diarrhea; most respond well to discontinuation of the implicated antibiotic ± metronidazole (250 mg qid or 500 mg tid x 10 days). Other GI side effects include nausea, vomiting, and anorexia. Rash – generalized morbilliform is most common; less common is urticaria, pruritus, Stevens-Johnson syndrome.

DRUG INTERACTIONS: Loperamide or diphenoxylate HCl with citropine sulfate (*Lomotil*) increases risk of diarrhea and *C. difficile*-associated colitis.

PREGNANCY: Category B

CLOFAZIMINE

TRADE NAME: *Lamprene* (Novartis)

This drug is no longer used for *M. avium* infections because it does not improve outcome and is associated with high rates of side effects and increased mortality (*N Engl J Med* 1996;335:377).

CLOTRIMAZOLE

TRADE NAMES: *Lotrimin* (Schering-Plough), *Mycelex* (Bayer), *Gyne-Lotrimin* (Schering-Plough), *FemCare* (Schering), or generic

FORMS AND PRICES

- Troche 10 mg at $1.68
- Topical cream (1%) 15 g at $5.29; 30 g at $8.29
- Topical solution/lotion (1%) 10 mL at $7.40; 30 mL at $15.52

- Vaginal cream (1%) 45 g at $8.00
- Vaginal tablets 3-200 mg at $7.53
- Vaginal tablets 500 mg at $13.88 (single dose)

CLASS: Imidazole (related to miconazole)

INDICATIONS AND DOSES

- **Thrush:** 10 mg troche 5x/day; must be dissolved in the mouth. Clotrimazole troches are only slightly less effective than fluconazole for thrush and are often preferred to avoid azole resistance (*HIV Clin Trials* 2000;1:47). The problem is the need for 5 doses/day, although treatment with lower doses is often successful.

- **Dermatophytic infections and cutaneous candidiasis:** Topical application of 1% cream, lotion, or solution to affected area bid x 2 to 8 weeks; if no improvement, reevaluate diagnosis.

- **Candidal vaginitis:** Intravaginal 100 mg tab bid x 3 days (preferred); alternatives: 100 mg tabs qd x 7; 500 mg tab x 1. Vaginal cream: One applicator (about 5 g) intravaginally at hs x 7 to 14 days.

ACTIVITY: Active against *Candida* species and dermatophytes.

PHARMACOLOGY

- **Bioavailability:** Lozenge (troche) dissolves in 15 to 30 minutes; administration at 3-hour intervals maintains constant salivary concentrations above MIC of most *Candida* strains. Topical application of 500 mg tab intravaginally achieves local therapeutic levels for 48 to 72 hours. Small amounts of drug are absorbed with oral, vaginal, or skin applications.

SIDE EFFECTS: Topical to skin (rare) – erythema, blistering, pruritus, pain, peeling, urticaria; topical to vagina (rare) – rash, pruritus, dyspareunia, dysuria, burning, erythema; lozenges – elevated AST (up to 15% – monitor LFTs); nausea and vomiting (5%)

PREGNANCY: Category C. Avoid during first trimester.

CRIXIVAN – see Indinavir (p. 226)

CYTOVENE – see Ganciclovir (p. 217)

DALMANE – see Benzodiazepines (p. 160)

5 Drugs: Clotrimazole

DAPSONE

TRADE NAME: Generic

FORMS AND PRICES: Tabs: 25 mg at $0.19, 100 mg at $0.20

- **Comparison prices for PCP prophylaxis:**
  - □ Dapsone (100 mg/day): $6.00/month
  - □ TMP-SMX (1 DS/day): $5.40/month
  - □ Aerosolized pentamidine: $138/month (plus administration costs)
  - □ Atovaquone (1500 mg/day): $738/month

CLASS: Synthetic sulfone with mechanism of action similar to sulfonamides – inhibition of folic acid synthesis by inhibition of dihydropteroate synthetase.

■ TABLE 5-12: **Dapsone Indications and Dose Regimens**

Indication	Dose Regimen
PCP prophylaxis	100 mg PO qd
PCP treatment (mild to moderately servere)	100 mg PO qd (plus trimethoprim 15 mg/kg/day PO) x 3 weeks
PCP + toxoplasmosis prophylaxis	50 mg PO qd (plus pyrimethamine 50 mg/week plus folinic acid 25 mg/week) or dapsone 200 mg (+ pyrimethamine 75 mg + leucovorin 25 mg) once weekly

EFFICACY: A review of 40 published studies found dapsone (100 mg/day) to be slightly less effective than TMP-SMX for PCP, prophylaxis, but comparable with aerosolized pentamidine and highly cost-effective (*Clin Infect Dis* 1998;27:191). For PCP treatment, dapsone/trimethoprim is as effective as TMP-SMX for patients with mild or moderately severe disease (*Ann Intern Med* 1996;124:792).

PHARMACOLOGY

- **Bioavailability:** Nearly completely absorbed except with gastric achlorhydria (dapsone is insoluble at neutral pH).
- **T½:** 10 to 56 hours (average 28 hours)
- **Elimination:** Hepatic concentration, enterohepatic circulation, maintains tissue levels 3 weeks after treatment is discontinued.
- **Dose modification in renal failure:** None

SIDE EFFECTS

- **Most common in AIDS patients:** Rash, pruritus, hepatitis, hemolytic anemia, and/or neutropenia in 20% to 40% receiving dapsone prophylaxis for PCP at a dose of 100 mg/day.

Drugs: Dapsone

- **Most serious reaction:** Dose-dependent hemolytic anemia, with or without G6-PD deficiency, and methemoglobinemia; rare cases of agranulocytosis (0.2-0.4%) and aplastic anemia. Suggested monitoring includes screening for G6-PD deficiency prior to treatment, especially in high-risk patients, including African-American men and men of Mediterranean extraction. G6-PD deficiency is not a contraindication to dapsone in the case of the African variant but enhances need for monitoring; dapsone should not be used with the Mediterranean variant of G6-PD deficiency. Hemolysis and Heinz body formation are exaggerated in patients with a G6-PD deficiency, methemoglobin reductase deficiency, or hemoglobin M. Asymptomatic methemoglobinemia independent of G6-PD deficiency has been found in up to two thirds of patients receiving 100 mg dapsone/day plus trimethoprim (*N Engl J Med* 1990;373:776). Acute methemoglobinemia is uncommon, but the usual features are dyspnea, fatigue, cyanosis, deceptively high pulse oximetry, and chocolate-colored blood (*J Acquir Immune Defic Syndr* 1996;12:477). Methemoglobin levels are related to the dose and duration of dapsone therapy; TMP increases dapsone levels, so TMP may precipitate methemoglobinemia. Methemoglobin levels are usually <25%, which is generally tolerated except in patients with lung disease. Patients with glutathione or G6-PD deficiency are at increased risk. The usual laboratory findings are increased indirect bilirubin, haptoglobin <25 mg/dL, elevated LDH, and a smear showing spherocytes and fragmented RBCs. For G6-PD deficiency elevation, see p. 37. Treatment consists of oxygen supplementation, transfusion for anemia, and discontinuation of the implicated drug. This is usually adequate if the methemoglobin level is <30%. Activated charcoal (20 mg qid) may be given to reduce dapsone levels. Treatment for severe cases in the absence of G6-PD deficiency is IV methylene blue (1-2 mg/kg by slow IV infusion). In less emergent situations methylene blue may be given orally (3-5 mg/kg q4h-q6h); methylene blue should not be given with G6-PD deficiency because methylene blue reduction requires G6-PD; hemodialysis also enhances elimination.

- **GI intolerance:** Common; may reduce by taking with meals.

- **Infrequent ADRs:** Headache, dizziness, peripheral neuropathy. Rare side effect is "sulfone syndrome" after 1 to 4 weeks of treatment, consisting of fever, malaise, exfoliative dermatitis, hepatic necrosis, lymphadenopathy, and anemia with methemoglobinemia (*Arch Dermatol* 1981;117:38).

DRUG INTERACTIONS: Decreased dapsone absorption – buffered ddI, H_2 blockers, antacids, omeprazole, and other proton pump inhibitors. Dapsone levels decreased 7- to 10-fold by rifampin; use alternative. Trimethoprim – increases levels of both drugs; monitor for methemo-globinemia. Coumadin – increased hypoprothrombinemia;

pyrimethamine – increased marrow toxicity (monitor CBC); probenecid – increases dapsone levels; primaquine – hemolysis due to G6-PD deficiency.

RELATIVE CONTRAINDICATIONS: G6-PD deficiency – monitor hematocrit and methemoglobin levels if anemia develops.

PREGNANCY: Category C. No data in animals; limited experience in pregnant patients with Hansen's disease shows no toxicity. Hemolytic anemia with passage in breast milk reported (*Clin Infect Dis* 1995; 21[suppl 1]:S24).

DARAPRIM – see Pyrimethamine (p. 278)

DAUNORUBICIN CITRATE LIPOSOME INJECTION

TRADE NAME: *DaunoXome* (Gilead Sciences)

NOTE: Liposomal doxorubicin (*Doxil*), 20 mg/M^2 every 2 weeks, is equally as effective.

FORM AND PRICE: Vials containing equivalent of 50 mg daunorubicin at $442.19/50 mg vial

CLASS: Daunorubicin encapsulated within lipid vesicles or liposomes

INDICATIONS AND DOSES (FDA labeling): First-line cytotoxic therapy for advanced HIV-associated Kaposi's sarcoma (KS). Usual indications in trials are symptomatic visceral KS, >25 skin lesions, "B" symptoms, or lymphedema. Administer IV over 60 minutes in dose of 40 mg/M^2; repeat every 2 weeks. CBC should be obtained before each infusion and therapy withheld if absolute leukocyte count is <750/mL. Treatment is continued until there is evidence of tumor progression with new visceral lesions, progressive visceral disease, >10 new cutaneous lesions, or 25% increase in the number of lesions compared with baseline. Dose adjustment for hepatic impairment: bilirubin 1.2-3 mg/dL: 3/4 of a normal dose; bilirubin >3 mg/dL: 1/2 of normal dose.

CLINICAL TRIALS: Controlled trials comparing liposomal doxorubicin (*Doxil*) or liposomal daunorubicin vs chemotherapy show better response and less toxicity with *Doxil* and *DaunoXome*, which are considered equivalent (*J Clin Oncol* 1996;14:2353; *J Clin Oncol* 1998;16:2445; *J Clin Oncol* 1998;16:683).

PHARMACOLOGY: Mechanism of selectively targeting tumor cells is unknown. Once at the tumor, daunorubicin is released over time.

SIDE EFFECTS

- **Granulocytopenia** is the most common toxicity requiring monitoring of the CBC.

- **Cardiotoxicity** is the most serious side effect. It is most common in patients who have previously received anthracyclines or who have preexisting heart disease. Common features of cardiomyopathy are decreased left ventricular ejection fraction (LVEF) and usual clinical features of congestive heart failure. Cardiac function (history and physical examination) should be evaluated before each infusion, and LVEF should be monitored when the total dose is 320 mg/M^2, 480 mg/M^2, and every 160 mg/m^2 thereafter.
- **The triad of back pain, flushing, and chest tightness** is reported in 14%; this usually occurs in the first 5 minutes of treatment, resolves with discontinuation of the infusion, and does not recur with resumption of infusion at a slower rate.
- Care should be exercised to avoid drug extravasation, which can cause tissue necrosis.

DRUG INTERACTIONS: Additive bone marrow suppression with AZT, ganciclovir, and pyremethamine; monitor closely with co-administration.

PREGNANCY: Category D. Studies in rats showed severe maternal toxicity, embryolethality, fetal malformations, and embryotoxicity.

ddC – see Zalcitabine (p. 321)

ddl – see Didanosine (p. 180)

DELAVIRDINE (DLV)

TRADE NAME: *Rescriptor* (Pfizer)

CLASS: NNRTI

FORMULATIONS AND REGIMENS
- **Forms:** Tabs, 100 and 200 mg
- **Regimens:** 100 mg tabs – 400 mg tid, dispersed in ≥3 oz water (slurry). 200 mg tabs – 400 mg tid, take intact

FOOD EFFECT: None

ANTACIDS AND BUFFERED DDI: Separate dosing by ≥1 hr

RENAL FAILURE: Standard dose

HEPATIC FAILURE: No recommendation; uses with caution

PATIENT ASSISTANCE PROGRAM: 888-777-6637

ADVANTAGES: Virtually none

5 Drugs: Delavirdine

DISADVANTAGES: Limited efficacy data; requires tid dosing; limited experience

CLINICAL TRIALS

- **Study 0071** showed equivalence between DLV + ddl vs ddl monotherapy with regard to CD4 response and viral load. ACTG 261 found DLV/AZT, DLV/ddl, and AZT/ddl to be equivalent with respect to VL suppression. In an as-treated analysis of **protocol 0021-2** at 52 weeks, 70% of patients receiving DLV/AZT/3TC had viral loads <400/mL accompanied by CD4 cell count increases of 49-135/mm^3. The viral load results were significantly superior to those achieved with AZT/3TC or DLV/AZT. In **protocol 0073** DLV (600 mg bid) + NFV (1250 mg bid) + ddl ± d4T produced a good virologic response at 40 weeks. **Protocol 0081** was a pilot study of DLV/AZT/3TC/SQV using varying doses of DLV (600 mg bid or 400 mg tid) and SQV (1400 mg bid or 1000-1200 mg tid). Pharmacokinetic and virologic studies favored DLV 600 mg/SQV 1400 mg bid; at 24 weeks viral load was <400 c/mL in 83% of 24 patients receiving this combination (8th CROI, Chicago, Illinois, February 2001, Abstract 331).

PHARMACOLOGY

- **Bioavailability:** Absorption is 85%; there are no food restrictions. Food reduces absorption by 20%. Antacids, buffered ddl, and gastric achlorhydria decrease absorption. Separate buffered medications and antacids by ≥1 hour.

- **Distribution:** CSF: Plasma ratio=0.02

- **T½:** 5.8 hours

- **Elimination:** Primarily metabolized by hepatic cytochrome P450 (CYP3A4) enzymes. DLV inhibits cytochrome P450 CYP3A4, indicating that it inhibits its own metabolism as well as that of IDV, NFV, RTV, and SQV. Excretion is in urine (50%) and stool (44%). The standard dose is recommended in renal failure.

- **Dose reduction in renal or hepatic failure:** None; consider empiric dose reduction with severe liver disease.

SIDE EFFECTS: Rash noted in about 18%; 4% require drug discontinuation. Rash is diffuse, maculopapular, red, and predominantly on upper body and proximal arms. Erythema multiforme and Stevens-Johnson syndrome have been reported. Duration of rash averages 2 weeks and usually does not require dose reduction or discontinuation (after interrupted treatment). Rash accompanied by fever, mucous membrane involvement, swelling, or arthralgias should prompt discontinuation of treatment. Hepatotoxicity – less frequent and severe than with NVP. Other side effects include headache.

DRUG INTERACTIONS: Inhibits cytochrome P450 enzymes. The following drugs should not be used concurrently: Terfenadine (*Seldane*), rifampin, rifabutin, simvastatin, lovastatin, ergot derivatives, astemizole, cisapride, midazolam, alprazolam, triazolam, simvastatin, lovastatin, H_2 blockers, and proton pump inhibitors. Other drugs that either probably or definitely have increased half-life when given with DLV: Clarithromycin, quinidine, amiodirone, bepridil, lidocaine, propafenone, sirolimus, tacorolimus, cyclosporine, flecainide, atorvastatin, warfarin, quinidine, sildenafi, and other ED medicationsl; sildenafil should not exceed 25 mg/48 hours; vardenafil should not exceed 2.5 mg/24 hours. Ethinyl estradiol levels decrease 20%; use alternative or additional method of birth control. Ketoconazole levels increase 50%. There is no change in DLV with methadone. Drugs that decrease levels of DLV: Carbamazepine, phenobarbital, phenytoin, rifabutin and rifampin. Absorption of DLV is decreased with antacids, buffered ddl (administer ≥1 hour apart), H_2 blockers, and proton pump inhibitors.

■ TABLE 5-13: **DLV Combined with PIs**

Drug	AUC	Regimen
IDV	IDV ↑>40% DLV no change	IDV 600 mg q8h DLV 400 mg tid; limited data
RTV	RTV ↑70% DLV no change	No data
SQV (*Fortovase*)	SQV ↑5x DLV no change	*Fortovase* 800 mg tid DLV 400 mg tid (monitor transaminase levels)
NFV	NFV ↑2x DLV ↓50%	NFV 1250 mg bid DLV 600 mg bid (limited data); not recommended
APV	APV ↑125% DLV ↓60%	Not recommended
LPV/r	LPV ↑8% to 134% DLV no change	Limited data
ATV	No data	No data; not recommended
FPV	No data	No data; not recommended
TPV	No data	No data; not recommended

PREGNANCY: Category C. Ventricular septal defects in rodent teratogenicity assay; placental passage studies show a newborn:maternal drug ratio of 0.15. DLV is not recommended for use in pregnancy due to concerns about teratogenicity in animals and lack of experience in patients.

d4T – see Stavudine (p. 295)

DESYREL – see Trazodone (p. 312)

Drugs: Delavirdine

5

DIDANOSINE (ddl)

TRADE NAMES: *Videx* and *Videx EC* (Bristol-Myers Squibb)

CLASS: Nucleoside analog

FORMULATIONS, REGIMENS AND PRICE

- **Forms**
  - Enteric coated caps (*Videx EC*): 125, 200, 250 and 400 mg
  - Buffered chewable tabs (*Videx*): 25, 50, 100, 150 and 200 mg
  - Buffered powder: 100, 167 and 250 mg

- **Regimens**
  - Enteric coated
    - For patients <60 kg: 250 mg qd; with TDF, 200 mg qd; see Warning.
    - For patients >60 kg: 400 mg qd; with TDF 250 mg qd; see Warning.
  - Buffered chewable tabs
    - For patients <60 kg: 250 mg qd or 125 mg bid; with TDF, 200 mg qd; see Warning.
  - Buffered powder: As above.

-----

* Videx EC: Generic form available and comparable EC formulation often preferred due to better tolerance, once-daily dosing and avoidance of buffer-related drug interactions (including ATV and IDV) and buffer-related side effects (diarrhea) (*J Infect Dis* 2001;28:150).

Warning: ddl/TDF: TDF increases levels of ddl, risking ddl toxicity, but adjusted ddl doses (*Videx EC* 250 mg qd) has been associated with excessive virologic failure, especially when combined with NNRTIs (see drug interactions). As a consequence the DHHS Guidelines panel has recommended avoidance of ddl/TDF/NNRTI (July 7, 2004). The European Agency for Evaluation of Medicinal Products recommends avoiding TDF/ddl completely (http://www.emea.eu.int/pdfs/human/press/pus/509403en.pdf).

- **AWP:** $260/month.

FOOD EFFECT: Food decreases ddl EC and buffered ddl levels 27% and 47%, respectively; must take >30 min before or >2 h after meal.

RENAL FAILURE

CrCl 30-59 mL/min	10-29 mL/min	<10 mL/min
>60 kg: 200 mg/d	125 mg/d	125 mg/d
<60 kg: 125 mg/d	100 mg/d	75 mg/d

Drugs: Didanosine

HEPATIC FAILURE: Standard dose

FINANCIAL ASSISTANCE: 800-272-4878

ADVANTAGES: Once daily therapy; extensive experience

DISADVANTAGES: Need for empty stomach; toxicity profile including pancreatitis, neuropathy, and other mitochondrial toxicities; restricted use with TDF and d4T, and contraindicated with ribavirin.

RESISTANCE: L74V and K65R are the most important resistance mutations. The L74V mutation results in cross-resistance to abacavir, and the K65R mutation causes cross-resistance with abacavir and tenofovir DF. Susceptibility to ddI is decreased with the accumulation of multiple TAMs. M184 results in a modest decrease in susceptibility to ddI, but it is not clinically significant unless combined with other mutations,

CLINICAL TRIALS: ddI has been included in numerous trials in combination with 3TC, d4T, FTC, and AZT.

- **ACTG 384** is one of the few studies that defined a significant difference between NRTI combinations in HAART (*N Engl J Med* 2003;349:2293). The trial compared AZT/3TC vs ddI/d4T, each in combination with NFV or EFV. Results with 980 participants at a median follow-up of 2.3 years showed superior virologic outcomes with EFV/AZT/3TC compared with EFV/ddI/d4T or to either NRTI combination with NFV. Treatment-limiting toxicity, especially peripheral neuropathy, was significantly greater with ddI/d4T. The conclusion is that ddI should not be paired with d4T based on this and other studies demonstrating excessive rates of peripheral neuropathy, lactic acidosis and pancreatitis (BMS warning letter to providers 1/5/01).

- **Jaguar:** ddI intensification after virologic failure produced a median decrease in VL of 0.5 $\log_{10}$ c/mL at week 4 (*J Infect Dis* 2005;191:840). The decrease in VL correlated with TAMs: 0-1, 0.8-1.0 $\log_{10}$ c/mL; 2, 0.7 $\log_{10}$ c/mL; ≥3, no significant response. L74V mutation also predicted failure to respond. Clinical cut-offs were defined in this study using the *PhenoSense* assay. Those with a fold-change (FC) ≤1.3 had the best response to addition of ddI; those with FC between 1.3 and 2.2 had an intermediate response; and those with FC ≥2.2 had minimal response (12th CROI, Boston, 2005, Abstr. 105).

PHARMACOLOGY

- **Bioavailability:** Tablet – 40%; powder – 30%; food decreases bioavailability by 47% with buffered ddI, 27% with ddI EC. Take all formulations on an empty stomach.

- **T½:** 1.5 hours

- **Intracellular T½:** 25 to 40 hours

5 Drugs: Didanosine

- **CNS penetration:** CSF levels are 20% of serum levels (CSF: plasma ratio=0.16-0.19).

- **Elimination:** Renal excretion: 40% unchanged in urine. Renal failure: p. 180.

CAUTION: FDA warning for ddI + ribavirin based on 23 cases of pancreatitis and/or lactic acidosis; use with caution. Tenofovir increases levels of ddI; dose reduction to 250 mg/day (for >60 kg) or 200 mg/day (for <60 kg). The combination of d4T + ddI is contraindicated in pregnant women and should be avoided in all patients.

SIDE EFFECTS

- **Pancreatitis (Black box FDA warning):** Reported in 1% to 9% (7%-9% in the pre-HAART era; it is <1% in the HAART era). ddI-associated pancreatitis is fatal in 6% (*J Infect Dis* 1997;175:255). The frequency of pancreatitis is dose-related. The drug should be discontinued if there is clinical evidence of pancreatitis. In November 1999, Bristol-Myers Squibb issued a warning about pancreatitis as a result of four deaths ascribed to this complication in an ACTG trial. Analysis of these cases and those reported to the FDA MedWatch showed that most cases were associated with ddI/d4T with or without hydroxyurea. Risk factors for ddI-associated pancreatitis include renal failure, alcohol abuse, morbid obesity, history of pancreatitis, hypertriglyceridemia, cholelithiasis, endoscopic retrograde cholangio-pancreatography (ERCP), and concurrent use of d4T, hydroxyurea, allopurinol, or pentamidine.

- **Peripheral neuropathy** with pain, numbness, and/or paresthesias in extremities. Frequency is 5% to 12%; it is increased significantly when ddI is given with d4T, hydroxyurea, or both (*AIDS* 2000;14:273). Onset usually occurs at 2 to 6 months of ddI therapy and may be persistent and debilitating if ddI is continued despite symptoms.

- **GI intolerance** with buffered tablets and powder are common. For that reason, *Videx EC* is the preferred formulation because it causes fewer GI side effects. If the buffered ddI preparation is used, an alternative is to use ddI pediatric powder reconstituted with 200 mL water and mixed with 200 mL *Mylanta DS* or *Maalox* extra strength with anti-gas suspension in patient's choice of flavor. The final concentration is 10 mg/mL, and the usual dose is 25 mL.

- **Hepatitis** with increased transaminase levels

- **Miscellaneous:** Rash, marrow suppression, hyperuricemia, hypokalemia, hypocalcemia, hypomagnesemia, optic neuritis, and retinal changes

- **Sodium load in buffered formulations:** 11.5 mEq/tab and 60 mEq/powder packet. Mg^{++} load: 8.6 mEq/tab (may be problematic in renal failure).

Drugs: Didanosine

- **Class adverse effect:** Lactic acidosis and severe hepatomegaly with hepatic steatosis caused by mitochondrial toxicity. This complication should be considered in patients with fatigue, abdominal pain, nausea, vomiting, and dyspnea. Laboratory studies show elevated serum lactate (>2 mmol/L), CPK, ALT, and/or LDH and low bicarbonate. CT scan or liver biopsy may show steatosis. This is a life-threatening reaction, and NRTIs should be stopped if the serum lactate level is >2 mmol/L with typical symptoms; most cases are associated with lactate levels >5 mmol/L. The most frequent cause is ddI/d4T. This combination should be avoided, especially in pregnancy (Black box FDA warning), based on reports of at least two fatal cases. Didanosine can presumably cause lipoatrophy, which is also believed to be mediated by mitochondrial toxicity.

DRUG INTERACTIONS

- **Tenofovir:** Concurrent use of TDF and ddI results in a 28% increase in the ddI AUC. This occurs whether given with food or in a fasting state, whether administered simultaneously or separately, and whether ddI is given in buffered or EC formulation. The risk is ddI-associated side effects including lactic acidosis and pancreatitis. The recommendation is to prevent overexposure to ddI, but this has been complicated by suspiciously high failure rates, especially when used with NNRTI-based HAART. This combination should be avoided completely in NRTI-naïve patients and patients without TAMs because of their high risk for selection of K65R and high rates of virologic failure (*AIDS* 2005;19:1695; *AIDS* 2005;19:1183; *Antiviral Ther* 2005;10:171). There is also concern about several reports of blunted CD4 response with this combination (*AIDS* 2005;19:569; *AIDS* 2005;19:1107; *AIDS* 2005;19:569).

- **Buffered formulation:** Drugs that require gastric acidity for absorption, including IDV, TPV, DLV, ATV, ketoconazole, tetracyclines, and fluoroquinolones, should be given 1 to 2 hours before or after ddI if the buffered formulation is used. (This limitation does not apply to NFV, APV, SQV, EFV, or NVP, and it does not apply when using *Videx EC*).

- **Alcohol:** The package insert states that patients taking ddI should avoid alcohol because it may increase the risk of pancreatitis or liver damage. However, there is no evidence that moderate alcohol consumption increases the risk of ddI-induced pancreatitis or hepatotoxicity.

- **Drugs that cause peripheral neuropathy** should be used with caution or avoided: EMB, INH, vincristine, gold, disulfiram, or cisplatin. Concurrent use of d4T and/or hydroxyurea potentiates the risk of peripheral neuropathy and pancreatitis. Co-administration of ddI and ddC is contraindicated due to anticipated high rates of peripheral neuropathy and pancreatitis.

5 Drugs: Didanosine

- **Atazanavir:** buffered ddI reduces ATV AUC 87%; use ddI-EC. The combination of ATV and any form of ddI requires separate administration, since ddI is taken on an empty stomach and ATV is taken with food. If using buffered formulation, give ATV 2 hours before or 1 hour after buffered ddI.
- **Tipranivir:** Separate administration by 2 h.
- **Methadone** reduces AUC of buffered ddI by 41%; ddI has no effect on methadone levels (*J Acquir Immune Defic Syndr* 2000;24:241). Use ddI EC (not affected by methadone).
- **Allopurinol** increases ddI concentrations. Avoid co-administration.
- **Oral ganciclovir** increases ddI AUC by 100% when administered 2 hours after ddI or concurrently. Monitor for ddI toxicity and consider dose reduction.
- **Ribavirin** increases intracellular levels of ddI and may cause serious toxicity; avoid combination (*Antiviral Ther* 2004;9:133).

PREGNANCY: Category B. No lifetime harm in rodent teratogen and carcinogenicity studies; placental passage in humans shows newborn:maternal drug ratio of 0.5; no controlled studies have been performed in humans. Pharmacokinetics are not altered in pregnancy (*J Infect Dis* 1999;180:1536). ddI appears safe, but the combination of ddI and d4T should be avoided in pregnancy due to excessive rates of lactic acidosis and hepatic steatosis.

DIFLUCAN – see Fluconazole (p. 206)

DOXYCYCLINE

TRADE NAMES: *Vibramycin* (Pfizer), *Doryx* (Warner Chilcott), or generic

FORMS AND PRICES: 50 mg cap, 100 mg tab at $1.10. IV form 100 mg at $14.80

CLASS: Tetracycline

INDICATIONS AND DOSE: 100 mg PO bid
- ***C. trachomatis:*** 100 mg PO bid x 7 days. Common respiratory tract infections (sinusitis, otitis, bronchitis) – 100 mg PO bid x 7 to 14 days
- **Bacillary angiomatosis:** 100 mg PO bid x ≥3 months; lifelong with relapse
- **Syphilis (primary, secondary, and early latent) in patients with contraindication to penicillin:** 100 mg bid x 14 days + close monitoring
- **Respiratory tract infections (sinusitis, pneumonia, otitis):** 100 mg bid x 7 days

PHARMACOLOGY

- **Bioavailability:** 93%. Complexes with polyvalent cations (Ca^{++}, Mg^{++}, Fe^{++}, Al^{+++}, etc.), so milk, mineral preparations, cathartics, and antacids with metal salts should not be given concurrently.
- **T½:** 18 hours
- **Elimination:** Excreted in stool as chelated inactive agent independent of renal and hepatic function.
- **Dose modification with renal or hepatic failure:** None

SIDE EFFECTS: GI intolerance (10% and dose-related, reduced with food), diarrhea; deposited in developing teeth – contraindicated from mid-pregnancy to term and in children <8 years of age (Committee on Drugs, American Academy of Pediatrics); photosensitivity (exaggerated sunburn); *Candida* vaginitis; "black tongue;" rash.

DRUG INTERACTIONS: Chelation with cations to reduce oral absorption; half-life of doxycycline decreased by carbamazepine (*Tegretol*), cimetidine, phenytoin, barbiturates; may interfere with oral contraceptives; potentiates oral hypoglycemics, digoxin, and lithium.

PREGNANCY: Category D. Use in pregnant women and infants may cause retardation of skeletal development and bone growth; tetracyclines localizes in dentin and enamel of developing teeth to cause enamel hypoplasia and yellow-brown discoloration. Tetracyclines should be avoided in pregnant women and children <8 years unless benefits outweigh these risks.

DRONABINOL

TRADE NAME: *Marinol* (Unimed Pharmaceuticals)

FORMS AND PRICES: Gel-caps: 2.5 mg at $5.05, 5 mg at $10.52, 10 mg at $19.32

CLASS: Psychoactive component of marijuana

INDICATION AND DOSE: For anorexia associated with weight loss (also used in higher doses as antiemetic in cancer patients). Long-term therapy with dronabinol has led to significant improvement in appetite but no significant weight gain in two controlled trials (*J Pain Sympt Manage* 1995;10:89; *AIDS Res Hum Retroviruses* 1997;13:305). When weight gain is achieved, it is primarily due to an increase in body fat (*J Pain Symptom Manage* 1997;14:7; *AIDS* 1992;6:127). Based on these observations, dronabinol is not recommended in federal guidelines or nutrition in HIV management (*Clin Infect Dis* 2003;36[suppl 2]:S69).

- 2.5 mg bid (before lunch and before dinner)
- CNS symptoms (dose-related mood high, confusion, dizziness, somnolence) usually resolve in 1 to 3 days with continued use. If

5 Drugs: Dronabinol

these symptoms are severe or persist, reduce dose to 2.5 mg before dinner and/or administer at hs.

- If tolerated and additional therapeutic effect desired, increase dose to 5 mg bid.
- 10 mg bid is occasionally required, especially for control of nausea.

PHARMACOLOGY
- **Bioavailability:** 90% to 95%
- **T½:** 25 to 36 hours
- **Elimination:** First-pass hepatic metabolism and biliary excretion; 10% to 15% in urine.
- **Biologic effects post dose**
  - Onset of action: 0.5 to 1.0 hour, peak 24 hours
  - Duration of psychoactive effect: 4 to 6 hours; appetite effect: ≥24 hours

SIDE EFFECTS (dose-related)
- 3% to 10%: CNS with "high" (euphoria), somnolence, dizziness, paranoia, GI intolerance, anxiety, emotional lability, confusion
- Others: Depersonalization, confusion, visual difficulties, central sympathomimetic effects, hypotension, palpitations, vasodilation, tachycardia, and asthenia

DRUG INTERACTIONS: Sympathomimetic agents (amphetamines, cocaine) – increased hypertension and tachycardia; anticholinergic drugs (atropine, scopolamine), amitriptyline, amoxapine, and other tricyclic antidepressants – tachycardia, drowsiness.

WARNINGS: Dronabinol is a psychoactive component of *Cannabis sativa* (marijuana).

- **Schedule II (CII):** Potential for abuse. Use with caution in patients with psychiatric illness (mania, depression, schizophrenia), with cardiac disorder (hypotension), and in elderly patients. Caution should also be exercised in patients concurrently receiving sedatives and/or hypnotics and in patients with history of or current substance abuse.
- **Warn patient of the following:**
  - CNS depression with concurrent use of alcohol, benzodiazepines, barbiturates.
  - Avoid driving, operating machinery, etc. until safety and tolerance is established.
  - Mood and behavior changes.

PREGNANCY: Category C

EFAVIRENZ (EFV)

TRADE NAME: *Sustiva* (Bristol-Myers Squibb), *Stocrin* (Merck)

CLASS: NNRTI

FORMULATIONS, REGIMENS AND PRICE

- **Forms:** Caps 50, 100 and 200 mg; tabs 600 mg
- **Regimens:** 600 mg qd
- **AWP:** $420/month

FOOD EFFECT: Take on empty stomach or with a low-fat meal; a concurrent meal increases AUC 20% and peak level 40-50%, which may increase side effects. Take on empty stomach for initial 2-3 wks to minimize CNS side effects.

RENAL FAILURE: Standard dose

HEPATIC FAILURE: No recommendations; use with caution

PATIENT ASSISTANCE PROGRAM: 800-272-4878

INDICATIONS AND DOSE: EFV-based HAART is a favored regimen for treatment-naïve patients without pregnancy potential (Chapter 4). The standard dose is 600 mg/day, usually in combination with two nucleosides, taken in the evening to reduce the CNS side effects that are common in the first 2 to 3 weeks. Patients should be warned of these side effects and of the possibility of rash. When changing from a PI-containing regimen to EFV, consider overlapping the PI and EFV by 1-2 weeks because this is the time required to reach therapeutic levels. When discontinuing antiretrovirals, discontinue EFV 1-2 weeks earlier than NRTIs to account for the long "washout," thus avoiding monotherapy (11th CROI, San Francisco, Feb. 2004, Abstr. 131). Alternatively, substitute a PI for EFV for 1 to 4 weeks before discontinuing regimen. A high fat/caloric meal increases peak concentration 40% to 80%, so some advocate avoidance of concurrent food, especially in the first 2-3 weeks, to reduce CNS toxicity. May be taken with food if tolerated after CNS side effects have resolved.

- **Time:** EFV is usually taken at hs, presumably so that major CNS effects go unnoticed during sleep. Morning dosing is safe, effective and sometimes preferred due to sleep disturbances (3rd IAS Conf, Rio, 2005, Abstr. WePe 12.3 C03).

ADVANTAGES: EFV-based HAART is superior or comparable to all comparators for initial treatment in multiple clinical trials; sustained activity with 5-year follow-up; once daily therapy; low pill burden; minimal food effect.

DISADVANTAGES: High rate of CNS effects in first 2-3 weeks; single mutation confers high-level resistance to NNRTI class; potential for teratogenicity if used in first trimester of pregnancy.

Drugs: Efavirenz

5

Comparative Trials of EFV-based HAART in Treatment-naïve Patients

Study	Comparison	N	Dur (wk.)	VL <50	VL <200-400
DuPont 006 (*N Engl J Med* 1999;341:1865)	EFV/3TC/AZT	154	48	64%*	70%
	IDV/AZT/3TC	148		43%	48%
	IDV/EFV	148		47%	53%
ACTG 384 (*N Engl J Med* 2003;349:2293)	EFV/3TC/AZT	155	48		88%
	EFV/ddI/d4T	155			63%
	NFV/3TC/AZT	155			67%
	NFV/ddI/d4T	155			68%
	NFV/EFV/3TC/AZT	182			84%
	NFV/EFV/ddI/d4T	178			81%
Gilead 903 (*JAMA* 2004;292:191)	EFV/TDF/3TC	299	48	78%	82%
	EFV/d4T/3TC	301		74%	78%
CLASS (XIV Internal Aids Conf, 07/04, Abst TuOrB1189)	APV/r /3TC/ABC	96	48	59%	75%
	d4T/3TC/ABC	98		60%	81%
	EFV/3TC/ABC	97		72%	80%
2NN (*Lancet* 2004;363:180)	EFV/3TC/d4T	400	48	70%	—
	NVP/3TC/d4T	387		65%	—
Gilead FTC 301A (*JAMA* 2004;292:180)	EFV/FTC/ddI	286	60	78%*	81%
	EFV/d4T/ddI	285		59%	68%
INITIO (12th CROI 2/05, Abst 165 LB)	EFV/ddI/d4T	915	192	74%	
	NFV/ddI/d4T			62%	
	EFV/NFV/ddI/d4T			62%	
ACTG 5095 (*N Engl J Med* 12004;350:1850)	EFV/3TC/AZT ± ABC	765	32	83%*	89%
	AZT/3TC/ABC	382		61%	74%
BMS 034 (*J Acquir Immun Defic Syndr* 2004;36:1011)	ATV/AZT/3TC	286	98	32%**	70%
	EFV/AZT/3TC	280		37%	64%
GS 934 (3rd IAS, 2005, WeOa0202)	TDF/FTC/EFV	255	48	77%*	81%*
	AZT/3TC/EFV	254	48	68%	70%
ESS 30009 (*JAMA* 2001;285:1155)	ABC/3TC/TDF	102	12**		51%†
	ABC/3TC/EFV	169	48	71%*	75%*

*Superior to comparator arm (*P*<0.05)

**Low value compared to other studies attributed to failure to use optimal transport medium.

† Arm terminated early due to high failure rate.

Drugs: Efavirenz

- **Comparison with NVP**
  - **2NN.** The trial randomized 1147 treatment-naïve patients to receive EFV, NVP qd, NVP bid, or EFV/NVP, each in combination with 3TC/d4T. By ITT analysis at 48 weeks, the frequency of VL <50 c/mL was: EFV – 70%, NVP bid – 65.4%, NVP once daily – 70% and NVP/EFV – 62.7% EFV and NVP were comparable but did not meet equivalency criteria (*Lancet* 2004;350:1850). The only significant difference was between EFV and EFV/NVP. The median increase in CD4 count was 150-170/mm^3 in all four groups.

- **Treatment-experienced patients**
  - **DuPont 020** included 327 NRTI-experienced patients with a CD4 cell count >50/mm^3, viral load >10,000 c/mL, and no prior treatment with NNRTIs or PIs randomized to EFV/IDV + one to two NRTIs vs IDV + one to two NRTIs. At 24 weeks, 60% in the EFV arm had an undetectable viral load (<400 c/mL) compared with 50% in the IDV arm without EFV (*P* <0.05) (*J Infect Dis* 2001;183:392).
  - **M98-957** was a salvage trial involving 57 patients who failed more than two PI-containing regimens (40th ICAAC, Toronto, Canada, September 2000, Abstract 697). Participants received LPV/r in two doses, each in combination with EFV. At 48 weeks VL was <400 c/mL in 71% who received high-dose LPV/r (533/133 mg bid) vs 59% in the group that received 400/100 mg bid by ITT analysis.
  - **ACTG 364** enrolled 195 patients who failed treatment with NRTIs but were naïve to PIs and NNRTIs. Participants received one to two NRTIs + NFV, EFV, or NFV/EFV. VL was <50 c/mL in 22%, 44%, and 67%, respectively at 40-48 wks. The superior results with EFV vs NFV were statistically significant (*N Engl J Med* 2001;345:398).
  - **HIV-NAT 009:** Open-label trial of EFV (600 mg qd)/IDV (800 mg bid)/RTV (100 mg bid) in 61 patients with virologic failure with a nucleoside regimen (10 CROI, Boston, MA, 2003, Abstr 566). At 48 weeks 53 (87%) had viral load <50 c/mL, a median VL decrease of -2.3 log$_{10}$ c/mL and a median CD4 increase of 116/mm^3.

- **Switch studies**
  - **DMP 049** was a study of patients who were responding well to PI-containing HAART regimens with viral load <20 c/mL and were randomized to continue the PI-based regimen or switch to EFV (8th CROI, Chicago, 2001, Abstract 20). At 48 weeks, VL was <50 c/mL in 97% of the EFV arm and 85% of the PI continuation arm.
  - **ALIZE – ANRS 099** was a randomized trial of switch to EFV/FTC/ddl qd vs continued PI-based HAART in patients with viral suppression. At 12 months outcomes were comparable among the 355 patients for viral suppression (*J Infect Dis* 2005;191:830).

□ **A5116** examined the relative merits of LPV/r (533/133 mg bid) + EFV 600 mg qd vs. EFV alone to simplify treatment in patients with viral suppression on IDV-based HAART. Among 236 participants, EFV alone was superior in terms of viral suppression and tolerance (12th CROI, Boston, Feb. 2005, Abstr. 162).

□ **Other "Switch Studies:"** There are multiple studies that address the issue of lipodystrophy complicating PI-based HAART to determine the effect of changing to EFV-based HAART vs continuation of the original regimen. A review of 14 such studies with 910 patients (*Topics HIV Med* 2002;10:47) showed virologic failure in only 6 patients. Effects on triglycerides and cholesterol were variable, and lipodystrophy was rarely changed (see Table 4-25, p. 97). One report showed pravastatin was a more effective strategy (12th CROI, Boston, Feb. 2005, Abstr. 859).

- **NRTI-sparing regimen:** The combination most extensively studied is EFV (600 mg qd) + IDV (1000 mg q8h). In trial DMP-003, 74% had <50 c/mL at 48 weeks; in trial DMP-024, 53% had <50 c/mL at 24 weeks. These results are inferior to those achieved with EFV + two NRTIs, but may be useful in patients who cannot take nucleosides. Other NRTI-sparing options containing EFV are EFV/ATV/r and EFV/LPV/r (EFV 600 mg qd + LPV/r 533/133 mg bid or 4 tabs bid) (*Antimicrob Ag Chemother* 2003;47:350).

RESISTANCE: The K103N mutation causes high-level resistance to EFV as well as NVP and DLV. This mutation is associated with high levels of resistance to all currently available NNRTIs and does not reduce HIV fitness. This is a major concern with discontinuation of EFV-containing regimens, since it results in a period of EFV monotherapy due to the long half-life of EPV (see p. 79). Other RT mutations associated with reduced susceptibility are RT codons 100I, 106M, 108I, 181C/I, 188L, 190S/A, and 225H. The 181C/I mutation is not selected by EFV, but this mutation contributes to low-level EFV resistance; clinical significance is not known. One study of 29 patients who failed NNRTI failure showed 70% had persistence of mutations 103N and 181C/I at 1 year (*Antimicrob Agents Chemother* 2004;48:172). NNRTIs are not active against HIV-2.

PHARMACOLOGY

- **Oral bioavailability:** 40% to 45% without food; high-fat meals increase absorption of both capsule and tablet forms by 39% and 79%, respectively, should be avoided in patients who are experiencing CNS side effects. Serum levels are highly variable for reasons that are unclear (*AIDS* 2001;15:71) and this variation explains some of the variations in virologic response (*Antimicrob Agents Chemother* 2004;48:979).

- **T½:** 36-100 hr (11th CROI, San Francisco, 2004, Abstr. 131)

Drugs: Efavirenz

- **Distribution:** Highly protein-bound (>99%); CSF levels are 0.25% to 1.2% plasma levels, which is above the IC_{95} for wild-type HIV (*J Infect Dis* 1999;180:862). Virologic failure correlates with levels <1.1 mg/L (12th CROI, Boston, Feb. 2005, Abstr. 80).
- **Elimination:** Metabolized by cytochrome P450 (CYP3A4 and CYP2B6); 14% to 34% excreted in the urine as glucuronide metabolites and 16% to 61% in stool.
- **Dose modification with renal or hepatic disease:** No dose modification (*AIDS* 2000;14:618; *AIDS* 2000;14:1062). More frequent monitoring is advocated when given with hepatic disease.

SIDE EFFECTS

- **Rash:** Approximately 15% to 27% develop a rash, which is usually morbilliform and does not require discontinuation of the drug. More serious rash reactions that require discontinuation are blistering and desquamating rashes, noted in about 1% to 2% of patients, and Stevens-Johnson syndrome, which has been reported in 1 of 2,200 recipients of EFV. The median time of onset of the rash is 11 days, and the duration with continued treatment is 14 days. The frequency with which the rash requires discontinuation of EFV is 1.7% compared with 7% given NVP and 4.3% given DLV.
- **CNS** side effects have been noted in up to 52% of patients but are sufficiently severe to require discontinuation in only 2% to 5%. Symptoms are noted on day 1 and usually resolve after 2 to 4 weeks. They include confusion, abnormal thinking, impaired concentration, depersonalization, abnormal dreams, and dizziness. Other side effects include somnolence, insomnia, amnesia, hallucinations, and euphoria. Patients need to be warned of these side effects before starting therapy and should also be told that symptoms improve with continued dosing and rarely persist longer than 2 to 4 weeks. It is recommended that the drug be given in the evening on an empty stomach during the initial weeks of treatment. This reduces side effects but does not eliminate them because of the long half-life of EFV. There is a potential additive effect with alcohol or other psychoactive drugs. Patients need to be cautioned to avoid driving or other potentially dangerous activities if they experience these symptoms.
- Serious psychiatric disorders have been reported in recipients of EFV, including severe depression in 2.4% (Bristol-Myers Squibb letter to providers, March 2005).
- **Hyperlipidemia:** The D:A:D study showed that EFV is associated with increased triglyceride and total cholesterol levels; these effects were greater for EFV compared to NVP (*J Infect Dis* 2004;189:1056). One study of 636 patients given IDV-based HAART vs EFV-based HAART showed no significant difference in lipid profiles (*HIV Clin Trials* 2003;4:29).

5 Drugs: Efavirenz

- **False-positive urine cannabinoid (marijuana) test:** This occurs with the screening test only, and only with the Microgenic's *CEDIA DAU* Multilevel THC assay.
- **Increased transaminase levels:** Levels >5 x ULN in 2% to 8% (*Hepatology* 2002;35:182; *HIV Clin Trials* 2003;4:115). Frequency is increased with hepatitis C or with concurrent hepatotoxic drugs. Hepatotoxicity is less frequent and less severe than seen with NVP – grade 3-4 in 12% given NVP vs 4% given EFV in one study of 298 patients (*HIV Clin Trials* 2003;4:115). The mechanism is unknown. Discontinuation of EFV is recommended if hepatotoxicity is symptomatic (infrequent) or ascribed to hypersensitivity, or if the transaminase levels are >10x ULN in the absence of other causes (grade IV) (*Clin Liver Dis* 2003;7:475). Some authorities recommend discontinuation with transaminase levels >5x ULN.

DRUG INTERACTIONS: EFV both induces and, to a lesser extent, inhibits the cytochrome P450 CYP3A4 enzymes. Enzyme induction has been observed in the majority of PK studies.

CONTRAINDICATED DRUGS FOR CONCURRENT USE: Astemizole, terfenadine, midazolam, triazolam, cisapride, ergot alkaloids, St. John's wort, and voriconazole

OTHER DRUGS WITH SIGNIFICANT INTERACTIONS: Drugs contraindicated for concurrent use are **astemizole**, **terfenadine**, **cisapride**, **midzolam**, **trizolam**, **ergot derivatives**, **voriconazole** and **St. John's wort**. EFV may reduce concentrations of **phenobarbital**, **phenytoin**, and **carbamazepine**; monitor levels of anticonvulsant. **Rifampin** decreases EFV levels by 25%; rifampin levels are unchanged: Use standard dose of rifampin and increased dose of EFV (800 mg qd). **Rifabutin** has no effect on EFV levels, but EFV reduces levels of rifabutin by 35%; with concurrent use, the recommended dose of rifabutin is 450-600 mg/day or 600 mg 3x/week plus the standard EFV dose (*MMWR* 2002;51[RR-7]:48). Concurrent use with **ethinyl estradiol** increases levels of the contraceptive by 37%; implications are unclear, but a second form of contraception is recommended. EFV reduces **methadone** levels by 52%; titrate methadone levels to avoid opiate withdrawal. EFV also decreases levels of **buprenorphine** but may be preferred to methadone in opiate-dependent patients since no withdrawal symptoms were observed (12th CROI, Boston, Feb. 2005, Abstr. 653). EFV ↓ simvastatin AUC by 58%, and ↓ **atorvastatin** AUC by 43%, and an increase in statin dose may be needed, but do not exceed the maximum dose. **Atorvastatin**, **pravastatin**, **rosuvastatin**, or **fluvastatin** may be preferred. Monitor carefully when using **warfarin** with EFV. There is a 46% incidence of rash reactions when combining EFV and **clarithromycin**, and levels of clarithromycin are decreased 39%; consider **azithromycin**. Interactions and dose recommendations for EFV in combination with PIs are listed in Table 5-15, p. 193.

Drugs: Efavirenz

■ TABLE 5-15: **PI Interactions and Dose Recommendations**

PI	PI AUC	EFV AUC	Recommendation
IDV	↓31%	No change	IDV 1000 mg q8h + EFV 600 mg qhs or IDV 800 mg bid + RTV 200 mg bid + EFV 600 mg qd
RTV	↑18%	↑21%	RTV 500-600 mg bid + EFV 600 mg qhs
NFV	↑20%	No change	NFV 1250 mg bid + EFV 600 mg qhs
SQV	↓62%	↓12%	Not recommended when SQV is used as single PI
APV	↓36%	No change	APV 1200 mg tid + EFV 600 mg qhs or APV 600 mg bid + RTV 100 mg bid + EFV 600 mg qhs
SQV/RTV	No change	No change	Standard doses; qd dosing not recommended
LPV/r	↓40%	No change	LPV/r 533/133 mg (4 caps) bid + EFV 600 mg qhs
ATV	↓74%	No change	ATV 300 mg qd + RTV 100 mg qd + EFV 600 mg qd; unboosted ATV not recommended
FPV	No change	No change	FPV 700 mg bid + RTV 100 mg bid + EFV 600 mg qhs or FPV 1400 mg qd + RTV 300 mg qd + EFV 600 mg qd
TPV	No change	No change	TPV 500 mg/RTV 200 mg bid + EFV 600 mg qhs

COMBINATION OF 2 PIs/EFV

- EFV 600 mg qd/SQV 400 mg bid + RTV 400 mg bid
- EFV 600 mg qd/APV 600-1200 mg bid/RTV 100-200 mg bid
- EFV/RTV/IDV combination is under study. Consider EFV 600 mg qd + IDV 800 mg bid + RTV 200 mg bid.
- EFV/APV/LPV/r under study with EFV 600 mg qd + APV 750 mg bid + LPV/r 4 caps bid.
- EFV 600 mg qd/ATV 300 mg/RTV 100 mg qd
- EFV 600 mg qd/FPV 700 mg bid/RTV 100 mg bid or EFV 600 mg qd + FPV 1400 mg qd + RTV 300 mg qd

PREGNANCY: Category D. This drug caused birth defects (anencephaly, anophthalmia, and microphthalmia) in 3 of 20 gravid cynomolgus monkeys. There have been four cases of neural tube defects in infants born to women with first-trimester exposures to EFV, including three with meningomyeloceles and one with Dandy-Walker syndrome (Bristol-Myers Squibb letter to providers, March 2005). The Antiretroviral Pregnancy Registry shows birth defects in 5 of 188 live births associated with EFV exposures, all in the first trimester. None was a neural tube defect. EFV should be avoided in the first trimester, and women with childbearing potential should be warned of this. Safety in the second or third trimester is not established but should be safe since the neural tube has closed. Pregnant women exposed to EFV should be reported to the Antiretroviral Pregnancy Registry, 800-258-4263.

5 Drugs: Efavirenz

EMTRICITABINE (FTC)

TRADE NAME: *Emtriva* (Gilead Sciences)

CLASS: NRTI

FORMULATIONS, REGIMENS AND PRICE

- **Forms:** FTC – caps 200 mg; TDF/FTC (*Truvada*) – tab 300/200 mg
- **Regimens:** FTC, 200 mg qd; TDF/FTC, 1 tab qd
- **AWP:** FTC, $280/month; TDF/FTC, $800/month

FOOD EFFECTS: None

RENAL FAILURE: Adjust dosing of FTC as follows for CrCl (mL/min) levels: 30-49, 200 mg q 48 h; 15-29, 200 mg q 72 h; <15 or dialysis, 200 mg q 96 h. Adjust *Truvada* as above for CrCl levels ≥30 mL/min, but avoid at <30 mL/min.

HEPATIC FAILURE: No dose adjustment

PATIENT ASSISTANCE: 1-800-445-3235

ADVANTAGES: Potent antiretroviral activity, well tolerated, no food effect, longer intracellular half-life than 3TC, once-daily dosing. Delays TAMs.

DISADVANTAGES: Rapid selection of 184V RT mutation in non-suppressive regimen with substantial loss of activity. Active against HBV, but clinical experience is limited. 3TC has an advantage in co-formulations with AZT (*Combivir*) and AZT/ABC (*Trizivir*). Cutaneous hyperpigmentation (usually palms and soles) noted in some patients, especially dark skinned individuals. **Note:** Most authorities consider 3TC and FTC to be very comparable.

INDICATIONS: Similar to 3TC in activity against HIV, loss of most activity and rapid selection of M184V mutation, prolonged intracellular half-life and activity against HBV (*Antimicrob Agents Chemother* 2004;48: 3702). 3TC has been more extensively used and studied. FTC has a longer intracellular half-life.

CLINICAL TRIALS

- **Gilead 301A** was the FDA registration trial using FTC (200 mg qd) vs d4T, each in combination with ddI/EFV in 571 treatment-naïve patients. At 60 weeks, VL <50 c/mL was achieved in 76% of FTC recipients compared to 54% in the d4T group (P <0.001), and the CD4 cell count at 48 wks was greater with FTC, a mean of 156/mm³ vs. 119/mm³ (P = 0.01) (*JAMA* 2004;292:180).

- **Gilead 303** was a 3TC equivalence open label trial in which 440 patients receiving 3TC as a component of HAART were randomized to continue bid 3TC or to switch to qd FTC. VL was <50 c/mL in 72% and 67%, respectively at 48 weeks (p = NS) (*AIDS* 2004;18:2269).

Protocol 350, a continuation study, showed equivalent rates of viral suppression for these two groups for an additional 48 wks (*AIDS* 2004;18:2269).

- **ALIZE-ANRS 99:** Switch study in 335 patients randomized to continue PI-based HAART or switch to FTC/ddI/EFV qd. At 48 wks, 87% and 95% had VL <50 c/mL, respectively (*p* <0.05) (*J Infect Dis* 2005;191:830).

- **Abbott 418:** 190 treatment naïve patients were randomized to receive LPV/r 800/200 qd or LPV/r 400/100 bid, each with TDF 300 mg qd + FTC 200 mg qd. At 48 weeks 70% in the qd arm and 64% in the bid arm had a VL <50 c/mL (*p*=NS).

- **GS 934:** 517 treatment-naïve patients were randomized to receive co-formulated AZT/3TC + EFV or TDF + FTC + EFV. At 48 wks, more patients experienced virologic suppression in the TDF arm by ITT analysis, 81% vs. 70% <400 c/mL, 77% vs. 68% <50 c/mL. The difference was explained primarily by the higher proportion of discontinuations due to adverse events in the AZT/3TC arm (9% vs. 4%), most of which were due to anemia (3rd IAS, 2005, #WeOa0202).

RESISTANCE: Non-suppressive therapy with FTC results in the rapid selection of the M184V mutation, which confers high-level resistance to 3TC and FTC, modest decreases in susceptibility to abacavir and ddI. and increased susceptibility to TDF, AZT, and d4T. K65R, and multiple TAMS reduce activity of FTC 3- to 7-fold. All of these changes apply to 3TC as well (12th CROI, Boston, Feb. 2005, Abstr. 713).

PHARMACOLOGY

- **Bioavailability:** 93%, not altered by meals
- **Levels:** C_{max} 1.8 ± 0.7 µg/mL; C_{min} 0.09 µg/mL
- **Distribution:** Protein-binding <4%, concentrated in semen
- **T½:** plasma, 10 hours; intracellular, 39 hours (*Antimicrob Agents Chemother* 2004;48:1300).
- **Elimination:** 13% metabolized to sulfadioxide and glucoronide metabolites. Unchanged drug and metabolites are renally eliminated.

SIDE EFFECTS: Generally well tolerated with minimal toxicity. Occasionally, patients note nausea, diarrhea, headache, asthenia, or rash; about 1% discontinue the drug due to adverse effects. Lactic acidosis and steatosis, including fatal cases, have been reported with nucleosides. Skin hyperpigmentation has been noted primarily on palms and soles and almost exclusively in Africans and African-Americans. FTC is active against HBV, so discontinuation may result in HBV exacerbation **(FDA black box warning)**.

DRUG INTERACTIONS: None of clinical consequence are known.

PREGNANCY: Category B

5 Drugs: Emtricitabine

ENFUVIRTIDE (ENF, T20)

TRADE NAME: *Fuzeon* (Roche-Trimeris)

ADULT DOSE: 90 mg (1mL) SC q 12h into upper arm, anterior thigh or abdomen with each injection given at a site different from the preceding injection site. Prior to administration reconstitute with 1.1 mL of sterile water for injection, yielding a final volume of 1.2 mL.

FORMULATION: Enfuvirtide is packaged in a 30-day kit containing: 60 (90 mg) single-use vials of enfuvirtide, 60 vials of sterile water for injection, 60 reconstitution syringes (3 cc), 60 administration syringes (1 cc), and alcohol wipes. Enfuvirtide kit can be stored at room temperature. However, once enfuvirtide powder has been reconstituted, it must be refrigerated and used within 24 hours.

COST: 60-90 mg vials at $2,082 or $24,984/yr (AWP). Cost-effective analysis is estimated at $69,500/life-year saved (*J Acquir Immune Defic Syndr* 2005;39:69).

ADVANTAGE: New mechanism of action, potent antiviral activity, virtually no resistance in patients not previously treated with this drug, well studied in treatment-experienced patient.

DISADVANTAGES: Requirement for twice daily subcutaneous injections, local reactions at injection sites, need for concurrent use of at least one active drug to avoid monotherapy.

MECHANISM OF ACTION: Enfuvirtide binds to HR1 site in the gp41 subunit of the viral envelope glycoprotein and prevents conformational change required for viral fusion and entry into cells.

CLINICAL TRIALS: T-20-301 and T-20-302 (a.k.a. TORO 1-North America and Brazil, and TORO 2-Europe and Australia): Pooled data presented these to the FDA are from two randomized, controlled, open-label studies involving 995 treatment-experienced HIV-infected patients with virologic failure (*N Engl J Med* 2003;348:2175; *N Engl J Med* 2003; 348:2186). Enfuvirtide plus an individualized background regimen was superior to an optimized background regimen (OBR) only. Patients had a baseline viral load of 5.2 $\log_{10}$ c/mL, a mean of 12 prior antiretroviral agents, and 80% to 90% had ≥5 resistance mutations to NRTIs, NNRTIs, or PIs. The viral load change from baseline to week 24 was -1.52 $\log_{10}$ c/mL for patients in the enfuvirtide plus background regimen arm compared to -0.73 $\log_{10}$ for patient receiving only the OBR (P<0.0001). As expected, patients with two or more active antiretrovirals, based on history and genotype or phenotype resistance testing, were more likely to achieve a viral load <400 c/mL.

■ TABLE 5-16: **PI Interactions and Dose Recommendations**

Study	Regimen	No.	Dur (wks)	VL <50	VL <200-500
TORO 1 (*N Engl J Med* 2003;348:2175)	ENF/Optomized regimen	491	24	20%*	32%*
	Optomized Regimen Only (ORO)	165		7%	16%
TORO 2 (*N Engl J Med* 2003;348:2186)	ENF/Optomized regimen	335	24	12%*	28%*
	Optomized Regimen Only (ORO)	169		5%	14%
RESIST 1 (ICAAC 11/04 Abst 3726)	TPV/r/2 NRTIs/ENF	577	24	33%*	47%*
	CPI†/r/2 NRTIs			14%	22%

* Significantly better than comparator.

† Comparator PI

DRUG RESISTANCE AND CROSS-RESISTANCE: Resistance to ENF occurs rapidly with a nonsuppressive regimen (12th CROI, Boston, Feb. 2005, Abstr. 717). Resistance is correlated with mutations in the first heptad repeat (HR1) region of gp41 at codons 36, 38, 40, 42, 43 and 45 (*J Virol* 2005;79:4991). These mutations reduce fusion efficiency, resulting in reduced fitness. They do not cause cross-resistance with other entry inhibitors such as CCR5 and CXCR5 inhibitors. Discontinuation of ENV in patients with ENV-resistant strains results in a moderate increase in VL (12th CROI, Boston, Feb. 2005, Abstr. 680).

PHARMACOKINETIC

- **Absorption:** Well absorbed from subcutaneous (SC) site with an absolute bioavailability of 84.3%. Following 90 mg SC, the mean C_{max} was 5.0 mcg/mL, C_{min} was 3.3 mcg/mL, and AUC was 48.7 mcg/mL • hr. Virologic failure is associated with C trough levels <2.2 mcg/mL (12th CROI, Boston, Feb. 2005, Abstr. 643).

- **Distribution:** Vd=5.5. Levels in CSF are nil (12th CROI, Boston, Feb. 2005, Abstr. 402).

- **Protein binding:** 92%

- **Metabolism:** After SC injection, the drug is completely absorbed and largely catabolized, but about 17% is converted to an active deaminated form. Metabolism is not influenced by cytochrome P450 (*Clin Pharmacokinet* 2005;44:175).

- **T½:** 3.8 hours

DOSING WITH RENAL FAILURE: No dose adjustment (*Clin Infect Dis* 2004;39:119).

Drugs: Enfuvirtide

5

DOSING WITH HEPATIC INSUFFICIENCY: No data

DOSING WITH RENAL INSUFFICIENCY: Estimate CrCl>35 mL/min: 90 mg SC q12; CrCl <35 mL/min: A single case with modest renal insufficiency showed no change in pharmacokinetics (*Clin Infect Dis* 2004;39:119). Usual dose likely.

DRUG INTERACTIONS: None. *In vitro*, enfuvirtide did not inhibit or induce the metabolism of CYP3A4, CYP2D6, CYP1A2, CYP2C19 or CYP2E1 substrates. Does not interact with SQV/r, RTV, or rifampin [Boyd, et al. 10th CROI 2003, Abstract 541].

ADVERSE DRUG REACTIONS

- **Common ADRs:** A review by the FDA of 663 ENF recipients showed injection site reactions in 98%, including pain (96%; severe pain in 11%) induration (90%; severe in 57%), erythema (91%), nodules or cysts (80%) and/or pruritis (65%). Duration of the reaction was >3 days in 41% and >7 days in 24%. Treatment was discontinued in 7% due to these reactions (12th CROI, Boston, Feb. 2005, Abstr. 837). Successful desensitization has been reported (*Clin Infect Dis* 2004;39:110). Injection site reactions can be managed by rotating sites and massaging the area after injection. Excisional biopsies of these lesions show an excisional biopsy of the lesion, which demonstrated an inflammatory infiltrate consistent with drug hypersensitivity [Ball, et al. 10th CROI 2003, Abstract 714].

- **Occasional ADRs:** Bacterial pneumonia (event rate per 100 patients-years in trials was 4.68 in the treatment arm vs 0.61 in controls)

- **Rare ADRs:** Hypersensitivity with rash, nausea, vomiting, chills, fever, hypotension, and elevated transaminase, glomerulonephritis, thrombocytopenia, neutropenia, eosinophilia, fever, hyperglycemia, Guillain Barré syndrome, sixth nerve palsy, elevation in amylase and lipase (note that for rare ADRs, a causal relationship has not been established).

PREGNANCY/BREASTFEEDING RISKS: Category B. Not teratogenic in animal studies. There are no data concerning safety or pharmacokinetics in pregnancy. Breastfeeding not recommended.

ENTECAVIR (Baraclude)

CLASS: Guanosine nucleoside

FORMS: Tab 0.5 mg; oral solution 0.05 mg/mL (10 mL/day dose)

RECOMMENDED DOSE: 0.5 mg PO qd on empty stomach, 2 h before or after a meal. For patients who have failed lamivudine therapy for HBV or have known resistance to lamivudine, the dose is 1 mg qd on an empty stomach.

DOSE ADJUSTMENT FOR RENAL FAILURE: Usual adjustment at these CrCl (mL/min) levels: >50, 0.5 mg qd; 30-50, 0.25 mg qd; 10-30, 0.15 mg qd; <10 or dialysis, 0.05 mg qd. For lamivudine-resistant patients, adjust as follows: CrCl (mL/min) levels >50, 1 mg qd; 30-50, 0.50 mg qd; 10-30, 0.30 mg qd; <10 or dialysis, 0.1 mg qd.

HEPATIC FAILURE: No dose adjustment

INDICATIONS: Treatment of HBV infection in adults with evidence of viral replication + persistent elevations in ALT or AST or histologically active disease.

CLINICAL TRIALS

- Studies **A1463022** (HBeAg-neg) and **A1463027** (HBeAg-pos) included 430 patients with chronic HBV. Data at 48 wks showed 81% achieved a reduction in VL to <300 c/mL. No resistance to entecavir was detected.

■ TABLE 5-17: **Response of Chronic HBV to Entecavir Treatment (source: package insert)**

	A1463022 HBeAG Pos		A1463027 HBeAg Neg	
	Entecavir	Lamivudine	Entecavir	Lamivudine
Dose/d	0.5 mg	100 mg	0.5	100 mg
Sample size	314	314	296	287
Histologic Improvment	72%	62%	70%	61%
Fibrosis score improvement	39%	35%	36%	38%
	Lamivudine-refractory cases			
	Entecavir n=124		Lamivudine n=116	
Histologic improvement	55%*		28%	
Ishak fibrosis score improved	34%*		16%	
HBV DNA Undectectable (<300 c/mL)	19%*		1%	
Mean Viral load change (log_{10} c/mL)	-5.1%*		-0.5	
ALT normal (<1 x ULN)	61*		15%	
HBeAg seroconversion	8%		3%	

*Superior to treatment with 3TC (P <0.05)

- **Lamivudine-refractory infections:** There were 189 patients who received entecavir 1 mg/d. Genotypic analysis showed emergence of entecavir resistance in 13/189 (7%), including 3 who had virologic failure by week 48.

5 Drugs: Entecavir

RESISTANCE: In vitro tests show that lamivudine-resistant strains are 8- to 30-fold less sensitive to entecavir. Resistance to entecavir can emerge during treatment but is infrequent and requires additional reverse transcriptase mutations (*Antimicrob Agents Chemother* 2004;48:3498). HBV strains from patients who failed entecavir are resistant to lamivudine, but sensitive to adefovir.

PHARMACOLOGY

- **Bioavailability:** 100% for both oral solution and tablet forms when taken on an empty stomach. If taken with a fatty meal, the C_{max} is decreased 45% and AUC is decreased 18-20%.
- **T½:** 128-149 hrs
- **Elimination:** Entecavir does not induce or inhibit the P450 metabolic pathway. It is eliminated predominantly by renal clearance.

DRUG INTERACTIONS: None established

ADVERSE REACTIONS

- Similar to lamivudine in comparative trials for 48 wks
- Major severe reaction is lactic acidosis with steatosis, including fatalities
- Another serious adverse reaction is exacerbation of HBV when entecavir is discontinued

PREGNANCY: Category C

EPIVIR – see Lamivudine (3TC) (p. 241)

EPOGEN – see Erythropoietin (below)

ERYTHROPOIETIN (EPO)

TRADE NAME: *Procrit* (Ortho Biotech)

FORMS AND PRICES: Vials with 2000, 3000, 4000, 10,000, 20,000, and 40,000 units. Standard dose of 40,000 U/week costs $534.

PATIENT ASSISTANCE PROGRAM: 800-553-3851

PRODUCT INFORMATION: Recombinant human erythropoietin (rHU EPO) is a hormone produced by recombinant DNA technology. It has the same amino acid sequence and biologic effects as endogenous erythropoietin, which is produced primarily by the kidneys in response to hypoxia and anemia. Both forms act by stimulating the proliferation of red blood cells from progenitor cells found in the bone marrow.

Drugs: Entecavir

INDICATIONS: Serum erythropoietin level <500 milliunits/mL plus anemia ascribed to HIV infection, or to medications, including AZT in doses >600 mg/day (*Ann Intern Med* 1992;117:739; *J Acquir Immune Defic Syndr* 1992;5:847).

DOSE RECOMMENDATIONS: Although the FDA-approved dose for initial therapy is 10,000 U 3 times per week, the standard starting dose used in clinical practice is 40,000 U weekly, and trials investigating every-other-week dosing demonstrated good clinical efficacy (*Clin Infect Dis* 2004;38:1447). Onset of action is within 1 to 2 weeks, reticulocytosis is noted at 7 to 10 days, increases in hematocrit are noted in 2 to 6 weeks, and desired hematocrit is usually attained in 8 to 12 weeks. Response is dependent on the degree of initial anemia, baseline EPO level, dose, and available iron stores. Transferrin saturation should be ≥20%; serum ferritin should be ≥100 ng/mL. If levels are suboptimal, supplement with iron. (Some experts advocate routine iron supplementation in all patients taking EPO.) If after 4 weeks of therapy the Hb rise is <1 g/dL, dose may be increased to 60,000 U SQ weekly. After an additional 4 weeks, if Hb does not increase by at least 1 g/dL from baseline value, discontinue EPO therapy. After achieving the desired response (i.e., increased Hb/Hct level or reduction in transfusion requirements), titrate the dose for maintenance. If Hb >13 g/dL or Hct >40%, decrease EPO by 10,000-20,000 U/week or decrease dosing frequency (e.g., 40,000 U q 2 wks). When Hb is >15 g/dL, discontinue EPO, or adjust dose as above. With failure to respond or suboptimal response, consider iron deficiency, occult blood loss, folic acid or B12 deficiency, or hemolysis.

EFFICACY: A trial using EPO was performed in 1,943 patients with baseline serum EPO levels of <500 U/L and hematocrit <30%; including 75% receiving AZT at entry or at some point during the study period. The initial dose was 4,000 U SQ 6 days/week and the mean weekly doses ranged from 22,700-32,500 U/week (340-490 U/kg/week). Response to treatment, defined as an increase in baseline hematocrit by 6 percentage points (i.e., 30% to 36%) with no transfusions within 28 days, was achieved in 44%. Transfusion requirements were significantly reduced from 40% to 18% at 24 weeks and the average hematocrit increased from 28% to 35% at 1 year. Subset analysis demonstrated that this response was independent of AZT administration (*Int J Antimicrob Agent* 1997;8:189). In one study anemia was a risk factor for death, and this risk was decreased with EPO (*Clin Infect Dis* 1999;29:44).

PHARMACOLOGY

- **Bioavailability:** EPO is a 165-amino acid glycoprotein that is not absorbed with oral administration. IV or SC administration is required; SC is preferred.
- **T½:** 4 to 16 hours

- **Elimination:** Poorly understood but minimally affected by renal failure.
- **Dose adjustment in renal or hepatic failure:** None

SIDE EFFECTS: Generally well tolerated; adverse side effects reported in clinical trials are consistent with progression of HIV infection. Headache and arthralgias are most common; less common are flu-like symptoms, GI intolerance, diarrhea, edema, and fatigue. Hypertension is an uncommon complication that has been noted more frequently in patients with renal failure. EPO is contraindicated in patients with hypertension that is uncontrolled. The most common reactions noted in the therapeutic trial with 1,943 AIDS patients were rash, injection site reaction, nausea, hypertension, and seizures.

PREGNANCY: Category C. Teratogenic in animals; no studies in humans.

ETHAMBUTOL (EMB)

TRADE NAME: *Myambutol* (Lederle) or generic

FORM AND PRICE: 100 and 400 mg tab; 400 mg tabs at $1.78/tab

PATIENT ASSISTANT PROGRAM: 800-859-8586

INDICATIONS AND DOSE: Active tuberculosis or infections with *M. avium* complex or *M. kansasii* (see p. 360)

■ TABLE 5-18: **Ethambutol Dosing for Tuberculosis**

Dosing interval	Weight		
	40-55 kg	56-75 kg	76-90 kg
Daily	800 mg	1200 mg	1600 mg
2x/wk	2000 mg	2800 mg	4000 mg
3x/wk	1200 mg	2000 mg	2400 mg

PHARMACOLOGY
- **Bioavailability:** 77%
- **T½:** 3.1 hours
- **Elimination:** Renal
- **Dose modification in renal failure:** CrCl >50 mL/min – 15-25 mg/kg q24h; CrCl 10-50 mL/min – 15-25 mg/kg q24h-q36h; CrCl <10 mL/min – 15-25 mg/kg q48h

SIDE EFFECTS: Dose-related ocular toxicity (decreased acuity, restricted fields, scotomata, and loss of color discrimination) with 25 mg/kg dose (0.8%), hypersensitivity (0.1%); peripheral neuropathy (rare); GI intolerance

Drugs: Erythropoietin

WARNINGS: Patients to receive EMB in doses of 25 mg/kg should undergo a baseline screening for visual acuity and red-green color perception; this examination should be repeated at monthly intervals during treatment (*MMWR* 1998;47[RR-20]:31).

DRUG INTERACTIONS: Aluminum-containing antacids may decrease absorption.

PREGNANCY: Category C. Teratogenic in animals; no reported adverse effects in women with >320 case observations.

FAMCICLOVIR – see Acyclovir (p. 141)

FENOFIBRATE

TRADE NAME: *Tricor* (Abbott Laboratories), *Antara* (Reliant), *Lofibra* (Gate)

FORMS: Tricor tabs, 54 mg and 160 mg; Lofibra caps 67 mg, 134 mg, 200 mg, Antara caps, 43 and 130 mg

PRICES: 54 mg tab at $0.86, 160 mg tab at $2.58

CLASS: Fibrate

INDICATIONS AND DOSES: Hypertriglyceridemia, especially levels of >500-700 mg/dL. Starting dose 48 mg/day then increase if necessary at 4 to 8 week intervals; maximum dose – 145 mg/day. Take as a single daily dose with meal.

MONITORING: Triglyceride levels – discontinue use if response is inadequate after 2 months at 145 mg/day. Warn patients to report symptoms of myositis and obtain CPK if muscle tenderness, pain, or weakness. Monitor AST + ALT – discontinue if there is an otherwise unexplained increase to ≥3x ULN.

PRECAUTIONS: Avoid or use with caution with gallbladder disease, hepatic disease, renal failure with CrCl <50 mL/min.

PHARMACOLOGY

- **Bioavailability:** Good, improved 35% with food.
- **T½:** 20 hours
- **Elimination:** Renal – 60%; fecal – 25%
- **Renal failure:** 54 mg/day; increase with caution due to risk of myopathy, and monitor CPK.

5 Drugs: Fenofibrate

SIDE EFFECTS

- **Hepatic:** Dose-related hepatotoxicity with increased transaminase levels to >3x ULN in 6% receiving doses of 134-201 mg/day; most had return to normal levels with drug discontinuation or with continued treatment.
- **Influenza-like syndrome**
- **Rash, pruritus, and/or urticaria** in 1% to 3%
- **Myositis:** Warn patient regarding symptoms of muscle pain, tenderness, and/or weakness, especially with fever or malaise. Draw CPK and discontinue if significantly typical symptoms occur.
- **Rare:** Pancreatitis, agranulocytosis, cholecystitis, eczema, thrombocytopenia.

DRUG INTERACTIONS

- **Oral anticoagulants:** Potentiates warfarin activity.
- **Cholestyramine and colestipol:** These drugs bind fenofibrate – take fenofibrate >1 hour before or 4 to 6 hours after bile acid binding agent.
- **Statins:** Increased risk of rhabdomyolysis with renal failure.

PREGNANCY: Category C

FENTANYL

TRADE NAME: *Duragesic* (Janssen), *Fentanyl Oralet* (Abbott Laboratories)

FORMS AND PRICES

- Injection-fentanyl citrate, 50 µg/mL at $21
- Buccal (transmucosal) lozenge – 200, 300, 400 µg up to 4/day
- Transdermal
  - 25 µg/hour (10 cm^2) *Duragesic* 25: $12.80
  - 50 µg/hour (20 cm^2) *Duragesic* 50: $21.20
  - 75 µg/hour (30 cm^2) *Duragesic* 75: $33.80
  - 100 µg/hour (40 cm^2) *Duragesic* 100: $42.60

CLASS: Opiate; Schedule II controlled substance

INDICATIONS: Chronic pain requiring opiate analgesia

DOSING RECOMMENDATIONS

- Dose depends on desired therapeutic effect, patient weight, and most importantly, existing opiate tolerance. The initial dose in opiate-naïve patients is a system delivering 25 µg/hour.
- Cachectic patients should not receive a higher initial dose unless they have been receiving the equivalent of 135 mg of oral morphine. Most patients are maintained with patch applications at 72-hour

intervals. Adequacy of analgesia should be evaluated at 72 hours. The dose should be increased to maintain the 72-hour interval if possible, but application every 48 hours is another option. Supplemental opiates may be required with initial use to control pain and to determine optimal fentanyl dose. The suggested conversion ratio is 90 mg of oral morphine/24 hours to each 25 µg/hour labeled delivery. To convert patients who currently receive opiate therapy, the following daily doses are considered equivalent to 30-60 mg of oral morphine sulfate: Morphine sulfate, 10 mg IM; codeine 200 mg PO, heroin 5 mg IM or 60 mg PO, meperidine 75 mg IM, methadone 20 mg PO, and oxycodone 15 mg IM or 30 mg PO. The equivalent doses of fentanyl patches are listed in Table 5-19 below:

■ TABLE 5-19: **Equivalence of Fentanyl Patches and Oral Morphine Sulfate**

Oral MS/day	Fentanyl (µg/hour)	Oral MS	Fentanyl (µg/hour)
45-134 mg	25	495-584 mg	150
135-224 mg	50	675-764 mg	200
225-314 mg	75	855-994 mg	250
315-404 mg	100	1035-1124 mg	300

APPLICATION INSTRUCTIONS: The protective liner-cover should be peeled just prior to use. Application is to a dry, non-irritated, flat surface of the upper torso by firm pressure for 30 seconds. Hair should be clipped, not shaven, and the skin cleansed with water (not soaps or alcohol that could irritate skin) prior to application. Avoid external heat to the site because absorption is temperature-dependent. Rotate sites with sequential use. After removal, the used system should be folded so the adhesive side adheres to itself and flushed in the toilet.

NOTE: Buccal (transmucosal) form should be used only with monitoring in the hospital (OR, ICU, EW) due to life-threatening respiratory depression. Use in AIDS is primarily restricted to management of chronic pain in late-stage disease using the transdermal form. This drug should not be used for the management of acute pain.

PHARMACOLOGY: Transdermal fentanyl systems deliver an average of 25 µg/hour/10 cm^2 at a constant rate. Serum levels increase slowly, plateau at 12 to 24 hours, and then remain constant for up to 72 hours. The labeling indicates the amount of fentanyl delivered per hour. Peak serum levels for the different systems are the following: Fentanyl – 25: 0.3-1.2 ng/mL, 50: 0.6-1.8 ng/mL, 75: 1.1-2.6 ng/mL, and 100: 1.9-3.8 ng/mL. After discontinuation, serum levels decline with a mean half-life of 17 hours. Absorption depends on skin temperature and theoretically increases by one-third when the body temperature is 40° C. In acute pain models, the 100 µg/hour form provided analgesia equivalent to 60 mg of morphine IM.

5 Drugs: Fentanyl

- **Respiratory depression** with hypoventilation. This occurs throughout the therapeutic range of fentanyl concentration but increases at concentrations >2 ng/mL in opiate-naïve patients and in patients with pulmonary disease.

- **CNS depression** is seen with concentrations >3 ng/mL in opiate-naïve patients. At levels of 10-20 ng/mL there is anesthesia and profound respiratory depression.

- **Tolerance** occurs with extended courses, but there is considerable individual variation.

- **Local effects** include erythema, papules, pruritus, and edema at the site of application.

- **Drug interactions** include increased fentanyl levels with PIs and DLV given concurrently. Consider morphine with concurrent use with PIs.

PREGNANCY: Category C

FILGRASTIM – see G-CSF (p. 220)

FLAGYL – see Metronidazole (p. 255)

FLUCONAZOLE

TRADE NAME: *Diflucan* (Pfizer)

FORMS AND PRICE: Tabs: 50 mg, 100 mg at $9.78, 150 mg, 200 mg at $16.00. IV vials: 200 mg at $115.50, and 400 mg at $168.83

PATIENT ASSISTANCE PROGRAM: 800-207-8990

CLASS: Triazole related to other imidazoles – ketoconazole, clotrimazole, miconazole; triazoles (fluconazole and itraconazole) have three nitrogens in the azole ring.

DOSE: See Table 5-20, p. 208

RESISTANCE: Fluconazole is the preferred azole for systemic treatment of candidiasis, but the major concern with long-term use is azole-resistant *candidiasis*, which correlates with azole exposure and CD4 count <50/mm^3 (*J Infect Dis* 1996;173:219). All oral systemically active azoles predispose to resistance. Some cases involve evolution of resistance by *C. albicans*, and others reflect substitution with non-*albicans* species such as *C. glabrata* or *C. krusei* (*Antimicrob Agents Chemother* 2002;46:1723). Resistance is uncommon when fluconazole is used to treat vaginitis (*Clin Infect Dis* 2001;33:1069). Fluconazole-resistant strains of *Candida* can often be treated with caspofungin or amphoteracin B (*Antimicrob Agents Chemother* 2002;46:1723).

PHARMACOLOGY (see Table 5-20, p. 208

- **Bioavailability:** >90%
- **CSF levels:** 50% to 94% serum levels
- **T½:** 30 hours
- **Elimination:** Renal; 60% to 80% of administered dose excreted unchanged in the urine
- **Dose modification in renal failure:** CrCl >50 mL/min – usual dose; 10-50 mL/min – half dose; CrCl <10 mL/min – quarter dose

SIDE EFFECTS: GI intolerance (1.5% to 8%, usually does not require discontinuation); rash (5%); transient increases in hepatic enzymes (5%), increases of ALT or AST to >8x upper limit of normal requires discontinuation (1%); dizziness, hypokalemia, and headache (2%). Reversible alopecia in 10% to 20% receiving ≥400 mg/day at median time of 3 months after starting treatment (*Ann Intern Med* 1995;123:354).

DRUG INTERACTIONS: Inhibits cytochrome P450 (2C8/9 and 3A4) hepatic enzymes resulting in increased levels of atovaquone, some benzodiazepines, clarithromycin, opiate analgesics, warfarin, SQV, phenytoin, oral hypoglycemics, rifabutin, and cyclosoporine; cisapride (*Propulsid*), terfenadine and astemizole may cause life-threatening arrhythmias. Fluconazole levels are reduced with rifampin; with rifabutin there is no effect on fluconazole levels, but rifabutin AUC increases 80% – consider rifabutin dose of 150 mg/day. Can be used with PIs and NNRTIs without dose adjustments (unlike ketoconazole). Fluconazole increases AZT AUC 74% due to decreased AZT glucuronidation; monitor for AZT toxicity.

PREGNANCY: Category C. Animal studies show reduced maternal weight gain and embryolethality with dose >20x comparable to doses in humans; no studies in humans. Recommendation is for use only with systemic fungal infections. Avoid use for prophylaxis, thrush and vaginitis.

Drugs: Fluconazole

5

Indications	Dose Regimen*	Comment
CANDIDA		
Thrush		
Acute	100 mg PO x 7-14 days	Response rate 80% to 100%, usually within 5 days; may need up to 400-800 mg/day. Maintenance therapy often required in late-stage disease without immune reconstitution. Topical therapy (e.g., clotrimazole) preferred. Indication is severe or frequent recurrence. Risk of fluconazole resistance is increased (*Clin Infect Dis* 2000;30:749).
Prevention	100-200 mg PO qd	
Esophagitis		
Acute	200 mg/day PO or IV up to 800 mg/day x 14-21 days	Relapse rate is 85-90%. Relapse rate is >80% within 1 year in absence of maintenance therapy.
Prevention (maintenance)	100-200 mg PO qd	Maintenance generally is not recommended due to the risk of azole resistance.
Vaginitis	150 mg x 1 Multiple recurrences: Fluconazole 150 mg weekly	Response rate 90% to 100% in absence of HIV infection. Topical azoles generally preferred.
CRYPTOCOCCOSIS		
Non-meningeal, acute	200-400 mg/day PO or Amphotericin B	Fluconazole is recommended by the IDSA as the preferred treatment + flucytosine (100 mg/kg/day) for cryptococcal pneumonia (*Clin Infect Dis* 2000;3:710).
Meningitis		
Acute	400-800 mg/day PO x 10 to 12 wks, followed by maintenance	Acute treatment with amphotericin B x 2 weeks is preferred (*Clin Infect Dis* 2000;30:710). Alternative in patients with mild-to-moderate disease is fluconazole 400-800 mg/day x 10 to 12 weeks ± flucytosine (100 mg/kg/day x 6 weeks).
Consolidation (after Ampho induction)	400 mg PO qd x 8 weeks, followed by maintenance	Continue maintenance until immune reconstitution with CD4 >100-200/mm^3 x >6 months.
Maintenance	200 mg PO qd	
COCCIDIOIDOMYCOSIS		
Meningitis	400-800 mg IV or PO	Preferred for meningeal form.
Non-meningeal		
Acute	400-800 mg PO qd	Amphotericin B usually preferred, except with mild disease.
Maintenance	400 mg PO qd	Itraconazole considered equally effective.
HISTOPLASMOSIS		
Treatment	800 mg/day	Amphotericin B and itraconazole preferred.

Drugs: Fluconazole

FLUCYTOSINE (5-FC)

TRADE NAME: *Ancobon* (ICN Pharmaceuticals) or generic

FORMS AND PRICES: Caps: 250 mg at $4.53, 500 mg at $9.02

CLASS: Structurally related to fluorouracil

INDICATIONS AND DOSE: Used with amphotericin B or fluconazole to treat serious cryptococcosis. IDSA guidelines (*Clin Infect Dis* 2000;30: 710) recommend treating cryptococcal meningitis with amphotericin B + flucytosine 100 mg/kg/day in 4 doses for ≥2 weeks based on several studies showing benefit of this treatment (reduced rate of relapse and more rapid sterilization of CSF) compared with amphotericin B alone (*N Engl J Med* 1997;337:15; *N Engl J Med* 1992;326:83; *Ann Intern Med* 1990;113:183; *J Infect Dis* 1992;165:960; *Clin Infect Dis* 1999;28:291). The combination of fluconazole + flucytosine is also effective, but toxicity at higher doses may limit use of 5-FC (*Clin Infect Dis* 1994;19:741; *J Infect Dis* 1992;165:960). Flucytosine may also be combined with fluconazole for treatment of nonmeningeal cryptococcosis (*Clin Infect Dis* 2000;30:710).

- **Dose:** 25 mg/kg PO q6h (100 mg/kg/day)

PHARMACOLOGY

- **Bioavailability:** >80%
- **T½:** 2.4 to 4.8 hours
- **Elimination:** 63% to 84% unchanged in urine
- **CNS penetration:** 80% serum levels
- **Dose modification in renal failure:** CrCl >50 mL/min – 25.0-37.6 mg/kg q6h; 10-50 mL/min – 25-37 mg/kg q12h-q24h; <10 mL/min – 25 mg/kg q24h (use with close monitoring of CBC) and 5-FC serum level.
- **Therapeutic monitoring:** Measure serum concentration 2 hours post oral dose with goal of peak level of 50-100 mcg/mL.

SIDE EFFECTS: Dose-related leukopenia and thrombocytopenia, especially with levels >100 mcg/mL and concurrent use of other marrow-suppressing agents, and in patients with renal insufficiency, which can occur secondary to concurrent amphotericin B therapy; GI intolerance; rash; hepatitis; peripheral neuropathy.

PREGNANCY: Category C. Teratogenic in animals; no studies in human patients. Contraindicated in pregnancy except for serious systemic fungal infections after the first trimester.

Drugs: Flucytosine

FLUOROQUINOLONES

■ TABLE 5-21: **Fluoroquinolone Summary**

	Ciprofloxacin *Cipro*	Levofloxacin *Levaquin*	Gatifloxacin *Tequin*	Moxifloxacin *Avelox*
Oral form IV form	+ +	+ +	+ +	+ +
Price (AWP) oral formulation	$5.80 500 mg ($11.60/d)	$10.63 500-750 mg	$9.40 400 mg	$9.80 400 mg
T½	3.3 hours	6.3 hours	8 hours	12 hours
T½ renal failure	8 hours	35 hours	16 hours	12 hours
Oral bioavailability	65%	99%	96%	90%
Activity *in vitro** P. aeruginosa S. pneumoniae Mycobacteria Anaerobes	 +++(60% to 80%) + ++ —	 ++ ++ ++ +	 + ++ ++ ++	 + ++ ++ ++
Regimens (oral)	250-750 mg bid	500-750 mg qd	400 mg qd	400 mg qd

*All fluoroquinolones are active against most *Enterobacteriaceae,* enteric bacterial pathogens (except *C. jejuni* and *C. difficile*), methicillin-sensitive *S. aureus, Neisseria* spp., and pulmonary pathogens including *S. pneumoniae, H. influenzae, C. pneumoniae, Legionella,* and *M. pneumoniae.* Major advantages of newer fluoroquinolones are once-daily dosing, good tolerability, and activity against *S. pneumoniae,* including >98% of penicillin-resistant strains (*Antimicrob Agents Chemother* 2002;46:265). Class side effects include prolongation of QT interval when given to persons predisposed primarily by concurrent medications (macrolides, class IA and III anti-arrhythmics), tendon rupture (risk with age and steroids), and CNS toxicity including seizures. All are contraindicated in persons <18 years and in pregnant women. Divalent and trivalent cations reduce absorption – avoid concurrent antacids with Mg^{++} or Al^{++}, sucralfate, Fe^{++}, Zn^{++}, and buffered ddI. The major concern is abuse and resistance, with particular concern for *P. aeruginosa, S. pneumoniae, Staph aureus, C. jejuni,* and *Salmonella.*

FLUOXETINE

TRADE NAME: *Prozac* (Eli Lilly) or generic

FORMS AND PRICES: Caps: 10 mg at $2.60, 20 mg at $2.67, 40 mg at $5.33. Solution 20 mg/5 mL at $4.91/20 mg.

CLASS: Selective serotonin reuptake inhibitors (SSRI) antidepressant. Other drugs in this class include *Paxil, Zoloft, Celexa,* and *Lexapro.*

INDICATIONS AND DOSE

- **Major depression:** 10-40 mg/day usually given once daily in the morning. Onset of response requires 2 to 6 weeks. Doses of 5-10 mg/day may be adequate in debilitated patients.

- **Obsessive-compulsive disorder:** 20-80 mg/day

PHARMACOLOGY

- **Bioavailability:** 60% to 80%
- **T½:** 7 to 9 days for norfluoxetine (active metabolite)
- **Elimination:** Metabolized by liver to norfluoxetine; fluoxetine eliminated in urine.
- **Dose modification in renal failure:** None
- **Dose modification in cirrhosis:** Half-life prolonged – reduce dose

SIDE EFFECTS: Toxicity may not be apparent for 2 to 6 weeks. GI intolerance (anorexia, weight loss, nausea) – 20%; anxiety, agitation, insomnia, sexual dysfunction – 20%; less common – headache, tremor, drowsiness, dry mouth, sweating, diarrhea, acute dystonia, akathisia (sensation of motor restlessness).

NOTE: Case reports have suggested an association with suicidal ideation; reanalysis of data showed no significant difference compared with treatment with other antidepressants or placebo (*J Clin Psychopharmacol* 1991;11:166). Nevertheless, the FDA required manufacturers of SSRIs to add a warning label concerning increased risk of suicide with antidepressant initiation.

DRUG INTERACTIONS

- **MAO inhibitors:** Avoid initiation of treatment with fluoxetine until ≥14 days after discontinuing MAO inhibitor; avoid starting MAO inhibitor until ≥5 weeks after discontinuing fluoxetine (risk is "serotonergic syndrome").
- **Inhibits cytochrome P450:** Increased levels of tricyclic agents (desipramine, nortriptyline, etc.), phenytoin, digoxin, coumadin, terfenadine (ventricular arrhythmias; avoid), SQV, astemizole (avoid), theophylline, thioridazine, mesoridazine (contraindicated), haloperidol, carbamazepine.
- **Ritonavir:** Serotonin syndrome has been reported (*AIDS* 2001; 15:1281).
- **Linezolid:** Avoid co-administration. May increase risk of serotonin syndrome.

PREGNANCY: Category C

FLURAZEPAM – see Benzodiazepines (p. 160)

FOMIVIRSEN

TRADE NAME: *Vitravene* (Isis Pharmaceuticals); withdrawn from the market

5 Drugs: Fluoxetine

FORTOVASE – see Saquinavir (p. 291)

FOSAMPRENAVIR (FPV)

TRADE NAME: *Lexiva* (GlaxoSmithKline)

CLASS: Protease inhibitor (pro-drug of amprenavir)

PATIENT ASSISTANCE PROGRAM: 800-722-9294

FORMULATIONS, REGIMENS AND PRICE

- **Form:** FPV tab, 700 mg,
- **Regimen:** Dose is 1400 mg bid; FPV/r, dose is 700/100 bid or 1400/200 qd. Treatment-experienced patients should follow bid regimen.
- **AWP:** $1260/month

FOOD EFFECT: Not significant

EFV: With EFV, use RTV-boosted regimens. If using qd regimen, increase RTV dose to 300 mg qd.

RENAL FAILURE: Standard dose

HEPATIC FAILURE: Child-Pugh score: 5-8, FPV 700 mg bid without RTV boosting; >8, avoid FPV

STORAGE: Room temperature, 15-30°C

MAJOR TRIALS

■ TABLE 5-22: **Clinical Trials of FPV in Treatment-naïve Patients**

Trial	Regimen	No	Wks	VL (c/mL) <500	VL (c/mL) <50
SOLO Treatment-naïve (*AIDS* 2004;18:1529)	FPV/r 1400/200 mg qd/ABC/3TC	322	48	69%	55%
	NFV 1250 mg bid/ABC/3TC	327		68%	53%
NERT Treatment-naïve (*J Acquir Immun Defic Syndr* 2004;35:22)	FPV 1400 mg bid/ABC/3TC	166	48	66%*	58%*
	NFV 1250 mg bid/ABC/3TC	83		51%	42%
Context Failure 1-2 PI regimens (6th CROI 2003, Abstr. 178)	FPV/r 700/100 mg bid/2 NRTIs	315	48		46%*
	FPV/r 1400/200 mg qd/2 NRTI				37%
	LPV/r 400/100 mg bid/2 NRTIs				50%*
ACTG 5143 (*IDCP* 2004;12:191)	FPV vs LPV/r vs FPV + LPV/r — study stopped due to 69% decrease in C_{min} of LPV with FPV co-administration, but analysis of 56 of planned 216 subjects showed comparable efficiency (12th CROI, Boston, 2005, Abstr. 577).				

* Superior to comparator (P <0.05)

RESISTANCE: In trials of FPV in PI-naïve patients, the predominant mutations in patients experiencing virologic failure were 32I, L33F, 46I, 47V, and 54L/V/M, all mutations that cause minimal cross-resistance with other PIs. The primary PI mutations are I50V, which also confers resistance to LPV, and I84V, a multi-PI resistance mutation. Patients failing FPV/r in the SOLO trial had no PI mutations.

WARNINGS: Hepatic disease; see dose modification at p. 212.

ADVANTAGES: (1) Advantages over APV are reduced pill burden (4 vs 16); (2) no food requirement; (3) may be given qd; (4) Favorable resistance profile that may preserve PI options; (5) Less effect on serum lipids compared to smaller PIs unless boosted with RTV.

DISADVANTAGES: (1) Relatively new, so less is known about durability and long-term side effects; (2) once-daily therapy not recommended for PI-experienced patients.

PHARMACOLOGY

- **Absorption:** Not affected by food (unlike APV); bioavailability not established
- **Elimination:** APV is an inhibitor, inducer and substrate for P450 3A4
- **T½:** 7.7 hours

SIDE EFFECTS

- **Skin rash:** The most common adverse reaction is skin rash, seen in 12% to 33% of patients (package insert), that is sufficiently severe to result in discontinuation in <1%. FPV contains a sulfa moiety, so caution is advised with use in patients with a history of sulfa allergy, but no increase in rashes was noted in such patients in the registration trials.

- **GI intolerance** with nausea, vomiting, diarrhea and/or abdominal pain is reported in up to 40%, but severe in only 5% to 10%; compared to NFV (NEAT and SOLO trials), GI side effects were similar except for more diarrhea with NFV. GI intolerance rates appeared no more frequent or severe when FPV was combined with RTV 200 mg/day.

- **Hepatotoxicity:** ALT levels are increased >5x ULN in 6% to 8%
- **Lipids:** There appears to be no significant impact with FPV alone, but triglycerides are elevated to >750 mg/dL in 5% to 8% given RTV-boosted FPV.
- **Lipodystrophy:** Observed with FPV.

DRUG INTERACTIONS

- **The following drugs are contraindicated for concurrent use:** Astemizole, bepridil, cisapride, dihydroergotamine, ergotamine, midazolam, pimozide, terfenadine, triazolam, rifampin, simvastatin, and St. John's wort.

Drugs: Fosamprenavir

5

- **The following drugs should be given concurrently with caution:** Phenobarbital, phenytoin, and carbamazepine have potential to decrease APV levels and various effects on anticonvulsant levels – monitor anticonvulsant levels. Ethinyl estradiol/norethindrone decrease APV levels; alternative birth control methods should be used. Methadone levels decrease 35% and APV levels are decreased. Consider alternative antiretroviral agent; if used together, monitor for methadone withdrawal.

- **PIs:** See Table 5-6, p. 150

- **Other drug interactions:** Rifampin decreases APV AUC by 82% and should not be used concurrently. Rifabutin decreases APV AUC by 15% and APV increases rifabutin AUC by 193%; use standard APV dose and rifabutin at 150 mg qd or 300 mg 2-3x/week. Clarithromycin increases APV AUC by 18%; use standard doses of both drugs. Ketoconazole increases APV AUC by 32% and ketoconazole AUC increases 44%; use standard doses of both drugs. APV increases sildenafil AUC by 2-11x; do not exceed 25 mg/48 hours. Vardenafil AUC may also increase – limit dosage to 2.5 mg/24 hours (2.5 mg/72 hours with APV/RTV).

- TABLE 5-23: **Combination of FPV with Other PIs and with NNRTIs**

Combination recommended	Co-admin Drug	FPV	Comment
FPV/RTV 1400/200 mg qd 700/100 mg bid	ND	$\uparrow$100%	BID regimen recommended for treatment experienced
EFV + FPV/RTV 700/100 mg bid or 1400/300 mg qd	ND	C_{min} $\downarrow$36%	Note increased RTV dose with once daily regimen
ATV 300/FPV 1400/RTV 200 qd	1.9 µg/mL	8.9 µg/mL	Preliminary clinical and PK data good (3rd IAS, 7/05 Abstr. WePe 12.9 C14
NFV, IDV, SQV	ND	≠	Dose regimens not established
LPV/r 3 bid/FPV 700 mg bid + RTV 100 mg bid	C trough 66%	C trough 86%	Preliminary data support-uve (3rd IAS, 7/05 WePe 12.9 C12)

PREGNANCY: Category C. Animal studies showed no embryo-fetal developmental abnormalities. There are inadequate data on safety and pharmacokinetics in pregnancy to recommend use.

FOSCARNET

TRADE NAME: *Foscavir* (AstraZeneca)

FORMS AND PRICES: Vials: 6000 mg (250 mL) at $88.41 and 12,000 mg (500 mL)

INDICATIONS AND DOSING

■ TABLE 5-24: **Dose Recommendations for Foscarnet**

Indication	Dose Regimen
CMV retinitis	Induction: 60 mg/kg IV q8h or 90 mg/kg IV q12h x 14-21 days Maintenance: 90-120 mg/kg IV qd*
CMV (other)	60 mg/kg IV q8h or 90 mg/kg IV q12h x 14-21 days, indications for maintenance treatment are unclear
Acyclovir-resistant HSV	40 mg/kg IV q8h or 60 mg/kg q12h x 3 weeks
Acyclovir-resistant VZV	40 mg/kg IV q8h or 60 mg/kg q12h x 3 weeks

* Survival and time to relapse may be significantly prolonged with maintenance dose of 120 mg/day vs 90 mg/day (*J Infect Dis* 1993;168:444).

ACTIVITY: Active against herpesviruses including CMV, HSV-1, HSV-2, EBV (oral hairy leukoplakia), VZV, HHV-6, HHV-8 (KS-related herpes virus), most ganciclovir-resistant CMV, and most acyclovir-resistant HSV and VZV. Also active against HIV *in vitro* and *in vivo*. The frequency of CMV resistance *in vitro* is 20% to 30% after 6 to 12 months of foscarnet treatment (*J Infect Dis* 1998;177:770). Patients with CMV retinitis experienced a mean decrease of 0.5 $\log_{10}$ in HIV RNA/mL during foscarnet therapy (*J Infect Dis* 1995;172:225). The major clinical experience is with CMV retinitis, for which clinical effectiveness is equivalent to that of ganciclovir (*N Engl J Med* 1992;326:213; *Ophthalmology* 1994;101:1250). In two pre-HAART trials, foscarnet was associated with increased survival compared with ganciclovir (*N Engl J Med* 1992;326:213; *Am J Med* 1993;94:175) but had more treatment-limiting side effects. Many question the relevance of these data in the era of HAART. *In vitro* activity against HHV-8 is good, but results with foscarnet treatment of KS are variable; if KS is a true neoplasm, this treatment is of doubtful utility once malignant transformation has occurred (*Science* 1998;282:1837).

ADMINISTRATION: Controlled IV infusion using ≤24 mg/mL (undiluted) by central venous catheter or <12 mg/mL (diluted in 5% dextrose or saline) via a peripheral line. No other drug is to be given concurrently via the same catheter. Induction dose of 60 mg/kg is given over ≥1 hour via infusion pump with adequate hydration. Maintenance treatment with 90-120 mg/kg is given over ≥2 hours by infusion pump with adequate hydration. Many use 90 mg/kg/day for initial maintenance and 120 mg/kg/day for maintenance after re-induction for a relapse.

PHARMACOLOGY

- **Bioavailability:** 5% to 8% absorption with oral administration, but poorly tolerated

5 Drugs: Foscarnet

- **T½:** 3 hours
- **CSF levels:** 15% to 70% plasma levels
- **Elimination:** Renal exclusively

■ TABLE 5-24a: **Foscarnet Dose Adjustment in Renal Failure**

CrCl (mL/min/kg)	60 mg/kg Dose	90 mg/kg Dose	120 mg/kg Dose
>1.4	60	90	120
1.4-1.3	49	78	104
1.3-1.1	42	75	100
1.1-0.9	35	71	94
0.9-0.7	28	63	84
0.7-0.5	21	57	76

Hemodialysis: 60 mg/kg post-HD (consider serum level 500-800 mg M).

SIDE EFFECTS

- **Dose-related renal impairment:** 37% treated for CMV retinitis have serum creatinine increase to ≥2 mg/dL; most common in second week of induction and usually reversible with recovery of renal function within 1 week of discontinuation. Monitor creatinine 2 to 3x/week with induction and every 1 to 2 weeks during maintenance. Modify dose for creatinine clearance changes. Foscarnet should be stopped for creatinine clearance <0.4 mL/min/kg.

- **Changes in serum electrolytes** including hypocalcemia (15%), hypophosphatemia (8%), hypomagnesemia (15%), and hypokalemia (16%). Patients should be warned to report symptoms of hypocalcemia: Perioral paresthesias, extremity paresthesias, and numbness. Monitor serum calcium, magnesium, potassium, phosphate, and creatinine, usually ≥2x/week during induction and 1x/week during maintenance. If paresthesias develop with normal electrolytes, measure ionized calcium at start and end of infusion.

- **Seizures** (10%) related to renal failure and hypocalcemia

- **Penile ulcers**

- **Miscellaneous:** Nausea, vomiting, headache, rash, fever, hepatitis, marrow suppression

DRUG INTERACTIONS: Concurrent administration with IV pentamidine may cause severe hypocalcemia. Avoid concurrent use of potentially nephrotoxic drugs such as amphotericin B, aminoglycosides, and pentamidine. Possible increase in seizures with imipenem.

Drugs: Foscarnet

PREGNANCY: Category C. No adequate studies in animals or humans. Rcommended for treatment of life-threatening and site-threatening CMV infections.

FOSCAVIR – see Foscarnet (p. 214)

FUNGIZONE – see Amphotericin B (p. 147)

GANCICLOVIR AND VALGANCICLOVIR

TRADE NAME (IV AND ORAL FORMS)

- Ganciclovir: *Cytovene*, IV (Roche); *Vitrasert*, ocular implant (Bausch & Lomb)
- Valganciclovir: *Valcyte*, PO (Roche)

FORMS AND PRICES: Ganciclovir: 500 mg vial at $38.64. Valganciclovir: 450 mg at $31.46. Implant: $4,000/implant, $8,000/yr

Valganciclovir is the preferred oral formulation because it provides blood levels of ganciclovir comparable with those achieved with recommended doses of IV ganciclovir (*N Engl J Med* 2002;346:1119). Oral ganciclovir should no longer be used, and IV ganciclovir is reserved primarily for seriously ill patients and those who are unable to take oral medications.

PATIENT ASSISTANCE PROGRAM: 800-282-7780

CLASS: Synthetic purine nucleoside analog of guanine

ACTIVITY: Active against herpes viruses including CMV, HSV-1, HSV-2, EBV, VZV, HHV-6, and HHV-8 (KS). About 10% of patients given ganciclovir ≥3 months for CMV will excrete resistant strains that are sensitive to foscarnet (*J Infect Dis* 1991;163:716; *J Infect Dis* 1991;163:1348). The frequency of ganciclovir resistance at 9 months in patients receiving maintenance IV ganciclovir therapy for CMV retinitis is 26% (*J Infect Dis* 1998;177:770). Ganciclovir is active *in vitro* against HHV-8, but the clinical experience with ganciclovir treatment of KS is variable; if KS is a true neoplasm, it may be necessary to treat HHV-8-seropositive patients prior to malignant transformation (*Science* 1998;282:1837).

INDICATIONS AND DOSE REGIMEN

- **CMV Retinitis:** A controlled trial of 141 patients randomized to receive IV ganciclovir (5 mg/kg/bid x 3 weeks followed by 5 mg/kg) vs oral valganciclovir (900 mg bid x 3 weeks followed by 900 mg/day) showed comparable response rates (77% vs 72% at 4 weeks) and median time to progression (125 vs 160 days) (*N Engl J Med* 2002;346:1119). Oral valganciclovir is now the standard for ganciclovir treatment. Multiple trials show that IV ganciclovir, IV foscarnet, IV cidofovir, oral valganciclovir, and the ganciclovir implant are all effective, although time to relapse is longest with the implant (*N Engl J Med* 1997;337:83; *N Engl J Med* 1999;340:1063). Many authorities now prefer the sustained-release ganciclovir implant (*Vitrasert*), usually in combination with valganciclovir, to prevent systemic CMV disease and contralateral retinitis (*N Engl J Med* 1997;337:83;337:105; *Am J Ophthalmol* 1999;127:329). Current guidelines for initial management of CMV retinitis reflect this preference and are modified based on the probability of rapid vision loss and anticipated benefit from HAART as summarized in pp. 341-344. For early relapse, the options include reinduction with the same drug or combination treatment (*Ophthalmology* 1994;101:1250; *Arch Ophthalmol* 1996;114:23). Switching drugs for early relapse is usually not more effective than reinduction with the same drug (*Ophthalmology* 1994;101:1250). However, ganciclovir resistance rates increase to 26% by 9 months, so a foscarnet substitution is more likely to be effective in late relapses. The intraocular ganciclovir implant must be replaced every 6 to 8 months.

Discontinuation of maintenance therapy can be considered in the setting of immune reconstitution with a CD4 count >150/mm³ for 3 to 6 months (*JAMA* 1999;282:1633). The specific CDC/IDSA recommendation is to make this decision in consultation with an ophthalmologist based on magnitude and duration of the CD4 response, anatomic location of the lesion, vision in the other eye, and feasibility of ophthalmologic monitoring.

- **Other Forms of Disseminated CMV:** Ganciclovir or foscarnet are the standard agents to treat CMV esophagitis, colitis, pneumoniitis and neurologic disease (see Table 5-23 below and p. 314) (*AIDS* 2000;14:517; *Clin Infect Dis* 2002;34:101). Recommendations for suspending maintenance therapy with immune reconstitution are unclear for non-ocular CMV, but most will follow the guidelines for CMV retinitis using a CD4 threshold of 100-150 cells/mm³ x ≥3 months (*AIDS* 2001;15:F1). Failures ascribed to lack of CMV-specific CD4 responses with recurrent CMV retinitis have been reported (*J Infect Dis* 2001;183:1285).

PHARMACOLOGY

- **Bioavailability:** Valganciclovir – 60% absorption with food vs 6%-9% for oral ganciclovir. The valganciclovir formulation is rapidly hydrolyzed to ganciclovir after absorption.
- **Serum level:** Mean peak concentration with IV induction doses is 11.5 µg/mL (MIC$_{50}$ of CMV is 0.1-2.75 µg/mL).

Mean AUC with Valganciclovir Compared with IV Ganciclovir in Standard Doses (*N Engl J Med* 2002;346:1119)

	AUC (µg/hr/mL)	
	Valganciclovir	IV Ganciclovir
Induction	32.8	28.6
Maintenance	34.9	30.7

- **CSF Concentrations:** 24% to 70% of plasma levels; intravitreal concentrations: 10% to 15% of plasma levels – 0.96 µg/mL (*J Infect Dis* 1993;168:1506).

- **T½:** 2.5 to 3.6 hours with IV administration; 3 to 7 hours with oral administration. Intracellular T½ – 18 hours.

- **Elimination:** IV form: 90% to 99% excreted unchanged in urine. Oral form: 86% in stool and 5% recovered in urine.

- **Renal failure:** Hemodialysis removes 50% of ganciclovir (*Clin Pharmacol Ther* 2002;72:142).

■ TABLE 5-26: **Ganciclovir and Valganciclovir Dose Modification in Renal Failure (Induction Dose)**

Creatinine Clearance			
Ganciclovir (IV Form)		**Valganciclovir* (Oral Form)**	
>80 mL/min	5 mg/kg q12h	>60 mL/min	900 mg bid
50-79 mL/min	2.5 mg/kg q12h	40-59 mL/min	450 mg bid
25-49 mL/min	2.5 mg/kg q24h	25-39 mL/min	450 mg qd
10-24 mL/min	1.25 mg/kg q24h	10-24 mL/min	450 mg qod (induction); 450 biw (maintenance)
<10 mL/min	1.25 mg/kg tiw	<10 mL/min	Not recommended

*Hemodialysis: 1.25 mg/kg tiw; give post-dialysis.
 Maintenance dose = 50% of induction dose.

SIDE EFFECTS, IV FORM

- **Neutropenia** with ANC <500/mm³ (25% to 40%) requires discontinuation of drug in 20%. Alternative is administration of G-CSF. Discontinuation or reduced dose will result in increased ANC in 3 to 7 days. Monitor CBC 2 to 3x/week and discontinue if ANC <500/mm³ or platelet count <25,000/mm³.

- **Thrombocytopenia** in 2% to 8%

- **CNS toxicity** in 10% to 15% with headaches, seizures, confusion, coma

- **Hepatotoxicity** in 2% to 3%

- **GI intolerance** 2%

5 Drugs: Ganciclovir

- **Note:** Neutropenia (ANC <500/dL) or thrombocytopenia (<25,000/dL) are contraindications to initial use.

SIDE EFFECTS, ORAL FORM: Of 212 patients with CMV retinitis followed for a median of 272 days, 10% developed neutropenia with ANC <500/mm³, hemoglobin <8 g/mL in 12%, diarrhea in 35%, nausea in 23%, and fever in 18% (*J Acquir Immune Defic Syndr* 2002;30:392). This is similar to the side effects with oral or IV ganciclovir.

DRUG INTERACTIONS: AZT increases the risk of neutropenia, and concomitant use is not recommended. Other marrow-toxic drugs include interferon, sulfadiazine, hydroxyurea, pyrimethamine, and TMP-SMX. Oral and IV ganciclovir increase AUC of ddI by 100% – monitor for adverse effect of ddI or consider dose reduction of ddI. (Studies with enteric coated ddI have not been performed.) (*MMWR* 1999;48[RR-10]:48). Probenecid increases ganciclovir levels by 50%. Additive or synergistic activity with foscarnet *in vitro* against CMV and HSV. Use with caution with drugs that inhibit replication or rapidly dividing cells: dapsone, pentamidine, pyrimethamine, flucytosine, cytotoxic antineoplastic drugs (vincristine, vinblastine, doxorubicin), amphotericin B, TMP-SMX, and nucleoside analogs.

PREGNANCY: Category C. Teratogenic in animals in concentrations comparable to those achieved in humans; should be avoided unless need justifies the risk.

G-CSF (Filgrastim)

TRADE NAME: *Neupogen* (Amgen)

FORMS AND PRICE: 300 µg in 1 mL vial at $165.30 and 480 µg in 1.6 mL vial

REIMBURSEMENT ASSISTANCE/APPEAL: 800-272-9376

NOTE: 300 µg vial and 480 µg vial are the only forms available. Pharmacists commonly instruct patients to discard unused portion; the cost-effective alternative is to retain the unused portion in refrigerated syringes for later use. For example, a 75 µg dose = 1 immediate dose and 3 syringes with subsequent doses.

PATIENT INSTRUCTIONS: Subcutaneous injections are usually self administered into the abdomen or upper thighs or in the back of upper arms if injected by someone else. Injection sites should be rotated. The drug should be stored in a refrigerator at 36°F to 46°F.

PRODUCT INFORMATION: A 20-kilodalton glycoprotein produced by recombinant technique that stimulates granulocyte precursors.

INDICATIONS: Neutropenia with ANC <500-750/mm³ ascribed to 1) AZT (*Blood* 1991;77:2109), 2) Other drugs such as ganciclovir, foscarnet,

Drugs: Ganciclovir

ribavirin, flucytosine, pyrimethamine, TMP-SMX, hydroxyurea, and interferon, 3) Cancer chemotherapy (lymphoma or KS), or 4) HIV infection *per se*. Indications are arbitrary. Some authorities conclude that AIDS patients may tolerate low ANC levels better than cancer patients do in terms of infectious complications (*Arch Intern Med* 1995;155:1965; *Infect Control Hosp Epidemiol* 1991;12:429), and G-CSF is "not routinely indicated" for neutropenic patients with HIV infection, according to the guidelines of USPHS/IDSA (*MMWR* 1999;48[RR-10];*Clin Infect Dis* 2000;30[suppl 1]:S29). Nevertheless, the incidence of bacterial infections appears to be increased 2- to 3-fold in patients with an ANC <500/mL (*Lancet* 1989;2:91; *Arch Intern Med* 1995;155:1965), and most HIV infected patients respond. A therapeutic trial in 258 HIV infected patients with ANC of 750-1000/mm^3 found G-CSF recipients had 31% fewer bacterial infections, 54% fewer severe bacterial infections and 45% fewer hospital days for these infections, but no mortality benefit (*AIDS* 1998;12:65). A review of the 719 G-CSF recipients with neutropenia ascribed to ganciclovir treatment of CMV retinitis in three multicenter trials showed that G-CSF use reduced the incidence of neutropenia-associated bacteremia and death, but this benefit was not statistically significant when adjusted for confounding variables (*AIDS* 2002;16:757).

- **GM-CSF (sargramostim):** May also be used for neutropenia in AIDS patients and is available as leukine (*Immunex*). There has been concern that stimulation of the monocyte/macrophage cells would enhance HIV replication, but this has not been a problem in studies where viral load was monitored (*AIDS Res Hum Retroviruses* 1996;12:1151). Another possible application is the use of GM-CSF to restore allostimulatory function of accessory cells (*HIV Clin Trials* 2002;3:219). The dosing recommendation is 250 µg/m^2 IV over 2 hours qd. Note: Round off to nearest vial size of 250 or 500 mcg to reduce wastage.

DOSE: Initial dose of G-CSF is 5-10 µg/kg/day subcutaneously (based on lean body weight), usually 5 µg/kg/day. For practical purposes, the dose can be a convenient approximation of the calculated dose using a volume of 1 cc (300 µg), 0.5 cc (150 µg), 0.25 cc (75 µg) or 0.2 cc (60 µg). This may be increased by 1 µg/kg/day after 5 to 7 days up to 10 mcg/kg/day or decreased 50%/week and given either daily, every other day, or 2-3 times per week. Monitor CBC 2x/week and keep ANC >1,000 to 2,000/mL (*N Engl J Med* 1987;317:593). If unresponsive after 7 days at 10 µg/kg/day, treatment should be discontinued. Usual maintenance dose is 150-300 µg given 3 to 7x/week.

PHARMACOLOGY

- **Absorption:** Not absorbed with oral administration. G-CSF must be given IV or SQ; SQ is usually preferred.
- **T½:** 3.5 hours (SQ injection)

- **Elimination:** Renal

SIDE EFFECTS: Medullary bone pain is the only important side effect, noted in 10% to 20%, and usually manageable with acetaminophen.

RARE SIDE EFFECTS: Mild dysuria, reversible abnormal liver function tests, increased uric acid, and increased LDH.

DRUG INTERACTIONS: Should not be given within 24 hours of cancer chemotherapy. Lithium may ↑ leukocytosis. Vincristine ↑ peripheral neuropathy (*J Clin Oncol* 1996;14:935).

PREGNANCY: Category C. Caused abortion and embryolethality in animals at 2-10x dose in humans; no studies in humans.

GEMFIBROZIL

TRADE NAME: *Lopid* (Pfizer) or generic

FORM AND PRICE: 600 mg tab at $1.24/tab

CLASS: Antihyperlipidemic; fibric acid derivative (like clofibrate)

INDICATIONS AND DOSE: Elevated serum triglycerides; may increase LDL cholesterol and cholesterol levels. 600 mg bid PO >30 minutes before meal.

MONITORING: Blood lipids, especially fasting triglycerides and LDL cholesterol; if marked increases in LDL cholesterol, discontinue gemfibrozil and expect return of LDL cholesterol to pretreatment levels in 6 to 8 weeks. Gemfibrozil should be discontinued if there is no decrease in triglyceride or cholesterol level at 3 months. Obtain liver function tests and CBC at baseline, at 3 to 6 months, and then yearly. Discontinue gemfibrozil for otherwise unexplained abnormal liver function tests.

PHARMACOLOGY
- **Bioavailability:** 97%
- **T½:** 1.3 hour
- **Elimination:** renal – 70%, fecal – 6%
  - Hepatic failure: Reduce dosage; use with caution
  - Renal failure: Consider reducing dose

PRECAUTIONS: Contraindicated with gallbladder disease, primary biliary cirrhosis, and severe renal failure.

SIDE EFFECTS
- **Blood lipids:** May increase LDL cholesterol and cholesterol by a mechanism that is poorly understood.

- **Gallbladder:** Gemfibrozil is similar to clofibrate and may cause gallstones and cholecystitis ascribed to increased biliary excretion of cholesterol.
- **Miscellaneous:** GI intolerance, decreased hematocrit, and/or WBC

DRUG INTERACTIONS

- **Gemfibrozil and "statins"** have resulted in rhabdomyolysis and renal failure; possible increased risk of myositis when used with other statins; monitor closely for evidence of myositis with concurrent use. Rosuvastatin AUC ↑ 90%; use fenofibrate instead.
- **Oral anticoagulants:** May potentiate activity of warfarin.

PREGNANCY: Category C

GROWTH HORMONE, HUMAN (Somatropin)

TRADE NAME: *Serostim* (Serono)

FORMS AND PRICES: Vials of 4 mg (about 12 IU), 5 mg (about 15 IU), and 6 mg (about 18 IU) at $42/mg. The average cost is $252/day or $21,000 for a 12-week course.

PATIENT ASSISTANCE PROGRAM: 888-628-6673 for compassionate use and for support above the cap of $36,000/calendar year for each qualified patient.

CLASS: Human growth hormone produced by recombinant DNA technology.

INDICATIONS AND DOSES: Treatment of AIDS-associated wasting or cachexia (FDA labeling). Administer SQ at bedtime in the following doses:

- >55 kg – 6 mg SQ daily
- 45-55 kg – 5 mg SQ daily
- 35-45 kg – 4 mg SQ daily
- <35 kg – 0.1 mg/kg SQ daily

Assess at 2 weeks.

CLINICAL TRIALS: Benefits of growth hormone in AIDS patients include increased body weight, lean body mass, and body fitness (*Am J Managed Care* 2000;6:1003).

- In a therapeutic trial in 178 AIDS patients with wasting, those receiving 12 weeks of somatropin treatment had a mean 3.0 kg increase in body weight and a mean 1.6 kg increase in lean body mass compared with placebo recipients. The growth hormone recipients also had a 13% increase in median treadmill work output. There was no significant survival benefit (*Ann Intern Med* 1996;125:873).

- Another trial in 60 patients with wasting showed similar results (*Ann Intern Med* 1996;125:865). Drug cost was over $1000/week, raising questions about cost-effectiveness (*Ann Intern Med* 1996;125:932). One option to reduce cost is to limit use to 2 weeks during periods of OIs to reduce OI-associated weight loss (*AIDS* 1999;13:1195) or to use a lower dose, 1-4 mg/d (*Ann Intern Med* 1996;125:865).

- The most definitive study of growth hormone for lipodystrophy was an observational trial of 30 patients with HAART-associated visceral fat accumulation. They were given growth hormone 6 mg/day x 6 months, followed by a wash-out period, and then an optional maintenance course of 4 mg qod. There was an average reduction in visceral fat of 42% with the 6 mg/day dose, but visceral fat returned when therapy was discontinued. The effect on blood lipids was variable: 4 patients developed diabetes, and many patients had joint pains and poor quality of life (*J Acquir Immune Defic Syndr* 2002;30:379).

CONCLUSION: A consensus statement from multiple federal agencies addressing nutritional issues in HIV infection concluded that growth hormone or other protein anabolic agents may play a role in preventing or attenuating rapid weight loss that often occurs with acute infections (*Clin Infect Dis* 2003;36:S69).

PHARMACOLOGY

- **Bioavailability with SQ injection:** 70% to 90%
- **T½:** 3.9 to 4.3 hours
- **Elimination:** Metabolized primarily in renal cells; also metabolized in the liver.
- **Dose in liver or renal failure:** Decreased clearance but clinical significance and specific guidelines for dose modification are unknown.

SIDE EFFECTS: Growth hormone may cause dose-related fluid and sodium retention with edema (primarily in extremities), arthralgias, myalgias, and hypertension. The most common side effects are musculoskeletal discomfort (20% to 50%) and increased tissue turgor with swelling of hands and feet (25%); both usually subside with continued treatment. Fat atrophy and insulin resistance are noted above. Other side effects include flu-like symptoms, rigors, back pain, malaise, carpal tunnel syndrome, chest pain, nausea, and diarrhea. Side effects may be reduced by reduction in daily dose or by reduction in the number of doses per week.

DRUG INTERACTIONS: Not studied

PREGNANCY: Category C. Limited data suggest that growth hormone does not transfer across the placenta to the fetus.

HALCION –
see Benzodiazepines (p. 160)

HUMATIN – see Paromomycin (p. 269)

HYDROXYUREA (HU)

TRADE NAME: *Hydrea, Droxia* (Bristol-Myers Squibb), or generic

FORM AND PRICE: *Hydrea* caps: 500 mg at $1.27. *Droxia* caps: 200, 300, and 400 mg.

CLASS: HU is used primarily for sickle cell disease and is not FDA-approved for treatment of HIV. HU inhibits cellular ribonucleotide reductase, resulting in decreased intracellular deoxynucleoside triphosphates that are required for DNA synthesis (*AIDS* 1999;13: 1433). This makes ddl a more potent inhibitor of HIV, and *in vitro* studies show synergistic activity when HU is combined with ddl against HIV in resting lymphocytes (*Proc Natl Acad Sci USA* 1994;91:11017). Synergy was not demonstrated with concentrations that can be achieved clinically using hydroxyurea with AZT and ddC. The cytostatic property causes blunting of the CD4 response. The combination of HU with ddl + d4T appears to magnify nucleoside-associated mitochondrial toxicity.

DOSE: Optimum dose is not known. Usual dose is 500 mg bid or 1000 mg qd (with ddl + additional agents), but is no longer recommended.

CLINICAL TRIALS

- Some studies have shown that the addition of HU to a ddl-containing regimen improves virologic outcome and reduces viral load by an additional 0.2-0.6 $\log_{10}$ c/mL (*J Acquir Immune Defic Syndr* 1995;10:36; *HIV Clin Trials* 2000;1:1; *J Infect Dis* 1997;175:801), but these results are inconsistent. The CD4 count is usually not significantly increased due to the cytotoxic effect of HU, and ddl-associated complications are more frequent (*J Acquir Immune Defic Syndr* 2002;29:368).

- Conclusions about efficacy are limited by the lack of well-controlled trials or consistency in results of trials. More importantly, there is increasing concern about toxicity.

- **ACTG 5025** was discontinued prematurely after three deaths ascribed to pancreatitis were observed in the ddl/d4T/IDV/HU arm (7th CROI, San Francisco, 2000, Abstr. 456), and the FDA reported a possible increase in hepatotoxicity with HU (8th CROI, Chicago, 2001, Abstr. 617).

5 Drugs: Hydroxyurea

PHARMACOLOGY

- **Bioavailability:** Well absorbed
- **T½:** 2 to 3 hours
- **Penetration:** Highly diffusible with good CNS penetration (*Science* 1994;266:801)
- **Elimination:** Half is degraded by the liver and excreted as respiratory CO_2 and in the urine as urea.

SIDE EFFECTS

- Dose-dependent bone marrow suppression with leukopenia, anemia, and thrombocytopenia in 5% to 7% (*AIDS* 1999;13:1433). Leukopenia is most common and usually occurs first. Recovery from marrow depression is usually rapid with discontinuation of treatment. In sickle cell anemia patients receiving 25-35 mg/kg/day for painful crises, 10% had myelosuppression, and these patients had marrow recovery within 2 weeks following drug discontinuation. CBC should be monitored during therapy at regular intervals.

- Other side effects include GI intolerance, which may be severe, including stomatitis, nausea, vomiting, anorexia, altered taste, diarrhea, and constipation. Mild reversible dermatologic side effects are common and include a maculopapular rash, facial erythema, hyperpigmentation, oral ulceration, desquamation of the face and hands, and partial alopecia (*J Am Acad Dermatol* 1997;36:178). Chronic leg ulcers may complicate therapy that exceeds 3 years (*Ann Intern Med* 1998;29:128).

- HU potentiates ddI toxicity, with increased rates of ddI-associated peripheral neuropathy (*AIDS* 2000;14:273) and pancreatitis and hepatotoxicity (*AIDS* 2000;14:273; 8th CROI, Chicago, 2001, Abstrs. 617 and 620).

- Rare side effects include dysuria, neurologic complications (drowsiness, disorientation, hallucinations, convulsions), hyperuricemia, renal failure, fever, chills, and alopecia.

PREGNANCY: Category D. Contraindicated.

INDINAVIR (IDV)

TRADE NAME: *Crixivan* (Merck)

FORMULATIONS, REGIMENS, PRICE

- **Forms:** IDV caps 200, 333 and 400 mg
- **Regimens:** IDV 800 mg q 8h; IDV/r, 800/100 or 800/200 mg bid
- **AWP:** $500/month

FOOD: Unboosted, take 1 hr before or 2 hrs after meal, or take with light, low-fat meal. No food restrictions for IDV/r.

FLUIDS: Must take ≥1.5 L/day

RENAL FAILURE: No restrictions

STORAGE: Room temperature, 15-30°C

PATIENT ASSISTANCE PROGRAM: 800-850-3430

CLASS: Protease inhibitor

INDICATIONS AND DOSE: The standard dose without RTV boosting is 800 mg q8h in fasting state (1 hour before or 2 hours after a meal), or with a light, nonfat meal, such as dry toast with jelly, juice, coffee (with skim milk and sugar) or corn flakes with skim milk. Patients should drink ≥48 oz fluids daily; 6-8 oz glasses of fluids/day, preferably water, to prevent IDV-associated renal calculi. Most now use RTV-boosted IDV regimens, which permit bid dosing and eliminate the food effect. Standard regimens are IDV/RTV 800 mg/100 mg bid or 800 mg/200 mg bid (increased risk of renal calculi) or 400 mg/400 mg (increased RTV side effects).

ADVANTAGES: Extensive experience with long-term follow-up

DISADVANTAGES: Need for q8h dosing on empty stomach if used without RTV boosting; risk of nephrolithiasis and need for large fluid intake with or without RTV boosting; dermatologic side effects, including dry skin, alopecia, and paronychia with or without RTV boosting.

CLINICAL TRIALS

■ TABLE 5-27: **Clinical Trials of IDV for Treatment-naïve Patients**

Trial	Regimen	No.	Dur (wks)	VL <50	VL <200-500
ACTG 320 (*N Engl J Med* 1997;537:725)	IDV 800 mg q 8h/AZT 3TC	577	24		60%*
	AZT/3TC	579			9%
Merck 035 (*N Engl J Med* 1997;337:734)	IDV/AZT/3TC	32	24		90%*
	IDV	28			43%
	AZT/3TC	31			0
Dupont 006 (*N Engl J Med* 1999;341:1865)	EFV/3TC/AZT	154	48	64%*	70%*
	IDV/3TC/AZT	148		43%	48%
	IDV/EFV	148		47%	53%
Merck 060 (*AIDS* 2000;14:367)	IDV/AZT/3TC	52	52		60%*
	AZT/3TC	50			46%
Atlantic (*AIDS* 2003;17:987)	IDV/ddl/d4T	417	48	55%	57%
	NVP/ddl/d4T	394		54%	58%
	3TC/ddl/d4T	396		46%	59%
CNAAB 3005 (*JAMA* 2001;285:1155)	ABC/3TC/AZT	282	48	40%	51%
	IDV/3TC/AZT	280		46%	51%
CNA 3014 (*Curr Med Res J* 2004;20:103)	ABC/3TC/AZT	169	48	59%*	64%
	IDV/3TC/AZT	173		48%	50%
START-1 (*AIDS* 2000;14:1481)	IDV/3TC/d4T	424	48	49%	53%
	IDV/3TC/3TC	422		47%	52%

* Superior to comparator (*P* <0.05)

5 Drugs: Indinavir

- **Salvage regimen:** Indinavir combined with NVP has been reported as a successful "rescue regimen" in 59% of patients who failed amprenavir-based HAART in ACTG 373 (*J Infect Dis* 2001;183:715). IDV may also be combined with EFV for "rescue" (*J Infect Dis* 2001;183:392).

- **Boosted IDV:** Trials combining IDV with RTV have demonstrated favorable pharmacokinetics with 2- to 5-fold increases in IDV trough levels permitting bid dosing (6th CROI, Chicago, Illinois, 1999, Abstracts 362, 363, 364, 631, and 677). The optimal dose regimen is not known. The regimen of 400 mg bid of both drugs is associated with trough IDV levels that are 3- to 4-fold higher and with lower peak levels, which would be expected to reduce the risk of nephrolithiasis. However, the dose of 400 mg bid of RTV is poorly tolerated and may be complicated by higher blood lipids (*J Acquir Immune Defic Syndr* 2001;26:218). The alternative is to use IDV 800 mg bid + RTV 100-200 mg bid; this is better tolerated but is associated with higher peak levels of IDV and higher rates of nephrotoxicity. One study using the 800/100 mg bid regimen showed a good virologic response, but 23% had nephrolithiasis by week 24 (*HIV Clin Trials* 2000;1:13). Results from a trial involving RTV intensification in patients with detectable virus in IDV-containing regimens demonstrated increased IDV trough levels; 38% of patients achieved a viral load <50 c/mL at 48 weeks (*Antimicrob Agents Chemother* 2002;46:3907).

RESISTANCE: Mutations 10I/R/V, 20M/R, 24I, 32I, 36I, 54V, 71V/T, 73S/A, 77I, 82A/F/T, 84V and 90M correlate with reduced *in vitro* activity (*Antimicrob Agents Chemother* 1998;42:2775; *Topics HIV Med* 2003;11:94). Substitutions at codons 46, 82, and 84 are major mutations that predict resistance but are not necessarily the first mutations. In general, at least three mutations are necessary to produce phenotypic resistance. Overlap with RTV is extensive, so that strains resistant to one are usually resistant to both. (The rationale for the RTV-IDV combination is pharmacologic enhancement with improved IDV trough levels that permit twice-daily administration.) The overlap with other PIs is less extensive, but multiple mutations generally confer class resistance (*Nature* 1995;374:569).

PHARMACOLOGY

- **Bioavailability:** Absorption is 65% in fasting state or with only a light, nonfat meal. Full meal decreases IDV levels 77%; give 1 hour before or 2 hours after meal, with light meal or with RTV. Food has minimal effect on IDV when it is coadministered with RTV.

- **T½:** 1.5 to 2.0 hours (serum)

- **C$_{max}$:** Peak >200 nm; 8 hours post dose – 80 nm (95% inhibition *in vitro* at 25-100 nm). Peak levels correlate with nephrotoxicity and trough levels correlate with efficacy, but levels seem somewhat unpredictable when IDV is boosted with RTV (*J Acquir Immune Defic*

Syndr 2002;29:374). This suggests a possible role for therapeutic drug monitoring, although results are highly variable (*Antimicrob Agents Chemother* 2001;45:236; 8th CROI, Chicago, Illinois, 2001, Abstracts 730 and 734). Penetration into CSF is moderate (CSF: serum=0.06-0.16) but is superior to that of other PIs and adequate to inhibit IDV-sensitive strains (*Antimicrob Agents Chemother* 2000;44:2173), since levels achieved are above the IC_{95} for most HIV isolates (*AIDS* 1999;13:1227). CSF trough levels of IDV are increased >5-fold when IDV is combined with RTV (7th CROI, San Francisco, California, 2000, Abstract 312).

- **Elimination:** Metabolized via hepatic glucoronidation and cytochrome P450 (CYP3A4)-dependent pathways. Urine shows 5% to 12% unchanged drug and glucuronide and oxidative metabolites.

- **Dose in renal failure:** Standard dose. This also applies to hemodialysis and peritoneal dialysis (*Nephrol Dial Transplant* 2000;15:1102).

SIDE EFFECTS

- **Asymptomatic increase in indirect bilirubin** to ≥2.5 mg/dL without an increase in transaminases noted in 10% to 15% of patients. Clinically inconsequential, and rarely associated with jaundice or scleral icterus.

- **Mucocutaneous:** Paronychia and ingrown toenails, alopecia, dry skin, mouth, and eyes (common).

- **Class adverse effects:** Insulin-resistant hyperglycemia, lipodystrophy, hyperlipidemia (increased triglyceride, cholesterol, LDL levels), and possible increased bleeding with hemophilia (*AIDS* 2001;15:11). Use of IDV is generally not recommended in patients with hemophilia due to the availability of many alternative PIs.

- **Nephrolithiasis ± hematuria** in 10% to 28%, depending on duration of treatment, age, and fluid prophylaxis (*J Urol* 2000;164:1895). The major cause is crystallization of the drug with high serum levels and/or dehydration; IDV crystals can be detected in urine of up to 60% of IDV recipients. The frequency of nephrolithiasis with renal colic, flank pain, hematuria and/or renal insufficiency in the ATHENA cohort with 1219 IDV recipients was 8.3/100 patient-years; risk factors included low weight, low mean body mass, regimens with >1000 mg IDV, and warm climate (*Arch Intern Med* 2002;162:1493). Factors that do not appear to influence risk are CD4 cell count and urine pH. Patients should drink 48 oz of fluid daily to maintain urine output at ≥150 mL/hour during the 3 hours after ingestion; stones are crystals of IDV ± calcium (*Ann Intern Med* 1997;349:1294). Nephrolithiasis usually reflects peak plasma concentrations >10 µg/mL (*AIDS* 1999;13:473). This is most likely with IDV in standard doses or ritonavir-boosted IDV regimens, with the 800/100 mg or 800/200 mg bid IDV/RTV regimen (*J Acquir Immune Defic Syndr* 2002;29:374).

5 Drugs: Indinavir

- **Nephrotoxicity:** In a prospective study of 184 IDV recipients, routine urinalysis indicated pyuria in 35%; this was often accompanied by proteinuria, hematuria, and IDV crystals (*J Acquir Immune Defic Syndr* 2003;32:135). About 25% with persistent pyuria developed elevated serum creatinine that persisted ≥3 months after IDV was discontinued. Interstitial nephritis with pyuria and renal insufficiency was previously reported in about 2% of IDV recipients (*Clin Infect Dis* 2002;34:1033).

- **Alopecia:** May involve all hair-bearing areas (*N Engl J Med* 1999; 341:618)

- **GI intolerance:** Primarily nausea, with occasional vomiting, epigastric distress

- **Less common:** Increased transaminase levels, headache, diarrhea, metallic taste, fatigue, insomnia, blurred vision, dizziness, rash, and thrombocytopenia. Rare cases of fulminant hepatic failure and death. Fulminant hepatitis has been associated with steatosis and an eosinophilic infiltrate, suggesting a drug-related injury (*Lancet* 1997;349:924). Gynecomastia has been reported (*Clin Infect Dis* 1998;27:1539).

DRUG INTERACTIONS

■ TABLE 5-28: **Recommendations for IDV in Combination with Other PIs or with NNRTIs**

Agent	AUC	Concurrent Use Regimen
RTV*	IDV ↑2-5x	RTV 100 mg bid + IDV 800 mg bid or RTV 400 mg bid + IDV 400 mg bid
SQV	SQV ↑4-7x; IDV No effect	No data; possible *in vitro* antagonism (*J Infect Dis* 1997;176:265)
NFV	NFV ↑80%; IDV ↑50%	IDV 1200 mg bid + NFV 1250 mg bid (limited data)
NVP	NVP no effect; IDV ↓28%	IDV 1000 mg q8h or IDV/RTV + NVP standard
DLV	DLV no effect; IDV ↑40%	DLV 400 mg tid + IDV 600 mg q8h
EFV	EFV no effect; IDV ↓31%	EFV 600 mg qhs + IDV 1000 mg q8h or IDV/RTV 800/200 mg bid + EFV 600 mg qhs
APV	APV ↑33%; IDV ↓38%	APV 800 mg tid + IDV 800 mg tid (limited data)
LPV/r	LPV no change; IDV ↑3x	IDV 600 or 666 mg bid + LPV/r 400/100 mg bid
ATV	Combination contraindicated, since both drugs cause indirect bilirubinemia	
FPV	No data	No data

* It is possible that IDV/RTV could be given once daily (IDV/RTV 1200/400), but data are limited (7th CROI, San Francisco, California, 2000, Abstract 512). Note that the IDV/r 400/400 mg bid regimen is often associated with GI intolerance and the IDV/r 800/100-200 mg regimen is associated with increased rates of nephrotoxicity (*J Acquir Immune Defic Syndr* 2002;29:374).

Drugs: Indinavir

- **Contraindicated for concurrent use:** Rifampin, astemizole, terfenadine, cisapride, midazolam, triazolam, ergotamines, simvastatin, lovastatin, atazanavir, St. John's wort, and pimozide.
- **Antimycobacterial agents:** Rifabutin – IDV levels decreased 32% and rifabutin levels increased 2x – reduce rifabutin dose to 150 mg/day or 300 mg 3x/week and increase IDV dose to 1000 mg tid with IDV/RTV use standard PI dose and rifabutin 150 mg qod or 150 mg 3x/wk.
- **Didanosine (buffered):** Use *Videx EC* formulation or separate doses by ≥2 hours if using buffered formulation.
- **Other interactions**
  - Ketoconazole and itraconazole increase IDV levels 70%; decrease IDV dose to 600 mg q8h.
  - Voriconazole – no interaction unless combined with RTV
  - Clarithromycin levels increase 53% – no dose change.
  - Grapefruit juice reduces IDV levels 26%.
  - Oral contraceptives: Norethindrone levels increase 26% and ethinylestradiol levels increase 24% – no dose change.
  - Carbamazepine markedly decreases IDV levels; consider alternative.
  - IDV increases sildenafil (*Viagra*) AUC 340% (*AIDS* 1999;13:F10). The maximum recommended dose is 25 mg/48 hours. Vardenafil AUC increased 16x IDV AUC ↓ 30% and should be limited to 2.5 mg qd or use alternative; with IDV/RTV it should be limited to 2.5 mg/3 days. Tadalafil AUC increased; use 5 mg initially and do not exceed 10 mg/72 hours.
  - Methadone: There is no change in levels of methadone.
  - St. John's wort reduces IDV AUC by 57% (*Lancet* 2000;355:547); contraindicated.
  - Vitamin C (≥1 gm/d): Decreases IDV C_{min} 32%

PREGNANCY: Category C. Negative rodent teratogenic assays; placental passage studies show high newborn:maternal drug levels in rats, low ratio in rabbits. Pharmacokinetic studies in PACTG 358 showed that mean levels at 30-32 wks gestation were 74% lower than at 6 wks postpartum; the manufacturer does not recommend use of IDV in pregnancy (Merck letter to providers, Dec. 27, 2004).

INTERFERON – see also Pegylated Interferon (p. 270)

TRADE NAME: *Roferon* (Roche), *Intron* (Schering-Plough), *Infergen* (InterMune)

NOTE: Interferon has been largely supplanted by pegylated interferon due to easier administration and superior outcome for treatment of

HCV genotype 1. The drug is included here because some ADAP and other plans will not pay for the pegylated form due to higher cost.

FORMS AND PRICES

- Interferon alfa-2a (*Roferon*): Vials of 3, 6, 9, 18, and 36 million units at $38.18
- Interferon alfa-2b (*Intron*): Vials of 3, 5, 10, 18, 25, and 50 million units at $48.83

PATIENT ASSISTANCE PROGRAMS: *Intron*: 800-521-7157; *Roferon*: 800-443-6676; cap program (983 million units ≤ year)

CLASS: Interferon-alfa is a family of highly homogeneous species-specific proteins of human origin (using donor cells, cultured human cell lines, or recombinant techniques with human genes) possessing complex antiviral, antineoplastic, and immunomodulating activities. The alfa-2a and alfa-2b refer to similar subtypes prepared by recombinant techniques.

INDICATIONS AND DOSES (Interferon alfa-2b)

- **Hepatitis C:** The usual interferon dose is 3 million units IM or SQ 3x/week x 12 to 18 months (*N Engl J Med* 1995;332:1457). This interferon formulation has become antiquated with the approval of pegylated interferon, which has a more convenient dosing schedule (once vs 3x/week) and better efficacy (*Lancet* 2001;358:958). However, the cost differential is large: $18,000/48 weeks for interferon + ribavirin vs $26,000/48 weeks for peg-interferon + ribavirin. Efficacy was comparable between Peg-interferon + RBV and interferon for genotype 2 and 3. However, for genotype 1, peg-interferon 1.5 mg/kg + RBV 800 mg was superior to IFN + RBV 1000-1200 mg, with 42% vs 33% achieving SVR (*Lancet* 2001;358:958). A pivotal study of *Pegasys* + ribavirin found the pegylated formulation superior to interferon alfa-2b + ribavirin regardless of genotype (*N Engl J Med* 2002;347:975). Results are superior when interferon is given with ribavirin (*Lancet* 1998;351:83). See ribavirin for dosing instructions, p. 260. The 2002 guidelines from the NIH HCV Consensus Conference are available at http://consensus.nih.gov/cons/116/116cdc_intro.htm. All registration studies and most trials have excluded HIV-infected patients.

- **Hepatitis B:** 5 million units IM or SQ daily or 10 million units 3x/week x 16-24 weeks (HBeAg+) or >12 months (HBeAg–). (Alternative drugs are lamivudine, adefovir, tenofovir DF, and entecavir; pegylated interferon should work as well as interferon but has not been formally evaluated or FDA-approved for HBV.)

- **Kaposi's sarcoma:** 30 to 36 million units IM or SQ (3 to 7x/week) until KS lesions resolve; toxicity or rapid progression of KS (average

7 months) precludes further treatment. Optimal response (40-50%) is observed in patients with CD4 counts >200/mm^3 and no B symptoms.

ACTIVITY: Broad-spectrum antiviral agent with *in vitro* activity against HIV, HPV, HBV, HCV, HSV-1 and 2, CMV, and VZV

PHARMACOLOGY

- **Bioavailability:** Protein with 165 amino acids and molecular weight of 18,000-20,000; no absorption after oral administration is nil; bioavailability with SQ or IM administration is 80%.
- **T½:** 2.0 to 5.1 hours
- **CSF level:** None detected
- **Elimination:** Metabolized by kidney

SIDE EFFECTS: All patients have side effects, especially with doses ≥18 million units. Most side effects diminish in frequency and severity with continued administration. Side effects include:

- **Flu-like syndrome** (50% to 98%): Fever, chills, fatigue, headache, and arthralgias, usually within 6 hours of administration, lasting 2 to 12 hours (reduced with NSAIDs)
- **GI intolerance** (20% to 65%): Anorexia, nausea, vomiting, diarrhea, metallic taste, and abdominal pain
- **Neuropsychiatric toxicity** with irritability, depression, or confusion (20% to 50%)
- **Marrow suppression** with neutropenia, anemia, or thrombocytopenia
- **Hepatotoxicity** (10% to 50%) with increased transaminase levels
- **Dyspnea and cough**
- **Rash ± alopecia** (25%)
- **Proteinuria** (15% to 20%)

DRUG INTERACTIONS: AZT and other marrow suppressants (ganciclovir, pyrimethamine, 5FC) – increased hematologic toxicity, especially aneuria; increased levels of theophylline, barbiturates

PREGNANCY: Category C. Abortifacient in animals with doses 20x to 500x doses in humans. No data for humans. Use in pregnancy only when need justifies the risk.

INTRON – see Interferon (above)

INVIRASE – see Saquinavir (p. 291)

ISONIAZID (INH)

TRADE NAMES: *Nydrazid, Laniazid, Teebaconin*, or generic; combination with rifampin: *Rifamate*, with rifampin and pyrazinamide: *Rifater* (Aventis)

FORMS AND PRICES: 50, 100, and 300 mg tabs; $0.16 per 300 mg tab. *Hydrazid* IV – Injections 100 mg/mL 10 mL vial $20; INH liquid – $1.25 per 300 mg; *Rifater* – $1.90/tab

COMBINATIONS: Caps with rifampin: 150 mg INH + 300 mg rifampin (*Rifamate*) and tabs with 50 mg INH + 120 mg rifampin and 300 mg PZA (*Rifater*)

INDICATIONS AND DOSES: Prophylaxis and treatment of tuberculosis (see p. 361)

■ TABLE 5-29: **INH Dosing Regimens: 2003 Recommendations of CDC/ATS/IDSA** (*Am J Resp Crit Care Med* 2003;167:603)

	Daily	DOT	Pyridoxine (Vitamin B6)
Prophylaxis x 9 months	300 mg	900 mg 2x/week	50 mg/day or 100 mg 2x/week
Treatment x 6-9 months	300 mg	900 mg 2 to 3x/week*	50 mg/day or 100 mg 2x/week

*Continuation phase should be 3x/week for patients co-infected with HIV with CD4 <100 mm³.

- Treatment of active TB with *Rifamate*: 2 caps/day
- Treatment of active TB with *Rifater*: <65 kg – 1 tab/10 kg/day; >65 kg – 6 tabs/day. Take 1 h before or 2 h after meals.

COMPLIANCE: Compliance concerns have resulted in a preference for DOT in all patients treated for active tuberculosis and sometimes for treatment of latent TB with HIV-coinfection. Many studies in the coinfected population show poor adherence that is improved with DOT (*Br Med* J 2003;325:1282)

PHARMACOLOGY

- **Bioavailability:** 90%
- **T½:** 1 to 4 hours; 1 hour in rapid acetylators
- **Elimination:** Metabolized and eliminated in urine. Rate of acetylation is genetically determined. Slow inactivation reflects deficiency of hepatic enzyme N-acetyltransferase and is found in about 50% of whites and African-Americans. Rate of acetylation does not affect efficacy of standard daily or DOT regimens.

- **Dose modification in renal failure:** Half dose with creatinine clearance <10 mL/min in slow acetylators.

SIDE EFFECTS

- **Hepatitis:** ALT elevations are noted in 10% to 20%, clinical hepatitis in 0.6%, and fatal hepatitis in 0.02% (*Am Rev Respir Crit Care Med* 2003;167:603). The risk of hepatitis increases with increased age, alcoholism, prior liver disease, pregnancy, and concurrent rifampin. One report showed hepatotoxicity rates (defined as an ALT >5 ULN) of 0.15% in 11,141 patients treated for latent TB. It was 1% in those receiving multiple antituberculosis drugs for active TB (*JAMA* 1999;281:1014). CDC/ATS/IDSA 2003 guidelines for management of TB recommend monitoring INH recipients for clinical evidence of hepatitis by requiring monthly INH prescriptions contingent on this review. LFTs, primarily transaminase levels, should be monitored in most patients only if there are symptoms; patients with baseline liver disease or abnormal LFTs that develop during treatment should have monthly LFTs. INH should be stopped if transaminase levels increase to >5 times upper limit of normal.

- **Peripheral neuropathy** due to increased excretion of pyridoxine, which is dose-related and rare (0.2%) with usual doses; it is prevented by use of concurrent pyridoxine (10-50 mg/day), which is recommended for diabetics, alcoholics, pregnant patients, AIDS patients, and malnourished patients. The usual dose is 25 mg/d.

- **Miscellaneous Reactions:** Rash, fever, adenopathy, GI intolerance. Rare reactions: Psychosis, arthralgias, optic neuropathy, marrow suppression.

DRUG INTERACTIONS

- Increased effects of warfarin, benzodiazepines, carbamazepine, cycloserine, ethionamide, phenytoin, theophylline
- INH absorption decreased with aluminum-containing antacids
- Ketoconazole: Decrease ketoconazole levels
- Food: Decreases absorption
- Tyramine (cheese, wine, some fish): Rare patients develop palpitations, sweating, urticaria, headache, and vomiting

PREGNANCY: Category C. Embryocidal in animals; not teratogenic. Large retrospective studies have shown no pattern of congenital abnormalities; small studies suggest possible CNS toxicity (*Clin Infect Dis* 1995;21[suppl 1]:S24). American Thoracic Society recommendation is that pregnant women with positive PPD plus HIV infection should receive INH to begin after first trimester if possible.

5 Drugs: Isoniazid

ITRACONAZOLE

TRADE NAME: *Sporanox* (Janssen)

FORMS AND PRICES: 100 mg caps at $9.63; 150 mL oral solution with 10 mg/mL at $10.71/100 mg; 200 mg vials for injection at $211.91

PATIENT ASSISTANCE PROGRAM: 800-652-6227

CLASS: Triazole (like fluconazole) with three nitrogens in the azole ring; other imidazoles have two nitrogens.

ACTIVITY AND PERSPECTIVE: *In vitro* activity against *H. capsulatum, B. dermatitidis, Aspergillus, Cryptococcus, Candida* spp. Strains of *Candida* that are resistant to fluconazole may be sensitive to itraconazole (*Antimicrob Agents Chemother* 1994;38:1530). Compared with fluconazole, itraconazole appears to be equivalent for non-meningeal coccidioidomycosis (*Ann Intern Med* 2000;133:676), superior for penicilliosis (*Am J Med* 1997;103:223), inferior for cryptococcosis (*Clin Infect Dis* 1999;28:291), and equivalent for most candidiasis (*HIV Clin Trials* 2000;1:47). Major concerns are somewhat erratic absorption, multiple drug interactions, and recently described cardiotoxicity (*FDA Health Advisory*, 5/09/02).

DOSE REGIMENS: See Table 5:30 p. 237

PHARMACOLOGY

- **Bioavailability:** Caps require gastric acid for absorption; average is 55% and improved when taken with food. Acidic drinks such as colas and orange juice may increase absorption in patients with gastric achlorhydria (*Antimicrob Agents Chemother* 1995;39:1671). Follow serum levels to ensure absorption. The usual therapeutic level anticipated with a standard dose is ≥ 1 µg/mL and < 10 µg/mL. The liquid formulation is better absorbed and should be taken on an empty stomach. The supplier recommends a dose adjustment of one half of that recommended for capsules. Some consider the liquid formulation to be preferred for all oral itraconazole therapy. However, nearly all studies were performed using the capsule formulation, and bioavailability studies have shown substantial variation. Based on these concerns, some authorities prefer the liquid formulation only for thrush, where its topical effect may improve efficacy, for patients with known achlorhydria, and for patients with inadequate serum levels.

- **Reference laboratories for serum levels:**
  - Dr. Michael Rinaldi, Dept. of Pathology, University of Texas Health Science Center, 7703 Floyd Curl Drive, San Antonio, TX 78284-7750; telephone 210-567-4131. Cost is $59.
  - Specimen should be serum or plasma. Volume >0.5 mL (2-4 mL preferred) sent in frozen state. Specimen can be obtained about 2

■ TABLE 5-30: **Itraconazole Dose Regimens** (*Clin Infect Dis* 2000;30:652)

Usual Doses

- **Loading dose:** 200 mg tid x 3 days for serious infections
- **Capsules:** 100-200 mg PO qd or bid *with food* (200-400 mg/day)
- **Oral liquid formulation:** 100 mg PO qd or bid *on empty stomach* (100-200 mg/day)
- **IV:** 200 mg IV bid x 4 (loading), then 200 mg IV qd

Treatment by Pathogens		
Pathogen	**Dose (oral)**	**Comment**
Aspergillosis	200-400 mg/day (caps)	Voriconazole preferred
Blastomycosis	200 mg qd or bid (caps)	
Candidiasis ■ Thrush ■ Esophagitis ■ Vaginal	■ 200 mg/day (liquid) swish & swallow (S&S) ■ 200 mg/day (liquid) S&S ■ 200 mg/day x 3 days or 200 mg bid x 1 (caps)	■ As effective as fluconazole, but absorption more erratic and there are more drug interactions (*HIV Clin Trials* 2000;1:47) ■ For fluconazole resistant *Candida*, options include itraconazole (PO or IV), voriconazole (PO or IV), caspofungin (IV), or amphotericin (IV). Voriconazole is the most predictably active triazole.
Coccidioido-mycosis	■ Acute non-meningeal, mild: 200-400 mg PO bid ■ Chronic suppressive treatment: itraconazole 200 mg PO bid	Non-meningeal form. (For meningeal form, fluconazole 400-800 mg/d is preferred.)
Cryptococcosis	200 mg qd (caps) bid x 8 weeks, then 200 mg qd maintenance	■ For patients with meningeal form who cannot tolerate fluconazole and for non-meningeal cryptococcosis ■ Fluconazole preferred
Dermatophytes	200 mg qd (caps)	■ *Tinea corporis* and *T. cruris*: 15 days ■ *T. pedis, T. manum*: 30 days ■ *T. capitis*: 4 to 8 weeks
Histoplasmosis	■ Acute: 400 mg IV/day ■ Continuation: 200 mg PO tid x 3 days then 200 mg bid (caps) ■ Maintenance: 200 mg PO bid (caps)	■ Preferred azole ■ Amphotericin B preferred for initial treatment of severe disseminated histoplasmosis; itraconazole is appropriate for acute phase treatment of those with mild illness
Onychomycosis ■ Fingernails ■ Toenails	200 mg/day (caps) ■ 1 week/month x 2 mos. ■ 1 week/month x 4 mos.	Warn patients of and monitor for cardiotoxicity and hepatotoxicity.
Penicilliosis	■ Acute: 200 mg PO bid + amphotericin B 0.7 mg/kg/d x 1-2 weeks ■ Maintenance: 200 mg PO bid	Preferred azole
Sporotrichosis	200 mg bid	

5 Drugs: Itraconazole

hours post dosing, after ≥5 days of treatment to assure steady state has been reached. Results are available in 3 days. Goal is level of ≥1 µg/mL.

- **T½:** 64 hours
- **Elimination:** CYP 3A4 inhibitor and substrate; metabolites include hydroxyitraconazole, which is active *in vitro* against many fungi. Renal excretion is 0.03% of parent drug and 40% of administered dose as metabolites.
- **Dose modification with renal failure:** None
- **Dose modification with liver disease:** No data. Manufacturer suggests monitoring serum levels.

SIDE EFFECTS

- **Cardiotoxicity:** The negative inotropic effect was noted in animal toxicity studies and in clinical trials combined with 58 cases of CHF reported to the FDA "Drug Watch," which is an anecdotal series of cases reported to the FDA and reported by that agency through May, 2001.
- **Hepatoxicity:** Elevation of hepatic enzymes is seen in 4%, but clinically significant hepatitis is rare (*Lancet* 1992;340:251). Hepatic enzymes should be monitored in patients with prior hepatic disease, and patients should be warned to report symptoms of hepatitis.
- **Other:** Most common side effects are GI intolerance (3% to 10%) and rash (1% to 9% and most common in immunosuppressed patients).
- **Rare:** Infrequent dose-related toxicities include hypokalemia, adrenal insufficiency, impotence, gynecomastia (at doses >600 mg/d), hypertension, and edema. Ventricular fibrillation due to hypokalemia has been reported (*J Infect Dis* 1993;26:348).

DRUG INTERACTIONS: Impaired absorption of caps with buffered ddl, H_2 blockers, proton pump inhibitors, antacids, or sucralfate. Give itraconazole 2-4 hours before buffered ddl or use *Videx EC* or take with cola to decrease gastric pH. Itraconazole is a CYP3A4 inhibitor and substrate, resulting in bidirectional inhibition with increased levels of itraconazole and the following interacting drugs: clarithromycin, erythromycin, DLV, and PIs, especially RTV-boosted PIs. Reduce IDV dose to 600 mg q8h and do not exceed 400 mg/d of itraconazole. NVP and EFV may ↓ itraconazole levels; monitor levels. With TPV/r, do not exceed itraconazole 200 mg. Should not be given concurrently with terfenadine (*Seldane*), cisapride, astemizole, triazolam (*Halcion*), lovastatin (*Mevacor*), simvastatin (*Zocor*), rifampin, rifabutin, phenytoin, carbomazapine, or phenobarbital. Itraconazole increases levels of cyclosporine, sirolineus, tacrolineus, oral hypoglycemics, calcium channel blockers, and digoxin.

PREGNANCY: Category C. Teratogenic to rats. Generally not recommended in pregnancy, but some studies have found it to be safe (*Am J Obstet Gynecol* 2000;183:617).

KALETRA – see Lopinavir/Ritonavir (p. 245)

KETOCONAZOLE

TRADE NAME: *Nizoral* (Janssen)

FORMS AND PRICES: Tabs: 200 mg at $3.09; 2% cream: 15 g at $19.19, 30 g at $28.32, and 60 g; 2% shampoo: 120 mL at $27.75

PATIENT ASSISTANCE PROGRAM: 800-652-6227

CLASS: Azole antifungal agent

INDICATIONS AND DOSES: Infrequently used due to erratic absorption, multiple drug interactions, and availability of many alternative agents. Main justification is low cost compared to other azoles.

- **Thrush:** 200 mg PO 1 to 2x/day
- ***Candida* esophagitis:** 200-400 mg PO bid. Note: Fluconazole (200 mg/day) is superior, but initial treatment with ketoconazole may be cost-effective (*Ann Intern Med* 1992;117:655).
- ***Candida* vaginitis:** 200-400 mg/day PO x 7 days or 400 mg/day x 3 days

PHARMACOLOGY

- **Bioavailability:** 75% with gastric acid; decreased bioavailability with hypochlorhydria, which is common in AIDS patients.
- **Administration with hypochlorhydria:** Best alternative is to use an azole that does not require gastric acid, such as fluconazole. Alternatives are concurrent administration of 580 mg glutamic acid hydrochloride or 240 mL acidic drinks such as colas, ginger ale, or orange juice (*Antimicrob Agents Chemother* 1995;39:1671).
- **T½:** 6 to 10 hours
- **Elimination:** Metabolized by liver, but half-life is not prolonged with hepatic failure.
- **Dose modification in renal failure:** None

SIDE EFFECTS: Gastrointestinal intolerance; temporary increase in transaminase levels (2% to 5%); dose-related decrease in steroid and testosterone synthesis with impotence, gynecomastia, oligospermia, reduced libido, menstrual abnormalities (usually with doses ≥600 mg/day for prolonged periods); headache, dizziness, asthenia; rash; hepatitis (more common compared to other azoles); abrupt hepatitis

5 Drugs: Ketoconazole

with hepatic failure (1:15,000); rare cases of hepatic necrosis; marrow suppression (rare); hypothyroidism (genetically determined); hallucinations (rare).

DRUG INTERACTIONS

- **Important interactions:** Increase in gastric pH impairs ketoconazole absorption: Antacids, H_2 blockers, proton pump inhibitors, and buffered ddI should be taken ≥2 hours apart, use alternative antifungal agent, (*MMWR* 1999;48[RR-10]:47) or use *Videx EC*. INH decreases ketoconazole effect; rifampin – decreased activity of both drugs; terfenadine (*Seldane*), cisapride, quinidine, and pimozide – ventricular arrhythmias (avoid concurrent use). Other interactions listed under itraconazole also apply to ketoconazole.

- **PI and NNRTIs:** See Table 5-31.

■ TABLE 5-31: **Ketoconazole Interactions with Antiretroviral Agents**

Agent	PI/NNRTI	Ketoconazole	Dose
IDV	↑68%	—	IDV 600 mg q 8 hour
RTV	—	↑3x	Ketoconazole dose ≤200 mg/day
SQV	↑3x	—	Standard doses. Monitor for ketaconazole toxicity with dose >200 mg/d
NFV	↑35%	—	Standard doses
APV	↑31%	↑44%	Consider dose reduction if dose >400 mg/d
LPV/r	↑13%	↑3x	Ketoconazole dose ≤200 mg/day
NVP	↑15% to 30%	↓63%	Not recommended
EFV	—	May ↓	Dose implications unclear; consider another azole
ATV	Not affected	—	Standard doses
FPV	↑	↑	Presumed to be same as APV; with FPV/r – do not exceed 200 mg/d
TPV	May ↑	May ↑	Do not exceed 200 mg/d ketoconazole

- **Other:** Alcohol – possible disulfiram-like reaction; oral anticoagulants – increased hypoprothrombinemia; corticosteroids – increased levels of methylprednisolone; cyclosporine – increased cyclosporine activity; phenytoin – may ↓ ketoconazole and ↑ phenytoin; theophylline – increased theophylline levels.

PREGNANCY: Category C. Embryotoxic and teratogenic in experimental animals with large doses; no studies in humans; use with caution.

LAMIVUDINE (3TC)

TRADE NAME: *Epivir* (GlaxoSmithKline)

FORMULATIONS, REGIMENS AND PRICE

- **Forms and regimens**
  - □ 3TC: 150 mg and 300 mg tabs; 10 mg/mL solution (24-oz. bottle). Regimen: 150 mg bid or 300 mg qd
  - □ AZT/3TC: 300/150 mg (*Combivir*). Regimen: 1 bid
  - □ AZT/3TC/ABC: 300/150/300 mg (*Trizivir*). Regimen: 1 bid
  - □ 3TC/ABC: 300/600 mg (*Epzicom*). Regimen: 1 qd
- **AWP**
  - □ 3TC: Tabs or solution: $300/mo
  - □ AZT/3TC: $640/mo
  - □ AZT/3TC/ABC: $1,020/mo
  - □ 3TC/ABC: $760/mo

FOOD: No effect

RENAL FAILURE: Lamivudine – at CrCl (mL/min) level: 30-49, 150 mg qd; 15-29, 150 mg, then 100 mg qd; 5-14, 150 mg, then 25 mg qd <5 or dialysis, 50 mg, then 25 mg qd. Combivir, Trizivir, Epzicom – avoid when CrCl <50 mL/min.

HEPATIC FAILURE: No recommendation; usual dose likely

HEPATITIS B: Standard dose is 100 mg/day; coinfected patients should receive the HIV dose of 300 mg/day

PATIENT ASSISTANCE: 800-722-9294

CLASS: Nucleoside analog

INDICATIONS AND DOSES

- **HIV:** 3TC or FTC are recommended as components of all initial regimens in the 2005 DHHS guidelines. The standard dose is 150 mg bid or 300 mg qd without regard for meals. 3TC is coformulated as *Combivir*, *Trizivir*, and *Epizicom* which improve convenience.

- **Hepatitis B:** 3TC is a potent inhibitor of HBV replication (*N Engl J Med* 2004;350:1118). Several studies have verified activity with HBeAg seroconversion and loss of HBV DNA (*Ann Intern Med* 1996;125:705: *Lancet* 1995;345:396), elimination of HBeAg (*N Engl J Med* 1998;339:61), improved ALT levels (*J Infect Dis* 1999;180:607), and improved hepatic histology (*N Engl J Med* 1998;339:61). Nevertheless, a cost analysis showed 3TC to be inferior to interferon for chronic HBV infection (*Ann Intern Med* 2005;142:821). Mutations on the YMDD polymerase gene confer lamivudine resistance at a rate of 15-20% in year 1 and 60-70% by

Drugs: Lamivudine

year 4 (*Gastroenterology* 2000;119:172). These mutations result in HBV virologic failure and, in some cases, a hepatitis flare (*J Clin Virol* 2002;24:173; *Lancet* 1997;349:20; *Clin Infect Dis* 1999;28:1032). Such flares may result from lamivudine discontinuation or lamivudine resistance. The frequency of the YMDD mutation is substantially increased in HIV co-infected patients (*AIDS* 2003;17:1649). Other correlates of resistance are HBeAg, HBV DNA level >500 pg/mL and ALT <5x ULN (Chang ML, *J Hepatol* Apr. 26, 2005 e-pub). Tenofovir DF, entecavir, and adefovir are active against lamivudine-resistant HBV (*Hepatology* 2002;36:507) and have much lower rates of resistance (<2%/year). The following recommendations have been made for HCV/HIV co-infected patients:

TREATMENT OF HIV ONLY: Consider withholding 3TC and FTC for future use or use TDF/FTC-containing regimen.

TREATMENT OF HBV ONLY: Consider adefovir, entecavir or pegylated interferon

TREATMENT OF HIV AND HBV: Consider TDF/FTC (*Truvada*) or TDF/3TC

ADVANTAGES: Potent against HIV, well tolerated, no food effect, may be taken once daily, co-formulated with AZT (*Combivir*), AZT/ABC (*Trizivir*), and ABC (*Epzicom*), active against HBV. 3TC resistance (M184V) increases susceptibility to AZT, d4T, tenofovir DF. Delays accumulation of TAMs, and may partially reverse their effects. 184V appears to be uniquely effective in reducing viral load as a single agent in patients who have multiply-resistant strains.

DISADVANTAGES: Single mutation (184V) confers high level resistance; use with HBV co-infection without other agents active against HBV likely to cause HBV resistance. Discontinuation in patients with chronic HBV may cause flare of hepatitis.

CLINICAL TRIALS: There is extensive experience with 3TC combined with AZT, TDF, d4T, and ddI, confirming antiviral potency, excellent long and short-term tolerability, but also early acquisition of the M184V resistance mutation if viral suppression incomplete.

- **ACTG 384** showed that AZT/3TC/EFV was superior to ddI/d4T/EFV in virologic suppression and tolerability (*N Engl J Med* 2003;349:2298).

- **Gilead 903** compared 3TC/TDF vs 3TC/d4T, each in combination with EFV, for initial therapy. Results at 144 weeks were similar, with 69-73% achieving viral load <50 c/mL by ITT (M = F) analysis (*JAMA* 2004;292:194).

- **CNA 30024** compared ABC/3TC vs. AZT/3TC, each with EFV, in 699 treatment-naïve patients. At 48 wks, VL was <50 c/mL in 69% and 70%, respectively by ITT analysis (*Clin Infect Dis* 2004;39:1038). This paved the way to coformulation as *Epzicom*.

Drugs: Lamivudine

- **ESS 30008** compared ABC/3TC twice daily vs. once daily in patients who had viral suppression with ABC/3TC twice daily combined with a PI or NNRTI. Results at 48 wks showed sustained viral suppression in 81% with once-daily therapy vs. 82% with twice-daily therapy. Toxicity rates and CD4 responses of the two groups were similar. There were no ABC hypersensitivity reactions. Adherence was better in the once-daily group (12th CROI, Boston, Feb. 2005, Abstr. 572).

- **Triple nucleoside regimens:** ACTG 5095 compared AZT/3TC/ABC vs EFV/3TC/AZT ± ABC. The study was discontinued prematurely due to higher rates of virologic failure in the triple nucleoside regimen (21% vs 10%) (*N Engl J Med* 2004;350:1850). ESS 30009 compared ABC/TDF/3TC and EFV/3TC/ABC. This study was also stopped prematurely due to greater rates of virologic failure in the triple nucleoside group (49% vs 5%). All patients with virologic failure had 184V mutations. Triple nucleoside regimens are not advocated for initial therapy unless PI or NNRTI-based HAART is not feasible. If used, the triple nucleoside regimen should include a thymidine analog (AZT or d4T).

RESISTANCE: Monotherapy with 3TC or non-suppressive therapy with 3TC-containing regimens result in the rapid selection of the M184V mutation, which confers high-level resistance to 3TC and FTC. Strains with the M184V mutation have enhanced susceptibility to AZT, d4T, and TDF and a modest decrease in susceptibility to ABC and ddI that is not clinically relevant in the absence of other NRTI mutations. The 184V mutation appears to be associated with reduced viral replication so that use with multiply-resistant HIV reduces VL a mean of 0.5 $\log_{10}$ c/mL. The mechanism may be reduced viral fitness (*New Microbiol* 2004;27 Suppl 2:31; *Expert Rev Anti Infect Ther* 2004;2:147). K65R and multiple TAMs reduce activity of 3TC 3- to 9-fold. The Q151M complex and the T69 insertion mutation are associated with 3TC resistance as well as with broad multinucleoside resistance. All of these changes are also found with FTC (12th CROI, Boston, Feb. 2005, Abstr. 713).

PHARMACOLOGY

- **Bioavailability:** 86%
- **T½:** 3 to 6 hours; Intracellular T½: 12 hours
- **CNS penetration:** 13% (CSF: Plasma ratio=0.11). These levels exceed the IC_{50} and have been shown to clear HIV RNA from CSF (*Lancet* 1998;351:1547).
- **Elimination:** Renal excretion accounts for 71% of administered dose.

SIDE EFFECTS: Experience with more than 25,000 patients given 3TC through the expanded access program showed minimal toxicity. Infrequent complications include headache, nausea, diarrhea, abdominal pain, and insomnia. Comparison of side effects in 251 patients given

Drugs: Lamivudine

5

3TC/AZT and 230 patients given AZT alone in four trials (A3001, A3002, B3001, and B3002) indicated no clinical or laboratory complications uniquely associated with 3TC. Pancreatitis has been noted in some pediatric patients given 3TC.

- **Class side effect:** Lactic acidosis and steatosis are listed as toxicities associated with the NRTI class, though it is not clear that these occur as a result of 3TC therapy. They are most often associated with d4T, AZT, and ddl (*Clin Infect Dis* 2002;34:838).

- **Hepatitis B:** In HIV-infected patients with HBV co-infection, discontinuation of 3TC may cause fulminant hepatic deterioration with increases in HBV DNA levels and increases in ALT levels (**FDA black box warning**). Monitor hepatic function and clinical course carefully for several months when 3TC is discontinued in patients with HIV/HBV co-infection. Immune reconstitution and development of HBV resistance may also cause a hepatitis B flare.

DRUG INTERACTIONS: TMP-SMX (1 DS daily) increases levels of 3TC; however, no dose adjustment is necessary due to the safety profile of 3TC.

PREGNANCY: Category C. Negative carcinogenicity and teratogenicity studies in rodents; placental passage studies in humans show newborn:maternal drug ratio of 1.0. Studies in pregnant women show that lamivudine is well tolerated and has pharmacokinetic properties similar to those of nonpregnant women (*MMWR* 1998;47[RR-2]:6). Use in pregnancy is extensive; safety is well established, and when combined with AZT, efficacy in preventing perinatal transmission is also well established (*Lancet* 2002;359:1178). AZT/3TC is recommended as the preferred NRTI backbone for HIV-infected pregnant women (DHHS guidelines, Apr. 7, 2005, p 93).

LAMPRENE – see Clofazimine (p. 172)

LEUCOVORIN (Folinic Acid)

TRADE NAME: Generic

FORMS AND PRICES

- Oral tabs: 5, 10, 15, and 25 mg tabs; 5 mg tab – $2.85
- Parenteral: 50, 100, and 350 mg; 3 mg/mL; 100 mg – $36.69

CLASS: Calcium salt of folinic acid

INDICATIONS: Antidote for folic acid antagonists

NOTE: Protozoa are unable to utilize leucovorin because they require p-aminobenzoic acid as a cofactor. It does not interfere with antimicrobial activity of trimethoprim or pyrimethamine. Usual use in HIV infected patients is to prevent hematologic toxicity of pyrimethamine and trimetrexate. Therapy is usually oral but should be parenteral if there is vomiting, or NPO status.

- **Toxoplasmosis treatment:** Pyrimethamine 50-75 mg/day + leucovorin 10-20 mg/day x 6 weeks; maintenance pyrimethamine 50 mg/day + leucovorin 15 mg/day
- **Toxoplasmosis prophylaxis:** Pyrimethamine/leucovorin, 25 mg every week (with dapsone + pyrimethamine)

PHARMACOLOGY: Normal folate levels are 0.005-0.015 µg/mL, levels <0.005 indicate folate deficiency, and levels <0.002 cause megaloblastic anemia. Oral doses of 15 mg/day result in mean level of 0.268 µg/mL.

SIDE EFFECTS: Nontoxic in therapeutic doses. Rare hypersensitivity reactions.

PREGNANCY: Category C

LOPINAVIR/RITONAVIR (LPV/r)

TRADE NAME: *Kaletra* (Abbott Laboratories)

CLASS: Protease inhibitor (boosted with coformulated ritonavir)

PATIENT ASSISTANCE: 800-659-9050

FORMULATIONS, REGIMENS AND PRICE

- **Forms:** LPV/r caps, 133/33 mg; LPV/r oral solution, 80/20 mg/mL. LPV/r tabs, 200/50 mg are expected early 2006; 2 PO bid or 4 PO qd.
- **Regimens:** 400/100 mg bid or 800/200 mg qd; oral solution 5 cc bid or 10 cc qd. Oral solution is sometimes preferred where there is GI intolerance; contains 42% alcohol. Once-daily therapy of 800/200 mg found therapeutically equivalent to standard bid therapy in treatment-naïve patients and is now FDA-approved. Nevertheless, in that setting, trough levels were lower and more variable (*J Infect Dis* 2004;189:265). Standard (twice-daily) therapy is preferred for treatment-experienced patients.
- **AWP:** $650/month
- **New formulation:** Expected in 2006, 200/50 mg tabs will offer a pill burden of 4/day plus more consistent bioavailability and less dependence on food effect (3rd IAS Conf, Rio, July 2005, Abstr. WeOa 0206).

FOOD: Take with food

RENAL FAILURE: Standard dose

HEPATIC FAILURE: No recommendation; use with caution

5 Drugs: Lopinavir/Ritonavir

STORAGE: Stable for 2 mos at room temperature (15-30°C); stable with refrigeration until expiration date on label; 200/150 mg formulation is more stable at room temperature.

ACTIVITY: LPV is approximately 10 times more potent than RTV against wild-type HIV. The protein binding-adjusted IC_{50} value for wild-type virus is 0.07 µg/mL. With bid dosing, the trough levels of LPV on average exceed the IC_{50} by >75-fold. LPV combined with other PIs showed an additive effect *in vitro* with IDV and APV and synergy with SQV (*Antimicrob Agents Chemother* 2002;46:2249).

ADVANTAGES: Potent antiretroviral activity; unbeaten in therapeutic trials; durability demonstrated with 5-year data; no evidence of PI resistance with virologic failure when used as first PI; co-formulated with RTV; frequently more active against PI-resistant virus than some other approved PIs with the exception of TPV/r.

DISADVANTAGES: Food requirement; need for bid dosing in PI-experienced patients. GI intolerance; hyperlipidemia and other PI-associated metabolic toxicities; limited experience in pregnant women.

CLINICAL TRIALS

- **Treatment-naïve patients**
  - **M97-720** was a dose-finding phase II trial of LPV/r + d4T/3TC in 100 treatment-naïve patients with viral load >5,000 c/mL. At 48 weeks, 82% given 400/100 mg bid had viral load <400 c/mL, and 78% had viral load <50 c/mL by ITT analysis (*AIDS* 2001;15:F1). At year 4, 70% still had <50 c/mL and the mean increase in CD4 count from baseline was 440/mm³. Among 6 patients with sustained viral load rebound to >400 c/mL, no protease inhibitor resistance mutations were seen (*AIDS* 2004;18:775).
  - **M98-863** was a phase III trial that compared LPV/r and NFV, each with d4T/3TC, in 653 treatment-naïve patients (*N Engl J Med* 2002;346:2039). By ITT analysis at 48 weeks, viral load was <400 c/mL in 75% of LPV/r recipients compared with 63% of NFV recipients (p=0.001) and <50 c/mL in 67% vs 52%, respectively (p<0.001). Both regimens were well tolerated. Among failures, PI resistance mutations were noted in 43 of 96 (45%) in the NFV arm and 0 of 51 in the LPV/r arm (*J Infect Dis* 2004;189:51). Resistance to 3TC was noted in 79/123 (82%) of NFV recipients who failed therapy compared to 19/74 (45%) who failed LPV/r treatment.
  - **Once daily vs twice daily LPV/r:** 38 treatment-naïve patients were randomized to receive LPV/r 400/100 mg bid or LPV/r 800/200 mg qd. Mean (± 1 SD) trough levels of LPV were 3.6 ± 3.4 µg/mL and 7.1 ± 2.9 µg/mL for qd vs bid regimens, respectively. The viral load decreases to <50 c/mL were 74% and 79% (*p* = 0.7) (*J Infect Dis* 2004;189:265). Pharmacology studies showed the two groups had similar AUCs and C_{max}, but trough levels were

lower and more available with qd dosing. Study 418 is an FDA registration study of TDV/FTC plus either LPV/r 800/200 qd or LPV/r 400/100 bid. Results at 96 weeks among 190 participants showed viral load <50 c/mL in 57% in the qd regimen and 53% in the bid regimen. Diarrhea was significantly more common in the qd regimen resulting in a higher dropout rate; 17% vs 9% (3rd IAS Conf, July 2005, Abstr. WePe 12.3 C12).

- **Treatment-experienced patients**

  ☐ **M98-957** was a salvage trial involving 57 patients who had failed at least two PI-containing regimens. The trial compared two doses of LPV/r (533/133 mg bid and 400/100 mg bid), each combined with EFV. At 72 weeks, viral load was <400 and <50 c/mL in 88% and 81% of patients, respectively (as-treated analysis). By ITT analysis, viral loads were <400 and <50 c/mL in 67% and 61%, respectively. Response was correlated with the number of PI mutations to LPV at baseline, with viral load <400 c/mL in 91% of those with 0 to 5 mutations, 71% with 6 to 7 mutations, and 33% with 8 to 10 mutations (*Antiviral Ther* 2002;7:165).

  ☐ **M97-765** was a phase II study in 70 NNRTI-naïve patients with a viral load of 1,000-100,000 c/mL (median viral load 10,000 c/mL and median CD4 349/mm³) on their PI regimen. Patients received LPV/r + NVP and 2 NRTIs. At 48 weeks, 60% had viral load <50 c/mL by ITT analysis (*J Virol* 2001;75:7462).

  ☐ **BMS 043** was an open-label randomized trial comparing unboosted atazanavir (ATV) with LPV/r, both in combination with two NRTIs selected by resistance testing, in 300 patients failing a PI-based regimen with HIV RNA ≥1,000 c/mL (2nd IAS, 2003, Abstract #117). Virologic suppression was superior in the LPV/r arm at 24 weeks (-2.11 vs. -1.57 $\log_{10}$ c/mL, *p* = 0.032). Virologic suppression to <50 c/mL occurred in 54% of those taking LPV/r vs. 38% of those taking ATV by ITT analysis (*p* = 0.008). Differences between LPV/r and ATV were more pronounced in those with greater antiretroviral experience or resistance.

- **RESIST:** Subset analysis of TPV/r vs. LPV/r in patients with 3 class failure showed a better virologic response (<400 c/mL) at 24 weeks in patients randomized to TPV/r (116/293, 40%) vs. LPV/r (62/290, 21%) (12th CROI, Boston, Feb. 2005, Abstr. 560).

- **ACTG 51250** was a switch study to determine the effect of LPV/r 533/133 mg bid + EFV 600 mg qd vs. continued HAART with two NRTIs. The NRTI-sparing regimen was associated with decreased lipoatrophy, increase in serum lipids and stable glucose metabolism (12th CROI, Boston, Feb. 2005, Abstr. 40).

- **A5116** was a randomized trial comparing LPV/r 533/133 mg bid + EFV 600 mg qd vs. EFV + two NRTIs in patients with HAART >18 mos and VL <200 c/mL. The latter regimen was superior to the NRTI-sparing regimen in terms of toxicity (17% vs. 5%; *P* <0.002), but

Drugs: Loprinavir/Ritonavir

5

there was a trend toward higher VL failure (*P* = 0.09, ITT) (12th CROI, Boston, Feb. 2005, Abstr. 162).

RESISTANCE: Major resistance mutations have not been defined. Treatment-naïve patients treated with LPV/r have not been shown to acquire PI resistance by genotypic or phenotypic testing. Resistance usually results from multiple PI resistance mutations, reflecting prior PI-containing regimens, at codons 10, 20, 24, 32, 33, 46, 47, 50, 53, 54, 63, 71, 73, 82, 84, and 90. Clinical trial data demonstrate reduced response rates with ≥4 mutations (8th CROI, Chicago, Illinois, 2001, Abstract 525). The I50V mutation selected by amprenavir causes significant loss of susceptibility to LPV. Consider phenotypic testing to facilitate interpretation. 63P is common without PI exposure; this mutation combined with other PI resistance mutations has been associated with LPV/r failure (*Topics in HIV Med* 2003;11:92).

PHARMACOLOGY

- **Bioavailability:** ~80% with food and 48% on an empty stomach. The addition of RTV results in a significant increase in LPV concentrations, AUC, and T½ due to inhibition of the cytochrome P450 CYP3A4 isoenzymes. The mean steady-state LPV plasma concentrations are 15- to 20-fold higher than those without RTV. Because RTV activity *in vitro* is 10-fold lower than that of LPV, RTV functions primarily as a pharmacologic enhancer and not as an antiretroviral agent. Protein binding is extensive, but there is sufficient CNS penetration to exceed the 50% IC (*AIDS* 2005;19:949).

- **T½:** 5 to 6 hours

- **Excretion:** Metabolized primarily by cytochrome P450 CYP3A4 isoenzymes. LPV/r inhibits CYP3A4 isoenzymes, but the effect is less than that of therapeutic doses of RTV, and similar to that of IDV. Based on PK data with APV, LPV/r appears to be an inducer of CYP3A4. Less than 3% excreted unchanged in urine.

- **Renal failure:** No data are available, but usual dose is recommended. LPV/r is not removed with hemodialysis (AIDS 2001;15:662).

- **Hepatic failure:** No dose modification recommendations are available. Use with caution in end-stage liver disease.

SIDE EFFECTS: The drug is generally well tolerated, with 2% discontinuing therapy due to adverse drug reactions in phase II and III clinical trials through 48 weeks.

- **Diarrhea:** The most common adverse reactions were gastro-intestinal, with diarrhea of at least moderate severity in 15% to 25%. Abdominal pain and nausea is also common and may improve with oral solution.

- **Transaminase levels:** Laboratory abnormalities through 72 weeks included transaminase increases (to >5x normal) in 10% to 12%.

- **Class adverse reactions:** Insulin resistance, fat accumulation, and hyperlipidemia. Clinical trials show triglyceride increases to >750 mg/dL in 12% to 22%, and cholesterol increases to >300 mg/dL in 14% to 22% of treatment-naïve patients receiving LPV/r. Trial M98-863, comparing LPV/r with NFV in 653 patients, showed comparable mean increases in cholesterol (about 50 mg/dL) and a mean triglyceride increase of about 100 mg/dL for LPV/r vs 25 mg/dL for NFV. In HIV-negative men given LPV/r for 10 days, the major effect was an increase in triglyceride levels averaging 83%; there was minimal effect on insulin sensitivity (*AIDS* 2004;18:641).

- Report of 7 cases of renal or parotid lithiasis (*AIDS* 2004;18:705).

DRUG INTERACTIONS: The major effect is due to the inhibition of CYP3A4 isoenzymes to prolong the half-life of drugs metabolized by the route. The inhibition is less than that seen with therapeutic doses of RTV.

- **Drugs contraindicated for concurrent use:** Astemizole, terfenadine, flecainide, propafenone, rifampin, simvastatin, lovastatin, midazolam, triazolam, cisapride, phenytoin, pimozide, ergot derivatives, St. John's wort, and rifapentine.

- **Drugs that require a modified dose**
  □ Rifabutin: C_{min} increased 3-fold; reduce rifabutin dose to 150 mg 3x/week with standard LPV dose.
  □ Phenytoin: LPV AUC ↓ 33% and phenytoin levels ↓ 31%; use with caution.
  □ Clarithromycin: Clari AUC increased 77%; reduce clarithromycin dose in renal failure.
  □ Methadone: AUC of methadone decreased by 26-36%; monitor for withdrawal (conflicting data on withdrawal symptoms).
  □ Atorvastatin: AUC increased 450%; use lowest dose (10 mg/d) or use alternative, such as pravastatin or fluvastatin, or rosuvastatin.
  □ Pravastatin: Levels increased 33%; no dose adjustment.
  □ Ketoconazole: Levels increased by 3x; limit to ≤200 mg/d.
  □ Oral contraceptives: Ethinyl estradiol AUC decreased by 42%; use additional or alternative methods.
  □ Drugs for erectile dysfunction: Sildenafil level increase anticipated; do not exceed 25 mg/48 hours. Vardenafil: no data; limit to 2.5 mg q72h. Tadalafil: Start with 5 mg dose and do not exceed 10 mg/72 hrs.
  □ Anticonvulsants: LPV and phenytoin decreased by 33% and 31%, respectively. Carbamazepine and phenobarbitol may decrease serum level of LPV. Consider TDM or use alternative anticonvulsants (i.e., valproic acid, lamotrigine, levetiracetam).
  □ Atovaquone: Levels of atovaquone may be decreased requiring dose adjustment.

Drugs: Loprinavir/Ritonavir

5

- Tenofovir DF: TDF levels increase 34%; clinical significance unknown; dose adjustment not recommended.
- Tacrolimus: Half-life of tacrolimus is increased 10-fold (12th CROI, Boston, Feb. 2005, Abstr. 662); sirolimus T½ may also be increased significantly.

■ TABLE 5-32: **Dose Adjustments for Concurrent Use with Other Antiretroviral Agents**

Drug	Effect on Coadministered Drug	Effect on LPV	Dose Recommendation
APV	↑ or ↓	No change or ↓	APV 750 mg bid + LPV/r 533/133 mg bid. Addition of EFV (600 mg/d) does not alter PI pharmacokinetics (12th CROI, Boston, Feb. 2005, Abstr. 79).
EFV	No change	C_{min} ↓39%	EFV 600 mg hs + LPV/r 533/133 mg bid
IDV	↑ C_{min} 3x	No change	IDV 600 or 666 mg bid + LPV/r 400/100 mg bid
NVP	No change	↓ C_{min} 55%	NVP standard + LPV/r 533/133 mg bid
SQV	↑ C_{min} 3.6x		SQV (*Invirase* or *Fortovase*) 1000 mg bid + LPV/r 400/100 mg bid*
NFV	↑25%	↓27%	Data insufficient; avoid coadministration
DLV	No change	↑8% to 134%	Limited data
ATV	↑	↔	Dose: ATV 300 mg qd/LPV 3 caps bid
FPV	↓64%	↓53%	No clear dose recommendation. FPV 1400 mg bid + LPV/r 533/133 mg still resulted in 42% ↓ in C_{min} compared to FPV 700/RTV 100 bid. Use with caution.

* Shows synergy *in vitro* (*Antimicrob Agents Chemother* 2002;46:2249).

PREGNANCY: Category C. Placental passage shown in rats (newborn: maternal ratio=0.08) Animal carcinogenicity studies incomplete. Rodent teratogenic studies negative (but delayed skeletal ossification and skeletal variations in rats at maternally toxic doses). There are limited data in pregnancy but increased dose may be required due to anticipated reduced LPV levels. DHHS guidelines (Oct. 6, 2005) recommend LPV/r as an alternative to preferred HAART regimens with NFV or SQV/r.

Drugs: Loprinavir/Ritonavir

LORAZEPAM

TRADE NAME: *Ativan* (Wyeth) or generic

FORMS AND PRICES: Tabs: 0.5 mg at $0.90, 1 mg at $1.17, 2 mg at $1.71. Vials: 2 mg, 4 mg, 20 mg, 40 mg

CLASS: Benzodiazepine, controlled substance category IV (see p. 136)

INDICATIONS AND DOSE REGIMENS: Preferred benzodiazepine with concurrent PIs and NNRTIs.

- Anxiety: 1-2 mg 2 to 3x/day; increase to usual dose of 2-6 mg/day in 2 to 3 divided doses
- IV administration: 2 mg
- Insomnia plus anxiety: 2-4 mg hs

PHARMACOLOGY

- **Bioavailability:** >90%
- **T½:** 10 to 25 hours
- **Elimination:** Renal excretion of inactive glucuronide metabolite. Not recommended with severe hepatic and/or renal disease.

SIDE EFFECTS: See Benzodiazepines (p. 185). Additive CNS depression with other CNS depressants including alcohol. Warn patient of prolonged sedation and decreased recall for ≥8 hours. Injected lorazepam may reduce physical coordination 24 to 48 hours.

PREGNANCY: Category D. Fetal harm: Contraindicated.

LOTRIMIN – see Clotrimazole (p. 172)

MARINOL – see Dronabinol (p. 185)

MEGACE – see Megestrol acetate (below)

MEGESTROL ACETATE

TRADE NAME: *Megace* (Bristol-Myers Squibb) or generic

FORMS AND PRICE: Tabs: 20 mg at $0.67, 40 mg at $1.15. Oral suspension: 40 mg/mL at $155/240 mL or $0.65/40 mg.

PATIENT ASSISTANCE: 800-272-4878

CLASS: Synthetic progestin related to progesterone

5 Drugs: Megestrol Acetate

INDICATIONS: Appetite stimulant to promote weight gain in patients with HIV infection or neoplastic disease (a concern is that most weight gain is fat. Hypogonadism in men may result.

USUAL REGIMEN

- **Oral suspension:** 400 mg/day (20 mL in one daily dose), up to 800 mg/day.
- **Tablets:** 400-800 mg/day (suspension usually preferred).

EFFICACY: A controlled trial of 271 patients with HIV-associated wasting showed those given 800 mg/day megestrol consumed a mean of 4 kg more than placebo recipients. (*Ann Intern Med* 1994;121:393). However, most of the gain is fat. Another study showed the increase in caloric intake was not sustained after 8 weeks (*Ann Intern Med* 1994;121:400). Published data are available only for men. Most authorities recommend use in combination with replacement dose of testosterone in men (200 mg q2wk) or anabolic steroids and resistance exercises (*N Engl J Med* 1999;340:1740).

PHARMACOLOGY

- **Bioavailability:** >90%
- **T½:** 30 hours
- **Elimination:** 60% to 80% excreted in urine; 87% to 30% excreted in feces.

SIDE EFFECTS

- **Most serious** are hypogonadism (which may exacerbate wasting), diabetes, and adrenal insufficiency.
- **Most common** are diarrhea, impotence, rash, flatulence, asthenia, hyperglycemia (5%), and pain.
- **Less common or rare** include carpal tunnel syndrome, thrombosis, nausea, vomiting, edema, vaginal bleeding, and alopecia; high dose (480 mg to 1600 mg/day) – hyperpnea, chest pressure, mild increase in blood pressure, dyspnea, congestive heart failure.
- A review of FDA reports of adverse drug reactions with megestrol showed 5 cases of Cushing syndrome, 12 new-onset diabetes cases, and 17 cases of possible adrenal insufficiency (*Arch Intern Med* 1997;157:1651).

DRUG INTERACTIONS: Not a substrate of CYP3A4. No interactions with rifabutin or AZT.

PREGNANCY: Category D. Progestational drugs are associated with genital abnormalities in male and female fetuses exposed during first 4 months of pregnancy.

MEPRON – see Atovaquone (p. 157)

Drugs: Megestrol Acetate

METHADONE

TRADE NAME: *Dolophine* (Roxane) or generic

FORMS AND PRICES: Tabs: 5 mg at $0.08, 10 mg at $0.14. Usual yearly cost of medication for methadone maintenance averages $180.

CLASS: Opiate schedule II. The FDA restricts physician prescribing for methadone maintenance to those licensed to provide this service and those attached to methadone maintenance programs. However, licensed physicians can prescribe methadone for pain control.

INDICATIONS AND DOSES

- **Detoxification** for substantial opiate abstinence symptoms: Initial dose is based on opiate tolerance, usually 15-20 mg; additional doses may be necessary. Daily dose at 40 mg usually stabilizes patient; when stable 2 to 3 days, decrease dose 20% per day. Must complete detoxification in <180 days or considered maintenance.

- **Maintenance** as oral substitute for heroin or other morphine-like drugs: Initial dose 15-30 mg depending on extent of prior use, up to 40 mg/day. Subsequent doses depend on response. Usual maintenance dose is 40-100 mg/day, but higher doses are sometimes required. Most states limit the maximum daily dose to 80 mg to 120 mg/day.

- **Note:** During first 3 months, and for all patients receiving >100 mg/day, observation is required 6 days/week. With good compliance and rehabilitation, clinic attendance may be reduced for observed ingestion 3 days/week with maximum 2-day supply for home administration. After 2 years, clinic visits may be reduced to 2x/week with 3-day drug supplies. After 3 years, visits may be reduced to weekly with a 6-day supply.

- **Pain control:** 2.5-10.0 mg PO, SQ or IM q3h-q4h or 5-20 mg PO q6h-q8h for severe chronic pain in terminally ill patients.

PHARMACOLOGY

- **Bioavailability:** >90% absorbed
- **T½:** 25 hours. Duration of action with repeated administration is 24 to 48 hours.

5 Drugs: Methadone

■ TABLE 5-33: **Drug Interactions with Methadone**

Drug	Effect on Methadone	Effect on Coadministered Drug	Comment
ABC	↓ levels	↓ Peak	Dose adjustment unlikely
APV (and FPV)	↓13% (active methadone)	↓25%	Monitor, may need methadone dose increase. No withdrawal symptoms observed.
ddI	None	Buffered ddI ↓63%; Videx EC – no change	ddI EC preferred
d4T	None	↓27%	No dose adjustment
TDF	No data	–	No data. Interaction unlikely.
DLV	No data	Not affected	Use standard DLV dose
EFV	↓52%	?	Likely to need ↑ methadone dose
Fluconazole	↑30%	–	No dose adjustment
IDV	None	No effect	No dose adjustment
LPV/r	↓26-36%	?	Monitor, may need methadone dose increase (conflicting data).
NFV	↓ inactive methadone	–	Monitor, may need methadone dose increase.
NVP	↓46-51%	No effect	Likely to need ↑ methadone dose
Rifampin	↓↓	–	Need ↑ methadone dose
Rifabutin	No effect	–	No dose adjustment
RTV	↓37%	No effect	Monitor, may need methadone dose increase. Stereoisomeres not measured.
AZT	None	–	No dose adjustment
Phenytoin	↓↓	–	May need ↑ methadone dose
SQV/RTV	↓20%	No effect	SQV/RTV 400/400 – no change in PI dose, monitor for methadone withdrawal (but no withdrawal symptoms observed).
ATV	No data	—	No data
TPV	↓50%	—	No dose adjustment; monitor for withdrawal symptoms

- **Elimination:** Metabolized by liver via CYP450 2B6>2C19>3A4. Parent compound excreted in urine with increased rate in acidic urine; metabolites excreted in urine and gut.

SIDE EFFECTS

- **Acute toxicity:** CNS depression (stupor or coma), respiratory depression, flaccid muscles, cold skin, bradycardia, hypotension

- **Treatment:** Respiratory support ± gastric lavage (even hours after ingestion due to pylorospasm) ± naloxone (but respiratory depression may last longer than naloxone duration of action (repeated dosing may be needed), and naloxone may precipitate acute withdrawal syndrome).
- **Chronic toxicity:** Tolerance/physical dependence with abstinence syndrome following withdrawal – onset at 3 to 4 days after last dose of weakness, anxiety, anorexia, insomnia, abdominal pain, headache, sweating, and hot-cold flashes.
- **Treatment:** Detoxification.

PREGNANCY: Category C. Avoid during first 3 months and use sparingly, in small doses, during last 6 months.

METRONIDAZOLE

TRADE NAME: *Flagyl* (Pharmacia & Upjohn); *Femazole, Metizol, MetroGel* (Galderma), *Metryl, Neo-Tric, Novonidazole, Protostat,* or generic

FORMS AND PRICES: Tabs: 250 mg at $0.43, 500 mg at $0.72. IV vials: $15.42/500 mg. Vaginal gel at $54.44/70 g.

CLASS: Synthetic nitroimidazole derivative

INDICATIONS AND DOSE REGIMENS
- **Gingivitis:** 250 mg PO tid or 500 mg PO bid
- **Intra-abdominal sepsis:** 1.5-2.0 g/day PO or IV in 2 to 4 doses
- **Amebiasis:** 750 mg PO tid x 5 to 10 days
- **Bacterial vaginosis:** 2 g x 1 or 500 mg PO bid x 7 days
- **Trichomoniasis:** 2 g x 1 or 250 mg PO tid x 7 days
- **C. difficile colitis:** 500 mg PO tid or 250 mg PO qid x 10 to 14 days
- **Giardiasis:** 250 mg PO tid x 5 to 10 days

ACTIVITY: Active against virtually all anaerobes (*Antimicrob Agents Chemother* 2001;45:1238), and selected enteric pathogens (*E. histolytica, Giardia*). Drug of choice for most anaerobic infections, gingivitis, *C. difficile*-associated diarrhea, amebiasis, giardiasis, and bacterial vaginosis. Mixed anaerobic infections need a companion antibiotic if aerobes are considered important because metronidazole is active against only anaerobes.

PHARMACOLOGY
- **Bioavailability:** >90%
- **Note:** Metronidazole is virtually completely absorbed with oral administration and should be given IV only if patient can take nothing by mouth.

Drugs: Metronidazole

5

- **T½:** 10.2 hours; serum level after 500 mg dose: 10-30 μg/mL
- **Elimination:** Hepatic metabolism; metabolites excreted in urine
- **Dose adjustment in renal failure:** None
- **Liver failure:** Half-life prolonged; consider reduced daily dose in severe liver disease

SIDE EFFECTS: Most common are GI intolerance and unpleasant taste. Less common are glossitis, furry tongue, headache, ataxia, urticaria, dark urine. Rare – seizures. Prolonged use may cause reversible peripheral neuropathy; disulfiram (*Antabuse*)-type reaction with alcohol.

DRUG INTERACTIONS: Increases levels of coumadin and lithium. Mild disulfiram-like reactions noted with alcohol (flushing, headache, nausea, vomiting, cramps, sweating). This is infrequent and unpredictable. Patients should be warned, and manufacturer recommends that alcohol be avoided. Concurrent use with disulfiram may cause psychoses or confusion; disulfiram should be stopped 2 weeks prior to use of metronidazole.

PREGNANCY: Category B. Fetotoxicity in animals. Contraindicated in first trimester, although 206 exposures during the first trimester showed no increase in birth defects. Use during the last 6 months is not advised unless essential. For trichomoniasis, CDC recommends 2 g x 1 after first trimester. Alternative agents are available for most other conditions.

MYCELEX – see Clotrimazole (p. 172)

MYCOBUTIN – see Rifabutin (p. 282)

MYCOSTATIN – see Nystatin (p. 267)

NEBUPENT – see Pentamidine (p. 273)

NELFINAVIR (NFV)

TRADE NAME: As above

CLASS: Protease inhibitor

FORMULATIONS, REGIMENS AND PRICE

- **Forms:** Tabs, 250 and 625 mg; oral powder, 50 mg/mL
- **Regimens:** 1250 mg bid or 750 mg tid (tabs); 25 cc bid (oral solution)
- **AWP:** $600/month

FOOD: Increases levels 2-3x; take with fatty food

RENAL FAILURE: Standard dose

HEPATIC FAILURE: No recommendation; use with caution

STORAGE: Room temperature, 15-30°C

PATIENT ASSISTANCE: 800-777-6637

ADVANTAGES: Extensive experience; well tolerated in pregnancy

DISADVANTAGES: Reduced potency compared to many other regimens; need for concurrent fatty meal; diarrhea; high pill burden (with 250 mg tab); inability to boost levels effectively with RTV

CLINICAL TRIALS

- **Pre-registration trials** demonstrated tolerability, with 4% of 696 patients discontinuing treatment due to side effects. The major side effect was diarrhea in 10% to 30%, which was sufficiently severe to require discontinuation of NFV in 1.6%.

- TABLE 5-34: **Clinical Trials in Treatment-naïve Patients**

Trial	Regimen	N	Duration (wks)	VL <50	VL <200-400
Combine (*Antiviral Ther* 2002;7:81)	NFV/AZT/3TC	70	48	50%	60%
	NVP/AZT/3TC	72		65%*	75%*
SOLO (*AIDS* 2004;18:1529)	FPV/r (1400/200 bid)/ AZT/3TC	322	48	56%	68%
	NFV (1250 bid/AZT/3TC	327		42%	65%
NEAT (*J Acquir Immune Defic Syndr* 2004;35:22)	FPV 1400 bid/AZT/3TC	166	48	58%	66%*
	NFP 1250 bid/AZT/3TC	83		42%	51%
ACTG 384 (*N Engl J Med* 2003;349:2293)	EFV/3TC/AZT	155	48		88%*
	NFV/3TC/AZT	155			67%
	NFV/EFV/3TC/AZT	178			84%
INITIO (12th CROI 2/05 Abst. 165 LP)	EFV/ddl/d4T	915	192	74%	
	NFV/ddl/d4T			62%	
	EFV/NFV/ddl/d4T			62%	
Abbott M98-863 (*N Engl J Med* 2002;346:2039)	LPV/r/d4T/3TC	326	48	67%*	75%*
	NFV/d4T/3TC	327		52%	63%
BMS 007 (*J Acquir Immune Defic Syndr* 2003;32:18)	ATV/d4T/ddl	103	48	36%	64%
	NFV/d4T/ddl	103		39%	56%
BMS 008 (*Reyataz* pkg. insert)	ATV/d4T/3TC	181	48	33%	67%
	NFV/d4T/3TC	91		38%	59%
Agouron 542 (*Viracept* pkg. insert)	NFV 750 tid/d4T/3TC	192	48	54%	58%
	NFV 1250 bid/d4T/3TC	323		51%	61%

* Superior to comparator (*p* <0.05)

5 | Drugs: Nelfinavir

RESISTANCE: The primary resistance mutation is D30N, which is associated with phenotypic resistance to NFV but not to other protease inhibitors (*Antimicrob Agents Chemother* 1998;42:2775). However, the L90M mutation can also occur and, unlike 30N, it confers cross-resistance to all PIs except TPV/r. Other less important or secondary mutations are 10F/I, 36I, 46I/L, 71V/T, 77I, 82A/F/T/S, 84V, 88D/S, 90M.

PHARMACOLOGY

- **Bioavailability:** Absorption with meals is 20% to 80%. Fatty meal substantially increases absorption 2- to 3-fold.
- **T½:** 5-6 hrs (serum)
- **CNS penetration:** No detectable levels in CSF (*J Acquir Immune Defic Syndr* 1999;20:39)
- **Excretion:** Primarily by cytochrome P450 CYP2C19 (major) and CYP3A4 (minor). Inhibits CYP3A4. Only 1% to 2% is found in urine; up to 90% is found in stool, primarily as a hydroxylated metabolite designated M8, which is as active as nelfinavir against HIV (*Antimicrob Agents Chemother* 2001;45:1086).
- **Dose modification in renal or hepatic failure:** None. NFV is removed with hemodialysis so that post dialysis dosing is important (*AIDS* 2000;14:89). The drug is not removed by peritoneal dialysis (*J Antimicrob Chemother* 2000;45:709).
- **Dose modification with hepatic failure:** With severe liver disease, consider therapeutic drug monitoring. It appears that autoinduction of NFV metabolism is blunted in severe liver disease, and there is also a reduction in the M8 active metabolite. Standard doses may yield high or low levels.

SIDE EFFECTS

- **Diarrhea:** About 10% to 30% of 1,500 recipients have reported diarrhea or loose stools. This is a secretory diarrhea, characterized by low osmolarity and high sodium, possibly due to chloride secretion (7th CROI, San Francisco, California, 2000, Abstract 62). Management strategies include use of several over-the-counter, inexpensive ($4 to $10/month) remedies, including oat bran (1500 mg bid), psyllium (1 tsp qd or bid), loperamide (4 mg, then 2 mg every loose stool up to 16/day), or calcium (500 mg bid). Some respond to pancreatic enzymes (1 to 2 tabs with meals) at a cost of $30-$111/month (*Clin Infect Dis* 2000;30:908).
- Class adverse effects: Lipodystrophy, increased levels of triglycerides and/or cholesterol, hyperglycemia with insulin resistance and type 2 diabetes, osteoporosis, and possible increased bleeding with hemophilia.

DRUGS THAT SHOULD NOT BE GIVEN CONCURRENTLY: Simvastatin, lovastatin, rifampin, astemizole, terfenadine, cisapride, pimozide, midazolam, triazolam, ergot derivatives, and St. John's wort

Drugs: Nelfinavir

DRUGS THAT REQUIRE DOSE MODIFICATIONS

- Oral contraceptives: Levels of ethinyl estradiol decreased by 47%; use alternative or additional birth control method.

- Anticonvulsants: Phenobarbital, phenytoin, and carbamazepine may decrease NFV levels substantially; monitor anticonvulsant levels. May need NFV levels.

- Drugs for erectile dysfunction: Sildenafil AUC increased 2- to 11-fold; do not exceed 25 mg/48 hours. Vardenafil: limit to 2.5 mg qd. Tadalafil: Start with 5 mg dose and limit to 10 mg/72 hrs.

- Rifabutin levels are increased 2-fold, and NFV levels are decreased by 32%; increase NFV dose to 1000 mg tid and decrease rifabutin dose to 150 mg/day or 300 mg 3x/week.

- NFV reduces levels of methadone, but in most cases no dose change is required (7th CROI, San Francisco, 2000, Abstr. 87).

- Statins: Atorvastatin levels increase 74%; start with lowest dose (10 mg/day) or use pravastatin, fluvastatin, or rosuvastatin.

- Ketoconazole: NFV AUC ↑35% (use standard dose).

- Clarithromycin: No data

- Voriconazole: Expect bidirectional inhibition with elevated levels of both drugs.

■ TABLE 5-35: **Combinations with PIs and NNRTIs**

Drug	AUC	Regimen
IDV	IDV ↑50% NFV ↑80%	IDV 1200 mg bid + NFV 1250 mg bid (limited data)
RTV	RTV No change NFV ↑1.5x	RTV 400 mg bid + NFV 500-750 mg bid (limited data)
SQV	SQV ↑3 to 5x (*Fortovase*) NFV ↑20%	SQV (*Fortovase*) 800 mg tid or 1200 bid + NFV 1250 bid or 750 mg tid; limited data
APV	APV ↑1.5x NFV ↑15%	NFV 750 mg tid or 1250 mg bid + APV 800 mg tid or 1200 mg bid (limited data)
NVP	NVP no change NFV ↑10%	Standard doses both drugs
EFV	NFV ↑20% EFV no change	Standard doses both drugs
DLV	DLV ↓50% NFV ↑2x	Avoid co-administration
LPV/r	LPV ↓27% NFV ↑25%	Data inadequate; avoid co-administration

PREGNANCY: Category B. Animal teratogenic studies – negative; long-term animal carcinogenicity studies – ↑ tumors in rats given ≥300 mg/kg; placental passage – not known. Experience to establish safety in pregnancy is extensive. The 750 tid dose produced variable levels in pregnant women that were generally lower than in non-pregnant women. The 1250 mg bid regimen produced adequate levels (*Clin Infect Dis* 2004;39:736). Many regard this as the preferred PI for use in pregnancy.

NEUPOGEN – see G-CSF (p. 220)

NEVIRAPINE (NVP)

TRADE NAME: *Viramune* (Boehringer Ingelheim)

CLASS: Non-nucleoside reverse transcriptase inhibitor

FORMULATIONS, REGIMENS AND PRICE

- **Forms:** Tabs, 200 mg; oral solution, 50 mg/mL (240 mL bottle)
- **Regimens:** 200 mg qd x 2 weeks, then 200 mg bid. After treatment interruption >7 days should restart with the 200 mg/d regimen. If rash appears during the lead-in period, delay dose escalation until after the rash has resolved, and rule out hepatitis. No dose escalation when switching from EFV to NVP; start with NVP 200 mg bid (*AIDS* 2004;18:572).

WARNINGS: 1) Avoid NVP as initial therapy in women with baseline CD4 count >250/mm³ due to high rates of symptomatic hepatitis. 2) See guidelines for discontinuing NVP at p. 79.

FOOD: No significant effect

RENAL FAILURE: Standard regimen

HEPATIC FAILURE: Avoid NVP in patients with moderate or severe liver disease

PATIENT ASSISTANCE: 800-556-8317

ADVANTAGES: Extensive experience; 2NN trial suggests antiviral potency comparable to EFV; no food effect. A safe and effective agent for perinatal transmission prevention in a resource-limited setting.

DISADVANTAGES: High rates of serious hepatotoxicity in treatment naïve women with baseline CD4 counts >250/mm³, high rates of rash, including TEN and Stevens-Johnson syndrome; single resistance mutation may result in loss of entire class; single dose for prevention of perinatal transmission may cause resistance. Efficacy data for EFV is more extensive.

Drugs: Nevirapine

CLINICAL TRIALS

■ TABLE 5-36: **Trials in Treatment-naïve Patients**

Trial	Regimen	N	Duration (wks)	VL <50	VL <200-400
Atlantic (*AIDS* 2000;15:2407)	NVP/ddl/d4T	89	48	54%*	58%
	IDV/ddl/d4T	100		55%*	57%
	3TC/ddl/d4T	109		46%	59%
Combine (*Antiviral Ther* 2002;7:81)	NVP/AZT/3TC	72	48	65%	75%
	NFV/AZT/3TC	70		50%	60%
2NN (*Lancet* 2004;363:1253)	NVP 400 mg qd/3TC/d4T	220	48	70%	
	NVP 200 mg bid/3TC/d4T	387		65%	
	EFV/3TC/d4T	400		70%	
	EFV/NVP/3TC/d4T	209		63%	

* Superior to comparators (P = <0.05)

- **2NN:** This is the pivotal study comparing EFV and NVP (see Table 5-36). ITT analysis at 48 weeks showed similar results for NVP bid and EFV, with VL <50 c/mL in 65% and 70%, respectively. The difference in efficacy was not statistically significant, but the trial did not show non-inferiority according to the FDA definition. There was more hepatotoxicity in NVP recipients (9.6% vs. 3.5%), and two deaths were attributed to NVP toxicity (*Lancet* 2004;363:1253). NVP given qd caused more hepatotoxicity (13.6%) and EFV/NVP was inferior virologically compared to EFV alone.

- **Treatment-experienced patients**
  - **NVP plus NFV** has been used as a salvage regimen (with full doses of each) with 52% achieving viral load <200 c/mL (*J Acquir Immune Defic Syndr* 2001;27:124). NVP has also been combined with IDV as a salvage regimen following failure of APV-based HAART, with 59% achieving viral load <500 c/mL at 48 weeks (*J Infect Dis* 2001;183:715).

- **Switch therapy**
  - Switch from a PI-containing regimen to NVP due to lipodystrophy is associated with good virologic control and rapid improvement in blood lipid changes and insulin resistance but minimal change in lipodystrophy (*AIDS* 1999;13:805; *J Acquir Immune Defic Syndr* 2001;27:229). Another similar trial also showed good virologic control but the opposite effect on metabolic changes, with half of the patients showing improved body shape changes but no changes in serum lipids (*AIDS* 2000;14:807).
  - **The ATHENA** study was a review of 125 patients who switched to NVP-based HAART compared with 321 who continued PI-based HAART. All participants had achieved viral load <500 c/mL on PI based HAART. Treatment failure due to toxicity requiring a

Drugs: Nevirapine

5

regimen change (36%) or virologic failure (6%) was greater in the PI continuation group (*J Infect Dis* 2002;185:1261).

- **NVP vs EFV switch:** Retrospective analysis of 162 patients on PI-based HAART were randomized to NVP or EFV for salvage or simplification. For simplification, 36/55 (66%) maintained virologic control at 48 weeks, and the two drugs were comparable. For salvage, virologic control was achieved in 15/58 (22%) of NVP recipients and 19/49 (38%) of EFV recipients (*HIV Clin Trials* 2003;4:244).

- **NEFA:** A randomized trial in which 460 patients receiving PI-based HAART were randomized to switch to ABC, NVP, or EFV (plus 2 NRTIs). At 48 weeks, virologic failure occurred in 13%, 10%, and 6% for these 3 groups, respectively ($P = 0.1$). Lipodystrophy did not change in any of the groups (*N Engl J Med* 2003;349:1036).

- **High baseline viral load:** In an analysis of six reports in 416 NVP recipients, viral suppression to <500 c/mL was observed in 83% and 89% of those with baseline viral loads above and below 100,000 c/mL, respectively (*HIV Clin Trials* 2001;2:317).

RESISTANCE: Monotherapy is associated with rapid and high-level resistance, with primary RT mutations 103N, 100I, 181C/I, and 190A resulting in an increase in the IC_{90} of >100-fold (*J Acquir Immune Defic Syndr* 1995;8:141; *J Infect Dis* 2000;181:904). There is cross-resistance with DLV; cross-resistance with EFV is more variable, and *in vitro* it is usually seen with K103N, which causes resistance to all currently available NNRTIs. NVP resistance is important in two distinct clinical settings, both related to the relatively long half-life and the low genetic barrier to resistance mutations:

The more extensive studies involve resistance associated with single-dose NVP for preventing perinatal transmission, which is a common strategy in developing countries. HIVNET 012 showed this was highly effective in perinatal transmission prevention, but resistance mutations were noted using standard assays in 19% of women (*J Infect Dis* 2002;186:181). Subsequent studies using real time PCR, with a detection limit of 0.2%, found that K103N was present in minority species in an additional 40% (*J Infect Dis* 2005;192:16). The frequency is clade-specific: clade C, 69%; clade D, 36%; clade A, 19% (12th CROI, Boston, Feb. 2005, Abstr. 799). Resistance mutations are also observed in the infants born to exposed mothers (12th CROI, Boston, Feb. 2005, Abstr. 800) and in strains recovered from breast milk (12th CROI, Boston, Feb. 2005, Abstr. 801). The clinical implications of these observations are unclear, but in one study, women with perinatal NVP exposure who were subsequently treated with NVP-based regimens had a poorer virologic response compared to women who had not been previously exposed to NVP (*N Engl J Med* 2004;351:217).

The second important application of these data pertains to discontinuation of NVP-based HAART. The concern is that the long half-life of NVP will result in a substantial exposure to monotherapy. Methods to deal with this theoretical concern have not been well studied, but the suggestion has been made to discontinue NVP and continue two NRTIs with a PI or boosted PI for 2-4 weeks before discontinuing the entire regimen.

PHARMACOLOGY

- **Bioavailability:** 93%; not altered by food, fasting, ddl, or antacids.

- **T½:** 25 to 30 hours

- **CNS penetration:** CSF levels are <45% peak serum levels (CSF: plasma ratio=0.45)

- **Metabolism:** Metabolized by cytochrome P450 (CYP3A4) to hydroxylated metabolites that are excreted primarily in the urine, which accounts for 80% of the oral dose. NVP autoinduces hepatic CYP3A4, reducing its own plasma half-life over 2 to 4 weeks from 45 hours to 25 hours (*J Infect Dis* 1995;171:537).

- **Dose modification with renal or hepatic failure:** NVP is extensively metabolized by the liver, and NVP metabolites are largely eliminated by the kidney with <5% unchanged in the urine. Usual doses are recommended in renal failure (*Nephro Dial Transplant* 2001;16:192). NVP is contraindicated in severe liver disease due to hepatotoxicity.

SIDE EFFECTS

- **Hepatotoxicity:** Early hepatotoxicity usually occurs in the first 6 weeks and appears to be a hypersensitivity reaction and may be accompanied by drug rash, eosinophilia, and systemic symptoms (DRESS syndrome). This reaction differs from "transaminitis" noted with PIs and EFV in that it (1) is symptomatic hepatitis, (2) may progress to liver necrosis and death even with early detection and drug discontinuation (3) occurs in the first 16 wks, and usually in the first 6 wks, (4) occurs primarily with high baseline CD4 counts, especially in women. The rate of symptomatic hepatitis in women a baseline CD4 count ≥250/mm³ is 11% compared to 0.9% in women with lower CD4 counts at baseline. Men also have an increased risk with a CD4 count ≥400/mm³, but the rates are lower, 6.4% vs 2.3%. The mechanism of this reaction is not known, but the association with high CD4 counts suggests an immune mechanism. There have been at least 6 deaths in pregnant women given continuous NVP-based HAART (*J Acquir Immune Defic Syndr* 2004;36:772). Many feel that NVP should not be given to treatment-naïve women with a CD4 count >250/mm³. Also, the CDC issued a warning against using NVP for PEP based on reports of two HCW with severe hepatitis, including one who required a liver transplant (*Lancet* 2001;357:687; *MMWR* 2001;49:1153). This concern does not apply to the single dose of NVP given at delivery to prevent perinatal transmission. NVP recipients may also develop hepatotoxicity later in the course of

Drugs: Nevirapine

5

treatment, a form of hepatitis that is more benign and similar to hepatitis seen with other anti-HIV drugs. This hepatitis is characterized by a elevation in transaminase levels, it is usually asymptomatic, the frequency is about 15% and is more common in those with chronic HBV or HCV. Management guidelines for the severe early form include frequent monitoring of hepatic function in the first 12-16 wks, warning the patient, and prompt discontinuation of NVP if this diagnosis is considered. Guidelines for the later asymptomatic transaminitis are unclear but many recommend discontinuation of NVP if the ALT is >5 or 10x the ULN (*Hepatology* 2002;35:182).

- **Rash:** Rash is seen in about 17%. It is usually maculopapular and erythematous with or without pruritus and is located on the trunk, face, and extremities. Some patients with rashes require hospitalization, and 7% of all patients require discontinuation of the drug, compared with 4.3% given DLV and 1.7% given EFV (package insert, PDR). Indications for discontinuation of an NNRTI due to rash are rash accompanied by fever, blisters, mucous membrane involvement, conjunctivitis, edema, arthralgias, or malaise. Steroids do not appear to be effective therapy (*J Acquir Immune Defic Syndr* 2003;33:41). Stevens-Johnson syndrome and TEN have been reported, and three deaths ascribed to rash have been reported with NVP (*Lancet* 1998;351:567). Patients with rash should always be assessed for hepatotoxicity, as the two may occur together.

DRUG INTERACTIONS: NVP, like rifampin, induces CYP3A4. Maximum induction takes place 2 to 4 weeks after initiating therapy.

- **Drugs that are contraindicated or not recommended for concurrent use:** Rifampin, ketoconazole, St. John's wort, rifapentine.

- TABLE 5-37: **Dose Recommendations for NVP + PI Combinations**

PI	PI Level	NVP Level	Regimen Recommended
IDV	↓28%	No change	IDV 1000 mg q8h (NVP standard)
RTV	↓11%	No change	Standard doses
SQV	↓25%	No change	Recommend SQV/RTV 1000 mg/100 mg
NFV	↑10%	No change	Standard doses
APV/FPV	No data	No data	No data. Consider FPV 700 mg/RTV 100 mg bid (NVP standard).
LPV/r	LPV ↓55%	No change	LPV/r 533/133 mg (4 caps) bid (NVP standard)
ATV	↓	No data	Expect ↓ATV levels. Consider ATV/RTV 300/100 mg qd. (NVP standard.)
TPV	↓	—	Standard: TPV/RTV 500/200 mg bid + NVP 200 mg bid

Drugs: Nevirapine

DRUGS THAT REQUIRE DOSE MODIFICATION WITH CONCURRENT USE

- **Oral contraceptives:** NVP decreases AUC for ethinyl estradiol by about 30% *(J Acquir Immune Defic Syndr* 2002;29:471); alternative or additional methods of birth control should be used.

- **Clarithromycin:** NVP reduces clarithromycin AUC by 30% but increases levels of the 14-OH metabolite, which has antibacterial activity that compensates for this reduction, so no dose adjustment is necessary. NVP levels increased 26%. Use standard doses and monitor or use azithromycin.

- **Ketoconazole** levels decreased 63% and NVP increases 15% to 30%; not recommended.

- **Voriconazole:** no data, but significant potential for decrease of voriconazole and/or increase of NVP serum level.

- **Rifabutin** levels are decreased by 16%; no dose alteration.

- **Phenobarbital, phenytoin, carbamazepine:** No data. Monitor anticonvulsant levels.

- **Methadone:** NVP reduces AUC of methadone by about 50%. Opiate withdrawal is a concern and has been reported; methadone dose increases are variable but average 15% to 25% *(Clin Infect Dis* 2001;33:1595).

- **Statins:** No known drug interaction.

PREGNANCY: Category C. Negative rodent teratogenicity assays; placental passage in humans shows a newborn:maternal ratio of 1.0. Pharmacokinetic studies show no important differences for women in the third trimester compared to non-pregnant women. Safety for the infant seems well established, but women with a baseline CD4 count >250/mm^3 should not receive NVP-based HAART based on high rates of severe hepatotoxicity as summarized above. This admonition does not apply to the single perinatal dose, which is highly effective for preventing transmission, but controversial due to the high probability of class resistance (see below).

- **Efficacy:** A study from Thailand compared AZT (076 protocol) + NVP (single intrapartum dose + single infant dose) reduced perinatal transmission rates in 636 women to 1.9%; the rate with AZT alone was 6.5% *(N Engl J Med* 2004;351:217).

- **The DHHS guidelines** include NVP as an option for prevention of perinatal transmission for HIV-infected women who present at term with no prior therapy. A single oral dose of 200 mg is given at the onset of labor, and a single dose (2 mg/kg) is given to the infant at 48 to 72 hours (http://www.aidsinfo.org).

- **WHO guidelines** include NVP as a preferred regimen for HIV-infected women who are pregnant or women for whom effective contraception cannot be assured in resource-limited areas *(Scaling Up Antiretroviral Therapy,* WHO, 2003). WHO guidelines to prevent

5 Drugs: Nevirapine

perinatal transmission are: AZT (076 protocol) + NVP 200 mg at onset of labor and a single infant dose of 6 mg at 48-72 h (*N Engl J Med* 2004;351:289).

- **Resistance:** The major concern with single-dose NVP is the high frequency of NVP resistance following exposure (see p. 120). This occurred in 19% in HIVNET 012 (*Lancet* 1999;354:795) and 15% in PACTG 316 (*J Infect Dis* 2002;186:181). Subsequent studies using single gene sequencing demonstrated much higher levels of resistance. In HIVNET 012 these mutations were not detected at 13-18 month postpartum (*AIDS* 2001;15:1951), but a subsequent study in Thailand showed patients who received a single intrapartum dose of NVP had a higher rate of virologic failure when NVP was used therapeutically (failure rates 49% vs. 68%, *p* <0.03; *N Engl J Med* 2004;351:229).

NIZORAL – see Ketoconazole (p. 239)

NORTRIPTYLINE – see also Tricyclic Antidepressants (p. 313)

TRADE NAMES: *Aventyl* (Eli Lilly), *Pamelor* (Mallinckrodt), or generic

FORMS AND PRICES: Caps: 10 mg at $0.41, 25 mg at $0.82, 50 mg at $1.52, 75 mg at $2.23. Oral suspension: 10 mg/5 mL, 480 mL at $45.68.

CLASS: Tricyclic antidepressant

INDICATIONS AND DOSE REGIMENS

- **Depression:** 25 mg hs initially; increase by 25 mg every 3 days until 75 mg, then wait 5 days, and obtain level with expectation of 100-150 ng/dL.
- **Neuropathic pain:** 10-25 mg hs; increase dose over 2 to 3 weeks to maximum of 75 mg hs. Draw serum levels if higher doses used.

PHARMACOLOGY

- **Bioavailability:** >90%
- **T½:** 13 to 79 hours, mean – 31 hours
- **Elimination:** Metabolized and excreted renally

SIDE EFFECTS: Anticholinergic effects (dry mouth, dizziness, blurred vision, constipation, urinary hesitancy), orthostatic hypotension (less compared with other tricyclics), sedation, sexual dysfunction (decreased libido), and weight gain.

DRUG INTERACTIONS: The following drugs should not be given concurrently: Adrenergic neuronal blocking agents, clonidine, other alpha-2 agonists, excessive alcohol, fenfluramine, cimetidine, MAO inhibitors, and any drugs that increase nortriptyline levels (cimetidine, quinidine, fluconazole). RTV, LPV/r, SQV, IDV, NFV may increase nortriptyline levels.

PREGNANCY: Category D. Animal studies are inconclusive, and experience in pregnant women is inadequate. Avoid during first trimester, and when possible limit use in the last two trimesters.

NORVIR – see Ritonavir (p. 287)

NYSTATIN

TRADE NAMES: *Mycostatin* (Bristol-Myers Squibb) or generic

FORMS AND PRICES (generic)
- **Lozenges:** 200,000 units at $1.03/lozenge
- **Cream:** 100,000 U/g, 15 g at $2.64; 30 g at $5.00
- **Ointment:** 100,000 U/g, 15 g at $2.64; 30 g at $5.00
- **Suspension:** 100,000 U/mL, 60 mL at $6.25; 480 mL at $82.63
- **Oral tabs:** 500,000 units at $0.69/tab
- **Vaginal tabs:** 100,000 units at $0.47/tab

PATIENT ASSISTANCE PROGRAM (*Bristol-Myers Squibb*): 800-272-4878

CLASS: Polyene macrolide similar to amphotericin B

ACTIVITY: Active against *C. albicans* at 3 µg/mL and other *Candida* species at higher concentrations.

INDICATIONS AND DOSES
- **Thrush:** 5 mL suspension to be gargled 4x/day x 14 days. Disadvantages: *Nystatin* has a bitter taste, causes GI side effects, must be given 4x/day, and does not work as well as clotrimazole troches or oral fluconazole (*HIV Clin Trials* 2000;1:47). Efficacy is dependent on contact time with mucosa.
- **Vaginitis:** 100,000 unit tab intravaginally 1-2x/day x 14 days

PHARMACOLOGY
- **Bioavailability:** Poorly absorbed and undetectable in blood following oral administration
- Therapeutic levels persist in saliva for 2 h after oral dissolution of two lozenges.

SIDE EFFECTS: Infrequent, dose-related GI intolerance (transient nausea, vomiting, diarrhea)

5 Drugs: Nystatin

OXANDROLONE

TRADE NAME: *Oxandrin* (BTG)

FORMS: Tabs, 2.5, 5 and 10 mg

PRICE: Per tab, $5.30 (2.5 mg), $10.60 (5 mg) and $18.88 (10 mg); cost per day (20 mg), $37.76 - $42.40 (Note: IM nandrolone is more cost-effective at $120/month vs $900/month.

PATIENT ASSISTANCE PROGRAM: 866-692-6374

CLASS: Anabolic steroid

INDICATION AND DOSES: Wasting. Prior studies showed a modest weight gain after 16 weeks with a dose of 15 mg/day (*AIDS* 1996;10:1657; *AIDS* 1996;10:745; *Br J Nutr* 1996;75:129). 2.5 mg 2 to 4x/day, up to 20 mg/day in 2 to 4 doses depending on response. Natural testosterone esters are preferred for hypogonadal men (*Clin Infect Dis* 2003;36[suppl 2]:S73).

TRIALS: In a placebo-controlled trial using oxandrolone at a dose of 15 mg/day, drug recipients had significant increases in weight (avg 1.8 kg), lean body mass (avg 2.0 kg), appetite, and physical activity (*AIDS* 1996;10:1657).

PHARMACOLOGY: Bioavailability is 97%

SIDE EFFECTS: Virilizing complications primarily in women, including deep voice, hirsutism, acne, clitoral enlargement, and menstrual irregularity. Some virilizing changes may be irreversible, even with prompt discontinuation. Men may experience increased acne and increased frequency of erections. Of particular concern is hepatic toxicity with cholestatic hepatitis; discontinue drug if jaundice occurs or abnormal liver function tests are obtained. Drug-induced jaundice is reversible. Peliosis hepatis (blood-filled cysts) has been reported and may result in life-threatening hepatic failure or intra-abdominal hemorrhage (reversible with drug discontinuation). Miscellaneous side effects: Nausea, vomiting, changes in skin color, ankle swelling, depression, insomnia, and changes in libido.

DRUG INTERACTIONS: Increase activity of oral anticoagulants and oral hypoglycemic agents

PREGNANCY: Category X. Teratogenic.

OXYMETHOLONE

TRADE NAME: *Anadrol-50* (Unimed Pharmaceuticals)

FORM AND PRICE: 50 mg tab at $17.11

CLASS: Anabolic steroid

INDICATIONS AND DOSES: Wasting. 1-5 mg/kg/day; see above (oxandra-lone) regarding indications. Oxandrolone and nandrolone preferred due to lower incidence of hepatotoxicity.

MONITOR: LFTs, x-ray for bone density every 6 months, blood lipids, CBC

PHARMACOLOGY

- **T½:** 1 to 2 days
- **Elimination:** Metabolized in liver; 20% to 25% excreted in urine

SIDE EFFECTS: Peliosis hepatis (blood-filled cysts in liver ± spleen with mildly abnormal LFTs), but may also cause cholestatic jaundice, overt liver failure, hepatic necrosis (rare), liver cancer (rare), or intra-abdominal hemorrhage. Decreased HDL with increased risk of cardiovascular disease. Virilization in women. GI: Nausea, vomiting, diarrhea. Osteoporosis, decreased TSH and T4, increased pro-time and blood glucose.

DRUG INTERACTION: *Coumadin* – increase prothrombin time

CONTRAINDICATIONS: Breast cancer, severe liver disease, nephrosis, prostate cancer

PREGNANCY: Category X. Animal studies show embryo toxicity, fetotoxicity, infertility, and masculinization.

PAMELOR – see Nortriptyline (p. 266)

PAROMOMYCIN

TRADE NAME: *Humatin* (Monarch Pharmaceuticals and Caraco), or generic

FORM AND PRICE: 250 mg cap at $3.21 ($539/21 day course)

CLASS: Aminoglycoside (for oral use)

INDICATIONS AND DOSE: Cryptosporidiosis. 1 g PO bid or 500 mg PO qid

EFFICACY: The drug is active *in vitro* and in animal models against *Cryptosporidia* but only at levels far higher than those achieved in humans. There are anecdotal reports of clinical response but controlled trials show marginal benefit and no cures (*Clin Infect Dis* 1992;15:726; *Am J Med* 1996;100:370). An uncontrolled trial showed good results with paromomycin 1 g bid + azithromycin 600 mg qd x 4 weeks, then paromomycin 1 g bid (alone) x 8 weeks (*J Infect Dis* 1998;178:900). At present, there is a consensus that there is no effective chemotherapy for cryptosporidiosis except immune

Drugs: Paromomycin

5

reconstitution with HAART. Even modest increases in CD4 counts are effective (*N Engl J Med* 2002;346:1723). Paromomycin probably doesn't work.

PHARMACOLOGY

- Not absorbed; most of oral dose is excreted unchanged in stool; lesions of the GI tract may facilitate absorption and serum levels may increase in presence of renal failure.

SIDE EFFECTS: GI intolerance (anorexia, nausea, vomiting, epigastric pain), steatorrhea, and malabsorption; rare complications include rash, headache; vertigo with absorption and serum levels. There could be ototoxicity and nephrotoxicity with systemic absorption as with other aminoglycosides.

PREGNANCY: Category C

PEGYLATED INTERFERON

TRADE NAMES: Peginterferon alfa-2a – *Pegasys* (Roche); peginterferon alfa-2b – *Peg-Intron* (Schering-Plough)

FORMS

- Peginterferon alfa-2a (*Pegasys*) is supplied as a solution ready for injection, which requires refrigeration and is available at a fixed dose of 180 µg per 1 mL solution at $364.
- Peginterferon alfa-2b (*Peg-Intron*) is supplied as lyophilized powder to be reconstituted with 0.7 mL saline; several strengths are available based upon body weight.

PRICE (AWP): *Pegasys* – $17,460/year and *Peg-Intron* – $17,892/year. AWP costs for 70 kg patient treated for 48 weeks: Peginterferon + ribavirin – approximately $30,216 to $40,152

PATIENT ASSISTANCE PROGRAM: 877-734-2797 (*Pegasys*) and 800-521-7157 (*Peg-Intron*)

PRODUCT: Recombinant alfa-interferon conjugated with polyethylene glycol (PEG), which decreases the clearance rate of interferon and results in sustained concentrations permitting less frequent dosing. The side effect profiles of pegylated and non-pegylated interferons appear to be similar.

INDICATIONS AND DOSE: FDA indications: Treatment of compensated chronic hepatitis C not previously treated with interferon alfa. HIV-HCV co-infected patients are candidates for anti-HCV therapy if they are considered at high risk for cirrhosis based on a liver biopsy showing bridging fibrosis and inflammation plus HCV RNA levels >50 IU/mL Cure rates with peginterferon + ribavirin in the absence of HIV co-infection are 42% to 46% for genotype 1 and 76% to 82% for

Drugs: Paromomycin

genotypes 2 and 3 (*Lancet* 2001;358:958; *N Engl J Med* 2002;347:975). HCV patients with or without HIV are not considered candidates for this treatment if there is active substance abuse, decompensated liver disease, severe, active psychiatric disease or refusal of therapy (*Ann Intern Med* 2002;136:288). All three clinical trials enrolled patients with a median CD4 count >500/mm^3. However, a subset analysis of 17 patients with a CD4 count <200/mm^3 given peginterferon + ribavarin showed HCV virologic response of 47% compared to 40% in patients with a higher baseline CD4 count (*N Engl J Med* 2004;351:2340).

- **Dose:** Pegylated interferon (alfa 2a 180 mg or alfa 2b 1.5 mg/kg) SC/week plus ribavirin 400 mg bid. (The ribavirin dose of 800 mg/d is the dose used in clinical trials of co-infected patients, but higher doses of RBV, 800 mg/d for <40 kg, 1000 mg/d for 45-75 kg, 1200 mg/d for >75 kg) may be more effective.) Usual duration is 48 weeks regardless of genotype. With CrCl <50 mL/min consider half dose interferon (*N Engl J Med* 2002;347:975).

■ TABLE 5-38: **Results of 3 Clinical Trials of PegIFN + Ribavirin for HCV in Patients with HIV Co-infection**

Source (11th CROI, 2004)	No. Pts	Regimen x 48 weeks	Rate of SVR	
			Gen 1	Gen 2/3
ACTG A5071 (*N Engl J Med* 2004;351:451)	66	PegIFN 180 mg/wk Ribavirin 600-1000 mg/d	14%	73%
APRICOT (*N Engl J Med* 2004;351:451)	289	PegIFN 180 mg/wk Ribavirin 800 mg/d	29%	62%
RIBAVIC (*JAMA* 2004;292: 2839)	205	PegIFN 180 mg/wk Ribavirin 800 mg/d	15%	—

MONITORING

- **Clinical response:** HCV RNA at 12 weeks (see Table 5-34). Patients without a ≥2 log$_{10}$ c/mL decrease in HCV RNA levels at 12 weeks are unlikely to achieve SVR, although this does not exclude the possibility of clinical benefit by other criteria. If HCV RNA is detectable after 12 weeks, consider discontinuation. Sustained virologic response is defined as undetectable HCV RNA at 24 weeks post therapy.

- **Toxicity:** CBC and comprehensive metabolic panel at baseline, at 2 weeks, then every 6 weeks. TSH at baseline and then every 12 weeks.

- **Patients with cardiac disease:** EKG at baseline and prn.

- **Women of childbearing potential:** Urine pregnancy testing every 4 to 6 weeks.

5 Drugs: Pegylated Interferon

PHARMACOLOGY

The differences between the two commercially available peg-IFN products are: 1) *Peg-Intron* (alfa–2b) is a linear chain PEG and *Pegasys* (alfa–2a) is a branched chain PEG. This structural difference results in higher serum level and more prolong T½ with *Pegasys*. Despite the PK difference, the two products appear to be clinically equivalent. 2) Clinical trials including HIV co-infected patients have all been performed with *Pegasys*.

- **Bioavailability:** Increases with duration of therapy – mean trough of peg-IFN alfa 26 with 1 µg/kg SQ at week 4=94 pg/mL, at week 48=320 pg/mL. C_{max} mean is 554 pg/mL at 15 to 44 hours and sustained up to 48 to 72 hours. Compared to non-pegylated interferon, peginterferon C_{max} is about 10x greater and AUC is 50x greater.

- **T½:** Peg-IFN alfa 2a = 77 h; Peg-INF alfa 2b = 40 hrs (compared with 8 h for non-pegylated interferon).

- **Elimination:** Renal 30% (7x lower clearance than non-pegylated interferon). Eliminated primarily in the bile.

SIDE EFFECTS: Similar to those of interferon; about 10% in clinical trials discontinue therapy due to adverse reactions (*N Engl J Med* 2004;351:438; *N Engl J Med* 2004;351:451).

- **Neuropsychiatric:** Depression, suicidal or homicidal ideation, and relapse of substance abuse. Should be used with extreme caution in patients with history of psychiatric disorders. Warn patient and monitor. Depression reported in 21% to 29%. Suicides reported. Active depression with suicidal ideation is a contraindication.

- **Marrow suppression:** ANC counts decrease in 70%, <500/mm³ in 1%, platelet counts decrease in 20%, <20,000/mm³ in 1%. Recommendation:

■ TABLE 5-39: **Marrow Toxicity: Criteria for Dose Reduction/Discontinuation**

Laboratory Measurement	Criteria for Dose Reduction to 0.5 µg/mL	Criteria for Discontinue
ANC*	<750/mm³	<500/mm³
Platelet count	<50,000/mm³	<25,000/mm³

* Leukopenia generally responds to G-CSF, which may be preferred to avoid dose reduction.

- **Flu-like symptoms:** Most common; about 50% will have fever, headache, chills, and myalgias/arthralgias. May decrease with continued treatment. May be treated with NSAIDS or acetaminophen; with liver disease acetaminophen dose should be <2 g/day.

- **Thyroid:** Thyroiditis with hyperthyroidism or hypothyroidism. TSH levels should be measured at baseline and during therapy every 12 weeks.

Drugs: Pegylated Interferon

- **Retinopathy:** Obtain baseline retinal evaluation in patients with diabetes, hypertension or other ocular abnormality.
- **Injection site reaction:** Inflammation, pruritus, pain (mild) in 47%
- **GI complaints:** Nausea, anorexia, diarrhea, and/or abdominal pain in 15% to 30%
- **Skin/hair:** Alopecia (20%), pruritus (10%), and/or rash (6%)
- **Miscellaneous:** Hyperglycemia, cardiac arrhythmias, elevated hepatic transaminase levels 2 to 5x, colitis, pancreatitis, autoimmune disorders, hypersensitivity reactions

DRUG INTERACTIONS: Avoid co-administration of marrow suppressive agents. (Note: clinically important interactions with ribavirin, see p. 259)

PREGNANCY: Category C. Abortifacient potential in primates. Ribavirin is a potent teratogen and must be avoided in pregnancy and used with caution in women of childbearing potential and their male sexual partners. Breastfeeding: No data.

PENTAM – see Pentamidine (below)

PENTAMIDINE

TRADE NAME: *Pentam* for IV use; *NebuPent* for inhalation (American Pharmaceutical Partners)

FORMS AND PRICE: 300 mg vial at $98.75

PATIENT ASSISTANCE PROGRAM: IV and aerosolized pentamidine 888-391-6300

CLASS: Aromatic diamidine-derivative antiprotozoal agent that is structurally related to stilbamidine

INDICATIONS AND DOSES

- ***P. jiroveci* pneumonia:** 3-4 mg/kg IV given over ≥1 hr x 21 days. The approved dose is 4 mg/kg, but some clinicians prefer 3 mg/kg. TMP-SMX is preferred (*Ann Intern Med* 1986;105:37; *AIDS* 1992;6:301).
- ***P. jiroveci* prophylaxis:** 300 mg/month delivered by a *Respirgard II* nebulizer using 300 mg dose diluted in 6 mL sterile water delivered at 6 L/min from a 50 psi compressed air source until the reservoir is dry. TMP-SMX preferred due to superior efficacy in preventing PCP, efficacy in preventing other infections, reduced cost, and greater convenience (*N Engl J Med* 1995;332:693). Aerosolized pentamidine should not be used for PCP treatment (*Ann Intern Med* 1990;113:203).

Drugs: Pentamidine

5

PHARMACOLOGY

- **Bioavailability:** Not absorbed orally. With aerosol, 5% reaches alveolar spaces via *Respirgard II* nebulizer. Blood levels with monthly aerosol delivery are below detectable limits.

- **T½:** Parenteral – 6 hours

- **Elimination:** Primarily nonrenal but may accumulate in renal failure

- **Dose modification of parenteral form with renal failure:** CrCl >50 mL/min – 4 mg/kg q24h; 10-50 mL/min – 4 mg/kg q24h-q36h; <10 mL/min – 4 mg/kg q48h.

SIDE EFFECTS

- **Aerosolized pentamidine:** Cough and wheezing – 30% (prevented with pretreatment with beta-2 agonist), sufficiently severe to require discontinuation of treatment in 5% (*N Engl J Med* 1990;323:769). Other reactions include laryngitis, chest pain, and dyspnea. The role of aerosolized pentamidine in promoting extrapulmonary *P. jiroveci* infection and pneumothorax is unclear. Risk of transmitting TB to patients and health care workers.

- **Systemic pentamidine:** In a review of 106 courses of IV pentamidine, 76 (72%) had adverse reactions; these were sufficiently severe to require drug discontinuation in 31 (18%) (*Clin Infect Dis* 1997;24: 854). The most common causes of drug discontinuation were nephrotoxicity and hypoglycemia. Nephrotoxicity is noted in 25% to 50%. It is usually characterized by a gradual increase in creatinine in the second week of treatment but may cause acute renal failure. Risk is increased with dehydration and concurrent use of nephrotoxic drugs. Hypotension is unusual (6%) but may cause death, most often with rapid infusions; drug should be infused over ≥60 minutes. Hypoglycemia, with blood glucose 25 mg/dL in 5% to 10%, can occur after 5 to 7 days of treatment, sometimes persisting several days after discontinuation. Hypoglycemia may last days or weeks and is treated with IV glucose ± oral diazoxide. Hyperglycemia (2% to 9%) and insulin-dependent diabetes mellitus may occur with or without prior hypoglycemia. Leukopenia and thrombocytopenia are noted in 2% to 13%. GI intolerance with nausea, vomiting, abdominal pain, anorexia, and/or bad taste is common. Local reactions include sterile abscesses at IM injection sites (no longer advocated) and pain, erythema, tenderness, and induration (chemical phlebitis) at IV infusion sites. Other reactions include hepatitis, hypocalcemia (sometimes severe), increased amylase, hypomagnesemia, fever, rash, urticaria, toxic epidermal necrolysis (TEN), confusion, dizziness (without hypotension), anaphylaxis, arrhythmias including Torsade de pointes.

MONITORING

- **Aerosolized pentamidine:** This is considered safe for the patient but poses risk of TB to healthcare workers and other patients. Patient should be evaluated for TB (PPD, X-ray, and sputum examination if indicated). Suspected or confirmed TB should be treated prior to aerosol treatments. Adequate air exchanges with exhaust to outside and appropriate use of particulate air filters are required. Some suggest pregnant HCWs should avoid environmental exposure to pentamidine until risks to fetus are better defined.

- **Parenteral administration:** Adverse effects are common and may be lethal. Due to the risk of hypotension, the drug should be given in supine position, the patient should be hydrated, pentamidine should be delivered over ≥60 minutes, and BP should be monitored during treatment and afterward until stable. Regular laboratory monitoring (daily or every other day) should include creatinine, potassium, calcium, and glucose; other tests for periodic monitoring include CBC, LFTs, and calcium.

DRUG INTERACTIONS: Avoid concurrent use of parenteral pentamidine with nephrotoxic drugs, including aminoglycosides, amphotericin B, and foscarnet and cidofovir. Amphotericin B – severe hypocalcemia.

PREGNANCY: Category C. Limited experience with pregnant women.

PRAVASTATIN

TRADE NAME: *Pravachol* (Bristol-Myers Squibb)

FORMS AND PRICES: Tabs: 10 mg at $2.78, 20 mg at $2.78, 40 mg at $4.34

CLASS: Statin (HMG-CoA reductase inhibitor)

INDICATIONS AND DOSES: Elevated total cholesterol, LDL cholesterol, and/or triglycerides and/or low HDL cholesterol. This is often a favored statin for dyslipidemia associated with PI-based HAART due to paucity of drug interactions with PIs (*Clin Infect Dis* 2003;37:613), although it may be less effective than other statins. Initial dose is 40 mg once daily. If desired cholesterol levels are not achieved with 40 mg daily, 80 mg once daily is recommended. A starting dose of 10 mg daily is recommended in patients with a history of significant hepatic or renal dysfunction. Can be administered as a single dose at any time of the day.

MONITORING: Blood lipids at 4-week intervals until desired results are achieved, then periodically. It is recommended that transaminases be measured prior to the initiation of therapy, prior to the elevation of the dose, and when otherwise clinically indicated. Patients should be warned to report muscle pain, tenderness, or weakness promptly, especially if accompanied by fever or malaise; obtain CPK for suspected myopathy.

PRECAUTIONS: Pravastatin (and other statins) are contraindicated with pregnancy, breastfeeding, concurrent conditions that predispose to

Drugs: Pravastatin

5

renal failure (sepsis, hypotension, etc.) and active hepatic disease. Alcoholism is a relative contraindication.

PHARMACOLOGY

- **Bioavailability:** 14%
- **T½:** 1.3 to 2.7 hours
- **Elimination:** Fecal (biliary and unabsorbed drug) – 70%; renal – 20%

SIDE EFFECTS

- **Musculoskeletal:** Myopathy with elevated CPK plus muscle tenderness, weakness, or pain + fever or malaise. Rhabdomyolysis with renal failure has been reported.
- **Hepatic:** Elevated transaminase levels in 1% to 2%; discontinue if otherwise unexplained elevations of ALT and/or AST are >3x ULN.
- **Miscellaneous:** Diarrhea, constipation, nausea, heartburn, stomach pain, dizziness, headache, skin rash (eczematous plaques), insomnia, and impotence (rare)

DRUG INTERACTIONS: PIs: Concurrent use considered appropriate with PIs and NNRTIs. RTV/SQV decreases pravastatin AUC 50%; EFV decreases pravastatin AUC 40%. Pravastatin dose may need to be increased. Possible interactions with spironolactone, cimetidine, and ketoconazole that reduce cholesterol levels and may effect adrenal and sex hormone production with concurrent use. Itraconazole increases pravastatin AUC and C_{max} 1.7x and 2.5x, respectively. Cholestyramine and colestipol decrease pravastatin AUC 40%; administer pravastatin 1 h before or 4 h after. Niacin and gemfibrozil: increased risk of myopathy. Rare cases of rhabdomyolysis with acute renal failure secondary to myoglobinuria have been reported with pravastatin and other drugs in this class.

PREGNANCY: Category X. Contraindicated.

PRIMAQUINE

TRADE NAME: Generic

FORM AND PRICE: 15 mg base tabs (26 mg primaquine phosphate) at $0.99

CLASS: Antimalarial

INDICATIONS AND DOSES: *P. jiroveci* pneumonia: Primaquine 15-30 mg (base)/day + clindamycin 600-900 mg q6-8h IV or 300-450 mg PO q6-8h. **Note:** The published experience and recommendation is for "mild to moderately severe" PCP (*Ann Intern Med* 1996;124:792; *Clin Infect Dis* 1994;18:905; *Clin Infect Dis* 1998;27:524). A meta-analysis of published reports of PCP patients who failed initial treatment showed the clindamycin-primaquine regimen was superior to all others with responses in 42 of 48 (87%) (*Arch Intern Med* 2001;161:1529).

PHARMACOLOGY

- **Bioavailability:** Well absorbed
- **T½:** 4 to 10 hours
- **Elimination:** Metabolized by liver

SIDE EFFECTS: Hemolytic anemia in patients with G6-PD deficiency; its severity depends on drug dose and genetics of G6-PD deficiency. In African Americans, the reaction is usually mild, self-limited and asymptomatic; in patients of Mediterranean or certain Asian extractions, hemolysis may be severe. Hemolytic anemia may also occur with other forms of hemoglobinopathy. Warn patient of dark urine as sign and/or measure G6-PD level prior to use in susceptible individuals. Other hematologic side effects: Methemoglobinemia, leukopenia. GI: Nausea, vomiting, epigastric pain (reduced by administration with meals). Miscellaneous: Headache, disturbed visual accommodation, pruritus, hypertension, arrhythmias.

PREGNANCY: Category C. Limited experience in pregnant women. There is a theoretical risk of hemolytic anemia if fetus has G6PD deficiency.

PROCRIT – see Erythropoietin (p. 200)

PYRAZINAMIDE (PZA)

TRADE NAME: Generic

FORM AND PRICE: 500 mg tab at $1.20 (usually 2 g/day at $4.48/day)

CLASS: Derivative of niacinamide

INDICATION AND REGIMEN: Tuberculosis, initial phase of three to four drug regimen, usually for 8 weeks (*MMWR* 1998;47[RR-20]; *MMWR* 2000;49:185). Treatment of latent tuberculosis: PZA + rifampin regimen (see rifampin p. 291). Note that the dose for PZA for treatment of latent infection is ≤20 mg/kg/day and not to exceed 2 g/day. For active TB, see Table 5-40.

■ Table 5-40: **PZA Doses for Active TB**

Weight	Daily*	2x/week*	3x/week*
40-55 kg	1 gm	2.0 gm	1.5 gm
56-75 kg	1.5 gm	3.0 gm	2.5 gm
76-90 kg	2.0 gm	4.0 gm	3.0 gm

*Patients with a CD4 count <100/mm³ should receive daily therapy or 3x/week therapy.

Drugs: Pyrazinamide

5

TREATMENT WITH *RIFATER* (tabs with 50 mg INH, 120 mg rifampin, and 300 mg PZA)

- <65 kg: 1 tab/10 kg/day
- >65 kg: 6 tabs/day

PHARMACOLOGY

- **Bioavailability:** Well absorbed; absorption is reduced about 25% in patients with advanced HIV infection (*Ann Intern Med* 1997;127:289).
- **T½:** 9 to 10 hours
- **CSF levels:** Equal to plasma levels
- **Elimination:** Hydrolyzed in liver; 4% to 14% of parent compound and 70% of metabolite excreted in urine.
- **Renal failure:** Usual dose unless creatinine clearance <10 mL/min – 12-20 mg/kg/day (increased risk of hyperuricemia).
- **Hepatic failure:** Contraindicated

SIDE EFFECTS: PZA appears to be the major cause of hepatotoxicity in patients with hepatitis as a complication of TB treatment (*Am J Respir Crit Care Med* 2003;167:1472). Hepatotoxicity occurs in up to 15% who receive >3 g/day: transient hepatitis with increase in transaminases, jaundice, and a syndrome of fever, anorexia, and hepatomegaly; rarely, acute yellow atrophy. Monitor LFTs monthly if there are abnormal baseline levels, symptoms suggesting hepatitis, or elevated levels during therapy that are not high enough to stop treatment (ALT <5x ULN). Hyperuricemia is common, but gout is rare. Nongouty polyarthralgia in up to 40%; hyperuricemia usually responds to uricosuric agents. Use with caution in patients with history of gout. Rare – rash, fever, acne, dysuria, skin discoloration, urticaria, pruritus, GI intolerance, thrombocytopenia, sideroblastic anemia.

PREGNANCY: Category C. Not teratogenic in mice, but limited experience in humans. Risk of teratogenicity is unknown, so INH, rifampin, and EMB are preferred. PZA is advocated for pregnant women if resistant *M. tuberculosis* is suspected or established and is acceptable outside the United States per WHO guidelines.

PYRIMETHAMINE

TRADE NAME: *Daraprim* (GlaxoSmithKline) or generic

FORM AND PRICE: 25 mg tab at $0.60

PATIENT ASSISTANCE PROGRAM: 800-722-9294

CLASS: Aminopyrimidine-derivative antimalarial agent that is structurally related to trimethoprim

INDICATIONS AND DOSE REGIMENS: Toxoplasmosis

■ Table 5-41: **Toxoplasmosis Treatment**

	Acute Phase (3 to 6 weeks)	Maintenance
First line	Pyrimethamine 200 mg x 1 then 50 mg (<60 kg) or 75 mg (>60 kg) + leucovorin 10-20 mg/d + sulfadiazine 1 g qid (<60 kg) or 1.5 g qid (>60 kg) x ≥6 weeks	Pyrimethamine at 50% acute dose and sulfadiazine at 50% acute dose + leucovorin 15 mg/day
Second line	Pyrimethamine + leucovorin + one of the following: ■ Clindamycin 600 mg PO or IV q 6 h or ■ TMP-SMX (5 mg TMP) IV or PO bid or ■ Atovaquone 1500 mg PO bid ■ Azithromycin 900-1200 mg PO qd	Pyrimethamine 25-50 mg qd + leukovorin 10-25 mg PO plus one of the following: ■ Clindamycin 300-450 mg PO q 6-8 h ■ Atovaquone 750 mg PO q 6-12 h
Other	■ Atovaquone 1500 mg PO bid + sulfadiazine 1.0-1.5 mg po q 6 h. ■ Atovaquone 1500 mg PO bid (without pyrimethamine/leukovorin)	■ Atovaquone 750 mg PO q 6-12 h (without pyrimethamine/leukovorin)

- **Primary prophylaxis:** Pyrimethamine 50 mg PO/week + dapsone 50 mg PO/day + leucovorin 25 mg/week or pyrimethamine 75 mg/week + dapsone 200 mg/week and leucovorin 25 mg/week or atovaquone 1500 mg/day ± pyrimethamine 25 mg/day + leucovorin 10 mg/day.

PHARMACOLOGY

- **Bioavailability:** Well absorbed
- **T½:** 54 to 148 hours (average 111 hours)
- **Elimination:** Parent compound and metabolites excreted in urine
- **Dose modification in renal failure:** None

SIDE EFFECTS: Reversible marrow suppression due to depletion of folic acid stores with dose-related megaloblastic anemia, leukopenia, thrombocytopenia, and agranulocytosis; prevented or treated with folinic acid (leucovorin).

- **GI intolerance:** Improved by reducing dose or giving drug with meals
- **Neurologic:** Dose-related ataxia, tremors, or seizures
- **Hypersensitivity:** Most common with pyrimethamine plus sulfadoxine (*Fansidar*) and due to sulfonamide component of combination

5 Drugs: Pyrimethamine

- **Drug interactions:** Lorazepam: hepatotoxicity. AZT, ganciclovir: assitive bone marrow suppression.

PREGNANCY: Category C. Teratogenic in animals, but limited experience has not shown association with birth defects in humans.

REBETOL – see Ribavirin (p. 281)

RETROVIR – see Zidovudine (AZT, ZDV) (p. 323)

RHO (D) IMMUNE GLOBULIN

TRADE NAME: *WinRho* (Univax)

FORMS AND PRICES: Vials of 600 IU at $103 and 1500 IU at $324. Cost of IVIG (1000 mg/kg): $3,570 to $4,569 (*Med Letter* 1996;38:8). Cost of *Win Rho* (AWP) is $972/4500 units.

INDICATION AND DOSES: Idiopathic thrombocytopenic purpura (ITP) in patient who is Rh-positive. Advantages over IVIG: Short infusion time, modest cost reduction and, in some cases, availability. Usual dose: 50 µg/kg or 3500 IU (70 kg). With hemoglobin levels <10 g/dL, give 25-50 µg/kg to reduce the severity of anemia. A disadvantage is the slow onset of action and a decrease in hemoglobin.

- **Note:** Patients must have intact spleen and be Rho(D)-positive for a biologic effect with treatment for ITP.

REGIMEN: Initial dose – 50 µg/kg IV over 3 to 5 minutes. May repeat at 3 to 4 days and may increase dose up to 80 µg/kg. Most patients require maintenance doses of 25-60 µg/kg.

MECHANISM: This product was developed to provide anti-D globulin to prevent Rh-isoimmunization in Rh-negative pregnant women with an Rh-positive fetus. Injection of anti-D into Rh-positive patients with ITP coats the patient's D+ RBCs with antibodies; this spares splenic clearance of antibody-coated platelets (*Trans Med Rev* 1992;6:17).

CLINICAL TRIALS: The average increase in platelets, including in patients with HIV-associated ITP, is 50,000/mm³ (*Am J Hematol* 1986;22:241; *Blood* 1991;77:1884). The response is somewhat delayed compared to IVIG. The effect lasts an average of 3 weeks.

SIDE EFFECTS: Hemolysis with decreases in hemoglobin of ≥2 g/dL in 5% to 10%. Monitor CBC. Fever and chills 1 to 2 hours after infusion (presumably due to hemolysis) in 10%; this can be avoided or reduced in severity with acetaminophen, antihistamines, or prednisone or by increasing infusion time to 15 to 20 minutes. Vial should not be shaken due to possible damage of protein or formation of aggregates.

RIBAVIRIN

TRADE NAME: *Rebetol* and *Rebetron* (combined *Rebetrol/Intron A*) (Schering-Plough); *Copegus* (Roche), *Virazole* (Valeant) inhalation

FORMS AND PRICES: 200 mg caps at $9.93 per cap; 200 mg tab (*Copegus*) at $7.60 per tab; $1575/6 gm vial (*Virazole*)

NOTE: Concurrent use with ddI is contraindicated due to increased risk of pancreatitis and/or lactic acidosis. Use with caution when given with AZT (additive anemia) or d4T (potentiation of mitochondrial toxicity).

INDICATION (FDA labeling): Ribavirin in combination with interferon is recommended for treatment of chronic hepatitis C in patients with compensated liver disease who have not previously been treated, and in patients who have relapsed after interferon monotherapy.

REGIMEN: Dose used in therapeutic trials was usually 400 mg bid, but dosage range 1000-1200 mg resulted in improved SVR (see p. 271). Standard dose in absence of HIV co-infection is: <75 kg – 400 mg in a.m., 600 mg in p.m.; >75 kg – 600 mg bid.

CLINICAL TRIALS: Several trials have tested the relative efficacy of HCV treatment using ribavirin + interferon vs interferon alone. The results with HIV-HCV co-infection show sustained viral suppression in 15-25% with genotype 1 and 70-80% with genotypes 2 and 3 (*N Engl J Med* 2004;351:451; *N Engl J Med* 2004;351:438; *JAMA* 2004;292:2909), see p. 270. Compared to patients with HCV without HIV, these rates of SVR are much lower for genotype 1 and comparable for genotypes 2 and 3 (*Lancet* 2001;358:958; *N Engl J Med* 2002;347:975).

PHARMACOLOGY

- **Oral bioavailability:** 64%; absorption increased with high-fat meal
- **T½:** 30 hours
- **Elimination:** Metabolized by phosphorylation and deribosylation; there are few or no cytochrome P450 enzyme-based drug interactions. Metabolites are excreted in the urine. The drug should not be used with severe renal failure.

SIDE EFFECTS: About 6% of patients receiving ribavirin/interferon discontinue therapy due to side effects. The main side effects are anemia, cough, and dyspepsia. Hemolytic anemia is noted in the first 1 to 2 weeks of treatment and usually stabilizes by week 4. In clinical trials without HIV co-infection, the mean decrease in hemoglobin was 3 g/dL, and 10% of patients had a hemoglobin <10 g/dL. Patients with a hemoglobin <10 g/dL or decrease in hemoglobin ≥2 g/dL *and* a history of cardiovascular disease should receive a modified regimen of ribavirin 600 mg/day + interferon 1.5 million units 3x/week. The drugs should be

Drugs: Ribavirin

5

discontinued if the hemoglobulin decreases to ≤8.5 g/dL or if the hemoglobin persists at <12 g/dL in patients with a cardiovascular disease. Erythropoietin (40,000 units SQ every week) is usually effective (*Am J Gastro* 2001;96:2802). Concurrent use of AZT should be avoided whenever possible. Ribavirin is a nucleoside that may cause mitochondrial toxicity, especially when combined with other NRTIs that cause mitochondrial toxicity, especially d4T; 2 of 15 patients given this combination developed lactic acidosis (*Lancet* 2001;357:280). Other side effects ascribed to ribavirin include leukopenia, hyperbilirubinemia, increased uric acid, and dyspnea.

NOTE: See pegylated interferon, p. 270, for side effects ascribed to that agent.

DRUG INTERACTION: Increased risk of anemia with AZT co-administration; monitor closely (*Antimicrob Agents Chemother* 1997;41:1231; *AIDS* 1998;14:1661). In combination with ddl, there is potentiation of ddl toxicity due to inhibition of mitochondrial DNA polymerase gamma, resulting in pancreatitis and lactic acidosis (*Antimicrob Agents Chemother* 1987;31:1613; *Lancet* 2001;72:177). This combination should be avoided.

PREGNANCY: Category X. Potent teratogen. Must be used with caution in women with childbearing potential and in their male sexual partners. Adequate birth control is mandatory.

RIFABUTIN

TRADE NAME: *Mycobutin* (Pharmacia)

FORM AND PRICE: 150 mg cap at $7.13

PATIENT ASSISTANCE PROGRAM: 800-242-7014

CLASS: Semisynthetic derivative of rifampin B that is derived from *Streptomyces mediterranei*

INDICATIONS AND DOSES

- **M. avium prophylaxis:** 300 mg PO qd. Efficacy established (*N Engl J Med* 1993;329:828); azithromycin or clarithromycin is usually preferred.

- **M. avium treatment:** Sometimes combined with clarithromycin or azithromycin and EMB using 300 mg/day, except in patients treated with PIs or NNRTIs where dose adjustment is recommended (see below).

- **Tuberculosis:** Preferred rifamycin for use in combination with most PIs or NNRTIs (*MMWR* 2004;53:37). Usual dose for TB treatment and prophylaxis: 300 mg/day, but dose must be adjusted for concurrent use with PIs and/or NNRTIs: See Table 6-2d, p. 367.

Drugs: Rifabutin

ACTIVITY: Active against most strains of *M. avium* and rifampin-sensitive *M. tuberculosis*; cross-resistance between rifampin and rifabutin is common with *M. tuberculosis* and *M. avium.*

PHARMACOLOGY

- **Bioavailability:** 12% to 20%
- **T½:** 30 to 60 hours
- **Metabolism:** Metabolized via CYP3A4 to 25-0-deacetyl-rifabutin (10% of total antimicrobial activity).
- **Elimination:** Primarily renal and biliary excretion of metabolites
- **Dose modification in renal failure:** None

SIDE EFFECTS: Common: Brown-orange discoloration of secretions; urine (30%), tears, saliva, sweat, stool, and skin. Infrequent: Rash (4%), GI intolerance (3%), neutropenia (2%). Rare: Flu-like illness, hepatitis, hemolysis, headache, thrombocytopenia, myositis. Uveitis, which presents as red and painful eye, blurred vision, photophobia, or floaters, is dose-related, usually with doses >450 mg/day, or with standard dose (300 mg/day) plus concurrent use of drugs that increase rifabutin levels: Most PIs, clarithromycin, and fluconazole (*N Engl J Med* 1994;330:868). Treated with topical corticosteroids and mydriatics. These patients should be evaluated by an ophthalmologist.

DRUG INTERACTIONS: Rifabutin induces hepatic microsomal enzymes (cytochrome P450 3AY), although the effect is less pronounced than for rifampin. Concurrent treatment with rifabutin reduces the levels of APV (14% decrease), coumadin, barbiturates, benzodiazepines, beta-blockers, chloramphenicol, clofibrate, oral contraceptives, cortico-steroids, cyclosporine, diazepam, dapsone, digitalis, doxycycline, haloperidol, oral hypoglycemics, voriconazole, ketoconazole, methadone, phenytoin, quinidine, theophylline, trimethoprim, and verapamil. Drugs that inhibit cytochrome P450 and prolong the half-life of rifabutin: PIs and DLV, erythromycin, clarithromycin (56% increase), and azoles (fluconazole, itraconazole, and ketoconazole). With concurrent rifabutin and fluconazole, the levels of rifabutin are significantly increased, leading to possible rifabutin toxicity (uveitis, nausea, neutropenia) or increased efficacy (*Clin Infect Dis* 1996;23;685).

COMMENTS

- Rifampin and rifabutin are related drugs, but *in vitro* activity and clinical trials show that rifabutin is preferred for *M. avium*, and rifampin is preferred for *M. tuberculosis.*
- Clarithromycin plus EMB without rifabutin may be the preferred regimen for treatment of disseminated *M. avium* infection due to the clarithromycin–rifabutin interaction.

5 Drugs: Rifabutin

- Drug interactions are similar for rifabutin and rifampin, although rifabutin is a less potent inducing agent of hepatic microsomal enzymes.
- Uveitis requires immediate discontinuation of drug and ophthalmology consult.
- All PIs and NNRTIs require a dose adjustment when given with rifabutin except for NVP (see Table 5-42, below).

■ TABLE 5-42: **Rifabutin Interactions and Dose Adjustments with Antiretroviral Drugs** (DHHS Guidelines for Use of Antiretroviral Agents in Adults and Adolescents, *MMWR* 2004;53:37)

| Agent | AUC for | | Comment |
	ART Agent	Rifabutin	
Nucleosides	NC	NC	Use standard doses[†]
APV/FPV	↓15%	↑193%	APV: standard; rifabutin: 150 mg/day or 300 mg 3x/week
DLV	↓80%	↑100%	Contraindicated
EFV*	NC	↓35%	EFV: standard; rifabutin: 450 mg/day or 600 mg 3x/week
IDV	↓32%	↑2x	IDV: 1000 mg q8h; rifabutin: 150 mg/day or 300 mg 3x/week
NVP*	NC	NC	NVP 200 mg bid; rifabutin 300 mg/day or 300 mg 3x/week
NFV	↓32%	↑2x	NFV: 1000 mg tid; rifabutin: 150 mg/day or 300 mg 3x/week
RTV	NC	↑4x	Rifabutin: 150 mg qod or 3x/week; RTV: standard
SQV (*Fortovase*)	↓40%		Not recommended without RTV
LPV/r	NC	↑3 fold	LPV/r: standard rifabutin: 150 mg qod or 3x/week
ATV	NC	↑2.5x	ATV standard; rifabutin: 150 mg qod or 3x/week
RTV boosted PI regimens (SQV, ATV, IDV, APV, FPV)	—	—	PI: standard; rifabutin 150 mg qod or 150 mg 3x/wk
TPV/r	NC	↑190%	TPV: standard; rifabutin 150 mg qod or 150 mg 3x/wk

[†] Regimens for 2 to 3x/week should be given 3x/week in patients with a CD4 count <100 cells/mm³ due to risk of rifampin resistance (*Am J Respir Crit Care Med* 2001;164:1319).
NC = No change

PREGNANCY: Category B. Not teratogenic in rats or rabbits.

RIFAMATE – see Isoniazid (p. 234) or Rifampin (p. 285)
(*Ann Intern Med* 1995;122:951)

RIFAMPIN

TRADE NAME: *Rifadin* (Aventis) or generic; Combination with INH: *Rifamate*. Combination with INH and PZA: *Rifater* (Aventis)

FORMS AND PRICES: Caps: 150 mg, 300 mg at $2.23. *Rifamate*: Caps with 150 mg INH + 300 mg rifampin at $2.57. *Rifater*: Tabs with 50 mg INH + 120 mg rifampin + 300 mg pyrazinamide at $1.90. IV vials: 600 mg at $90.00

INDICATIONS AND DOSE: Tuberculosis (with INH, PZA, and SM or EMB)

- **Dose:** 10 mg/kg/day (600 mg/day max) (see p. 333)
- **DOT:** 600 mg 2x to 3x/week (HIV-infected patients with CD4 counts <100/mm³ should receive DOT with 3x/week. The rationale is the observation of acquired rifamycin-resistance in trials of HIV-TB co-infected patients with CD4 counts <100/mm³ treated with rifapentine once weekly or rifabutin twice weekly, each in combination with INH (*Lancet* 1999;343:1843; *MMWR* 2002;51:214).
- **Prophylaxis (alone or in combination with PZA or EMB):** 10 mg/kg/day (600 mg/day max)
- **Antiretrovirals and TB treatment:** See Table 6-2, p. 364-367. Rifamycins should be included in any regimen for active TB. Options with HAART include:
  - □ Rifampin (standard dose) + EFV or full dose RTV. With EFV, consider increasing EFV dose to 800 mg/day.
  - □ Rifabutin with IDV, APV, NFV, LPV/r, SQV, ATV, or any RTV-boosted regimen in which the RTV dose is ≤200 mg bid.
  - □ Consider delay in antiretroviral therapy. See WHO guidelines.
- **Treatment of latent tuberculosis:** Rifampin (600 mg/day) + PZA (20 mg/kg/day with 2 g/day max) x 2 months was advocated as a preferred regimen for HIV infected patients with a positive PPD due to demonstrated efficacy comparable with the 12-month INH regimen and better compliance due to the abbreviated duration. In 2001, the CDC announced six hepatotoxic deaths with this regimen; none were known to have HIV Infection (*Am J Respir Crit Care Med* 2001;164:1319), and in 2003 the CDC announced it no longer advocated this regimen due to high rates of hepatotoxicity (*MMWR* 2003;52:735). A subsequent analysis showed no deaths or serious reactions among the 792 HIV-infected persons who took RIF/PZA; the rate of AST >250 U/l at 2 mos was 2.1% (*Clin Infect Dis* 2004;39:561).
- ***Rifater* treatment**
  - □ <65 kg – 1 tab/10 kg/day
  - □ >65 kg – 6 tabs/day

Drugs: Rifampin

5

- **Rifampin for:** *S. aureus* (with vancomycin, fluoroquinolones, or penicillinase-resistant penicillin): 300 mg PO bid

ACTIVE AGAINST: *M. tuberculosis, M. kansasii, S. aureus, H. influenzae, S. pneumoniae, Legionella,* and many anaerobes

PHARMACOLOGY

- **Bioavailability:** 90% to 95%, less with food. Absorption is reduced 30% in patients with advanced HIV infection; significance is unknown (*Ann Intern Med* 1997;127:289).
- **T½:** 1.5 to 5.0 hours, average – 2 hours
- **Elimination:** Excreted in urine (33%) and metabolized
- **Dose modification in renal failure:** None

SIDE EFFECTS

- **Common:** Orange-brown discoloration of urine, stool, tears (contact lens), sweat, skin.
- **Infrequent:** GI intolerance; hepatitis (in 2.7% given INH/RIF), usually cholestatic changes in first month of treatment; jaundice (usually reversible with dose reduction or continued use); hypersensitivity, especially pruritus ± rash (6%); flu-like illness in 0.4% to 0.7% given rifampin 2x/week with intermittent use – dyspnea, wheezing, purpura, leukopenia.
- **Rare:** Thrombocytopenia, leukopenia, hemolytic anemia, increased uric acid, and BUN. Frequency of side effects that require discontinuation of drug is 3%.

DRUG INTERACTIONS: Extensive, due to induction of hepatic cytochrome P450 (3A4, 2B6, 2C8, 2C9) enzymes (see www.cdc.gov/nchstp/tb/). Rifampin should be avoided with all PIs and NNRTIs except RTV (standard RTV dose), and EFV (800 mg hs). Limited experience suggests NVP at 200 or 300 mg bid is appropriate (*J Acquir Immune Defic Syndr* 2001;28:450; *AIDS* 2003;17:637). Rifampin should not be combined with LPV/r, but the CDC guidelines recommend an increased dose of RTV (LPV 3 caps bid + RTV 300 mg bid) when this combination is used (*MMWR* 2004;53:37). The following drugs inhibit cytochrome P450 enzymes and prolong the half-life of rifampin: clarithromycin, erythromycin, and azoles (fluconazole, itraconazole, and ketoconazole). EFV has no significant effect on rifampin levels, but rifampin reduces EFV levels by 20% to 26%; consider EFV 800 mg hs. CDC recommends standard doses of both rifampin and EFV; the recommendation is to avoid NVP combination or consider NVP 300 mg bid due to a 37-58% reduction in NVP levels (*MMWR* 2004;53:47).

Rifampin decreases levels of atovaquone, barbiturates, oral contraceptives, corticosteroids, cyclosporine, dapsone, fluconazole, ketoconazole, methadone, phenytoin, theophylline, and trimethoprim, and many other drugs that are 3A4 substrates. Rifampin should not be used concurrently with atovaquone, clarithromycin, or voriconazole. With fluconazole and itraconazole it may be necessary to increase the azole dose. The level of dapsone is decreased 7- to 10-fold – consider alternative.

PREGNANCY: Category C. Dose-dependent congenital malformations in animals. Isolated cases of fetal abnormalities noted in patients, but frequency is unknown. Large retrospective studies have shown no risk of congenital abnormalities; case reports of neural tube defects and limb reduction (*Clin Infect Dis* 1995:21[suppl 1]:S24). May cause postnatal hemorrhage in mother and infant if given in last few weeks of pregnancy. Must use with caution if used with INH and ethambutol.

RIFATER – see Isoniazid (p. 234) or Rifampin (above) or Pyrazinamide (p. 277) (*Ann Intern Med* 1995;122:951)

RITONAVIR (RTV)

TRADE NAME: *Norvir* (Abbott Laboratories)

FORMS AND PRICES: 100 mg soft-gel capsules at $10.71; Medicaid and ADAP price is $2.14/100 mg cap. Liquid formulation 80 mg/mL at $1800/240 mL.

PATIENT ASSISTANCE PROGRAM: 800-659-9050

CLASS: PI

Dose: 600 mg bid when used as a single PI or 100-400 mg qd or bid when used with another PI. Administration with food improves tolerability but is not required for absorption. Separate dosing with buffered ddl by ≥2 hours.

- **Recommended dose escalation regimen to improve GI tolerance:** When used as single PI: Days 1 and 2: 300 mg bid; days 3 to 5: 400 mg bid; days 6 to 13: 500 mg bid; day 14 and thereafter: 600 mg bid
- **Recommended regimens for PI-boosting** (DHHS Guidelines, April 7, 2005, p. 100) appear in the chart on the following page.

PI/r Regimen recommended		AUC PI (-fold increase)*
ATV/r	300/100 mg qd	2.5
APV/r	1200/200 mg qd 600/100 mg bid	2.5-3.5
FPV/r	1400/200 mg qd 700/100 mg bid	2
IDV/r	400/400 mg bid 800/100-200 mg bid	3-6
LPV/r	400/100 mg bid 800/200 mg qd	15-20
NFV/r	Not recommended	1.5
SQV/r	1000/100 mg bid	30-74
TVP/r	500/200 mg bid	29

*Based on data from Ogden RC and Flexner CW, eds, *Protease Inhibitors in AIDS Therapy* at 166-71, 173 (NY: M Dekker, 2001).

CLINICAL TRIALS: The activity of RTV has been extensively studied, alone initially as a single PI in HAART, and more recently in combination with other PIs to exploit RTV inhibition of the P450 metabolic pathway, which increases AUC values of PIs ranging from 1.5x for NFV to >20x for SQV. Combinations with the RTV dose of ≥400 mg generally achieve therapeutic levels for RTV; when used in doses of 100-200 mg qd or bid, RTV levels are subtherapeutic, meaning RTV is used only for pharmacologic enhancement of the companion PI. RTV as a single PI in HAART appears to be about as effective as IDV but is expensive, poorly tolerated, and rarely used (*AIDS* 2001;15:999).

RESISTANCE: Phenotypic resistance correlates with the following primary mutations on the protease genes 82A/F/T/S and 84V (*J Virol* 1995;69:701). Patients failing monotherapy have multiple mutations at codons 10, 20, 32, 33, 36, 46, 54, 71, 77, 82, 84, and 90 (*Nat Med* 1996;2:760; 7th CROI, 2000, Abstract 565). The initial mutation was at codon 82, which was consistently seen and appeared necessary for phenotypic resistance (*Antimicrob Agents Chemother* 1998;42:2775). This was followed by mutations at codons 54, 71, and 36; mutations at codons 84 and 90 occurred late and less frequently.

PHARMACOLOGY

- **Bioavailability:** 60% to 80% (not well determined). Levels increased 15% when taken with meals. CNS penetration: No detectable levels in CSF.
- **T½:** 3 to 5 hours
- **Elimination:** Metabolized by cytochrome P450 CYP3A4. RTV is a potent inhibitor of cytochrome P450 CYP3A4>2D6, and an inducer of CYP3A4 and CYP1A2.

Drugs: Ritonavir

- **Dose modification in renal or hepatic failure:** Use standard doses for renal failure. With hemodialysis, a small amount is dialyzed: dose post-hemodialysis (*Nephron* 2001;87:186). There are no data for peritoneal dialysis, but it is probably not removed and should be dosed post-dialysis. Consider empiric dose reduction in severe hepatic disease.

SIDE EFFECTS: The most frequently reported adverse events with full dose therapy are GI intolerance (nausea, diarrhea, vomiting, anorexia, abdominal pain, taste perversion), circumoral and peripheral paresthesias, and asthenia. GI intolerance is often severe (*J Acquir Immune Defic Syndr* 2000;23:236) and can improve with continued administration for ≥1 month. Side effects are less severe with the reduced doses used in boosted PI combinations. Hepatotoxicity with elevated transaminase levels is more frequent and more severe with full dose RTV than with other PIs; there does appear to be a modestly increased risk with hepatitis B or C co-infection (*JAMA* 2000;238:74; *J Acquir Immune Defic Syndr* 2000;23:236; *Clin Infect Dis* 2000;31:1234). This risk is reduced with the lower RTV doses used in dual-PI combinations. Laboratory changes include elevated triglycerides, cholestrol, transaminases, CPK, and uric acid.

- **Class adverse reactions:** Insulin-resistant hyperglycemia, fat accumulation, elevated triglycerides and cholesterol, and possible increased bleeding with hemophilia. The association between protease inhibitor therapy and osteonecrosis/avascular necrosis of the hips has not been determined. Hypercholesterolemia and triglyceridemia may be more frequent and severe with full dose RTV compared with other PIs (*J Acquir Immune Defic Syndr* 2000;23:236; *J Acquir Immune Defic Syndr* 2000;23:261).

DRUG INTERACTIONS: RTV is a potent inhibitor of cytochrome P450 enzymes, including CYP3A4 and 2D6, and can produce large increases in the plasma concentrations of drugs that are metabolized by that mechanism.

- **Use with the following agents is contraindicated:** Alfuzosin amiodarone, astemizole, bepridil, cisapride, encainide, flecainide, lovastatin, midazolam, ergot alkaloids, pimozide, propafenone, quinidine, simvastatin, terfenadine, triazolam, St. John's wort, rifapentine, and voriconazole (with ≥400 mg/d RTV).

- **Use with caution** in patients with ↑ QTc at baseline and with drugs that can ↑ QTc (cisapride, type I and III anti-arrhythmics, erythromycin).

- **Drugs that require dose modification**
  - Fluticasone (*Flonase*): RTV increased fluticasone AUC 350-fold, resulting in an 86% decrease in plasma cortisol AUC. Adrenal insufficiency reported. FDA warning: use concurrently only if benefit outweighs risk.

5 Drugs: Ritonavir

- Clarithromycin AUC increased 77% (*Clin Infect Dis* 1996;23:685); reduce clarithromycin dose for renal failure.
- Methadone levels are decreased by 36%; monitor for withdrawal.
- Desipramine levels are increased by 145%; decrease desipramine dose.
- ddl, buffered form, reduces absorption of RTV and should be taken ≥2 hours apart or use ddl EC.
- Ketoconazole levels are increased 3-fold; do not exceed 200 mg ketoconazole/day.
- Rifampin reduces RTV levels 35% (use standard dose RTV); limited data on combination use and concern for hepatotoxicity.
- Rifabutin levels increased 4-fold; rifabutin dose of 150 mg qod or 150 mg 3 days/week with standard RTV dose.
- Ethinyl estradiol levels decreased by 40%; use alternative or additional method of birth control.
- Theophylline levels decreased by 47%; monitor theophylline levels.
- Phenobarbital, phenytoin, and carbamazepine interaction anticipated; carbamazepine toxicity reported. Monitor anticonvulsant levels.
- Sildenafil AUC increased 2- to 11-fold; do not use >25 mg/48 hours; Vardenafil levels ↑49x , do not exceed 2.5 mg q72h.
- Trazodone: RTV may increase trazodone AUC causing nausea, dizziness, hypotension and syncope. Use with caution and consider lower dose of trazodone.
- A potentially fatal reaction has been reported with MDMA ("Ecstasy") (*Arch Intern Med* 1999;159:2221).
- Voriconazole AUC decreased 82% with RTV 400 mg bid; RTV AUC not changed. Avoid combination. Implications for low dose RTV (100-200 mg/d) unclear – alternative antifungal preferred.
- Atorvastatin levels increase 450% with RTV/SQV; use lower atorvastatin dose, or use pravastatin or fluvastatin or rosuvastatin.
- Tadalafil ↑ 129%; do not exceed 10 mg/72 h.

■ TABLE 5-43: **RTV Interactions with Antiretroviral Drugs**

Drug	Effect	Recommendation
SQV	SQV – ↑20 fold RTV – no change	SQV 1000 mg + RTV 100 mg bid *or* SQV 400 mg bid + RTV 400 mg bid (*Invirase* preferred)
NVP	RTV – ↓11% NVP – no change	Standard doses both drugs
TPV	↑TPV 2-fold	TPV 500 mg bid + RTV 200 mg bid (standard)
IDV	IDV – ↑2 to 5x RTV – no change	IDV 800 mg + RTV 100 mg bid *or* IDV 400 mg bid + RTV 400 mg bid. (Note increased nephrolithiasis with 800/100 regimen)
APV	APV – ↑2.5x - 3.5x RTV – no change	APV 600 mg bid + RTV 100 mg bid *or* APV 1200 mg qd + RTV 200 mg qd. With EFV/APV/RTV use: RTV 100 mg bid + APV 1200 mg bid + EFV 600 mg qhs
ATV	ATV ↑238%	ATV 300 mg qd + RTV 100 mg qd
FPV	FPV AUC ↑ 2-fold C_{min} ↑ 4-fold with qd C_{min} ↑ 6-fold with bid	FPV 700 mg bid + RTV 100 mg bid or FPV 1400 mg qd + RTV 200 mg qd. With EFV/APV/RTV use: RTV 100 mg + FPV 700 mg bid + EFV 600 mg qhs *or* RTV 300 mg qd + FPV 1400 mg qd + EFV 600 mg qhs

PREGNANCY: Category B. Negative rodent teratogenic assays; placental passage studies in rodents show newborn:maternal drug ratio of 1.15 at midterm and 0.15-0.64 at late term. Standard doses of SQV/RTV produced inadequate levels of SQV in pregnant women. The preferred regimen is 800 SQV/100 RTV bid (*HIV Clin Trials* 2001;2:460; *Antimicrob Agents Chemother* 2004;48:430).

ROFERON – see Interferon (p. 231)

SAQUINAVIR (SQV)

TRADE NAME: *Invirase* (hard-gel capsule) and *Fortovase* (soft-gel capsule) (Roche). The *Fortovase* formulation will be discontinued in February 2006.

FORMULATIONS AND REGIMENS

FORMS: *Invirase* (INV): caps, 200 and 500 mg; *Fortovase* (FTV): caps, 200 mg. INV is the preferred formulation.

REGIMENS: INV/r: Give only with RTV, 1000/100 mg bid or 2000/100 mg qd. Once-daily regimens are not FDA-approved.

FOOD: Take within 2 h of a meal

RENAL FAILURE: Standard regimen

HEPATIC FAILURE: In mild cases, standard regimen. No data for moderately severe or severe liver disease.

STORAGE: INV: store at room temperature, 15-30°C. FTV: store at <25°C (<77°F) for ≤3 mos or refrigerate.

NOTES: INV appears preferred for its better GI tolerance and 500-mg formulation. FTV will be discontinued in February 2006.

PATIENT ASSISTANCE PROGRAM: 800-282-7780

CLASS: PI. Note that most studies were done with the Fortovase formulation,

- **MaxC$_{min}$1:** The MaxC$_{min}$1 trial compared two boosted PI regimens, IDV/RTV (800/100 mg bid) and SQV/RTV (1000/100 mg bid) in naïve and experienced patients (*J Infect Dis* 2003;188:635). At 48 weeks, virologic suppression was similar in the two arms by as-treated analysis and intent-to-treat (ITT), switch-included analysis. However, by ITT switch=failure analysis, 68% of patients on SQV/RTV had viral loads <400 c/mL vs 53% on IDV/RTV. Treatment-related grade 3/4 adverse events were also significantly more common among IDV recipients, and lipid profiles were better in the SQV/RTV arm.

- **MaxC$_{min}$2:** This trial compared LPV/r with SQV/RTV (1000/100 mg bid) plus at least two NRTI/NNRTIs in 324 patients (2nd IAS, Paris, 2003, Abstr LB 23). The patient population was heterogeneous, and included treatment naïve patients as well as PI-naïve and PI-experienced patients. Time to virologic failure was longer in the LPV/r arm compared to the SQV/RTV arm (*p*=0.0006), and there were significantly more discontinuations in the SQV/RTV arm (29% vs. 14%, *p*=0.001).

- **FOCUS:** The FOCUS trial was an open-label trial comparing once-daily SQV/RTV (1600/100 mg) vs EFV, both in combination with 2 nucleoside analogs (41st ICAAC, 2001, Abstract I-670). The trial involved 161 treatment naïve patients. EFV was better tolerated: Eight patients discontinued therapy in the SQV/RTV arm vs one in the EFV arm. Nausea was seen in 22% vs 1%, and vomiting in 6% vs 0%. As a result, EFV was superior by intent-to-treat analyses, with 81% achieving viral loads <50 c/mL compared with 60% in the SQV/RTV arm (*p*=0.008). There was no difference in potency in either arm between patients with baseline viral loads <100,000 c/mL or those with >100,000 c/mL.

- **ATV/SQV:** Atazanavir (ATV) increases levels of other protease inhibitors through its inhibitory effect on the CYP 3A4 enzyme system (*AIDS* 2004;18:1291). In BMS 009, patients experiencing virologic failure on HAART (HIV RNA 2000-100,000 c/mL) received ATV/SQV at a dose of 400/1200 mg qd (*n*=34) or 600/1200 mg qd (*n*=28) or RTV/SQV at a dose of 400/400 mg bid (*n*=23) (*AIDS* 2003;17:1339). Patients in each arm experienced a 1-1.5 log drop in viral load at 24 weeks, but those on the ATV-based regimens had more favorable lipid profiles. A subsequent trial with 358 patients who failed ≥2 HAART regimens were randomized to receive LPV/r,

ATV/r or ATV/SQV (400/1200 mg qd). At 48 weeks there was a significantly greater frequency of virologic failure in recipients of ATV/SQV (62% vs 42%) (*Clin Infect Dis* 2004;38:1599).

Future trials will investigate ATV 300 mg/RTV 100 mg/SQV 1500 mg qd.

RESISTANCE: Major resistance mutations are L90M (most common; 3-fold decrease in sensitivity) and G48V (less common and 30-fold decrease in sensitivity). Minor mutations conferring resistance are at codons 10, 54, 63, 71, 73, 77, 82, and 84.

PHARMACOLOGY

- **Bioavailability:** Absorption of SQV requires a concurrent high-fat meal for therapeutic levels, but INV and FTV absorption are not influenced by food when taken with RTV. There is essentially no CNS penetration (CSF:serum ratio is 0.02). AUC and trough levels are significantly higher in women compared to men (*J Infect Dis* 2004;189:1176).

- **T½:** 1 to 2 hours

- **Elimination:** Hepatic metabolism by cytochrome P450 isoenzyme CYP3A4; 96% biliary excretion; 1% urinary excretion

- **Storage:** INV: Room temperature. FTV: 30 days at room temperature; long-term storage in refrigerator

- **Dose modification in renal or hepatic failure:** Use standard dose for renal failure. The drug is not removed by hemodialysis (*Nephron* 2001;87:186) and is unlikely to be removed by peritoneal dialysis. Consider empiric dose reduction for hepatic failure.

SIDE EFFECTS: Gastrointestinal intolerance with nausea, abdominal pain, diarrhea in 5% to 15% (INV), 20% to 30% (FTV); headache, and hepatic toxicity;case reports of hypoglycemia in patients with type 2 diabetes (*Ann Intern Med* 1999;131:980). Class adverse effects include fat accumulation, insulin resistance and type 2 diabetes, osteoporosis, and possible increased bleeding with hemophilia. SQV appears to have less effect on blood lipids compared to other PIs (*J Infect Dis* 2004;189:1056).

DRUG INTERACTIONS

- **Drugs that are contraindicated for concurrent use:** Terfenadine, astemizole, cisapride, triazolam, midazolam, rifampin, pimozide, rifabutin, ergot alkaloids, simvastatin, lovastatin, St. John's wort, and rifapentine.

- **Drugs that may require regimen modification**
  - Dexamethasone may decrease SQV levels.
  - Phenobarbital, phenytoin, and carbamazepine may decrease SQV levels substantially; monitor anticonvulsant levels.
  - Ketoconazole increases SQV levels 3x; standard dose. Monitor for SQV GI toxicity if ketoconazole dose is >200 mg/day.

5 Drugs: Saquinavir

- Clarithromycin increases SQV levels 177% and SQV increases clarithromycin levels 45%; standard dose.
- Oral contraceptives: No data. Recommend alternative form of contraception.
- Sildenafil AUC increased 2x; use 25 mg starting dose; Tadalafil – start with 5 mg dose and do not exceed 10 mg/72 hr; Vardenafil – start with 2.5 mg dose and do not exceed 2.5 mg/72 hrs.
- Rifampin reduces SQV levels by 80% and is contraindicated; with combination SQV/RTV (Roche letter to care providers, Feb. 2005).
- Rifabutin reduces SQV levels 40%. With any combination of SQV/RTV use rifabutin 150 mg qod or 150 mg 3x/wk.
- Voriconazole at subtherapeutic levels has potential for bidirectional interaction.
- Atorvastatin levels increase 450% with SQV/RTV; use lowest starting dose of atorvastatin, or use pravastatin, fluvastatin, or rosuvastatin.
- Methadone – With FTV there is a 8% to 10% reduction in methadone levels; no dose adjustment. This also applies to SQV/r 1600/100 qd (*J Clin Pharmacol* 2004;44:293).
- Other drugs that induce CYP3A4 (phenobarbital, phenytoin, NVP, dexamethasone, and carbamazepine) may decrease SQV levels; these combinations should be avoided if possible.
- Garlic supplements decrease SQV AUC, C_{max}, and C_{min} levels by about 50% (*Clin Infect Dis* 2002;34:234).
- Grapefruit juice increases SQV levels.

■ TABLE 5-44: **Combination Therapy with *Fortovase* Plus Second PI or an NNRTI**

Drug	AUC*	Regimen*
RTV	SQV ↑20x, RTV no change	SQV 1000 mg bid + RTV 100 mg bid *or* SQV 400 mg bid + RTV 400 mg bid *or* SQV 1600 mg qd + RTV 100 mg qd
IDV	IDV no change, SQV ↑4 to 7x	Insufficient data. In vitro antagonism
APV	APV ↓32%, SQV ↓19%	SQV 800 mg tid + APV 800 mg tid (limited data)
EFV	EFV ↓12%, SQV ↓62%	SQV 1000 mg bid + RTV 200 mg bid + EFV 600 mg hs
NVP	NVP no change, SQV ↓25%	Consider NVP standard dose plus SQV/RTV 400 mg/400 mg bid or 1000 mg/100 mg
DLV	DLV no change, SQV ↑5x	FTV 800 mg tid + DLV standard; monitor ALT
NFV	NFV ↑20%, SQV ↑3 to 5x	FTV 800 mg tid or 1200 mg bid + NFV standard
LPV/r	SQV ↑3 to 5x, LPV no change	SQV 1000 mg bid + LPV/r 400/100 mg bid
ATV	ATV (RTV effect); SQV ↑4.5x	ATV 300 mg + SQV 1500-1600 mg + RTV 100 mg qd

* RTV recommendation of SQV 1600 mg qd may change due to new SQV formulation.

Drugs: Saquinavir

PREGNANCY: Category B. Studies in rats showed no teratogenicity or embryotoxicity. There is substantial variation in SQV levels in pregnancy. The PK data suggests SQV/r at 800/100 mg bid is reasonable (*Antimicrob Agents Chemother* 2004;48:430).

SEROSTIM – see Growth Hormone, Human (p. 223)

SOMATROPIN – see Growth Hormone, Human (p. 223)

SPORANOX – see Itraconazole (p. 236)

SOMNOTE – see Chloral Hydrate (p. 165)

STAVUDINE (d4T)

TRADE NAME: *Zerit* and *Zerit XR* (Bristol-Myers Squibb)

CLASS: NRTI

FORMULATIONS, REGIMENS AND PRICE

FORMS: Caps, 15, 30 and 40 mg; oral solution, 1 mg/mL (200 mL bottle)

REGIMENS: For patients weighing >60 kg, 40 mg bid; <60 kg, 30 mg bid.

AWP: $320/month

FOOD: No effect

RENAL FAILURE: For CrCl 26-50 mL/min, 15 mg bid (wt <60 kg) or 20 mg bid (wt >60 kg); for CrCl 10-25 mL/min or hemodialysis, 15 mg qd (wt <60 kg) or 20 mg qd (wt >60 kg)

HEPATIC FAILURE: No dose recommendation

PATIENT ASSISTANCE: 800-272-4878

■ TABLE 5-45: **Trials in Treatment-Naïve Patients Comparing d4T with Other Antiretrovirals**

Study	Regimen	N	Dur (wks)	VL <50	VL <200-500
START 1 (*AIDS* 2000;14:1591)	d4T/3TC/IDV	101	48	49%	52%
	AZT/3TC/IDV	103		47%	52%
CLASS XV IAC 2004, Abstr. TuPeB4544	d4T/3TC/ABC	98	48	72%	81%
	FPV/3TC/ABC	96		59%	75%
	EFV/3TC/ABC	97		60%	80%
ACTG 384 (*N Engl J Med* 2003; 349:2293)	d4T/ddl/EFV	155	48		62%*
	d4T/ddl/NVP	155			63%
	AZT/3TC/EFV	155			89%*
	AZT/3TC/NVP	155			66%
FTC 301A (*JAMA* 2004;292:180)	FTC/ddl/EFV	386		78%†	81%
	d4T/ddl/EFV	324		59%	68%
Gilead 903 (*JAMA* 2004;292:180)	TDF/3TC/EFV	299	144	76%‡	90%
	d4T/3TC/EFV	301		80%	84%
AI 454-152 (*J Acquir Immune Defic Syndr* 2002;31:399)	d4T/ddl/NFV	258	48	33%	55%
	AZT/3TC/NFV	253		33%	56%

* Failure defined by VL >2000 c/mL at wk 24 or >200 c/mL at wk 48

† Superior to comparator (*p* <0.05)

‡ TDF/3TC significantly less toxic

CLINICAL TRIALS: There is extensive experience with d4T combined with 3TC and ddl. **ACTG 384** showed that EFV/AZT/3TC had greater activity and less toxicity compared with EFV/ddl/d4T (see Table 5-45) (*N Engl J Med* 2003;349:2293). **Gilead 903** compared d4T and TDF in 600 treatment-naïve patients who were randomized to receive TDF or d4T, each with 3TC and EFV. Both regimens were highly effective at 3 years, but d4T was associated with more neuropathy, hyperlipidemia, and lipodystrophy than TDF.

RESISTANCE: *In vivo* d4T resistance is mediated primarily by thymidine analog mutations (TAMs) (e.g., 41L, 67N, 70R, 210W, 215Y/F, 219Q/E), and d4T also selects for these mutations. As with AZT, the M184V mutation associated with 3TC resistance appears to increase susceptibility to d4T. The multinucleoside resistance mutations (Q151M complex and the T69-insertion mutation) also result in resistance to d4T. d4T can sometimes select for the K65R mutation, though it appears to have minimal effect on d4T susceptibility.

Drugs: Stavudine

PHARMACOLOGY

- **Bioavailability:** 86% and not influenced by food or fasting
- **T½:** (serum) 1 hour. Intracellular T½: 3.5 hours
- **CNS penetration:** 30% to 40% (*J Acquir Immune Defic Syndr* 1998;17:235) (CSF: plasma ratio=0.16-0.97)
- **Elimination:** Renal – 50%
- **Dose modification in severe liver disease:** No guidelines; use standard dose with caution.

SIDE EFFECTS

- **Mitochondrial toxicity:** d4T is an important cause of side effects attributed to mitochondrial toxicity, including hyperlactatemia or lactic acidosis with hepatic steatosis, peripheral neuropathy, and lipatrophy. In most studies of lactic acidosis, d4T is the most frequent NRTI (*Clin Infect Dis* 2001;33:1931; *Lancet* 2000;356:1423; *Ann Intern Med* 2000;133:192). A review of reported cases for 2000 to 2001 implicated d4T in 33 of 34 (*Clin Infect Dis* 2002;31:838).

  - □ **Lactic acidosis and steatosis:** Decreased mitochondrial DNA to DNA ratio is a marker of mitochondrial toxicity and is relatively common without abnormal function (*Antiviral Ther* 2004;9:47). Hyperlactatemia is also relatively common **(FDA black box warning)**. Lactic acidosis ± steatosis is an infrequent form of mitochondrial toxicity, reported in 1 to 14/1000 patient-years of NRTI exposure (*AIDS* 2001;15:717), but it is important to recognize due to the potential for lethal outcome. Patients present with nausea, vomiting, abdominal pain, fatigue, dyspnea, and/or weight loss, usually after 1 to 20 months of exposure (*Clin Infect Dis* 2003;36[suppl 2]:S96). Laboratory studies show elevated serum lactate (usually >5 mmol/L), sometimes combined with increased anion gap and elevated CPK, ALT, and LDH. CT scan, ultrasound, or liver biopsy may show hepatic steatosis. NRTIs should be stopped when this diagnosis is considered. In mild cases, switching to NRTIs that are less toxic to mitochondria (e.g., ABC, 3TC, FTC, TDF) may be considered, provided the patient can be closely monitored. d4T/ddI should be avoided, especially in pregnant women who have an increased risk of lactic acidosis **(FDA black box warning)**.

  - □ **Peripheral neuropathy:** Frequency is 5% to 15% but as high as 24% in some early trials. The presumed cause is depletion of mitochondrial DNA (*N Engl J Med* 2002;346:811). Risk appears to be substantially increased when d4T is combined with ddI or ddI plus hydroxyurea (*AIDS* 2000;14:273). Onset is usually noted at 2 to 6 months of treatment and usually resolves if d4T is promptly stopped, although the recovery is generally slow. Peripheral neuropathy due to HIV infection or alternative nucleoside analog treatment (ddI, ddC) represents a relative contraindication to d4T.

If it is necessary to resume d4T after resolution of neuropathy, some authorities recommend a decreased dose of 30 mg bid (12th CROI, Boston, Feb. 2005, Abstr. 851).

- □ **HIV-associated neuromuscular weakness syndrome:** A syndrome of ascending motor weakness is characterized by variable changes, including progressive sensorimotor polyneuropathy with areflexia and ascending neuromuscular weakness. EMG and pathology show changes in nerves, muscles or both. Of 69 cases reviewed, 61 were thought to be due to d4T, and many (36%) had onset of symptoms after d4T was stopped. Lactate levels are usually elevated (*AIDS* 2004;18:1403). The weakness was accompanied by lactic acidosis and is presumed to be a result of mitochondrial toxicity.

- □ **Lipodystrophy:** d4T is associated with lipoatrophy and hyperlipidemia. The lipoatrophy is a cosmetic effect that is most obvious in the malar (cheek) area, extremities and buttocks. These effects persist for prolonged periods after d4T is discontinued, although some studies show modest improvement after several months (12th CROI, Boston, Feb. 2005, Abstr. 860). Serum lipid changes ascribed to d4T are most significant for triglyceride elevations but also for LDL cholesterol (Gilead 903). Reversal of lipid effects are noted with switch to alternative NRTIs such as TDF or ABC (*J Acquir Immune Defic Syndr* 2005;38:263; *AIDS* 2005;19:15; 12th CROI, 2005, Abstr. 44LB).

- ■ **Other clinical side effects:** Complaints are infrequent and include headache, GI intolerance with diarrhea, or esophageal ulcers.

- ■ **Macrocytosis,** with MCV >100, which is inconsequential (*J Infect* 2000;40:160).

DRUG INTERACTIONS

- ■ **AZT:** Pharmacologic antagonism – avoid.

- ■ **Drugs that cause peripheral neuropathy** should be used with caution or avoided: ddC, ddI, ethionamide, EMB, INH, phenytoin, vincristine, glutethimide, gold, hydralazine, thalidomide, and long-term metronidazole.

- ■ **Methadone** reduces the AUC of d4T by 24%, but this is not thought to be sufficiently severe to require d4T dose adjustment; d4T has no effect on methadone levels (*J Acquir Immune Defic Syndr* 2000;24:241).

- ■ Use with caution when combined with **ribavirin.**

PREGNANCY: Category C. Rodent teratogenicity assay is negative; placental passage in rhesus monkeys showed a newborn:maternal drug ratio of 0.76. No studies in humans. Studies in pregnancy indicate good tolerability and pharmacokinetics (*J Infect Dis* 2004;190:2167). d4T + ddI

Drugs: Stavudine

should not be given to pregnant women due to possible lactic acidosis and hepatic steatosis (*Sex Trans Infect* 2002;78:58).

STOCRIN – see Efavirenz (p. 187)

SULFADIAZINE

TRADE NAME: Generic

FORMS: 500 mg tab at $1.44

CLASS: Synthetic derivatives of sulfanilamide that inhibit folic acid synthesis

INDICATIONS AND DOSES

- **Toxoplasmosis:** Initial treatment 1.0 g PO qid (<65 kg) or 1.5 gm PO qid (>65 kg); maintenance dose: half of prior dose
- **Nocardia:** 1 g PO qid x ≥6 months
- **UTIs:** 500 mg-1 g PO bid – qd x 3 to 14 days

PHARMACOLOGY

- **Bioavailability:** >70%
- **T½:** 7 to 17 hours
- **Elimination:** Hepatic acetylation and renal excretion of parent compound and metabolites
- **CNS penetration:** 40% to 80% of serum levels
- **Serum levels for systemic infections:** goal is 100-150 µg/mL
- **Dose modifications in renal failure:** CrCl >50 mL/min – 0.5-1.5 g q4h-q6h; CrCl 10-50 mL/min – 0.5-1.5 g q8h-q12h (half dose); CrCl <10 mL/min – 0.5-1.5 g q12h-q24h (one-third dose)

SIDE EFFECTS: Hypersensitivity with rash, drug fever, serum-sickness, urticaria; crystalluria reduced with adequate urine volume (≥1,500 mL/day) and alkaline urine – use with care in renal failure; marrow suppression – anemia, thrombocytopenia, leukopenia, hemolytic anemia due to G6-PD deficiency.

DRUG INTERACTIONS: Decreased effect of cyclosporine, digoxin; increased effect of coumadin, oral hypoglycemics, methotrexate(?), and phenytoin. Use with caution with ribavirin.

PREGNANCY: Category C. Competes with bilirubin for albumin to cause kernicterus – avoid near term or in nursing mothers.

SULFAMETHOXAZOLE-TRIMETHOPRIM –
see Trimethoprim-Sulfamethoxazole (p. 315)

Drugs: Sulfamethoxazole-Trimethoprim

5

SUSTIVA – see Efavirenz (p. 187)

3TC – see Lamivudine (p. 241)

TENOFOVIR DISOPROXIL FUMARATE (TDF)

TRADE NAME: *Viread* (Gilead Sciences). Combination with emtricitabine (FTC): *Truvada* (Gilead Sciences)

CLASS: Nucleotide analog reverse transcriptase inhibitor (NRTI)

PATIENT ASSISTANCE PROGRAM AND REIMBURSEMENT HOTLINE: 800-445-3235

FORMULATIONS, REGIMENS AND PRICE

FORMS: TDF – tab, 300 mg; TDF/FTC (*Truvada*) – tab, 300/200 mg

REGIMENS: TDF – 300 mg qd; TDF/FTC – 1 tab qd

AWP: TDF – $400/month; TDF/FTC – $800/month

FOOD: No substantial effect, but fatty meals increase absorption by 40%.

RENAL FAILURE: See table below.

CrCl	TDF	TDF/FTC (*Truvada*)
≥50	300 mg qd	1 tab qd
30-49	300 mg q 48 h	1 tab q 48 h
10-29	300 mg 2x/wk	not recommended
<10	not recommended	not recommended
hemodialysis	q 7 d after HD	not recommended

HEPATIC FAILURE: No dose recommendation

CLINICAL TRIALS

- **GS-97-901:** Dose-finding monotherapy study with 75, 150, and 300 mg qd x 28 days. Median decrease in viral load at 28 days with 300 mg dose was 1.2 $\log_{10}$/mL.

- **GS-98-902:** Dose finding/toxicity study using 75, 150, and 300 mg added to antiretroviral regimen in 189 treatment-experienced patients with viral load 400-100,000 c/mL. At 48 weeks, the mean viral load decrease was 0.62 $\log_{10}$ c/mL among 54 patients receiving 300 mg/day.

- **Gilead 907:** Placebo-controlled trial in treated patients with viral load 400-10,000 c/mL given 300 mg tenofovir. At 24 weeks (*n*=552), the mean decrease in viral load was 0.61 $\log_{10}$ c/mL among tenofovir recipients compared with 0.03 $\log_{10}$ c/mL in placebo recipients.

- **Gilead 903** was a randomized, placebo-controlled trial comparing TDF vs d4T, each in combination with 3TC and EFV for treatment of ART-naïve patients (*JAMA* 2004;292:191). By ITT (missing=failure) analysis at 144 weeks, 71% of TDF recipients and 61% of d4T recipients had a viral load <50 c/mL (*p*=NS) (*JAMA* 2004;292:191). The drop-out rate was low, but d4T recipients had higher rates of peripheral neuropathy, lipoatrophy and elevated fasting, total and LDL cholesterol and triglycerides.

- **ESS 30009** compared the triple NRTI regimen of TDF/ABC/3TC with EFV/ABC/3TC in a pilot study of 24 treatment-naïve patients that was stopped at 12 weeks due to high rates of virologic failure in the triple NRTI arm (49% vs 5%); resistance testing showed a high frequency of M184V (100%) and K65R (64%) in 36 with virologic failure (ICAAC 2003;Chicago, Abstr. 17229).

- **GS 934:** 517 treatment-naïve patients were randomized to receive co-formulated AZT/3TC + EFV or TDF + FTC + EFV. At 48 wks, more patients experienced virologic suppression in the TDF arm by ITT analysis, 81% vs. 70% <400 c/mL, 77% vs. 68% <50 c/mL. The difference was explained primarily by the higher proportion of discontinuations due to adverse events in the AZT/3TC arm (9% vs. 4%), most of which were due to anemia (3rd IAS, 2005, #WeOa0202).

- **TDF/ddI/3TC** also failed badly in a 24-week pilot study of 24 treatment-naïve patients using this once-daily triple NRTI regimen. At 12 weeks, 21/24 failed to decrease VL by ≥2 $\log_{10}$ c/mL; 95% had M184V mutations and 50% had K65R mutations (11th CROI, 2004, Abstr. 51).

- **HBV:** TDF is active against hepatitis B virus but is not FDA approved for that indication. In patients with HIV and a positive HBeAg, the inclusion of TDF in the HIV regimen results in a decrease of 4-5 $\log_{10}$ in HBV DNA levels, including those with lamivudine-resistant strains (*AIDS* 2003;17:F7; *J Infect Dis* 2003;186:1844; *J Infect Dis* 2004;189:1185; *Clin Infect Dis* 2004;38[suppl2]:S98; *Clin Infect Dis* 2003;37:1678; *J Infect Dis* 2004;189:1185). The addition of 3TC does not augment TDF activity against HBV, but the addition of TDF to 3TC protects against HBV resistance to 3TC (*J Infect Dis* 2004;189:1185).

RESISTANCE: Susceptibility is decreased in patients with three or more thymidine analog mutations (TAMs) that include the 41L and 210W mutations. Susceptibility is maintained with other TAM patterns and increased with 184V. TDF/ABC and TDF/ddI select for the 65R mutation which confers resistance to all three drugs, as well as to 3TC and FTC (*Antimicrob Agents Chemother* 2004;48:1413). There is substantial loss of susceptibility with the T69 insertion mutation

(*Antimicrob Agents Chemother* 2004;48:992), but it is maintained with Q151M complex. Partial phenotypic susceptibility may be maintained despite the presence at K65R when M184V is also present.

PHARMACOLOGY

- **Bioavailability:** 25% (fasting) to 40% (with food); improvement with food, especially high-fat meal
- **T½:** 12 to 18 hours; intracellular >60 hours
- **Elimination:** Renal

DRUG INTERACTION

- **ATV:** ATV AUC is decreased 25% and TDF AUC is increased 28%; use standard dose TDF plus ATV/r (300/100 mg) qd.
- **ddI:** ddI AUC is increased 40% to 60%, potentially causing increased rates of peripheral neuropathy and pancreatitis. Combination of TDF with lower doses of ddI (e.g., *Videx EC* 250 mg qd in patients >60 kg; Videx EC 200 mg qd <60 kg) should be used. Other concerns are possible reduced potency of ddI/TDF based on high failure rates when combined with EFV or NVP (*AIDS* 2005;19:695; *Antivir Ther* 2005;10:171; *AIDS* 2005;19:213). Another report showed TDF/ddI as the NRTI backbone in HAART was associated with viral suppression but a blunted CD4 response (*AIDS* 2005;19:569; *Clin Infect Dis* 2005;41:901; *AIDS* 2005;19:1107). Some of these effects may be ascribed to failure to adjust the dose of ddI when combined with TDF, but some are not.
- **Ganciclovir, valganciclovir, and cidofovir** compete for active tubular secretion with increased levels of either tenofovir or the companion drug; monitor for toxicities.
- **Lopinavir:** LPV increases levels of TDF 30% with co-administration, but this has not been associated with increased toxicity or need for dose adjustment in clinical trials.

SIDE EFFECTS

- **GI intolerance:** GI intolerance reported, but it is infrequent. Flatulence accurred more often in TDF-treated patients than placebo-treated patients.
- **Nephrotoxicity:** TDF and related drugs (adefovir and cidofovir) may cause renal injury with the characteristic features of the Fanconi syndrome, hypophosphatemia, hypouricemia, proteinuria, normo-glycemic glycosuria, and, in some cases, acute renal failure (*J Acquir Immune Defic Syndr* 2004;35:269; *AIDS* 2004;18:960; *Clin Infect Dis* 2003;37:e174). In the early stages this may be asymptomatic or cause myalgias; most resolve when the drug is discontinued (*J Acquir Immune Defic Syndr* 2004;35:269). Risk factors are low body weight and pre-existing renal disease (*Antimicrob Agents Chemother* 2001;45:2733). The incidence appears to be extremely low in patients with normal baseline renal function. Analysis of 600

participants in Gilead 903 with calculated creatinine clearances >60 mL/min and serum phosphorus ≥2.2 mg/dL showed no change in mean baseline creatinine and no difference compared to d4T in mean serum phosphorus levels at week 144 (*Nephrol Dial Transplant* 2005;20:743). Modest declines in creatine clearance have been observed in some clinical cohorts (*Clin Infect Dis* 2005;40:1194).

- **Other:** The incidence of laboratory and clinical adverse events has been similar to placebo in controlled clinical trials.

PREGNANCY: Category B. Studies in infant monkeys showed a significant reduction in growth and reduced bone porosity (*J Acquir Immune Defic Syndr* 2002;29:207). Studies in children show bone demineralization (*AIDS* 2002;16:1257). Due to concerns about bone abnormalities and limited experience it is recommended that TDF be used with caution in pregnancy.

TESTOSTERONE

SOURCE

- Testosterone cypionate (various generic manufacturers)
- Testosterone enanthate (various generic manufacturers)
- Testosterone scrotal patch (*Testoderm* patch, Alza Pharmaceuticals)
- Testosterone non-transscrotal patch (*Androderm*, Watson)
- Testosterone gel (*AndroGel,* Unimed, *Testim,* Auxilium)
- Testim 1% gel
- Testosterone buccal (*Striant,* Columbia Laboratories)

FORMS AND PRICES: Vials of 100 and 200 mg/mL at $18/200 mg

- *Androderm* patch at $2.97/2.5 or 5.0 mg 24-hour patch.
- *AndroGel* 5 g packet at $6.63
- *Striant*

INDICATIONS (for men only, except where noted)

- **Hypogonadism:** Normal testosterone levels in adult men are 300-1,000 ng/dL at 8 AM, representing peak levels with circadian rhythm. Prior studies show subnormal testosterone levels in 45% of patients with AIDS and 20-30% of HIV infected patients without AIDS (*Am J Med* 1988;84:611; *AIDS* 1994;7:46; *J Clin Endocrinol* 1996;81:4108). Testing should be performed in the morning and should measure free (unbound) levels or unbound levels (normal: 34-194 pg/mL). Replacement therapy is recommended for men with low or low-normal levels. Restoration of normal testosterone levels can be achieved with testosterone enanthate 200 mg IM every 2 weeks, a 5 mg *Androderm* patch applied nightly, a 5 mg *Testoderm TTS* patch applied each morning, 5 g of *AndroGel* or *Testim* per day, 30 mg of

Striant buccal bid. Therapeutic trials with testosterone treatment of hypogonadal men with HIV infection show substantial improvements in quality of life with increased libido, reduced fatigue, and reduced depression (*Arch Gen Psych* 2000;57:141). Benefit has also been shown in eugonadal HIV infected men receiving twice the physiological dose (200 mg every week), but long-term toxicity should be considered (*Ann Intern Med* 2000;133:348).

- **Wasting:** Testosterone is an anabolic steroid that may restore nitrogen balance and lean body mass in patients with wasting (*J Acquir Immune Defic Syndr* 1996;11:510; *J Acquir Immune Defic Syndr* 1997;16:254; *Ann Intern Med* 1998;129:18). A placebo-controlled trial of 51 hypogonadal men with AIDS-associated wasting showed replacement dosing (testosterone enanthate 300 mg IM q3wk) was associated with an average gain of 2.6 kg lean body mass over 6 months (*Ann Intern Med* 1998;129:18), and these results were sustained over 12 months in an open-label extension (*Clin Infect Dis* 1999;31:1240).

- **Lipodystrophy:** Testosterone may reduce visceral fat and reduce cholesterol; however, studies show minimal effect on body weight or muscle mass (*J Clin Eudocrinol Metals* 2005;90:1531) and risks include reduced HDL cholesterol, hepatotoxicity, and risk of prostatic cancer (*Clin Infect Dis* 2002;34:248).

- **Testosterone for wasting in women:** The following is based on a single report (*Arch Intern Med* 2004;164:897).
  - Indication: Free testosterone <3 pg/mL; weight <90% of ideal body weight or weight loss >10%.
  - Treatment: TTS patch (4.1 mg/patch) 2x/week
  - Results: Trial showed modest increase in muscle mass, no significant weight gain and no significant complications.

REGIMEN

- **Intramuscular:** 200-400 mg IM every 2 weeks. The dose and dosing interval may need adjustment; many use 100-200 mg IM every week given by self administration to avoid low levels in the second week; many initiate therapy for wasting with 300-400 mg every 2 weeks, with taper to 200 mg when weight is restored, or combine with other anabolic steroids. Replacement doses are 100 mg/week (*Clin Infect Dis* 2003;36:S73).

- **Transdermal systems:** Advantages are rapid absorption, controlled rate of delivery, avoidance of first-pass hepatic metabolism, avoidance of IM injections, and possibly less testicular shrinkage. Three delivery systems are available: Skin patches and a topical gel (*Androderm*) are available in 2.5-5 mg sizes to deliver 4 and 6 mg testosterone. Serum testosterone levels peak at 3 to 8 hours. After 1 month, a morning testosterone level should be obtained. *Androderm* consists of a liquid reservoir containing 12.2 g testosterone (delivers

2.5 mg/d of testosterone) or 24.3 mg (that delivers 5 mg/d testosterone). The usual dose is a system that delivers 5 mg/day. *AndroGel* or *Testim* is rubbed on to the skin starting with 5 mg qd and then has the notable advantage of permitting dose titration based on serum testosterone levels.

CONTROLLED SUBSTANCE: Schedule C-III

PHARMACOLOGY

- **Bioavailability:** Poor absorption and rapid metabolism with oral administration. The cypionate and enanthate esters are absorbed slowly from IM injection sites.

- **Elimination:** Hepatic metabolism to 17 ketosteroids that are excreted in urine.

SIDE EFFECTS: Androgenic effects include acne, flushing, gynecomastia, increased libido, priapism, and edema. Other side effects include aggravation of sleep apnea, salt retention, increased hematocrit, possible promotion of KS, and promotion of breast or prostate cancer. In women, there may be virilization with voice change, hirsutism, and clitoral enlargement. Androgens may cause cholestatic hepatitis. Patches are associated with local reactions, especially pruritus and occasionally blistering, erythema, and pain.

DRUG INTERACTIONS: May potentiate action of oral anticoagulants.

PREGNANCY: Category X

THALIDOMIDE

TRADE NAME: *Thalomid* (Celgene)

FORM AND PRICE: 50, 100, and 200 mg capsules; 100 mg cap at $53.44

AVAILABILITY: Thalidomide is FDA-approved for marketing through a restricted distribution program called "System for Thalidomide Education and Prescribing Safety" (STEPS). The STEPS Program is designed to eliminate the risk of birth defects by requiring registration of prescribing physicians, patients, and pharmacists, combined with informed consent, rigorous counseling, accountability, and a patient survey. Only physicians registered with STEPS may prescribe thalidomide. Call 888-423-5436 (option 1) to register and receive necessary forms. **Requirements for prescribing:** 1) Agreement to patient counseling as indicated in the consent form; 2) Patient consent form with one copy sent to Boston University; and 3) Completion of the physician monitoring survey. **Patients are registered if they** 1) agree to use two reliable methods of contraception; 2) have pregnancy tests performed regularly (females); 3) use latex condoms when having sex with women (males); and 4) agree to participate in mandatory and confidential patient survey. **Pharmacies must register to dispense**

5 Drugs: Thalidomide

thalidomide by agreeing to 1) collect and file informed consent forms; 2) register patients by phone or fax; 3) prescribe no more than a 28 day supply within 7 days of the prescription date; and 4) verify patient registry with refills.

PATIENT ASSISTANCE: 888-423-5436 (press 2)

FDA LABELING: Approved for moderate to severe erythema nodosum leprosum

REGIMEN: Usual dose is 50-200 mg/day, most commonly 100 mg/day at hs to reduce sedative side effect. Often start at 100-200 mg/day and titrate down to 50 mg/day or give intermittent dosing (*J Infect Dis* 2001;183:343). Doses above 200-300 mg/day are poorly tolerated (*N Eng J Med* 1997;336:1487; *Clin Infect Dis* 1997;24:1223).

MECHANISM: Presumed mechanism for HIV-associated wasting is the reduction in TNF-alpha production (*J Exp Med* 1991;173:699). Thalidomide also has numerous other anti-inflammatory and immunomodulatory properties (*Int J Dermatol* 1974;13:20; *Proc Natl Acad Soc USA* 1993;90:5974; *Mol Med* 1995;1:384; *J Exp Med* 1993;177:1675; *J Acquir Immune Defic Syndr* 1997;13:1047).

CLINICAL TRIALS

- **Aphthous ulcers:** In a placebo-controlled trial using thalidomide (200 mg/day) in patients with oral aphthous ulcers, 16/29 (53%) in the thalidomide arm responded compared with 2/28 (7%) in the placebo group (*N Engl J Med* 1997;336:1489). ACTG 251 was a placebo-controlled trial involving 45 patients given thalidomide (200 mg/day x 4 weeks followed by 100 mg/day for responders and 400 mg/day for nonresponders for oral or esophageal ulcers). Among 23 recipients of thalidomide, 14 (61%) had a complete remission in 4 weeks, and 21 (91%) had a complete remission or partial response. In another ACTG trial for patients with aphthous ulcers of the esophagus, thalidomide (200 mg/day) was associated with a complete response at 4 weeks in 8 of 11 (73%) (*J Infect Dis* 1999;180:61). Ulcers usually heal in 7 to 28 days. The usual dose for aphthous ulcers is 100-200 mg/day, with increases up to 400-600 mg/day if unresponsive; after healing, discontinue or use maintenance dose of 50 mg/day (*J Am Acad Dermatol* 1993;28:271).

- **Wasting:** Two placebo-controlled trials and three open-label studies demonstrated that thalidomide (daily doses of 50-300 mg/day) for 2 to 12 weeks was associated with significant weight gains. The largest trial showed a dose of 100 mg/day x 8 weeks was associated with a mean weight gain of 1.7 kg compared to placebo; half was lean body mass (*AIDS Res Hum Retroviruses* 2000;16:1345). The recommended dose is 100 mg/day because larger doses do not increase weight gain but cause more side effects (*Clin Infect Dis* 2003;36[suppl 2]:S74).

Drugs: Thalidomide

- **Chronic diarrhea due to microsporidia:** A trial in 18 HIV infected men with chronic diarrhea due to *E. bieneusi* that was unresponsive to albendazole were given thalidomide, 100 mg daily x 4 weeks. There was a complete response in 7 (38%) and a partial response in 3 (17%) (*Gastroenterology* 1997;112:1823).
- **Other possible uses in HIV infected patients:** Prurigo nodularis (200-400 mg/day), postherpetic neuralgia (100-300 mg/day), microsporiodosis (*Gastroenterology* 1997;112:1823), multicentric Castleman disease (*Am J Hematol* 2004;75:176) and AIDS-associated proctitis (300 mg/day) (*J Am Acad Dermatol* 1996;35:969)

PHARMACOLOGY (*Antimicrob Agents Chemother* 1997;41:2797)

- **Bioavailability:** Well absorbed
- **T½:** 6 to 8 hours. Peak levels with 200 mg dose are 1.7 µg/mL; levels >4 µg/mL are required to inhibit TNF-alpha (*Proc Natl Acad Sci USA* 1993;90:5974; *J Exp Med* 1993;177:1675; *J Am Acad Dermatol* 1996; 35:969). It is not known whether thalidomide is present in semen.
- **Elimination:** Nonrenal mechanisms, primarily nonenzymatic hydrolysis in plasma to multiple metabolites. There are no recommendations for dose changes in renal or hepatic failure.

SIDE EFFECTS

- **Teratogenic effects:** Major concern is in pregnant women due to high potential for birth defects, including absent or abnormal limbs; cleft lip; absent ears; heart, renal or genital abnormalities and other severe defects (*Nat Med* 1997;3:8). Maximum vulnerability is 35 to 50 days after the last menstrual period, when a single dose is sufficient to cause severe limb abnormalities in most patients (*J Am Acad Dermatol* 1996;35:969). It is *critical* that any woman of child-bearing potential not receive thalidomide unless great precautions are taken to prevent pregnancy (pills and barrier protection). Because thalidomide may be present in semen, condom use is recommended for men. Company records indicate that through January 2001, there were 26,968 patients treated, and there were no documented exposures during pregnancy. Several male exposures followed by conception were noted, but none resulted in birth defects.
- **Dose effect:** Teratogenic effects occur even with single dose. Neuropathy, rash, constipation, neutropenia, and sedation are common dose-related side effects found in up to 50% of AIDS patients and are more frequent with low CD4 cell counts (*Clin Infect Dis* 1997;24:1223; *J Infect Dis* 2002;185:1359).
- **Drowsiness:** Most common side effect is the sedation for which the drug was initially marketed. Administer at bedtime and reduce dose to minimize this side effect. There may be morning somnolence or "hangover."

5 Drugs: Thalidomide

- **Rash:** Usually pruritic, erythematous, and macular over trunk, back, and proximal extremities. TEN and Stevens-Johnson syndrome have been reported. Re-challenge following erythematous rash has resulted in severe reactions and should only be done with caution.
- **Neuropathy:** Dose-related paresthesias and/or pain of extremities, especially with high doses or prolonged use. This complication may or may not be reversible; it is not known whether the risk is increased by diabetes, alcoholism, or use of neurotoxic drugs including ddl, d4T, or ddC. Symptoms may start after the drug is discontinued. Neuropathy is a contraindication to the drug, and neurologic monitoring should be performed for all patients.
- **HIV:** Thalidomide may cause modest increase in plasma levels of HIV RNA (0.4 $\log_{10}$/mL) (*N Engl J Med* 1997:336:1487).
- **Neutropenia:** Discontinue thalidomide if ANC is <750/mm^3 without an alternative cause.
- **Constipation:** Common; use stool softener, hydration, milk of magnesia, etc.
- **Less common side effects** include dizziness, mood changes, bradycardia, tachycardia, bitter taste, headache, nausea, pruritus, dry mouth, dry skin, or hypotension.

DRUG INTERACTIONS: The greatest concern is in women of child-bearing potential who take concurrent medications, such as rifamycin and possibly PIs and NNRTIs, that interfere with the effectiveness of contraceptives. Concurrent use of drugs that cause sedation or peripheral neuropathy may increase the frequency and severity of these side effects.

PREGNANCY: Category X (contraindicated)

TIPRANAVIR (TPV)

TRADE NAME: *Aptivus* (Boehringer-Ingelheim)

CLASS: Protease inhibitor

FORMS AND PRICE: Caps, 250 mg

PATIENT ASSISTANCE: 800-556-8317; http://us.boehringer-ingelheim.com/about/philanthropy/Patient_Assistance_Program.html

STANDARD DOSE: TPV/r 500/200 mg bid with food
- **Advantages:** 1) Most active PI against PI-resistant HIV; 2) established efficacy in salvage therapy; 3) bid dosing
- **Disadvantages:** 1) Class adverse reactions of PIs including GI intolerance, elevated transaminase levels and hyperlipidemia; 2) reduced efficacy with extensive PI resistance (see "Resistance"); 3) multiple drug interactions, and inability to combine with other PIs.

Drugs: Thalidomide

308

INDICATION: The main advantage of TPV is activity versus HIV strains that are resistant to other PIs. It is indicated for patients with resistance to PIs who have genotypic or phenotypic evidence of susceptibility to TPV. It requires RTV boosting and has been most effective when combined with enfuvirtide (T20).

CLINICAL TRIALS

- **RESIST-1 and -2:** Phase 3 trials of patients who failed at least 2 PI-based regimens, had VL >1000 c/mL and had at least one primary PI mutation and no more than two at codons 33, 82, 84 and 90. RESIST-1 was conducted with 620 subjects in the U.S., Canada and Australia; RESIST-2 was conducted with 539 evaluable patients in Europe and South America. Participants were randomized to receive TPV/r or one of four alternative boosted PI regimens: LPV/r, IDV/r, SQV/r or APV/r. The 1159 participants had a median baseline VL of 4.8 $\log_{10}$ c/mL and median CD4 count of 155/mm³. Participants with no virologic response in control arm were allowed to roll over to trial 1182.17, which included TPV/r. The NRTI "backbone" was individualized. Response rates were reduced in patients with a higher "TPV score," determined by the number of the following PI mutations: 10V, 13V, 20M/R/V, 33F, 35G, 36I, 43T, 46L, 47V, 54A/M/V, 58E, 69K, 74P, 82L/T, 83D, 84V (12th CROI, Boston, 2005, Abstr. 104). Patients with 0-2 mutations had the best response (94% with mean 0.5 $\log_{10}$ drop in VL); those with 3-5 mutations had an intermediate response (84%); and those with ≥6 mutations had a poor response (72%). However, phenotypic testing is likely to provide a more accurate assessment of TPV susceptibility at present. The clinical cutoff for TPV using the *PhenoSense* assay is 4.0. Results at 24 wks are shown in the following table:

■ TABLE 5-46: **RESIST 1 and 2: Results at 24 Weeks**

	TPV/r (n = 582)	CPI/r (n = 577)
VL <400 c/mL	199 (34%)	86 (15%)*
VL <50 c/mL	139 (24%)	54 (9%)*
Increase CD4 count (median)	+34/mm³	+4/mm³*

*$P = <0.0001$

- **BI 1182.52:** This dose-finding study in 216 patients who failed ≥2 PI-based regimens (CROI 2003, Abstr. 596) showed that patients with ≥3 of 4 PRAMs (protease gene mutations at codons 33, 82, 84, and 90) had a reduced response. This accounts for the limitation of ≤2 PRAMs as an entry criterion for RESIST.

- **BI 1182.51:** This study enrolled simultaneously with RESIST but was restricted to the patients with 3 or 4 PRAMs. Patients were randomized to TPV/r (n = 61) or to LPV/r (n = 79), APV/r (n = 76), or SQV/r (n = 75). After 14 days TPV/r was added to the regimens of

5 Drugs: Tipranavir

patients in the other three arms. Patients on TPV/r had a median VL decrease of 1.2 $\log_{10}$ c/mL compared to <0.4 $\log_{10}$ c/mL in each of the other arms; the addition of TPV/r to the other regimens resulted in a substantial boost to viral suppression to a median total decrease of 1.2 $\log_{10}$ c/mL at 4 week. The suppression noted above was not sustained, indicating the need for additional active agents. Pharmacokinetic studies of the dual PI-boosted regimens showed that TPV reduced C_{min} of the concurrent PIs by 55% to 81%, presumably due to P450 induction. For this reason, dual-boosted PI therapy with these TPV combinations is not recommended.

- **TPV/r vs. LPV/r:** A subset analysis of RESIST-1 compared 24-week results for patients randomized to either TPV/r or LPV/r. Response was significantly better in the TPV/r recipients in terms of viral suppression (40% vs. 21%), proportion with VL <400 c/mL (34% vs. 25%) and mean CD4 response (+31/ mm^3 vs. +6/ mm^3) (12th CROI, 2005, Abstr. 560). Viral response was greater in both groups when ENF was used concurrently.

- **TPV/r + enfuvirtide:** Results in RESIST 1 and 2 showed viral response rates of 75% in those treated with enfuvirtide, 25% in those treated without enfuvirtide.

RESISTANCE: Mutations at 30N, 50V and 88D are associated with TPV hypersusceptibility (*HIV Clin Trials* 2004;5:371; *Expert Rev Anti-Infect Ther* 2005;3:9). Mutations that contribute to resistance are at codons 10, 13, 20, 33, 35, 36, 43, 47, 54, 58, 69, 74, 82, 38, and 84 (3rd IAS, Rio, 2005, Abstr. WeOa 0205).

PHARMACOLOGY

- **Bioavailability:** Oral absorption is substantially improved with a concurrent high-fat meal. A newer self-emulsifying drug delivery system doubles bioavailability and makes concurrent food unnecessary. RTV given concurrently increases TPV 29-fold and is always recommended for concurrent use.

- **T½:** 6 h

- **Excretion:** Most of TPV is eliminated in stool; minimal drug is found in urine.

- **Dose adjustment for renal failure:** None.

- **Dose adjustment for hepatic failure:** Not established.

DRUG INTERACTIONS

- **RTV:** RTV in doses of 200 mg bid increases TPV levels 29-fold and is required for TPV to achieve therapeutic levels.

- **NRTIs:** No clinically significant effect with concurrent d4T, TDF, 3TC. Must be dosed ≥4 h before or after ddI and ddI EC. AZT and ABC concentrations are decreased 40%-50%; dose adjustment is not established.

Drugs: Tipranavir

- **NNRTIs:** No interaction with EFV or NVP.
- **PIs:** Studies combining PIs with TPV/r showed that the drug induced P450, resulting in a 50%-80% reduction in the C_{min} levels of LPV, APV, and SQV. Therefore, these PIs should not be co-administered with TPV. There are no data for concurrent administration of ATV, NFV, or IDV, but the assumption is that these drugs will be affected in a similar way.
- Drugs contraindicated for concurrent administration: anti-arrhythmics (amiodirone, bepridil, flecainide, propafenone, quinidine), ergot derivatives, lovastatin, simvastatin, pimozide, midazolam, triazolam.
- **Other drugs:**
  - Alprazolam: increase alprazolam levels; consider lorazepam, temazepam, oxazepam
  - Antacids: decrease TPV AUC 25-30%; take ≥2 h apart
  - Atorvastatin: increase atorvastatin AUC 9x; use with caution starting with lowest dose and avoiding high doses (e.g. >40 mg/d) or use rosuvastatin or pravastatin
  - Benzodiazepines: Avoid clorazepate, estazolam, flurazepam; consider lorazepam, oxazepam or temazepan
  - Calcium channel blockers: cannot predict due to conflicting actions of TPV and RTV; monitor
  - Carbamazepine: consider valproic acid, lamotrigine, levetiracetam or topiramate
  - Clarithromycin: increases TPV levels; no dose adjustment necessary
  - Corticosteroids: decrease TPV levels, use with caution
  - Cyclosporine: increases cyclosporine levels; monitor levels
  - ddI EC: TPV increases ddI AUC 48-60%; use ddI in dose of 200 mg/d (<60 kg) or 250 mg/d (>60 kg)
  - Despiramine: Increase desiramine, reduce despiramine dose and monitor
  - Disulfiram/Metronidazole: TPV caps contain alcohol and may cause disulfiram-like reactions
  - Ethinyl estradiol: reduces hormone AUC; use alternative birth control
  - Flecainide: Increase flecainide levels; avoid or monitor levels
  - Fluconazole: TPV levels increased; clinical significance not known
  - Itraconazole and ketonazole: azole levels increased; consider fluconazole
  - Meperidine: Decrease meperidine levels and increase metabolite normeperidine, which has analgesic activity and may cause seizures

Drugs: Tipranavir

5

- Methadone: May need to increase methadone dose
- Nifedipine: increase levels nifedipine; avoid
- Paclitaxel: possible increase in paclitaxel levels; monitor closely
- Phenobarbital: may decrease TPV levels and increase or decrease phenobarbital levels; consider valproic acid, lamotrigine. Levetiracetam or topiramate
- Phenytoin: as with phenobarbital
- Rifampin: decrease TPV levels; avoid
- Rifabutin: RBT levels increased 20x; use reduced doses
- Sildenafil: increased sildenafil levels; limit to ≤25 mg in 48 h
- Tacrolimus: increased levels of tacrolimus; use reduced doses
- Theophylline: increased levels of theophylline; consider therapeutic monitoring
- Vardenafil: increased levels of vardenafil; do not exceed 2.5 mg q 72 h (with RTV)
- Voriconazole: may decrease voriconazole levels and increase TPV levels; avoid (use amphotericin or caspofungin) or monitor carefully

ADVERSE DRUG REACTIONS: TPV's side effects profile is similar to that of other PIs, except for high rates of elevated transminase and an FDA black box warning for clinical hepatitis. The most common side effects are GI intolerance and increases in transaminase levels (grade 3/4 increases in 8%). Hepatotoxicity is more common in patients with hepatitis B or C coinfection. Indications to discontinue TPV/r based on grade 3/4 transaminase increases are unclear. GI intolerance includes nausea (5%) and diarrhea (4-10%). Less frequent side effects are fatigue, headache, and abdominal pain. Rash reactions are more common in women (13% vs 8%). Increases in total cholesterol, LDL cholesterol, and triglycerides are common; serum lipid levels should be monitored.

TRAZODONE

TRADE NAME: *Desyrel* (Bristol-Myers Squibb) or generic

FORMS AND PRICES: Tabs: 50 mg at $0.40, 100 mg at $0.63, 150 mg at $1.41, 300 mg at $5.44

CLASS: Nontricyclic antidepressant (see Table 7-16, p. 440)

INDICATIONS AND DOSE REGIMENS

- **Depression**, especially when associated with anxiety or insomnia: 400-600 mg/day in two doses. If insomnia or daytime sedation, give as single dose at hs. Increase dose 50 mg every 3 to 4 days up to maximum dose of 400 mg/day for outpatients and 600 mg/day for hospitalized patients.

- **Insomnia:** 25-150 mg qhs

PHARMACOLOGY

- **Bioavailability:** >90%, improved if taken with meals
- **T½:** 6 hours
- **Elimination:** Hepatic metabolism, then renal excretion

SIDE EFFECTS: Adverse effects are dose- and duration-related and are usually seen with doses >300 mg/day; may decrease with continued use, dose reduction, or schedule change.

- **Major side effects:** Sedation in 15% to 20%; orthostatic hypotension (5%); nervousness; fatigue; dizziness; nausea; vomiting; and anticholinergic effects (dry mouth, blurred vision, constipation, urinary retention). Rare – priapism (1/6000); agitation; cardiovascular; and anticholinergic side effects are less frequent and less severe than with tricyclics.

DRUG INTERACTIONS: May increase levels of phenytoin and digoxin; alcohol and other CNS depressants potentiate sedative side effects; increase may trazodone levels with fluoxetine; may potentiate effects of antihypertensive agents.

PREGNANCY: Category C

TRICYCLIC ANTIDEPRESSANTS – see also Nortriptyline (p. 266)

Tricyclic antidepressants elevate mood, increase physical activity, improve appetite, improve sleep patterns, and reduce morbid preoccupations in most patients with major depression. The following principles apply:

INDICATIONS

- **Psychiatric indications:** Major depression – response rates are 60% to 70%. Low doses are commonly used for adjustment disorders including depression and anxiety.
- **Peripheral neuropathy:** Controlled trials have not shown benefit in AIDS-associated peripheral neuropathy, but clinical experience is extensive and results in diabetic neuropathy are good. If used, choice of agents depends on time of symptoms (*JAMA* 1998;280:1590). Night pain: Amitriptyline (sedating) 25 mg hs. Day pain: Nortriptyline (less sedating and less of an anticholinergic effect) 25 mg hs. Some recommend therapeutic drug monitoring for depression, but generally not for peripheral neuropathy.

5 Drugs: Tricyclic Antidepressants

DOSE: Initial treatment of depression is 4 to 8 weeks, which is required for therapeutic response. Much or all of the initial dose is given at hs, especially if insomnia is prominent or if sedation is a side effect. Common mistakes are use of an initial dose that is too high, resulting in excessive anticholinergic side effects or oversedation. The dose is increased every 3 to 4 days depending on tolerance and response. Treatment of major depression usually requires continuation for 4 to 5 months after response. Multiple recurrences may require long-term treatment.

SERUM LEVELS: Efficacy correlates with serum levels of nortriptyline when used as an antidepressant. Therapeutic monitoring of drug levels allows dose titration.

PHARMACOLOGY: Well absorbed, extensively metabolized, long half-life, variable use of serum levels (see below).

SIDE EFFECTS: Anticholinergic effects (dry mouth, dizziness, blurred vision, constipation, tachycardia, urinary hesitancy, sedation), sexual dysfunction, orthostatic hypotension, weight gain

RELATIVE CONTRAINDICATIONS: Cardiac conduction block, prostatism, and narrow angle glaucoma. Less common side effects – mania, hypomania, allergic skin reactions, marrow suppression, seizures, tardive dyskinesia, tremor, speech blockage, anxiety, insomnia, Parkinsonism, hyponatremia; cardiac conduction disturbances and arrhythmias (most common serious side effects are with overdosage).

TRIMETHOPRIM (TMP)

TRADE NAME: Generic

FORMS AND PRICES: Tabs: 100 mg at $0.68

INDICATIONS AND DOSE REGIMENS

- **PCP** (with sulfamethoxazole as TMP-SMX or with dapsone): 5 mg/kg PO tid (usually 300 mg tid or qid) x 21 days
- **UTIs:** 100 mg PO bid or 200 mg x 1/day x 3 to 14 days

PHARMACOLOGY

- **Bioavailability:** >90%
- **T½:** 9 to 11 hours
- **Excretion:** Renal
- **Dose modification with renal failure:** CrCl >50 mL/min – full dose; 10-50 mL/min – one-half to two-thirds dose; <30 mL/min – one-third to one-half dose

SIDE EFFECTS: Usually well tolerated; most common – pruritus and skin rash; GI intolerance; marrow suppression – anemia, neutropenia, thrombocytopenia; antifolate effects – prevent with leucovorin; reversible hyperkalemia in 20% to 50% of AIDS patients given high doses (*Ann Intern Med* 1993;119:291,296; *N Engl J Med* 1993;238:703).

DRUG INTERACTIONS: Increased activity of phenytoin (monitor levels) and procainamide; levels of both dapsone and trimethoprim are increased when given concurrently.

PREGNANCY: Category C. Teratogenic in rats with high doses; limited experience in patients shows no association with congenital abnormalities.

TRIMETHOPRIM-SULFAMETHOXAZOLE
(TMP-SMX, cotrimoxazole)

TRADE NAME: *Bactrim* (Roche), *Septra* (Monarch), or generic

FORMS AND PRICE: Trimethoprim/sulfamethoxazole 80/400 mg (SS) tabs at $0.73; 160/800 mg (DS) tabs at $1.21. For IV use: 10 mL vials with 16/80 mg/mL at $19.26/30 mL.

INDICATIONS AND DOSE REGIMENS

- **PCP prophylaxis:** 1 DS/day or 1 SS/day; alternative is 1 DS 3x/week. Discontinuation of PCP prophylaxis after HAART-associated immune reconstitution is safe and avoids significant toxicity (*Clin Infect Dis* 2001;33:1901; *MMWR* 2002;51[RR-8]:4).

- **Graduated initiation to reduce adverse effects** (ACTG 268) (*J Acquir Immune Defic Syndr* 2000;24:337): Oral preparation (40 mg trimethoprim and 200 mg sulfamethoxazole/5mL) – 1 mL/day x 3 days, then 2 mL/day x 3 days, then 5 mL/day x 3 days, then 10 mL/day x 3 days, then 20 mL x 3 days, then 1 TMP-SMX DS tab/day

- **Desensitization:** See Table 5-48, p. 318

- **PCP treatment:** 5 mg/kg (trimethoprim component) PO or IV q8h x 21 days, usually 5-6 DS/day

- **Toxoplasmosis prophylaxis:** 1 DS/day

- **Toxoplasmosis treatment:** Alternative to sulfadiazine – acute therapy (>6 weeks) TMP-SMX 5 mg/kg (TMP) PO or IV bid x ≥6 weeks, then maintenance at half dose (*Eur J Clin Microbiol Infect Dis* 1992;11:125; *Antimicrob Agents Chemother* 1998;42:1346).

- ***Isospora:*** 1 DS PO qid x 10 days; may need maintenance with 1-2 DS/day. IDSA recommendation: TMP-SMX 1 DS bid x 7 to 10 days, then 1 DS 3x/week or 1 *Fansidar* every week indefinitely.

- ***Salmonella:*** 1 DS PO bid x 5 to 7 days; treat >14 days if relapsing.

- ***Nocardia:*** 4-6 DS/day x ≥6 months

- **Urinary tract infections:** 1-2 DS/day x 3 to 14 days
- **Prophylaxis for cystitis:** ½ SS tab daily

ACTIVITY: TMP-SMX is effective in the treatment or prophylaxis of infections involving *P. jiroveci*, methicillin-sensitive *S. aureus*, *Legionella*, *Listeria*, and common urinary tract pathogens. Recent studies show increasing rates of mutations in the dihydropteroate synthase gene of *P. jerovici* that are associated with increased resistance to sulfonamides and dapsone (*J Infect Dis* 1999;180:1969); a meta-analysis found that this mutation is associated with prolonged exposure to sulfonamides, but the clinical significance of these mutations in terms of reduced response is unclear (*Emerg Infect Dis* 2004;10:1760). In a prospective trial, clinical outcome was not worse with DHPS mutation (*Lancet* 2001;358:545). Current rates of resistance of *S. pneumoniae* to TMP-SMX are about 15% to 30% (*Antimicrob Agents Chemother* 2002;46:2651; *N Engl J Med* 2000;343:1917).

PHARMACOLOGY

- **Bioavailability:** >90% absorbed with oral administration (both drugs)
- **T½:** Trimethoprim, 8 to 15 hours; sulfamethoxazole 7 to 12 hours
- **Elimination:** Renal; T½ in renal failure increases to 24 hours for trimethoprim and 22 to 50 hours for sulfamethoxazole
- **Renal failure:** CrCl >50 mL/min – usual dose; 10-50 mL/min – one-half to two-thirds dose; <10 mL/min – manufacturer recommends avoidance, but one-third to one-half dose may be used

SIDE EFFECTS: Noted in 10% of patients without HIV infection and about 50% of patients with HIV. The gradual initiation of TMP-SMX noted above results in a 50% reduction in adverse reactions (*J Acquir Immune Defic Syndr* 2000;24:337), suggesting that it is not a true hypersensitivity reaction. The prevailing opinion is that these side effects are usually due to toxic metabolites ascribed to altered metabolism of TMP-SMX with HIV infection. The presumed benefit from gradual initiation or desensitization is to permit time for enzyme induction.

- **Most common:** Nausea, vomiting, pruritus, rash, fever, neutropenia, and increased transaminases. Many HIV-infected patients may be treated despite side effects (GI intolerance and rash) if symptoms are not disabling; alternative with PCP prophylaxis is dose reduction usually after drug holiday (1 to 2 weeks) and/or "desensitization" (see below). The mechanism of most sulfonamide reactions is unclear, and cause of increased susceptibility with HIV is also unclear.
- **Rash:** Most common is erythematous, maculopapular, morbilliform, and/or pruritic rash, usually 7 to 14 days after treatment is started.

Drugs: Trimethoprim-Sulfamethoxazole

316

Less common are erythema multiforme, epidermal necrolysis, exfoliative dermatitis, Stevens-Johnson syndrome, urticaria, and Schönlein-Henoch purpura.

- **GI intolerance** is common with nausea, vomiting, anorexia, and abdominal pain; rare side effects include *C. difficile* diarrhea/colitis and pancretitis.

- **Hematologic side effects** include neutropenia, anemia, and/or thrombocytopenia. The rate of anemia is increased in patients with HIV infection and with folate depletion. Some respond to leucovorin (5-15 mg/day), but this is not routinely recommended.

- **Neurologic** toxicity may include tremor, ataxia, apathy, and ankle clonus that responds promptly to drug discontinuation.

- **Hepatitis** with cholestatic jaundice and hepatic necrosis has been described.

- **Hyperkalemia** in 20% to 50% of patients given trimethoprim in doses >15 mg/kg/day (*N Engl J Med* 1993;328:703)

- **Aseptic meningitis** (*Am J Med Sci* 1996;312:27)

PROTOCOL FOR ORAL "DESENSITIZATION" OR "DETOXIFICATION"

- **Rapid desensitization** (*Clin Infect Dis* 1995;20:849): Serial 10-fold dilutions of oral suspension (40 mg TMP, 200 mg SMX/5 mL) given hourly over 4 hours (see Table 5-47, below).

- **Note:** A prospective trial showed no difference in outcome with desensitization compared with rechallenge (*Biomed Pharmacother* 2000;54:45)

■ TABLE 5-47: **Rapid TMP-SMX Desensitization Schedule**

Time (hour)	Dose (TMP/SMX)	Dilution
0	0.004/0.02 mg	1:10,000 (5 mL)
1	0.04/0.2 mg	1:1,000 (5 mL)
2	0.4/2.0 mg	1:100 (5 mL)
3	4/20 mg	1:10 (5 mL)
4	40/200 mg	(5 mL)
5	160/800 mg	Tablet

- **8-day protocol:** Serial dilutions prepared by pharmacists using oral suspension (40 mg TMP, 200 mg SMX/5 mL). Medication is given 4 times daily for 7 days in doses of 1 cc, 2 cc, 4 cc, and 8 cc using the following dilutions:

5 Drugs: Trimethoprim-Sulfamethoxazole

Day	Dilution
1	1:1,000,000
2	1:100,000
3	1:10,000
4	1:1,000
5	1:100
6	1:10
7	1:1
8	Standard suspension – 1 mL 40 mg SMX – 8 mg TMP
≥9	1 DS tab/day

DRUG INTERACTIONS: Increased levels of oral anticoagulants, phenytoin, and procainamide. Risk of megaloblastic anemia with methotrexate.

PREGNANCY: Category C. Teratogenic in animals. No congenital abnormalities noted in 35 children born to women who received TMP-SMX in first trimester. Use with caution due to possible kernicterus, although no cases of kernicterus have been reported (*Clin Infect Dis* 1995;21[suppl 1]:S24).

TRUVADA – see Tenofovir, p. 300, and Emtricitabine (Gilead), p. 194

TRIZIVIR – see Zidovudine, p. 323; Lamivudine, p. 241; and Abacavir, p. 137 (GlaxoSmithKline)

VALACYCLOVIR – see Acyclovir (p. 141)

VALGANCICLOVIR – see Ganciclovir (p. 217)

VIBRAMYCIN – see Doxycycline (p. 184)

VIDEX – see Didanosine (p. 180)

VIRACEPT – see Nelfinavir (p. 256)

Drugs: Trimethoprim-Sulfamethoxazole

VIRAMUNE – see Nevirapine (p. 260)

VITRASERT – see Ganciclovir (p. 217)

VORICONAZOLE

TRADE NAME: *Vfend* (Pfizer)

FORMS AND PRICE: Tabs: 50 mg, 200 mg at $35; Vial for IV use: 200 mg at $109

CLASS: Triazole antifungal

REGIMENS

- **Oral:** 200 mg PO tid x 1 day (loading dose), then 200-300 mg PO bid on an empty stomach. Avoid high-fat meal. Usual dose for aspergillosis is 300 mg bid; use one-half dose for patients <40 kg.
- **IV:** 6 mg/kg IV q12h x 2 doses (loading dose), then 3-4 mg/kg IV q12h
- **Hepatic failure:** Use half-dose 6 mg/kg q12h x2 doses, then 2 mg/kg q12h
- **Renal failure:** Use standard oral dose

IN VITRO **ACTIVITY:** Active against most *Candida* species, including many fluconazole-resistant strains. Active against >98% of *C. albicans, C. krusei, C. tropicalis,* and *C. parapsilosis* (*Antimicrob Agents Chemother* 2002;46:1032; *J Med Microbiol* 2002;51:479; *J Clin Microbiol* 2002;40:852). Very active against most *Aspergillus;* more active *in vitro* than itraconazole (*J Infect Chemother* 2000;6:101; *Clin Infect Dis* 2002;34:563; *Clin Micro* 2002;40:2648; *Antimicrob Agents Chemother* 2002;46:1032). Zygomycetes (mucor) are less susceptible (*Antimicrob Agents Chemother* 2002;46:2708; *Antimicrob Agents Chemother* 2002;46:1581; *Antimicrob Agents Chemother* 2002;46:1032). Activity against *Scedosporium apiospermum* (*Pseudoallescheria boydii*) is variable (*Antimicrob Agents Chemother* 2002;46:62). Most dermatophytes are sensitive (*Antimicrob Agents Chemother* 2001;45:2524). *C. neoformans* is usually highly susceptible with *in vitro* activity superior to both fluconazole and itraconazole (*Eur J Clin Microbiol* 2000;19:317; *Antimicrob Agents Chemother* 1999;43:1463; *Antimicrob Agents Chemother* 1999;43:169). Also active *in vitro* vs *H. capsulatum, B. dermatitidis,* and *C. neoformans.*

FDA APPROVAL: Voriconazole is approved for treatment of invasive aspergillosis and serious infections caused by *Scedosporium apiospermum* and *Fusarium* spp.

CLINICAL TRIAL: Major clinical trial compared voriconazole (6 mg/kg IV q12h x 2 doses, then 4 mg/kg IV q 12 x ≥7 days, then oral voriconazole 200 mg bid) with amphotericin B (1.0-1.5 mg/kg/day IV) in 277 patients with invasive *Aspergillus*. Voriconazole showed a significantly better response rate (53% vs 32%), better 12-week survival (71% vs 58%), and less toxicity (*N Engl J Med* 2002;347:408).

PHARMACOLOGY

- **Oral bioavailability:** 96%; AUC reduced by 24% when taken with high-fat meal
- **CNS penetration:** Preliminary data suggest that effective levels are achieved in CSF (*Br J Haematol* 1997:97:663).
- **Loading dose:** Day 1; without loading dose, the maintenance dose requires 6 days to reach steady state.
- **Metabolism:** Metabolized primarily by P450 CYP2C19, 2C9, and 3A4 enzymes. >94% of metabolite is excreted in urine; metabolites have little or no antifungal activity; <2% parenteral formal is excreted in urine.
- **Hepatic failure:** AUC increases 2.3-fold – use 100 mg bid. T½ = 6-24 hr.
- **Levels:** Expect level ≥0.5 μg/mL.

DRUG INTERACTIONS: Based on induction or inhibition of P450 enzymes primarily CYP2C19 (*Antimicrob Agents Chemother* 2002;46:3091)

- **Contraindicated for concurrent use** (decrease voriconazole levels): Rifampin, rifabutin, carbamazepine, efavirenz, ritonavir (≥400 mg bid), and phenobarbital. (Voriconazole increases concurrent drug): Sirolimus, terfenadine, astemizole, cisapride, pimozide, quinidine, ergot derivatives
- **Alter dose**
    - ☐ Cyclosporine: Increase cyclosporine, use half dose cyclosporine and monitor levels.
    - ☐ Tacrolimus: Increase tacrolimus levels 3-fold; use ⅓ dose tacrolimus; monitor levels.
    - ☐ Warfarin: Increase prothrombin time, monitor.
    - ☐ Statins: Increase simvastatin lovastatin levels, consider pravastatin, rosuvastatin.
    - ☐ Benzodiazepines: Midazolam, triazolam + alprazolam increased levels expected, reduce benzodiazepine dose.
    - ☐ Calcium channel blocker: Felodipine level increase expected, may need dose decrease.
    - ☐ Methadone: Increases methadone AUC by 47%; monitor for withdrawal.

- Sulfonylureas: Tolbutamide, glipizide + glyburide level increases expected, monitor blood glucose.
- Vinca alkaloids: Vincristine + vinblastine levels increase expected, reduce dose to avoid neurotoxicity.
- Phenytoin: Decrease voriconazole and increase phenytoin. Recommended dose: Voriconazole 400 mg PO q12h or 5 mg/kg q12h. Monitor phenytoin levels.
- Omeprazole: Levels double; reduce omeprazole to half dose.

- **Protease inhibitors:** RTV (400 mg bid) decreases voriconazole AUC 82%; this combination is contraindicated. Implication for low dose RTV (100-200 mg/day) unclear; alternative antifungal preferred. IDV – no effect on either drug. Interaction with other PIs have not been studied.

- **NNRTI:** Voriconazole AUC decreased 77% by EFV and EFV AUC increased 44% – Avoid.

SIDE EFFECTS

- **Visual effects** are most common; 30% in clinical trials; these include altered visual perception, color change, blurred vision, and/or photophobia. Changes are dose related, reversible and infrequently require discontinuing therapy, but patients should be warned.

- **Rash** in 6%, including rare cases of Stevens-Johnson syndrome, erythema multiforme and toxic epidermal necrolysis.

- **Hepatotoxicity:** Elevated transaminases in 13%, usually resolves with continued drug administration. Serious hepatic toxicity is rare, but supplier recommends monitoring liver enzymes.

PREGNANCY: Category D. Teratogenic in rodents and congenital anomalies in rabbits.

WinRho –see Rho (D) immune globulin (p. 280)

XANAX – see Alprazolam (p. 146)

ZALCITABINE (ddC)

TRADE NAME: *Hivid* (Roche)

FORMS AND PRICES: Tabs: 0.375 mg at $2.27, 0.75 mg at $2.84 (cost per year is $2,989)

PATIENT ASSISTANCE: 800-282-7780

CLASS: Nucleoside analog reverse transcriptase inhibitor

INDICATIONS: In ACTG 155, the addition of ddC after ≥6 months treatment with AZT provided no clear benefit based on clinical parameters – delayed progression and prolonged survival (*Ann Intern Med* 1994;122:24). ACTG 175 confirmed this finding but also demonstrated that ddC + AZT was superior to AZT monotherapy in AZT-naïve patients with CD4 cell counts of 200-500/mm^3 (*N Engl J Med* 1996;335:1081).

DOSE: 0.75 mg PO tid; food – no effect

RESISTANCE: Mutations on the RT gene that confer resistance are 69D/N/A, 74V, and 184V. The 74 and 184V mutations suppress AZT resistance. Resistance to ddC appears to be uncommon during combination treatment (*J Acquir Immune Defic Syndr* 1994;7:135; *J Infect Dis* 1996;173:1354). In Delta 1, there were no detectable mutations conferring ddC resistance after 112 weeks of treatment (*Lancet* 1996;348:283). Susceptibility to ddC is also decreased by thymidine analog mutations (TAMs) and by multinucleotide resistance mutations (Q151M complex, T69 ins).

PHARMACOLOGY

- **Bioavailability:** 85%
- **T½:** 1.2 hours; intracellular: 10-50 hours
- **Distribution:** CSF levels: 20% serum levels (CSF: plasma ratio = 0.09-0.37)
- **Elimination:** Renal excretion – 70%
- **Dose adjustment in renal failure:** CrCl >50 mL/min – 0.75 mg PO tid; 10-50 mL/min – 0.75 mg PO bid; <10 mL/min – 0.75 mg PO qd. Dialysis – presumably 0.75 mg post dialysis.

SIDE EFFECTS

- **Neuropathy:** The major clinical toxicity is peripheral neuropathy, noted in 17% to 31% of patients in initial trials. It is more frequent than with ddI or d4T (*N Engl J Med* 1996;335:1099). Features are bilateral sensorimotor neuropathy with numbness and burning in distal extremities, usually after 2 to 6 months of therapy, followed by shooting or continuous pain. Symptoms usually resolve slowly if the drug is promptly discontinued; with continued use it may be irreversible and require narcotics. Frequency depends on dose and duration of ddC treatment. Pain requiring narcotics or progressive pain for ≥1 week represents a contraindication to future use; patients with less severe pain that resolves to mild intensity may be rechallenged with half dose.
- **Stomatitis and aphthous esophageal ulcers:** Seen in 2% to 4% (*Ann Intern Med* 1992;117:133) and usually resolve with continued ddC treatment.

- **Pancreatitis:** Noted in <1% of patients, but more frequently in those with a history of prior pancreatitis or elevated amylase levels at the time the treatment was started.
- **Rash** is common after 10 to 14 days of treatment; it is a red maculopapular rash over the trunk and extremities, and it usually resolves spontaneously.
- **Class adverse reactions:** NRTIs may cause lactic acidosis and hepatic steatosis. This drug may be associated with the highest degree of mitochondrial toxicity, though use of ddC waned prior to the recognition of the mechanism of this toxicity.

INTERACTIONS: Drugs that cause peripheral neuropathy should be used with caution or avoided: ddl, d4T, EMB, cisplatin, disulfiram, ethionamide, INH, phenytoin, vincristine, glutethimide, gold, hydralazine, and long-term metronidazole.

PREGNANCY: Category C. Teratogenic and embryolethal in doses >1000 x those used in patients; carcinogenicity studies – thymic lymphomas in rodents; placental passage in rhesus monkeys show newborn:maternal drug ratio of 0.3-0.5; no studies in humans. ddC is not generally recommended in pregnancy due to concerns about teratogenicity in animals and lack of safety data in patients.

ZERIT – see Stavudine (p. 295)

ZIAGEN – see Abacavir (p. 137)

ZIDOVUDINE (AZT, ZDV)

TRADE NAME: *Retrovir, Combivir* (AZT/3TC), *Trizivir* (AZT/3TC/ABC) (GlaxoSmithKline)

CLASS: Nucleoside analog

FORMULATIONS, REGIMENS AND PRICE
- **Forms**
  - AZT – 100 and 300 mg tabs; 10 mg/mL IV solution; 10 mg/mL oral solution.
  - AZT/3TC – 300/150 mg tabs (*Combivir*)
  - AZT/3TC/ABC – 300/150/300 mg tabs (*Trizivir*)
- **Regimens:** AZT – 300 mg bid or 200 mg tid; AZT/3TC or AZT/3TC/ABC – 1 tab bid.
- **AWP:** AZT, $350/month; AZT/3TC, $640/month; AZT/3TC/ABC, $1020/month. Generic AZT is now available at $0.50/300 mg tab (Roxane) or $30/mo.

Drugs: Zidovudine

5

- **Food:** No effect
- **Renal failure:** CrCl >15 – 100 mg tid. AZT/3TC (*Combivir*) and AZT/3TC/ABC (*Trizivir*): not recommended with CrCl <50 mL/min
- **Hepatic failure:** AZT, *Combivir, Trizivir* – standard dose; *Trivizir* contraindicated
- **ACTG 076 protocol:** Intrapartum regimen is 2 mg/kg IV over 1 h, then 1 mg/kg/h until delivery.

PATIENT ASSISTANCE PROGRAM: 800-722-9294

CLINICAL TRIALS: FDA-approved in 1987 based on a controlled clinical trial showing significant short-term benefit in preventing AIDS-defining opportunistic infections and death (*N Engl J Med* 1987;317:185). Early studies (ACTG 019, 076, 175, Concord, etc.) became sentinel reports. Despite 15 years of use, resistance in recently transmitted strains is only about 2% (*N Engl J Med* 2002;347:385). AZT is commonly paired with 3TC (*Combivir*), or ABC/3TC (*Trizivir*) as the nucleoside components of HAART regimens. Potency of these regimens is well established. ACTG 384 showed that AZT/3TC/EFV was superior to ddI/d4T/EFV, but this difference was not observed when nucleoside pairs were combined with NFV (*N Engl J Med* 2003;349:2293). In GS 934, the combination of TDF/FTC/EFV was superior to AZT/3TC/EFV at 48 wks by ITT analysis because of greater dropout due to adverse events, primarily anemia, in the AZT/3TC arm (3d IAS, 2005, Abstr. WeOa 0202).

RESISTANCE: The thymidine analog mutations (TAMs) are 41L, 67N, 70R, 210W, 215Y/F, and 219Q/E. A total of 3 to 6 mutations result in a 100-fold decrease in sensitivity. About 5% to 10% of recipients of AZT + ddI as dual nucleoside therapy develop the Q151M complex, and a larger number have the T69S insertion mutation, both of which confer high-level resistance to AZT, ddI, ddC, d4T, 3TC and ABC. The M184V mutation that confers high-level 3TC resistance delays resistance or improves susceptibility to AZT unless there are multiple TAMs. It may also prevent the emergence of multinucleoside mutations, which are now very uncommon. Analysis of patients with early HIV infection indicates that 2% to 10% have genotypic mutations associated with reduced susceptibility to AZT (*N Engl J Med* 2002;347:385).

PHARMACOLOGY

- **Bioavailability:** 60%; high-fat meals may decrease absorption. CSF levels: 60% serum levels (CSF:plasma ratio=0.3-1.35) (*Lancet* 1998;351:1547).
- **T½:** 1.1 hours; Renal failure: 1.4 hours; intracellular: 3 hours
- **Elimination:** Metabolized by liver to glucuronide (GAZT) that is renally excreted.
- **Dose modification in renal failure or hepatic failure:** Excreted in urine as active drug (14% to 18%) and GAZT metabolite (60% to

Drugs: Zidovudine

74%). In severe renal failure (CrCl <18 mL/min), AZT half-life is increased from 1.1 to 1.4 hours and GAZT half-life increased from 0.9 to 8.0 hours. Dosing recommendation: GFR >10 mL/min – 300 mg bid; GFR <10 mL/mm – 300 mg/day; hemodialysis and peritoneal dialysis – 300 mg/day. No dose modification with liver disease.

SIDE EFFECTS

- **Subjective:** GI intolerance, altered taste (dysgeusia), insomnia, myalgias, asthenia, malaise, and/or headaches are common and are dose related (*Ann Intern Med* 1993;118:913). Most patients can be managed with symptomatic treatment.

- **Marrow suppression:** Related to marrow reserve, dose and duration of treatment, and stage of disease. Anemia may occur within 4 to 6 weeks, and neutropenia is usually seen after 12 to 24 weeks. Marrow examination in patients with AZT-induced anemia may be normal or show reduced RBC precursors. Severe anemia should be managed by discontinuing AZT or giving erythropoietin concurrently (see pp. 360 and 214). With neutropenia, an ANC <750/mm³ should be managed by discontinuing AZT or giving G-CSF concurrently (see p. 232).

- **Myopathy:** Rare dose-related complication possibly due to mitochondrial toxicity. Clinical features are leg and gluteal muscle weakness, elevated LDH and CPK, muscle biopsy showing ragged red fibers, and abnormal mitochondria (*N Engl J Med* 1990;322: 1098); response to discontinuation of AZT occurs within 2 to 4 weeks.

- **Macrocytosis:** Noted within 4 weeks of starting AZT in virtually all patients and serves as crude indicator of adherence.

- **Hepatitis** with reversible increases in transaminase levels, sometimes within 2 to 3 weeks of starting treatment.

- **Class adverse reaction:** Lactic acidosis, often with steatosis, is a complication ascribed to all nucleoside analogs but primarily to d4T and ddC, and to a lesser degree, ddI and AZT. This complication should be considered in patients with fatigue, abdominal pain, nausea, vomiting, and dyspnea. Laboratory tests show elevated serum lactate, CPK, ALT and/or LDH, and reduced serum bicarbonate ± increased anion gap. Abdominal CT scan or liver biopsy may show steatosis. This is a life-threatening complication. Pregnant women and obese women appear to be at increased risk. NRTIs should be stopped or there should be a change to NRTIs that are unlikely to cause mitochondrial toxicity such as TDF, ABC. Lipoatrophy, also most commonly associated with d4T or d4T + ddI, also occurs with AZT therapy. In ACTG 384, lipoatrophy was observed in both the ddI + d4T and AZT + 3TC arms, but its onset was slower in the AZT + 3TC-treated patients.

- **Fingernail discoloration** with dark bluish discoloration at base of nail noted at 2 to 6 weeks.

Drugs: Zidovudine

5

- **Carcinogenicity:** Long-term treatment with high doses in mice caused vaginal neoplasms; relevance to humans is not known.

DRUG INTERACTIONS: Use with caution with ribavirin. Additive or synergistic against HIV with ddI, ddC, ABC, alpha interferon, and foscarnet *in vitro*; antagonism with ganciclovir and d4T. AZT and d4T should not be given concurrently due to *in vitro* and *in vivo* evidence of antagonism. Clinical significance of interaction with ganciclovir is unknown. Methadone increases levels of AZT 30% to 40%; AZT has no effect on methadone levels (*J Acquir Immune Defic Syndr* 1998;18:435). Marrow suppression usually precludes concurrent use with ganciclovir. Other marrow-suppressing drugs should be used with caution: TMP-SMX, dapsone, pyrimethamine, flucytosine, interferon, adriamycin, vinblastine, sulfadiazine, vincristine, amphotericin B, and hydroxyurea. Probenecid increases levels of AZT, but concurrent use is complicated by a high incidence of rash reactions to probenecid.

PREGNANCY: Category C. Advocated for pregnant women beyond first trimester to prevent vertical transmission.

Positive in rodent teratogen assay at near-lethal doses. Studies in humans show newborn:maternal ratio of 0.85. Prolonged high doses to pregnant rodents were complicated by the development of squamous epithelial vaginal tumors in 3% to 12% of female offspring (*Fund Appl Toxicol* 1996;32:148). The relevance of these studies to humans is questioned because the dose used in rodents was 10 to 12x higher and AZT in humans is largely metabolized, whereas unmetabolized AZT is excreted in urine of mice. A report from France found evidence of mitochondrial toxicity with neurologic consequences in 12 infants exposed to AZT *in utero* (*Lancet* 1999;354:1084). Subsequent reviews of ACTG 076 infants and several other cohorts with data on 20,000 infants exposed to AZT failed to show any neurologic, immunologic, oncologic, or cardiac complications (*N Engl J Med* 2000;343:759; *N Engl J Med* 2000;343:805; *AIDS* 1998;12:1805; *JAMA* 1999;281:151; *J Acquir Immune Defic Syndr* 1999;20:464). An expert NIH panel reviewed these data in January 1997 and concluded that the risk of perinatal transmission exceeded the hypothetical concerns of transplacental carcinogenesis. Nevertheless, they advised that pregnant women be warned of this risk. The Pregnancy Registry now has enough reports to detect a 2-fold increase in birth defects. The prevalence with AZT was 2.8% compared to 3.1% in the general U.S. population. AZT is considered the preferred NRTI, usually with 3TC, in pregnancy based on the extensive data on safety, tolerance and efficacy.

Extensive study and experience have clearly documented the efficacy and safety of AZT for reducing perinatal transmission (*N Engl J Med* 1994;331:1173). This benefit is related to the reduction in maternal viral load (*N Engl J Med* 1996;335:1621) and to other factors that are less well understood. More recent studies show that rates of perinatal transmission are far lower with HAART than with AZT monotherapy (0% vs 8.8%) (*J Acquir Immune Defic Syndr* 2002;29:484). Current USPHS recommendations are for HAART if the maternal viral load is >1,000 c/mL or the CD4 count is <350/mm³, and consideration of AZT monotherapy if the CD4 cell count is >350/mm³ and the viral load is <1000 c/mL. AZT/3TC is the preferred NRTI backbone for HAART in pregnant women (DHHS Guidelines, April 7, 2005, p. 100).

ZITHROMAX – see Azithromycin (p. 158)

ZOVIRAX – see Acyclovir (p. 141)

Drugs

6 | Management of Infections
(Pathogens are listed alphabetically)

Recommendations are based largely on Benson C., et al., U.S. Public Health Service (USPHS) – Infectious Disease Society of America (IDSA) Guidelines for the Treatment of Opportunistic Infections in Adults and Adolescents Infected with the Human Immunodeficiency Virus, *MMWR* 53(RR15):1 (December 17, 2004), available online at http://www.cdc.gov/mmwr/preview/mmwrhtml/rr5315a1.htm.

Aspergillus sp. (Aspergillosis)
Invasive Pulmonary or Disseminated Infection

PRESENTATION: Two recognized clinical forms in AIDS patients: (1) **Pulmonary** – invasive pseudomembranous tracheitis or pneumonia that presents with cough, fever, dyspnea, wheezing or stridor. With tracheitis, bronchoscopy shows exudative pseudomembrane. With pneumonitis there is a diffuse pulmonary infiltrate or a wedge-shaped pulmonary infection, usually at the pleural base. (2) **Febrile, diffuse meningoencephalitis** – risk factors include CD4 count <50/mm^3, neutropenia, corticosteroid use, and broad spectrum antibiotic exposure. Common features include vessel invasion with infarction in the lung or brain. Diagnostic criteria from the National Mycosis Study Group are as follows: Definite = positive histology + positive culture, or positive culture from a normally sterile site. Probable = two positive cultures of sputum or one positive bronchoscopy + appropriate host (AIDS, prednisone, ANC <500) (*Clin Infect Dis* 2001;33:1824). Halo sign on CT scan is highly suggestive (*Lancet* 2000;355:423).

TREATMENT

- **Preferred regimen:** (invasive disease) Voriconazole, 6 mg/kg IV q12h x 2, then 4 mg/kg IV q12h ≥1 week, then 200 mg bid (*N Engl J Med* 2002;347:408). (See comment for voriconazole + RFV or EFV.)

  Note: CDC/IDSA guidelines favor amphotericin B for invasive aspergillosis in AIDS patients because voriconazole has not been studied in that setting (*MMWR 2004*;55RR-15, p 36).

- **Alternative regimens**
  - Amphotericin B 1.0 mg/kg/day or lipid formulation of amphotericin: *Amphotec, Abelcet,* or *AmBisome.* Doses of 5.0 mg/kg have been used (*Antimicrob Agents Chemother* 2001;45:3487).
  - Voriconazole (above doses) plus caspofungin 70 mg IV day 1, then 50 mg IV qd (*Lancet* 2002;359:1135).

6 Management of Infections

□ Voriconazole AUC ↓ 80% by EFV or RTV (400 mg bid): Monitor closely, or use higher dose voriconazole, or add AmBisome or caspofungin.

- **Comments**

  □ Randomized trial in 277 patients with invasive *Aspergillus* demonstrated that voriconazole was significantly better than amphotericin (1-1.5 mg/kg/day) in rates of response and survival (*N Engl J Med* 2002;347:408).

  □ Promising investigational azoles include posaconazole + ravuconazole (*Clin Microbiol Rev* 1999;12:40).

  □ There is no evidence that combination therapy is more effective (*Lancet* 2002;359:1135).

  □ *In vitro* sensitivity tests have not been standardized for *Aspergillus* (*J Antimicrob Chemother* 2001;47:333).

  □ Predisposing factors: Corticosteroids: Reduce dose or discontinue; neutropenia: G-CSF and avoid 5-FC + AZT, avoid marijuana.

RESPONSE: Prognosis with invasive pulmonary disease is poor without immune reconstitution (*Clin Infect Dis* 1992;14:141; *Clin Microbiol Rev* 1999;12:310). A report of 277 patients without HIV infection demonstrated a good response in 52% given voriconazole and 20% given amphotericin B (*N Engl J Med* 2002;347:408). Median survival in a review of 110 cases in patients with AIDS was 3 months (*Clin Infect Dis* 2000;31:1253). A review of 33 reported cases of CNS aspergillosis in AIDS patients showed all were fatal; amphotericin was uniformly unsuccessful (*Medicine* 2000;79:269).

Bartonella henselae and *quintana*
Bacillary Angiomatosis, Trench Fever and Peliosis Hepatitis

PRESENTATION: *B. henselae* and *B. quintana* cause bartonellosis, which may involve every organ. Most common is bacillary angiomatosis with red papular skin lesions that resemble Kaposi sarcoma in patients with a CD4 count <50/mm^3. Less common are lytic bone lesions, peliosis hepatitis, endocarditis and bacteremia presenting as FUO typically in homeless persons with low CD4 counts (*Clin Infect Dis* 2003;37:559). Diagnosis is established with tissue histology using silver stain to detect *Bartonella*. Serology is available from the CDC (*Clin Infect Dis* 2003;37:559; *Lancet* 1992;339:1443) and PCR is available for experimental use. The organism is hard to grow but can be recovered from blood with lysis centrifugation and incubation for >3 weeks (*Clin Infect Dis* 2003;37:559; *N Engl J Med* 1992;327:1625).

TREATMENT

- **Preferred regimen (oral, skin involvement):** Erythromycin 500 mg PO or IV qid or doxycycline 100 mg PO or IV x >3 months

- **Alternative:** Azithromycin 600 mg qd or clarithromycin 500 mg bid

- **IV therapy (bone, parenchymal tissue, endocarditis, or neurologic syndrome):** Erythromycin, doxycycline, or azithromycin (± rifampin or rifabutin)
- **CNS infection:** Doxycycline 100 mg IV bid
- **Comments**
  - Prevention: Macrolide for MAC prophylaxis is protective.
  - Duration: Patients who relapse should be treated with life-long therapy.
  - *In vitro* sensitivity does not predict response. Lesions develop in presence of TMP-SMX, betalactams, fluoroquinolones.

RESPONSE: The role of antibiotic therapy is often unclear, but it is usually recommended for the immunosuppressed host and for parenchymal involvement or bacteremia. Treatment rapidly reduces microbial load. Clinical response is slow and relapse is common.

Candida spp.
Thrush (Oral Candidiasia)

PRESENTATION: Most common is pseudomenbraneous candidiasis with white painless plaques on the buccal or pharyngeal mucosa or tongue surface that can easily be scraped off plus a risk factor: CD4 <250 cells/mm³, antibiotics, chronic steroids, etc. If lab confirmation is necessary, use KOH prep. Culture is best used for speciation and sensitivity testing (*Medicine* 2003:82:39) but not for diagnosis due to high rates of colonization.

TREATMENT: INITIAL INFECTION
- **Preferred regimen**
  - Clotrimazole oral troches 10 mg 5x/day *(HIV Clin Trials* 2000;1:47) until lesions resolve, usually 7-14 days.
  - Nystatin 500,000 units (4-6 mL) gargled 4-5x day or 1 to 2 flavored pastilles 4-5x/day x 7-14 days.
  - Fluconazole 100 mg/day PO x 7-14 days.
- **Alternative regimens for refractory infections**
  - Itraconazole 200 mg/day oral suspension swished and swallowed, empty stomach.
  - Amphotericin B oral suspension 1-5 mL qid swish and swallow. No longer available commercially but can be prepared by pharmacist with 100 mg/mL. (Note: Standard recommendation is 1 mL dose, but patients cannot easily gargle 1 mL.)
  - Amphotericin B IV 0.3 mg/kg/day.

6 Management of Infections

- **Comments**
  - ◻ Tolerability: Nystatin has a bitter taste, many GI side effects, must be taken 4x to 5x daily and is significantly less effective than fluconazole for rates of response and relapse. Clotrimazole is easier to take and more effective (*HIV Clin Trials* 2000;1:47).
  - ◻ Fluconazole is preferred over itraconazole and ketoconazole due to more predictable absorption (*HIV Clin Trials* 2000;1:47; *Am J Med* 1998;104:33).
  - ◻ *In vitro* azole resistance is most common with prolonged prior azole exposure and late-stage HIV infection with CD4 count <50 cells/mm^3 (*Clin Infect Dis* 2000;30:749). Definition of *in vitro* resistance is often arbitrary (*Lancet* 2002;359:1135). Molecular typing shows a single strain of *C. albicans* that becomes progressively more resistant (*Eur J Clin Microbiol Infect Dis* 1997;16:601) and/or high rates of non-*albicans* species (*Lancet* 2002;359:1135; *HIV Clin Trials* 2000;1:47, *Clin Rev Microbiol* 2000;26:59). Some report high rates of response (48/50) to fluconazole despite *in vitro* resistance (*J Infect Dis* 1996;174:821).

RESPONSE: Most respond within 7-14 days, except with extensive prior azole exposure and CD4 count <50/mm^3 (*Clin Infect Dis* 2000;30:749; *Clin Infect Dis* 1997;24:28). Failure of fluconazole: 1) Use empiric treatment (see above) or 2) Culture to determine *in vitro* sensitivity; empiric therapy with itraconazole solution is favored by CDC/IDSA guidelines. Relapses within 3 months after treatment are common and require intermittent therapy, maintenance therapy, or immune reconstitution.

MAINTENANCE (Not generally recommended)

- **Preferred regimens**
  - ◻ Topical clotrimazole or nystatin prn.
  - ◻ Fluconazole 100 mg/day PO or 200 mg 3x week.
  - ◻ Itraconazole solution 100-200 mg/day on empty stomach.
- **Comments**
  - ◻ Immune reconstitution is highly effective (*AIDS* 2000;14:979).
  - ◻ Itraconazole and ketoconazole are considered second-line drugs due to variable absorption.
  - ◻ Problems with use of continuous or intermittent fluconazole include azole resistance, drug interactions, and cost. Risks for azole resistant *Candida* infections are prolonged azole exposure, use of TMP/SMX prophylaxis for PCP, and low CD4 cell count (*J Infect Dis* 1996;173:219). Most authorities try to avoid continued use of fluconazole except where necessary, such as in cases of cryptococcal meningitis (*Clin Infect Dis* 2000;30:749), recurrent

esophagitis, or severe and refractory oropharyngeal candidiasis (*J Infect Dis* 1998;27:1291).

Esophagitis

PRESENTATION: Main symptoms are diffuse retrosternal pain, dysphagia, and odynophagia, usually without fever. Thrush is usually noted and the CD4 count is <100/mm^3. Cases with typical features are usually treated empirically; rapid response to standard treatment strongly supports this diagnosis.

TREATMENT: INITIAL INFECTION

- **Preferred regimen:** Fluconazole 100-400 mg/day PO or IV x 14-21 days.
  - □ Itraconazole solution 200 mg PO x 14-21 days.
- **Alternative regimens**
  - □ Amphotericin B IV 0.3-0.7 mg/kg/day.
  - □ Amphotericin lipid formulations: 3 to 5 mg/kg/day.
  - □ Caspofungin IV 70 mg day 1, then 50 mg/day.
  - □ Voriconazole 200 mg PO bid or 6 mg/kg IV q 12 h x2, then 4 mg/kg IV q 12 h.
- **Comments**
  - □ Fluconazole is preferred over ketoconazole and itraconazole due to more predictable absorption. It is preferred over voriconazole and caspofungin due to greater experience in HIV-infected persons.
  - □ Caspofungin was superior to amphotericin (0.5 mg/kg/day) in one comparative trial (*Antimicrob Agents Chemother* 2002;46:451) and comparable to fluconazole in another (*Clin Infect Dis* 2001;33: 1529).
  - □ Voriconazole 200 mg/day is equivalent to fluconazole (*Clin Infect Dis* 2001;33:1447).
  - □ Relapse rate within 1 year is high in absence of either immune reconstitution or maintenance therapy.
  - □ Resistance: See oropharyngeal candidiasis, below.

RESPONSE: Most (85-90%) patients respond within 7-14 days (*Clin Infect Dis* 2004;39:842). For refractory cases: 1) Perform endoscopy to establish diagnosis ± fungal culture for *in vitro* sensitivity tests, or 2) Change therapy: increase fluconazole dose, use alternative azole (voriconazole or itraconazole), or IV treatment (caspofungin, amphotericin or fluconazole). Fluconazole-resistant *Candida* esophagitis will often respond to itraconazole at least temporarily. Many patients relapse after therapy and require maintenance or immune reconstitution.

6 Management of Infections

MAINTENANCE: Only with relapsing disease

- **Preferred regimen:** Fluconazole 100-200 mg/day PO.

- **Comment:** Consider maintenance therapy in patients with recurrent esophagitis, although this increases the possibility of resistance (*J Infect Dis* 1996;173:219). Best treatment is immune reconstitution (*J Infect Dis* 1998;27:1291; *AIDS* 2000;14:23).

Vaginitis (*MMWR* 2002;51[RR-6]:45)

DIAGNOSIS: Typical symptoms are mucosal burning and pruritis combined with a creamy yellow-white discharge. Examination shows erythema and yellow-white adherent discharge; 10% KOH prep or gram stain show yeast or pseudohyphae. Most cases are in immunocompetent women. Culture is rarely necessary except to detect a non-*albicans* species (rare) or fluconazole resistance (also rare).

TREATMENT

- **Preferred Regimens: Intravaginal azoles, usually 3-7 days**
  - Butoconazole 2% cream 5 g/day x 3 days* or clotrimazole 1% cream 5 g/day x 7 to 14 days* 100 mg vaginal tab/day x 7 to 14 days, 100 mg vaginal tab bid x 3 days, 500 mg vaginal tab x 1.
  - Miconazole 2% cream 5 g/day x 7 days* 100 mg vaginal supp/day x 7 days*, 200 mg supp/day x 3 days.*
  - Tionazole 6.5% ointment 5 g x 1*, 0.4% cream 5 g/day x 7 days, 0.8% cream 5 g/day x 3 days 80 mg supp/day x 3 days.
  - Nystatin 100,000 units/day x 14 days

  * Available over-the-counter

- **Preferred systemic azoles**
  - Fluconazole 150 mg PO x 1.
  - Itraconazole 200 mg PO bid or 200 mg qd x 3 days

- **Comments**
  - Treatment is identical for women with and without HIV infection.
  - Clotrimazole, tioconazole and miconazole are available over the counter. Self administration advised only if prior diagnosis and typical symptoms.
  - Azole-resistant strains of *Candida* are rare causes of vaginitis.
  - Severe disease: Topical azole x 7 to 14 days or oral fluconazole 150 mg PO x 2 separated by 72 hours.
  - Pregnancy: Topical azole only.

Management of Infections

334

RESPONSE: Uncomplicated vaginitis (90% of all cases) responds rapidly. Complicated cases are prolonged or refractory, account for 10% of cases and are treated for >7 days.

MAINTENANCE (with ≥4 episodes/year): Clotrimazole 500 mg supply every week, or fluconazole 100-150 mg PO every week or ketoconazole 200 mg PO every week or itraconazole 400 mg every month or 100 mg every week, all x 6 months. (Based on recommendations for women without HIV infection.)

Coccidioides immitis

Coccidioidomycosis (*Clin Infect Dis* 2005;41:1174)

DIAGNOSIS: The usual presentation is disseminated disease (90%) or meningitis (10%), most commonly in patients with a CD4 count <250/mm^3. Clinical features of disseminated disease include fever, generalized adenopathy, skin nodules or ulcers, hepatitis, bone/joint lesions, or peritonitis. The diagnosis is established by 1) positive culture from any clinical specimens; 2) histopathology of tissues showing typical spherules; and 3) positive *C. immitis* complement fixation (CF) serology; titer >1:16 indicates disseminated disease. With meningitis the usual presentation is fever, lethargy, headache, nausea, and vomiting. CSF shows a mononuclear pleocytosis, glucose <50 mg/dl, and protein that is normal or slightly elevated. The diagnosis is established by positive CF serology in CSF.

INITIAL TREATMENT

- **Preferred regimen**
  - □ Diffuse pulmonary or disseminated (non-meningeal): Amphotericin B 0.5-1 mg/kg/day IV until clinical improvement, usually 500 to 1000 mg total dose amphotericin.
  - □ Mild disease: Fluconazole 400-800 mg/day PO or itraconazole 200 mg capsule bid PO.
  - □ Meningitis: Fluconazole 400-800 mg/day IV or PO.

- **Comments**
  - □ Therapeutic trial of fluconazole 400 mg/day vs itraconazole 200 mg bid in 198 patients with non-meningeal cocci showed no significant difference, but the trend favored itraconazole (*Ann Intern Med* 2000;133:676).
  - □ Fluconazole is preferred for meningitis (*Ann Intern Med* 1993; 119:28).
  - □ Intrathecal amphotericin B should be added for coccidioidomycosis meningitis that fails to respond to fluconazole.
  - □ There is no reported experience with lipid amphotericin B. Dose recommendations are unknown.

6 Management of Infections

◻ Focal lesions often require debridement or drainage.

RESPONSE: Response is slow (weeks) and relapses are common. Options for non-response include increasing the fluconazole dose, alternative azole, amphotericin, and/or surgical debridement or drainage. Treatment is continued for life, even with immune reconstitution. Criteria have been recommended for stopping maintenance therapy.

MAINTENANCE

- **Preferred regimen:** Fluconazole 400 mg/day or itraconazole 200-400 mg PO bid.

- **Comments:** Fluconazole is preferred due to better absorption and fewer drug interactions (*Antimicrob Agents Chemother* 1995; 39:1907).

Cryptococcus neoformans
Cryptococcal Meningitis

PRESENTATION (NIAID Mycosis Study Group Recommendations, *Clin Infect Dis* 2000;30:710): The usual portal of entry is the lung, and many have pneumoniitis. The usual presentation is subacute meningitis with fever, headache and malaise in a patient with a CD4 count <100/mm³. Some patients are asymptomatic and many have non-meningeal sites of involvement, especially the skin, with vesicular or papular lesions that may resemble molluscum. CSF analysis should be performed whenever there is evidence of cryptococcal infection. The diagnosis of cryptococcal meningitis is usually easy, with positive blood cultures in 50 to 70%, positive serum cryptococcal antigen in >95%, positive CSF culture in >95%, positive CSF cryptococcal antigen in >95%, and positive India ink in 60% to 80%. CSF usually shows elevated opening pressure (>200 mm H_2O in 75%) increased protein (50-150 mg/dL) and mononuclear pleocytosis (5-100 mg/dL) (*N Engl J Med* 1992;329:83; *N Engl J Med* 1997;337:15).

TREATMENT

- **Preferred regimen:** Amphotericin B 0.7 mg/kg/day IV + 5-FC PO 100 mg/kg/day x 14 days ("induction phase"), then fluconazole 400 mg/day x 8 weeks or until CSF is sterile ("consolidation phase"), then maintenance therapy, fluconazole 200 mg/day ("suppressive phase"). See comments regarding management of elevated intracranial pressure.

- **Elevated intracranial pressure:** With focal neurologic signs or obtundation, obtain CNS imaging before LP to define lesions that contraindicate LP.

  ◻ Occasional patients have very high pressure (>400 mm H_2O) and may require a lumbar drain or a V-P shunt.

□ Elevated pressure persists: Lumbar drain or ventricular-peritoneal shunt.

- **Alternative regimens** (induction and consolidation stages)
  - □ Amphotericin B 0.7-1.0 mg/kg/day V (without 5-FC) x 14 days, then fluconazole 400 mg/day x 8 to 10 weeks.
  - □ Fluconazole 400-800 mg/day PO + 5-FC 100 mg/kg/day PO x 6 to 10 wks.
  - □ *AmBisome* 4 mg/kg/day IV x 14 days, then fluconazole 400 mg/day x 8 to 10 weeks.
  - □ Consolidation: Itraconazole 200 mg PO bid

- **Comments**
  - □ Repeat LP is indicated only to control elevated intracranial pressure or if there is failure to respond with new symptoms after 2 weeks of therapy.
  - □ Management of increased intracranial pressure is critical (*Clin Infect Dis* 2000;30:47). Increased intracranial pressure accounts for >90% of deaths in first 2 weeks and 40% of deaths in weeks 3-10 (*Clin Infect Dis* 2000;30:47).
  - □ Patients with renal failure receiving fluconazole should have fluconazole blood levels monitored; 2 h post-dose level should be <100 mg/mL.
  - □ Amphotericin B + flucytosine is superior to amphotericin B alone in preventing relapse but does not improve immediate outcome (*N Engl J Med* 1997;337:15; *Ann Intern Med* 1990;113:183). There may be no need for flucytosine in patients with anticipated response to HAART.
  - □ *Abelcet* (5 mg/kg) showed clinical response equivalent to amphotericin B but slower CSF sterilization in a small trial (*Clin Infect Dis* 1996;22:315).
  - □ Fluconazole + flucytosine is effective but toxic, possibly due to higher 5-FC doses used (*Clin Infect Dis* 1994;19:741; *Clin Infect Dis* 1998;26:1362).
  - □ Lipid amphotericin: Best data are for *AmBisome* at 4 mg/kg/day (*AIDS* 1997;11:1463).
  - □ Amphotericin B + flucytosine will sterilize CSF at 2 weeks in 60% to 90% (*N Engl J Med* 1987;317:334).
  - □ Serum cryptococcal antigen is not useful in following response to treatment; CSF antigen may be (*HIV Clin Trials* 2000;1:1).
  - □ Resistance: Amphotericin B resistance is rare or hard to demonstrate (*Antimicrob Agents Chemother* 1993;37:1383; *Clin Microbiol Rev* 2001;14:643; *Antimicrob Agents Chemother* 1999;43:1463). Resistance develops rapidly with flucytosine monotherapy (*Lancet* 2002;359:1135). Fluconazole resistance is

6 Management of Infections

rare (*Antimicrob Agents Chemother* 1999;43:1856; *Antimicrob Agents Chemother* 2001;45:420).

RESPONSE: The major early concern is elevated intracranial pressure, which can lead to cranial nerve deficits or herniation. Management of elevated intracranial pressure with lumbar drainage is critical *(Clin Infect Dis* 2000;30:47). Most deaths are associated with increased intracranial pressure (*Clin Infect Dis* 2000;30:47). CSF culture at 2 weeks is negative in 70% (*Clin Infect Dis* 2000;30:710). A repeat LP at 2 weeks is indicated if there are new symptoms or signs. Serum cryptococcal antigen is not useful in following response to treatment; CSF antigen may be (*HIV Clin Trials* 2000;1:1).

TREATMENT FAILURE: Treatment failure is defined as failure to achieve clinical response in 2 weeks. Recommendations are to (1) continue the same treatment, (2) use higher doses of fluconazole in combination with flucytosine, (3) use alternative drugs such as voriconazole. Serum antigen titers are not useful in the following course (*HIV Clin Trials* 2000;1:1). Immune reconstitution Syndrome must be excluded as a cause of an apparent failure (*J Infect Dis* 2005;51:165).

MAINTENANCE

- **Preferred regimen:** Fluconazole 200 mg/day PO.
- **Alternative regimens**
  - Amphotericin B 1.0 mg/kg/week or twice weekly for patients with multiple relapses on azoles.
  - Fluconazole: May increase maintenance dose to 400 mg/day.
  - Itraconazole 200 mg caps PO qd (for patients who failed fluconazole or could not tolerate it).
- **Comments**
  - Fluconazole maintenance (200 mg/day) is superior to amphotericin B maintenance (*N Engl J Med* 1992;326:793) and superior to itraconazole at a dosage of 200 mg/day PO (*Clin Infect Dis* 1999; 28:291).
  - Immune reconstitution: Discontinue treatment (secondary prophylaxis) when CD4 cell count is >100-200/mm³ per month for >6 months, initial therapy is completed, and patient is asymptomatic (*Clin Infect Dis* 2003;36:1329).

Pulmonary, Disseminated, or Antigenemia

DIAGNOSIS: Positive cultures of blood, urine, and/or respiratory secretions virtually always indicate cryptococcal disease and mandate lumbar puncture to exclude meningitis. Serum antigenemia suggests cryptococcosis, especially with titer >1:8; this test should be confirmed with positive culture.

TREATMENT

- **Preferred regimen:** Fluconazole 200-400 mg/day PO indefinitely unless immune reconstitution is achieved.

- **Alternative regimen:** Itraconazole 200 mg PO bid as caps with meal + acidic drink or 200 mg/day bid oral suspension on empty stomach indefinitely unless immune reconstitution is achieved.

- **Comments**
  - Goal of treatment is to prevent meningitis.
  - Refractory lung and bone lesions may require surgery.
  - Non-meningeal sites include lungs, skin, joints, eye, adrenal gland, GI tract, liver, pancreas, prostate, and urinary tract.
  - Antigenemia: Obtain chest x-ray, LP, urine and blood culture. If no focus identified and antigenemia at >1:8 confirmed, treat with fluconazole (*Clin Infect Dis* 1996;23:827).

MAINTENANCE (Need for maintenance therapy with non-meningeal cryptococcosis is not established.)

- **Preferred regimen:** Fluconazole 200 mg/day PO.

- **Alternative regimens:** Itraconazole 200 mg/day as caps with meal + acidic drink or 100-200 mg/day oral suspension on empty stomach or amphotericin B 0.6-1 mg/kg IV weekly or twice/week.

Cryptosporidia parvum

Cryptosporidiosis (See *Clin Microbiol Rev* 1999;12:554; *Clin Infect Dis* 2001;32:331; *N Engl J Med* 2002;346:1723)

PRESENTATION: Typical symptoms are acute, subacute or chronic profuse watery diarrhea often associated with cramps, nausea and vomiting; about one-third have fever (*Ann Intern Med* 1996;124:429; *Clin Infect Dis* 2003;36:903). Stool assays with acid fast stain, IFA or EIA are sensitive, specific, and nearly equal in diagnostic utility with watery stools (*N Engl J Med* 2002;346:1723). IFA is preferred for formed stool. A single specimen is adequate with severe diarrhea. Repeat sampling is recommended for less severe disease. Patterns of disease with AIDS: 1) asymptomatic carriage (4%); 2) self-limited diarrhea <2 months (29%); 3) chronic diarrhea >2 months (60%); 4) fulminant diarrhea with >2 k/day (8%) (*N Engl J Med* 2002;346:1723). The chronic and fulminant form are seen almost exclusively with CD4 counts <100 cells/mm^3.

TREATMENT

- **Preferred regimens**
  - HAART with immune reconstitution is the only treatment that controls persistent cryptosporidiosis. Resolution usually occurs with CD4 >100/mm^3 and may improve with only minor increases.

Management of Infections

6

- Symptomatic treatment: Fluids (sports rehydration beverages such as *Gatorade*, bouillon, oral rehydration; see comments below), nutritional supplements and anti-diarrheal agents: *Lomotil*, loperamide, paregoric, bismuth subsalicylate (*Pepto-Bismol*), and deodorized tincture of opium.

- **Regimens that are infrequently effective**
  - Paromomycin 500 mg PO qid or 1000 mg PO bid with food x 14 to 28 days, then 500 mg PO bid.
  - Nitazoxanide (*Alinia* Unimed Pharmaceuticals, Buffalo Grove, Ill.) 500 mg PO bid (*Curr Opin Infect Dis* 2004;17:557)
  - Paromomycin 1 g bid + azithromycin 600 mg qd x 4 weeks, then paromomycin alone x 8 weeks.
  - Octreotide (*Sandostatin*) 50-500 µg tid SQ or IV at 1 µg/hour.
  - Azithromycin 1200 mg PO x 2 first day, then 1200 mg/day x 27 days, then 600 mg/day.
  - Atovaquone 750 mg PO suspension bid with meal.

- **Comments**
  - Antimicrobials: Over 95 drugs have been tried, and none is consistently successful. (*N Engl J Med* 2002;346:1723; *J Infect Dis* 2001;184:103; *Clin Infect Dis* 2000;31:1084; *Lancet* 2002;360:1375). This includes paromomycin, azithromycin, and nitazoxanide. One randomized trial of paromomycin (a nonabsorbable aminoglycoside) showed a modest but statistically significant improvement in symptoms and oocyte shedding (*Clin Infect Dis* 2000;31:1084); another randomized trial showed no benefit (*J Infect Dis* 1995;170:419).
  - Oral rehydration (severe diarrhea): NaCl 3.5 g (3/4 tsp), $NaHCO_3$ 2.5 g (1 tsp baking soda), KCl 1.5 g (1 cup orange juice or bananas) in 1 liter water. Packets of pre-mixed salts available from Cera Products (888-237-2598) and Jianas Brothers (816-421-2880).
  - Nitazoxanide is FDA-approved for cryptosporidiosis in immunocompetent children. Usual adult dose regimen is 500 mg q 6-12 h or 1 gm bid.
  - Clarithromycin or rifabutin prophylaxis for MAC prophylaxis may reduce risk of cryptosporidiosis (*JAMA* 1998;279:384).

RESPONSE: Cryptosporidiosis in patients with CD4 count >100 cells/mm^3 usually resolves spontaneously after 2 to 8 weeks, as it does with immunocompetent hosts. For AIDS patients with fulminant or chronic, persistent cryptosporidiosis, the goal is immune reconstitution: even modest elevations in CD4 count may result in resolution of symptoms and pathogen elimination (*J Acquir Immune Defic Syndr* 1998;12:35; *J Acquir Immune Defic Syndr* 2000;25:124).

Cytomegalovirus (CMV)

CMV Retinitis

PRESENTATION: May be asymptomatic or present with floaters, field defects, scotomata or decreased acuity. CD4 count is usually <50/mm^3. Funduscopic exam shows perivascular yellow-white retinal infiltrates ± intraretinal hemorrhage ("cottage cheese and ketchup"). Blood cultures and antigen assays are often not helpful due to lack of specificity (*J Clin Microbiol* 2000;323:563), but blood cultures may be useful for *in vitro* sensitivity tests in reference labs for patients with relapses. The diagnosis is usually made by funduscopic exam by an experienced ophthalmologist. CMV PCR is often positive in vitreous and aqueous humor and is highly specific (*Ophthalmolgia* 2004;218: 43). The diagnosis is usually based on findings on funduscopic exam.

TREATMENT

- **Preferred regimens**
  - Vision threatening lesion: Intraocular ganciclovir implant (*Vitrasert*) every 6-8 months + valganciclovir 900 mg PO bid with food x 14-21 days, then 900 mg/day.
  - Peripheral lesions: Oral valganciclovir (above doses). Some would not treat small peripheral lesions if immune recovery is anticipated but risk of immune reconstitution uveitis.

- **Alternative regimens for peripheral lesions**
  - Ganciclovir 5 mg/kg IV q12 h x 14 to 21 days, then valganciclovir 900 mg PO qd
  - Foscarnet 60 mg/kg IV q8h or 90 mg/kg IV q12h x 14 to 21 days then 90-120 mg/kg IV q12h.
  - Ganciclovir 5 mg/kg IV bid x 14 to 21 days then 5 mg/kg/day IV.
  - Valganciclovir 900 mg PO bid x 21 days, then 900 mg/day.
  - Cidofovir 5 mg/kg IV x 2 weeks, then 5 mg/kg every other week (+ probenecid)

- **Comments**
  - Intraocular ganciclovir implant requires replacement every 6 to 8 months in absence of immune reconstitution.
  - Some would not treat small peripheral lesions if immune recovery is anticipated, but risk of immune reconstitution uveitis may be greater in absence of anti-CMV therapy (*Arch Ophthalmol* 2003;121:466; *J Infect Dis* 1999;179:179; *Am J Ophthalmol* 2000;130:49).
  - Valganciclovir is a prodrug of ganciclovir and provides serum levels comparable with IV ganciclovir in standard doses (*N Engl J Med* 2002;346:1119).

6 Management of Infections

□ *Vitrasert* (intraocular ganciclovir release device) was superior to IV ganciclovir in time to relapse (220 days vs 71 days), but there is increased risk of involvement of the other eye and increased risk of extraocular CMV disease without concomitant systemic anti-CMV therapy (*N Engl J Med* 1997;337:83). Thus, local therapy should be accompanied by systemic anti-CMV therapy such as valganciclovir.

PROGRESSION OR RELAPSE

- **Preferred regimens**

  □ Intraocular ganciclovir implant if not used previously, even with relapse on ganciclovir, since intraocular levels are high with implant, plus systemic treatment with ganciclovir, foscarnet, cidofovir or valganciclovir, with drug selection based on anticipated or measured CMV resistance.

  □ Induction dose of the same agent (ganciclovir 10 mg/kg/day, foscarnet 180-240 mg/kg/day, or valganciclovir 900 mg bid). Switching to alternative drug for first relapse is generally not advocated unless resistance is suspected (see below) or toxicity is the reason.

  □ Late relapse: switch to alternative agent (see below).

  □ Fomivirsen, 330 mg by intravitreal injection day 1 and 15, then monthly.

- **Comments**

  □ Relapse is expected in the absence of immune recovery.

  □ Early relapse (<3 months) is usually not due to drug resistant CMV; late relapse (>6 months) usually is.

  □ Resistance rates are similar for ganciclovir, foscarnet, and cidofovir. For ganciclovir it is <10% at 3 months and 25% to 30% at 9 months (*J Infect Dis* 1998;177:770; *Antimicrob Agents Chemother* 1998;42:2240; *J Infect Dis* 1991;163:716; *J Infect Dis* 2001;183:333; *Am J Ophthalmol* 2001;132:700; *Antimicrob Agents Chemother* 2005;49:873). Low-level ganciclovir resistance is due to CMV UL97 phosphotransferase gene, high level resistance is due to UL97 and UL54 DNA polymerase genes. High-level resistance shows cross-resistance to cidofovir and sometimes foscarnet (*J Infect Dis* 2001;183:333; *J Infect Dis* 2000;182:1765). Low-level resistance may be overcome with the ganciclovir implant; high-level resistance requires use of an alternative regimen.

  □ Monitoring CMV (*AIDS* 1998;12:615). Sequencing the CMV gene for UL97 mutations also predicts resistance (*J Clin Infect* 1995;95:257).

□ Time to relapse varies with definition, use of retinal photographs, and treatments summarized above. Subsequent relapses occur more rapidly.

RESPONSE: Goals of therapy are to prevent further vision loss with anti-CMV drugs and to control disease control with immune reconstitution using HAART. Vision loss prior to therapy is typically irreversible. Evaluation of response is by ophthalmological examination. Most patients stabilize, but most eventually relapse unless there is immune recovery. Early relapse (<3 months) is usually not associated with ganciclovir resistance; relapse at >6 months usually is. Resistance testing on blood isolates of CMV performed using by CMV DNA PCR with sequencing for CMV UL97 mutations or a point mutation assay (*Am J Ophthalmol* 2002;133:467; *J Clin Invest* 1995;95:257). Relapse after immune recovery is ascribed to lack of CMV specific CD4 cell response and is rare (*J Infect Dis* 2001;183:1285).

MAINTENANCE
- **Preferred regimens**
  - □ Valganciclovir 900 mg/day PO.
  - □ Intraocular ganciclovir implant every 6 months + oral valganciclovir 900 mg/day.
- **Alternative regimens**
  - □ Foscarnet 90-120 mg/kg/day IV.
  - □ Cidofovir 5 mg/kg IV every other week.
- **Immune reconstitution:** Discontinue maintenance therapy when the CD4 cell count is >100-150/mm^3 for ≥6 months, there is no evidence of active disease, and there will be regular ophthalmologic exams. Restart prophylaxis when CD4 count is <50-100 cells/mm^3. Relapses occur when the CD4 count decreases to <50 cells/mm^3 (*AIDS* 2000;14:173). Safety of these recommendations has been shown (*AIDS* 2001;15:23), but rare patients have relapses with CD4 counts >100 cells/mm^3 x 3 months due to lack of CMV-specific immunity (*J Infect Dis* 2001;183:1285).

IMMUNE RECOVERY VITRITIS
- Clinical features: Inflammation in the anterior chamber and/or vitreous, usually at 4 to 12 weeks after initiating HAART (*Arch Ophthalmol* 2003;121:466; *Am J Ophthalmol* 2000;129:634). Incidence is highly variable, from 0.11/person-years to 0.86/person-years (*Am J Ophthalmol* 2000;129:634; *J Infect Dis* 1999;179:697). Lower rate may be due to better CMV suppression before HAART started. CMV PCR on aqueous humor and vitreous is usually negative (*Ophthalmalgia* 2004;218:43).

Management of Infections

6

- **Preferred regimen:** Systemic or periocular corticosteroids. About 50% respond.

CMV Extraocular Disease – Gastrointestinal (Usually esophagitis or colitis)

DIAGNOSIS: CMV esophagitis is characterized by fever, odynophagia ± retrosternal pain that is often well localized in patients with a CD4 count <50/mm³. The diagnosis is established by endoscopic visualization of shallow ulcers in the distal esophagus and biopsies showing characteristic intranuclear and intracytoplasmic inclusions. CMV colitis is characterized by fever, abdominal pain, weight loss and diarrhea in patients with a CD4 count <50/mm³. Major complications include hemorrhage or perforation. The diagnosis is established by endoscopic evidence of mucosal ulcers and biopsies showing typical intranuclear and intracytoplasmic inclusions.

TREATMENT

- **Preferred regimens**
  - Valganciclovir 900 mg PO bid with food x 3 to 4 weeks (if symptoms do not interfere with oral meds).
  - Ganciclovir 5 mg/kg IV bid x 3 to 4 weeks.
  - Foscarnet 60 mg/kg q8h or 90 mg/kg IV q12h x 3 to 4 weeks.
  - Indication for maintenance therapy: Relapse on or after therapy.

- **Comments**
  - All patients with symptomatic CMV esophagitis should be treated; indications to treat CMV colitis are less clear due to poor response.
  - Ganciclovir and foscarnet are equally effective for CMV colitis (*Am J Gastroenterol* 1993;88:542).
  - Duration of treatment is usually 21-28 days or until signs and symptoms have cleared.
  - Valganciclovir provides ganciclovir serum levels comparable with IV ganciclovir and is generally preferred in patients who can swallow.
  - Patients should have ophthalmoscopic screening.

RESPONSE: CMV esophagitis usually responds within 1 to 2 weeks with decrease in fever and odynophagia. Patients with colitis respond poorly – abdominal pain and diarrhea may not improve or may improve only modestly; viral shedding is markedly reduced.

CMV Neurological Disease

DIAGNOSIS: CMV neurologic disease includes dementia, ventriculo-encephalitis and ascending polyradiculomyelopathy. *Dementia* presents with: 1) lethargy, confusion and fever and 2) CSF with mononuclear cells and elevated protein. Patients with *polyradiculomyelopathy* present with: 1) progressive leg paresis, then bladder and bowel dysfunction; 2) CSF shows polymorphonuclear cells and increased protein. *Encephalitis* presents with (1) rapidly progressing delirium, cranial nerve defects, ataxia and nystagmus; (2) CSF with increased protein and a mononuclear pleocytosis; (3) MRI showing periventricular enhancement. The diagnosis of CMV CNS disease is established by a compatible clinical syndrome plus detection of CMV, usually by PCR, in CSF or brain. The sensitivity of CSF PCR is 80% with specificity of 90% (*Clin Infect Dis* 2002;34:103). Brain biopsy with histopathology or culture is diagnostic. With radiculomyelopathy CSF shows PMNs.

TREATMENT

- **Preferred regimen**
  - Ganciclovir 5 mg/kg IV bid x 3 to 6 weeks + foscarnet 90 mg/kg IV bid x 3 to 6 weeks, then maintenance with ganciclovir/valganciclovir + foscarnet.
  - Immune reconstitution is most important.
- **Alternative regimen:** Ganciclovir 5 mg/kg IV bid x 3 to 6 weeks, then maintenance with ganciclovir IV or valganciclovir PO.
- **Comments**
  - Ganciclovir + foscarnet is probably optimal, but tolerability is poor, and response is limited. In one report of 36 patients treated with this combination, the median survival was 3 months (*AIDS* 2000;14:517). This combination is associated with poor quality of life (*J Infect Dis* 1993;167:1184). The most important factor is immune reconstitution with HAART.
  - Cidofovir: There is minimal experience with neurologic disease.
  - Treatment does not significantly prolong survival, and irreversible damage is often present when treatment is started (*Neurology* 1996;46:444; *Clin Infect Dis* 2002;34:103).

RESPONSE

- CMV encephalitis: A trial of ganciclovir + foscarnet for CMV encephalitis showed a median survival of 94 days vs 42 days in historic controls (*AIDS* 2000;14:517).
- CMV polyradiculopathy: Improvement occurs within 2 to 3 weeks (*Neurology* 1993;43:493).
- Induction therapy may need to be continued for several months in severe cases (*Clin J Infect Dis* 1993;17:32). Maintenance therapy is lifelong. It is unclear if valganciclovir is adequate for induction.

6 Management of Infections

CMV Pneumonitis

DIAGNOSIS: Symptoms include fever, cough, dyspnea and interstitial infiltrates. Minimum diagnostic criteria include all of the following (*Clin Infect Dis* 1996;23:76): 1) pulmonary infiltrates; 2) characteristic intracellular inclusions in lung tissue; and 3) absence of another pulmonary pathogen.

INDICATIONS TO TREAT: CMV pneumonitis in patients with histologic evidence of CMV disease plus failure to respond to treatment of other pathogens.

TREATMENT: Ganciclovir 5 mg/kg IV bid > 21 days, foscarnet 60 mg/kg q8h or 90 mg/kg IV q12h >21 days, or valganciclovir 900 mg PO bid x 21 days.

- **Comments**
  - □ Response to ganciclovir is >60% (*Clin Infect Dis* 1996;23:76).
  - □ Indications are unclear for long-term maintenance therapy.

Entamoeba histolytica (*Clin Infect Dis* 2001;32:331)

DIAGNOSIS: Stool always shows blood with invasive disease; fecal leukocytes are usually not present. O&P examination x 3 has 85% to 95% sensitivity. Antigen assay with monoclonal antibody distinguishes pathogenic *E. histolytica* from *E. dispar*, which is non-pathogenic, more common, and looks the same on smear (*J Clin Microbiol* 1993; 31:2845).

TREATMENT

- **Preferred regimens:** Metronidazole 750 mg PO or IV tid x 5 to 10 days, plus diiodohydroxyquin 650 mg tid x 20 days or metronidazole plus paromomycin 500 mg tid x 7 days.
- **Alternative regimen:** Paromomycin 500 mg PO tid x 7 days.
- **Comments:** Pathogen distinction: *E. histolytica* is responsible for amebiasis – dysentery and liver abscesses. *E. dispar* accounts for over 90% of stool isolations; most laboratories do not use the serologic or stool EIA tests that distinguish between the two (*Clin Infect Dis* 2000;30:959; *Clin Infect Dis* 2000;30:955). Only *E. histolytica* causes disease and requires therapy.

RESPONSE: Cure rate with metronidazole x 10 days is 90%; second agent is given to assure elimination of intraluminal encysted organism.

Haemophilus influenzae

TREATMENT

- **Preferred regimen:** Cefuroxime.

- **Alternative regimens**
  - ▢ TMP-SMX.
  - ▢ Cephalosporins, 2nd and 3rd generation.
  - ▢ Fluoroquinolones.
- **Comments**
  - ▢ Standard therapy is usually adequate (*Clin Infect Dis* 2000;30:461).
  - ▢ *H. influenzae* vaccine is not recommended for adults because most infections involve non-encapsulated strains that are not covered by the vaccine.

Hepatitis viruses – see pp. 404-407

Herpes Simplex (*MMWR* 2002;51[RR-6]:13, *MMWR* 2004;53[RR-15]:21)

PRESENTATION: Orolabial and genital HSV are similar in presentation, diagnosis and management, except for anatomical site of infection. The usual presentation starts with a sensory prodrome at the involved site, followed by rapid evolution of lip/genital papule → vesicle → ulcer → crust. Lesions with advanced AIDS are more severe, more likely to disseminate, more likely to be refractory to therapy and more likely to have acyclovir-resistant HSV. The diagnosis is made on the basis of appearance. With atypical presentation or lesions that do not respond to therapy, the diagnosis can be confirmed by swabs of lesions submitted for viral culture, HSV antigen detection and/or Tzanck prep. The Tzanck prep show has a sensitivity of 60-80%; viral culture, DFA stains and viral PCR are more sensitive (*MMWR* 2002;51[RR-6]:13). Culture with sensitivity tests is necessary to detect resistance to acyclovir.

TREATMENT

- **Preferred regimen**
  - ▢ Orolabial herpes and initial or recurrent genital lesions: Acyclovir 400 mg PO tid x 7 to 10 days or famciclovir 500 mg PO bid x 7 to 10 days valacyclovir 2 gm PO bid x 1 day or valacyclovir 1 g PO bid x 7 to 10 days.
  - ▢ Severe disease: Acyclovir 5 mg/kg IV q8h until lesions regress, then use oral regimen above and continue until lesions heal.
  - ▢ Acyclovir-resistant HSV: Foscarnet 120-200 mg/d in 2-3 doses until resolution or cidofovir 5 mg IV weekly until clinical response, or topical treatment with trifluridine or cidofovir gel 1% applied once daily x 5 days (must be compounded by pharmacy). Note: Topical treatment to resolution often requires 3-4 weeks of treatment.
  - ▢ Genital, pregnancy: Herpetic lesions or prodrome symptoms at onset of labor is indication for cesarean section to prevent neonatal

herpes. Safety of acyclovir, famciclovir, and valacyclovir is not clearly established; the most experience is with acyclovir which appears safe and is preferred. Some advocate acyclovir for pregnancy with first episode, or severe recurrent HSV. Famciclovir exposures during pregnancy should be reported to 1-888-669-6682.

□ Severe disease with pneumonitis, esophagitis, disseminated infection, or hepatitis: Acyclovir 5-10 mg/kg IV q8h for 2 to 7 days or until improvement, then valacyclovir 1 g PO bid to complete ≥10 days, then oral treatment with famciclovir, acyciclovir or valacyciclovir.

□ Encephalitis: Acyclovir 10 mg/kg IV q8h x 14 to 21 days.

□ Herpes keratitis: Trifluridine, 1 drop q2h up to 9x/day for ≤21 days.

RESPONSE: Early treatment shortens duration of mucocutaneous lesions, reduces systemic symptoms, and reduces viral shedding (*Arch Int Med* 1996;156:1729); it does not change probability of recurrence (*Med Letter* 1995;37:117). With refractory disease plus HIV infection, suspect acyclovir resistance (*N Engl J Med* 1991;325:551). Acyclovir-resistant strains are resistant to famciclovir, valacyclovir and (usually) ganciclovir. Treatment options are topical cidofovir or IV foscarnet (*J Infect Dis* 1997;17:862, *N Engl J Med* 1993;327:968) or topical trifluridine (Viroptic 1%) (*J Acquir Immune Defic Syndr* 1996;12:147).

SUPPRESSION

- **Indication:** ≥6 recurrences/year; alternative is to treat each episode.
- **Suppressive regimens:** Acyclovir 400 mg bid, famciclovir 250 mg bid, or valacyclovir 0.5 or 1 g qd.
- **Comments**

  □ Acyclovir, famciclovir and valacyclovir are clinically equivalent (*Sex Transur Dis* 1997;24:481; *J Infect Dis* 1998;178:603; *JAMA* 2001; 144:818; *Br J Dermatol* 2001;144:188).

  □ Patient information services recommended by CDC: 800-227-8922, http://www.ashastd.org.

  □ Allergy to acyclovir is rare but will contraindicate famciclovir and valacyclovir. Desensitization has been described (*Ann Allergy* 1993;70:386).

  □ Acyclovir registry for exposure in first trimester of pregnancy does not indicate risk (*Am J Obstet Gynecol* 2000;182:159).

  □ Prophylactic acyclovir beginning at 36 weeks gestation reduces the risks of genital HSV recurrence at delivery. Cesarean section is indicated for active genital lesion at time of delivery (*Obstet Gynecol* 2003;102:1396).

  □ Control of HSV genital ulcers appears to be an important factor in reducing HIV transmission and HIV acquisition (*J Acquir Immune*

Defic Syndr 2004;35:435; *J Infect Dis* 2003;187:19; *J Infect Dis* 2003;187:1513).

- □ Suppressive therapy may decrease the rate of HIV progression (*J Infect Dis* 2002;186:1718).

Herpes Zoster

PRESENTATION: About 95% of healthy adults are seropositive for VZV and about 5% of healthy adults develop zoster. Risk factors are advanced age and immunosuppression. The risk with HIV infection is 15x to 25x greater and does not correlate with CD4 count (*J Acquir Immune Defic Syndr* 2005;38:111; *J Acquir Immune Defic Syndr* 2004;37:1604). The usual presentation is a painful prodrome in the region of a dermatone that then evolves within days to a characteristic dermatomal vesicular rash. The diagnosis is usually made on the basis of clinical presentation, but culture and/or DFA stain of a swab taken from a vesicle can be diagnostic; Tzanck prep is about 60% sensitive. PCR is experimental and probably most useful with CSF. Most cases include pain syndromes, often severe and sometimes requiring narcotics for pain relief. There are no residual defects except scars.

- ■ **Major complications:**
  - □ Progressive outer retinal necrosis is associated with rapid vision loss (*Ophthalmology* 1994;101:1488; *AIDS* 2002;16:1045). Most patients have CD4 counts <50/mm³, the disease is characterized by dermatomal zoster and multifocal retinal opacification. Immediate evaluation by an ophthalmologist and high-dose IV acyclovir plus foscarnet are required.
  - □ Acute retinal necrosis with peripheral necrotizing retinitis and vitritis and a high rate of vision loss is sometimes due to retinal detachment. This may be seen with any CD4 count.
  - □ Neurologic VZV syndromes seen rarely in AIDS patients include transverse myelitis, encephalitis and vasculitic stroke. Caution is necessary in the interpretation of CSF findings, since a mononuclear pleocytosis, with increased protein and positive VZV PCR, may also characterize uncomplicated shingles.

TREATMENT
- ■ **Preferred regimens**
  Dermatomal zoster (localized)
  - □ Famciclovir 500 mg PO tid or valacyclovir 1 g PO tid x 7 to 10 days.
  - □ Severe cutaneous or visceral disease: Acyclovir 10 mg/kg IV q 8 h followed by valacyclovir, 1 gm PO tid until all lesions are cleared.
  - □ Acute retinal necrosis: Acyclovir 10 mg/kg IV q 8 h followed by valacyclovir.

- Progressive outer retinal necrosis: Acyclovir 10 mg/kg IV q 8 h plus foscarnet 60 mg/kg IV q 8 h.
- Suspected resistance: Foscarnet IV 120-200 mg/kg/d.

Pain control

- Gabapentin, tricyclics, carbamazepine, lidocaine patch, narcotics (effective and underutilized).
- Chicken pox: IV acyclovir 30 mg/kg/day x 7 to 10 days until afebrile, then valacyciclovir 1 g tid or famciclovir 500 mg po tid.

- **Comments**
  - Some authorities recommend corticosteroids to prevent post-herpetic neuralgia (*Ann Intern Med* 1996;125:376), but this is not recommended in HIV infection.
  - Postherpetic neuralgia is uncommon in persons <55 years, including AIDS patients.
  - Foscarnet preferred for acyclovir-resistant cases (*N Engl J Med* 1993;308:1448).
  - Comparative trial of oral acyclovir vs valacyclovir showed slight advantage of valacyclovir (*Antimicrob Agents Chemother* 1995;39: 1546).

RESPONSE: Antiviral therapy of zoster reduces the duration of lesions, reduces the number of new lesions, and reduces systemic complaints, but the benefits are modest and largely limited to those receiving therapy within 24 hours of onset (*N Engl J Med* 1991;325:1539). For most patients the main concern is pain, and for older patients it is post-herpetic neuralgia.

PREVENTION

- **Indication:** Exposure to chickenpox or shingles plus no history of either and, if available, negative anti-varicella IgG. Preventive treatment must be initiated within 96 hours of exposure and preferably within 48 hours.
- **Preferred regimen:** Varicella zoster immune globulin (VZIG) 5 vials (6.25 mL) within 96 hours of exposure.
- **Alternative regimen:** Acyclovir 800 mg PO 5x/day x 3 weeks. Note: Acyclovir has been removed from the 1999 USPHS/IDSA guidelines for prophylaxis due to lack of documented efficacy.

Histoplasma capsulatum
Histoplasmosis, Disseminated

PRESENTATION: The usual presentation with disseminated disease is a CD4 count <150/mm³ plus multiorgan disease with constitutional symptoms including fever, weight loss and fatigue, often with lung, marrow, GI tract ± CNS involvement (*Medicine* 1990;69:361; *Clin Infect Dis* 2005;40:1122). Cultures of blood, respiratory tract secretions, marrow or focal infections are positive in 85% but take 2 to 4 weeks. The usual method to detect *H. capsulatum* is by stain of tissue or by detection of capsular polysaccharide in urine (sensitivity 90%) and blood (sensitivity 85%) (*Trends Microbiol* 2003;11:488). Relative sensitivities with disseminated disease reported by MiraVista Diagnostics are: antigen detection, 92%; culture, 86%; histopathology, 43%; serology, 71%. The antigen level falls with treatment and rises with relapse. The antigen assay is often positive in BAL fluid with pulmonary involvement and in CSF with meningitis (*Ann Intern Med* 1991;115:936). This test is available from Dr. Joe Wheat at 866-MIRAVISA, 317-856-2681, or http://www.miravistalabs.com.

INITIAL TREATMENT

- **Preferred regimens**
  - □ Severe, acute infection: Amphotericin B IV 0.7 mg/kg/day or *AmBisome* IV 4 mg/kg/day, 3 to 10 days.

    Continuation phase: Itraconazole 200 mg capsule PO bid x 12 weeks, then maintenance treatment with itraconazole 200 mg PO bid or fluconazole 800 mg PO qd.

  - □ Mild to moderate illness: Itraconazole, above doses for 12 weeks.
  - □ Meningitis: Amphotericin B or *AmBisome* 3 mg/kg/day x 12 to 16 weeks, then itraconazole capsule 200 mg qd.

- **Alternative regimen**
  - □ Itraconazole 400 mg IV/d
  - □ Acute infection: Itraconazole 400 mg IV/d
  - □ Mild disease: Fluconazole 800 mg PO/d (less effective than itraconazole)

- **Comments**
  - □ Severe disseminated disease is defined by one or more of: the following temp >39º C, systolic BP <90 systolic, PO_2 <70 torr, weight loss > 5%, Karnofsky <70, hemoglobin <10 gm/dL, neutrophil count <1000/mL, ALT >2.5 ULN, creatinine >2x ULN, albumin <3.5 gm/mL or other organ dysfunction (*Clin Infect Dis* 2000;30:688; *Ann Intern Med* 2002;137:154).

  - □ Itraconazole may be used for initial treatment of mild to moderate histoplasmosis without CNS involvement, or it may be used for maintenance after induction with amphotericin B (*Am J Med* 1995;98:336).

  - □ *AmBisome* may be more effective than amphotericin B deoxycholate (*Ann Intern Med* 2002;137:154).

  - □ Fluconazole is inferior to itraconazole *in vitro* and in a controlled clinical trial (*Clin Infect Dis* 2001;33:1910). This study showed a

6 Management of Infections

correlation between *in vitro* resistance and clinical response; fluconazole resistant strains were sensitive *in vitro* to itraconazole.

□ A therapeutic trial of amphotericin B vs *AmBisome* in AIDS patients showed more rapid defervescence and fewer adverse reactions in the *AmBisome* group (*Antimicrob Agents Chemother* 2001;45:2354). The AWP is $1200/day as compared with $12/day for amphotericin B.

□ Itraconazole levels: Some recommend measurement of serum levels to assure levels of >1 μg/mL or 2 μg/mL for free, plus the hydroxylated metabolite, which also has antifungal activity. This should be measured after >5 days of itraconazole (San Antonio Lab, 210-567-4131). Inadequate levels: Make sure caps are given with meal ± acidic drink, avoid drugs that neutralize gastric acid or interact with itraconazole (PIs and NNRTIs), or use liquid formulation with food.

□ Some authorities discontinue chronic therapy if (1) disease is in remission, (2) serum and urine *Histoplasma* antigen assay is <4 units, (3) patient has completed >1 year of therapy and (4) CD4 count is >150/mm^3.

RESPONSE: Most patients show subjective and objective response within 1 week. The rate of response with *AmBisome* or itraconazole is 85%, with negative blood cultures at 2 weeks in 50% (itraconazole) to 85% (*AmBisome*) (*Antimicrob Agents Chemother* 2001;45:2354). Antigen titer in blood and urine correlate with clinical response and usually decrease after 2 to 4 weeks; blood and urine assays are recommended at 3 to 6 month intervals during maintenance therapy to detect relapse. Clinical failure correlates with *in vitro* sensitivity test results, especially with fluconazole, which is far less active than itraconazole (*Clin Infect Dis* 2001;33:1910). Some authorities recommend routine monitoring of itraconazole levels to assure absorption.

MAINTENANCE

- **Preferred regimen:** Itraconazole 200 mg/day (*see Comment*).

- **Alternative regimens:** Fluconazole 800 mg/day PO lifelong (use only if itraconazole is not tolerated).

- **Comment:** Immune reconstitution: No criteria recommended for stopping (CDC/IDSA Guidelines, *MMWR* 2002;51[RR-8]:16). CDC/IDSA treatment guidelines recommend lifelong treatment. However, a more recent report indicates regimen can be safely stopped under the following conditions: 1) >12 months of treatment; 2) CD4 >150/mm^3; 3) HAART ≥6 months; and 4) urine and serum antigen <4.1 units (*Clin Infect Dis* 2004;38:1485).

Isospora belli

Isosporiasis

PRESENTATION: The usual presentation is watery diarrhea ± fever, abdominal pain, vomiting and wasting. The diagnosis requires detection of oocysts in stool with acid fast stain, which is specific and reasonably sensitive, but several stool specimens may be required. There are no commercial antigen detection methods.

TREATMENT

- **Acute Infection**
  - Preferred regimen: TMP-SMX 1 DS PO bid (or equivalent IV) x 10 days (CDC/IDSA 2004)
  - Alternative regimen: Pyrimethamine 50-75 mg/day PO + leucovorin acid 5-10 mg/day x 10 days
  - Ciproflaxin 500 mg PO bid x 10 days
  - Other fluoroquinolone
  - Support: Fluid and nutritional management; HAART

- **Comment**
  - Immunocompetent patients usually have self-limited diarrhea lasting 2 to 3 weeks. AIDS patients may have severe or persistent diarrhea and are usually treated. Duration of therapy is not well defined.
  - The response with TMP-SMX or TMP + sulfamethoxazole is rapid, but relapses are common with CD4 counts <200/mm^3 (*N Engl J Med* 1989;320:1044; *Ann Intern Med* 2001;132:885)
  - Pyrimethamine may be as effective as TMP-SMX, but experience is less extensive (*Ann Intern Med* 1988;109:474).

RESPONSE: AIDS patients usually respond to TMP-SMX within 2-3 days (*N Engl J Med* 1986;315:87; *N Engl J Med* 1989;320:1024). Stool examination may show continued shedding after clinical response.

SUPPRESSIVE THERAPY

- **Preferred regimen:** TMP-SMX 1-2 DS/day or 3x/week.
- **Alternative regimens**
  - Pyrimethamine 25 mg + sulfadoxine 500 mg/week PO (1 *Fansidar/* week).
  - Pyrimethamine 25 mg + folinic acid 5 mg/day.
- **Duration:** Consider discontinuation of TMP-SMX when CD4 >200/mm^3 for ≥3 months (CDC/IDSA 2004 guidelines).

6 Management of Infections

JC Virus
Progressive Multifocal Leukoencephalopathy (PML)

DIAGNOSIS: Most healthy persons (70%) harbor JC virus. PML is the only disease caused by JC virus and occurs most frequently as a devastating neurologic syndrome with insidious onset and progression over weeks or months. Common features are (1) cognitive dysfunction, dementia, seizures, aphasia, cranial nerve deficits, ataxia, hemiparesis; (2) CSF that shows no cells and normal protein; (3) no fever; (4) CD4 count that is usually <100/mm^3 but may be >200/mm^3 in up to one-third; (5) a head CT or MRI that shows hypodense white matter disease and (6) a course that is inevitably progressive over weeks or months (*Clin Infect Dis* 2003;36:1047; *Clin Infect Dis* 2002;34:103; *Lancet* 1997;349:1534) A definitive diagnosis requires compatible clinical history and MRI findings plus a brain biopsy positive by DFA stain for JC virus and typical inclusions in oligodendrocytes. PCR in CSF for JCV has a sensitivity of 80%, specificity of 90%.

TREATMENT

- **Preferred regimen:** There is no effective treatment. With HAART some improve, some stabilize and some progress.

- **Comments**

  □ Positive PCR plus typical clinical and MRI findings constitute presumptive PML. If PCR is negative, consider brain biopsy depending on probability of a treatable alternative diagnosis.

  □ Prognosis: Median survival after PML diagnosis is 2 to 4 months (*J Acquir Immune Defic Syndr* 1992;5:1030; *N Engl J Med* 1998; 338:1345; *Clin Infect Dis* 2002;34:103).

  □ HAART: One of the largest series (n=57) showed neurologic improvement in 26%, and there was eradication of JCV DNA in CSF in 57%. New PML lesions developed in nine patients after response to HAART (*J Infect Dis* 2000;182:1077). Others have shown variable clinical and virologic responses to HAART, including clinical deterioration in some (*AIDS* 1999;13:1881; *Clin Infect Dis* 1999;28:1152; *Clin Infect Dis* 2000;30:95).

  □ Treatment trials: No antiviral therapy is clearly effective, including cidofovir, interferon alfa, amantadine, adenosine, foscarnet, ganciclovir and cytosine arabinoside (*AIDS* 2002;16:1791; *J Neurovirol* 2001;7:364; *J Neurovirol* 2001;7:374; *J Neurovir* 1998;4:324; AIDS 2002;16:1791; *N Engl J Med* 1998;338:1345; *AIDS* 2000;14:517).

RESPONSE: Progressive neurologic disease with no good treatment. Progression can occur even with immune reconstitution, which should be attempted (*J Acquir Immune Defic Syndr* 2004;37:1268). HAART has been shown to improve survival but may also cause a fulminant imflammatory encephalitis due to immune reconstitution (*Acta Neuropathol* 2005;109:449).

Microsporidia

Microsporidiosis (*Clin Infect Dis* 2001;32:331)

PRESENTATION: Microsporidia are a broad group of microbes related to fungi that were implicated in 20-50% of AIDS-related chronic diarrhea in the pre-HAART era. The frequency now is much lower. The usual presentation is watery diarrhea in patients with a CD4 count <100/mm^3. The diagnosis is usually established by stool studies with light microscopy of stool specimens using calcofluor white, Chromatope 2R or Uvitex 2B to detect spores (*N Engl J Med* 1992;326:161; *Ann Trop Med Parasitol* 1993;87:99; *Adv Parasitol* 1998;40:351). These tests have sensitivity and specificity of about 100% and 80%, respectively (*J Clin Microbiol* 1998;36:2279). Microsporidia refers to a large group of microbes, of which only two are known to cause diarrhea: *Enterocytozoon* (*Septata*) *intestinalis*, which accounts for about 10-20% of microsporidiosis cases, and *E. bieneusi*, which accounts for 80-90%. Non-intestinal manifestations of microsporidiosis include encephalitis, ocular infections, myositis, sinusitis and disseminated infection (*Clin Infect Dis* 1994;19:517; *Adv Parasitol* 1998;40:321).

TREATMENT

- **Preferred regimens**
  - □ Optimal therapy: HAART with virologic control and CD4 count increase to >100/mm^3.
  - □ *E. bieneusi*: Fumagillin 60 mg/day x 14 days (this drug is associated with reversible thrombocytopenia; not available in U.S.).
  - □ *E. intestinalis*: Albendazole 400 mg PO bid until CD4 >200/mm^3. (See first comment below.)
  - □ Symptomatic treatment with nutritional supplements and anti-diarrheal agents (*Lomotil*, loperamide, paregoric, etc.).
  - □ Ocular: Fumidil B 3mg/mL saline (fumagillin 70 mg/mL) eye drops, forever. Add albendazole 400 mg PO bid for systemic infection.
  - □ Disseminated disease: Itraconazole 400 mg PO qd plus albendazole 400 mg PO bid (*Trachipleistophora* or *Brachiola*)

- **Comments**
  - □ Albendazole is recommended for disseminated (non-ocular) microsporidiosis caused by any microsporidia other than *E. bienuesi* (CDC/IDSA 2004).
  - □ Fumagillin proved effective in a controlled trial for microsporidiosis due to *E. bieneusi* (*N Engl J Med* 2002;346:1963).

6 **Management of Infections**

- Albendazole efficacy: Established only for infections involving *E. intestinalis*, which causes 10% to 20% of cases.
- Anecdotal success: Reported with itraconazole, fluconazole, nitazoxanide, nitrofurantoin, atovaquone, and metronidazole (*Infect Dis Clin N Amer* 1994;8:483).
- Immune reconstitution with CD4 >100/mm³: Best therapy, especially for the 80% to 90% of cases involving *E. bieneusi* (*Lancet* 1998;351:256; *AIDS* 1998;12:35; *J Clin Microbiol* 1999;37:421; *J Acquir Immune Defic Syndr* 2000;25:124).
- Extraintestinal: *E. bellum* – sinusitis and disseminated disease; *E. cuniculi* – CNS, conjunctiva, renal, lungs; *T. hominis* – myositis; *Braciola* – myositis.

RESPONSE: Symptoms resolve with CD4 count increase to >100/mm³. With fumagillin treatment of *E. bieneusi* there is response by week 4 as indicated by discontinuation of loperamide use and elimination of detectable Microsporidia in stool (*N Engl J Med* 2002;346:1963).

Molluscum Contagiosum

CAUSE: A poxvirus

PRESENTATION: Clinical presentation is with flesh-colored, pink, or whitish, dome-shaped papules with central umbilication (dimpling). It can occur anywhere on the body, except palms and soles. Most common areas are the face (beard area), neck, and genitals. Lesions are usually less than 5 mm in diameter; occasionally lesions are greater than 1 cm (giant molluscum). The diagnosis may be confirmed by KOH preparation, Tzanck smear, or biopsy that shows intraepidermal molluscum bodies. EM shows a large brick-shaped virus resembling smallpox.

TREATMENT: An individual lesion may be treated with curettage, cryotherapy, electrocauterization (*Sex Trans Infect* 1999;75[suppl 1]:S80), chemical cauterization (trichloroacetic acid, cantharidin, podophyllin, 5-FU, tretinoin, silver nitrate, phenol), imiquimod, topical cidofovir. Lesions usually disappear in patients responding to HAART (*Eur J Dermatol* 1999;9:211).

Mycobacterium avium Complex
Disseminated MAC

PRESENTATION: MAC is a ubiquitous mycobacterium found in environmental sources that is acquired by ingestion or inhalation. It is a relatively common cause of chronic pulmonary disease in otherwise healthy adults and of disseminated infection without pulmonary involvement in patients with AIDS. The incidence of disseminated MAC in patients with a CD4 count <100/mm³, no HAART and no MAC prophylaxis is 20-40%. With HAART and MAC prophylaxis, this is reduced to 2%.

- The usual symptoms in AIDS patients are fever, night sweats, weight loss, diarrhea and abdominal pain typically occurring in patients with a CD4 count <50/mm³ (*Lancet Infect Dis* 2004;4:557) . The diagnosis is established by culture of MAC from a non-pulmonary, normally sterile site; blood cultures are 90% to 95% sensitive using Bactec 12B or 13A bottles but usually require 7 to 14 days. The diagnosis rarely requires biopsy of liver, bone marrow, or lymph nodes. Sputum and stool are insensitive and non-specific culture sources (*J Infect Dis* 1994;168:1045; *J Infect Dis* 1994;169:289).

- Pulmonary MAC (uncommon in HIV-infected patients): Infiltrate on X-ray and culture with ≥2+ growth and ≥1 positive AFB stain (*Am J Respir Crit Care Med* 1997;155:2041).

TREATMENT

- **Preferred regimens**
  - Clarithromycin 500 mg bid PO + ethambutol 15 mg/kg/day PO.
    Consider adding a third drug with CD4 count <50/mm³, high MAC load or absence of effective HAART: rifabutin 300 mg/day PO.
  - Start HAART simultaneously or within 1-2 weeks.

- **Alternative regimen:** Azithromycin 500-600 mg/day + ethambutol 15 mg/kg/day PO.

- Alternative "third drugs" are 1) levofloxacin 500 mg PO qd; 2) ciprofloxacin 500-750 mg PO bid; 3) Amikacin 15 mg/kg/d IV.

RESPONSE: Decrease in fever and in quantitative blood cultures is expected in 2-4 weeks. Obtain blood cultures if there is no clinical improvement within 4-8 weeks. Treatment failure is defined by positive blood cultures at 4 to 8 weeks. Sensitivity tests should be done and treatment should include at least two new drugs which show *in vitro* activity. Antibiotics to consider include ethambutol, rifabutin, ciprofloxacin, levofloxacin, and amikacin. Optimal HAART is always important (*Clin Infect Dis* 2000;31:1245; *Clin Infect Dis* 1998;27:1278). Care should be taken to distinguish MAC treatment failure from both MAC bacteremia and MAC reconstitution syndrome, which shows negative blood cultures and is discussed below.

- **Comments**
  - With severe disease use a 3-drug combination, but the best third drug is unclear. Studies with rifabutin as a third drug suggest improved survival and reduced resistance (*Clin Infect Dis*

1999;28:1080). Alternative third drugs are levofloxacin, ciprofloxacin, or amikacin, but data supporting benefit are sparse (*N Engl J Med* 1996;335:377; *Clin Infect Dis* 1997;25:621; *J Infect Dis* 1993;168:112).

- **Failure:** ≥2 new drugs; benefit of continuing clarithromycin or azithromycin if resistant *in vitro* is not known.

- **Macrolide resistance:** resistance to clarithromycin and azithromycin is unusual even in patients who develop MAC during use of these drugs for prophylaxis (*Clin Infect Dis* 1994;18:S237; *Ann Intern Med* 1994;121:905).

- **Clarithromycin drug interactions:** Clarithromycin AUC is increased with concurrent IDV (50%), RTV (75%), APV (18%), LPV/r (77%), ATV (94%), NVP (26%), and SQV (177%). The clarithromycin dose should be reduced 50% or should be avoided when used with ATV due to increased levels and concern for prolonged QTc; dose adjustments for the other drugs listed require no clarithromycin dose adjustment except when LPV/r or RTV are used with renal failure. With EFV, clarithromycin levels are decreased 39% – monitor response or use alternative drug (DHHS guidelines 11/04) (*N Engl J Med* 1996;335:428).

- **Rifabutin dose:** 300-600 mg/day, but should not exceed 300 mg/day if given with clarithromycin or fluconazole. Note interactions with PIs and NNRTIs (see Table 5-42, p. 284).

- ***In vitro* susceptibility:** Most useful for macrolides in patients with prior macrolide exposure (*N Engl J Med* 1996;335:392; *Clin Infect Dis* 1998;27:1369; *J Infect Dis* 2000;181:1289). Threshold for clarithromycin sensitivity is 32µg/mL and for azithromycin is 256µg/mL using Bactec radiometric susceptibility testing.

- **Clarithromycin vs azithromycin:** In a comparative trial for MAC bacteremia, clarithromycin was superior in time to negative blood cultures (*Clin Infect Dis* 1998;27:1278; see also *Antimicrob Agents Chemother* 1999;43:2869). Nevertheless, another large trial using azithromycin 600 mg/day vs clarithromycin 500 mg bid, each combined with EMB, showed comparable results (*Clin Infect Dis* 2000;31:1254).

- **3-drug combination:** Comparison of clarithromycin/EMB vs clarithromycin/EMB/rifabutin showed no clinical benefit to 3-drug regimen but a decreased rate of clarithromycin resistance (*Clin Infect Dis* 1999;28:1080).

- **ASA or NSAID** often effective for symptom relief.

- **Immune reconstitution:** Discontinue maintenance therapy when CD4 count >100 cells/mm³ x 6 months + ≥12 months treatment and asymptomatic.

MAC Immune Recovery Syndrome (IRS)

CHARACTERISTIC FEATURES: 1) Host and timing factors: most common in the first 8 months (usually at 1-3 months) after initiating HAART with baseline CD4 <50/mm³ and a good CD4 response to >100/mm³ and VL response (*Lancet* 1998;351:252; *J Acquir Immune Defic Syndr* 1999; 20:122; *Ann Intern Med* 2000;133:447; *Clin Infect Dis* 2004;38:1159). 2) Clinical expression with fever and usually a focal inflammatory lesion, usually cervical adenitis, but others include mediastinal adenitis, mesenteric adenitis, pericarditis, osteomyelitis, skin abscesses, bursitis, CNS infections, hepatic granuloma, etc. (*Ann Intern Med* 2000;133:447; *Clin Infect Dis* 2004;38:461; *Clin Infect Dis* 2004;38:1159).

TREATMENT

- Continue HAART
- Continue MAC therapy
- Treat IRS with NSAIDs; severe cases may need prednisone 20-40 mg/d x 4-8 weeks

Mycobacterium chelonae

TREATMENT

- **Preferred regimen:** Clarithromycin 500 mg bid x >6 months.
- **Alternative regimen:** Variable activity: Cefoxitin, amikacin, doxycycline, imipenem, tobramycin, erythromycin.
- **Comment:** *In vitro* susceptibility test results needed. Clinical: Skin and soft tissue, bone and joint.

Mycobacterium fortuitum

TREATMENT

- **Preferred regimen:** Amikacin 400 mg q12h + cefoxitin 12 g/day x 2 to 4 weeks, then oral agents based on *in vitro* tests – clarithromycin 1 g/day, doxycycline 200 mg/day, SMX 1 g tid, ciprofloxacin 500 mg bid.
- **Comments**
  - Duration: >3 months for cutaneous lesions and >6 months for bone lesions in non-HIV infected patients.
  - Clinical: Skin and soft tissue, bone, CNS, disseminated.

Mycobacterium genavense

(*Am J Clin Pathol* 2001;116:225)

TREATMENT

- **Preferred regimen:** Clarithromycin/EMB/rifampin.
- **Alternative regimen:** Other possible agents: Ciprofloxacin, amikacin, and PZA.

6 Management of Infections

- **Comments**
  - □ Clarithromycin-containing regimens are most effective (*AIDS* 1993;7:1357).
  - □ Clinical: Similar to *M. avium* (*AIDS* 1995;9:659).

Mycobacterium gordonae
TREATMENT

- **Preferred regimen:** INH/rifampin/clofazimine or clarithromycin.
- **Alternative regimen:** SM may be useful.
- **Comments:** Validity: Most isolates are contaminants (*Dermatology* 1993;187:301; *AIDS* 1992;6:1217; *Antimicrob Agents Chemother* 1992;36:1987).

Mycobacterium haemophilum
TREATMENT

- **Preferred regimen:** INH/rifampin/EMB.
- **Alternative regimen:** Clarithromycin, doxycycline, ciprofloxacin, and amikacin are active *in vitro.*
- **Comment:** Clinical: Skin and disseminated disease (*Ann Intern Med* 1994;120:118). Experience is limited (*Eur J Clin Microbiol Infect Dis* 1993;12:114; *Tuberculosis* 2004;84:341).

Mycobacterium kansasii
TREATMENT

- **Preferred Regimen:** INH 300 mg/day PO + rifampin 600 mg/day PO + EMB 25 mg/kg/day x 2 months, then 15 mg/kg/day x 18 months (total) to life long therapy ± SM 1 g IM 2x/week x 3 months (*Am J Respir Crit Care Med* 1997;156:S1).
- **Alternative Regimen:** Also consider ciprofloxacin 750 mg PO bid and clarithromycin 500 mg PO bid.
- **Comments**
  - □ Experience in HIV infected patients (*J Acquir Immune Defic Syndr* 1991;4:516; *Ann Intern Med* 1991;114:861; *HIV Med* 2004;5:431; *Clin Infect Dis* 2003;37:584).
  - □ *In vitro* sensitivity data is needed.
  - □ Duration is arbitrary – many physicians treat HIV-infected patients for life.
  - □ Most strains are resistant to INH, but it is usually included in the regimen with little supporting data. All are resistant to PZA.

□ Immune reconstitution: Reports of cervical and mediastinal adenopathy, osteomyelitis and arthritis due to *M. kansasii* during the first 3 months of HAART.

Mycobacterium malmoense

TREATMENT

- **Preferred regimen:** Clarithromycin or azithromycin, rifabutin, ethambutol, and ciprofloxacin.
- **Comment:** Clinical: Cavitary pulmonary, CNS (*Clin Infect Dis* 1993; 16:540; *J Clin Microbiol* 1996;34:731; *Eur Respir J* 2003;21:478).

Mycobacterium scrofulaceum

TREATMENT

- **Preferred regimen:** Surgical excision.
- **Alternative regimen:** Clarithromycin, azithromycin, rifabutin ± streptomycin, cycloserine + sulfonamides.
- **Comments:** Cervical adenitis.

Mycobacterium tuberculosis (TB)

EPIDEMIOLOGY AND CLINICAL FEATURES: The risk of active TB with latent infection is increased 100-fold by HIV infection; primary TB is also common and accounts for one-third of cases (*MMWR* 2003;52RR-10:1). HIV promotes TB at all CD4 strata but clinical features vary according to CD4 count. With CD4 count >350/mm³ lung lesions are "typical," with upper lobe infiltrates ± cavitation. With CD4 count <50/mm³ extrapulmonary TB is far more common with pleuritis, pericarditis, meningitis and disseminated disease; chest X-rays typically show lower and middle lobe and miliary infiltrates, usually without cavitation. TB is associated with increased VL and more rapid progression of HIV infection (*Am J Respir Crit Care Med* 1995;151:129; *Am J Respir Crit Care Med* 1993;148:1293).

DIAGNOSIS: The standard test for pulmonary TB is morning expectorated sputa x 3 days for AFB smear and culture. Induced sputa and bronchoscopy are used if there is no sputum production. Sensitivity of AFB smear is about 50%, is similar for patients with and without AIDS, and is not better with induced sputum or bronchoscopy specimens compared with expectorated sputum (*Chest* 1992;101:1211; *Chest* 1992;102:1040; *Am J Respir Crit Care Med* 2000;162:2238). Specificity of the smear depends on prevalence of MAC (*J Clin Microbiol* 1998;36:1046), but most positive AFB smears of respiratory specimens in patients with AIDS indicate TB even in areas where MAC is common (*Clin Infect Dis* 1998;19:334). Nucleic acid amplification

6 Management of Infections

(Gen-Probe *Amplified MTD Test*; Roche *Amplicor MTB Test*) is more sensitive than AFB smear (80% vs 50%), is specific for *M. tuberculosis*, is 95% sensitive in AFB-smear positive cases, and hastens mycobacterial identification with culture and smear, but the tests are expensive ($50-100/assay). Current recommendation is that they be used with positive AFB smear or negative AFB smear plus high level of suspicion (*Am J Respir Crit Care Med* 2001;164:2020; *MMWR* 2000;49:593). With miliary TB, sputum cultures are positive in only 25%, but multiple other specimens are AFB smear or culture positive, including blood in 50% to 60%. PPD skin tests have high rates of false-negative results that correlate inversely with CD4 count – up to 65% false-negatives in AIDS patients with active TB (*J Infect Dis* 1992;166:194). Positive cultures for *M. tuberculosis* approach 100% for sensitivity and 97% for specificity (*Clin Infect Dis* 2001;31:1390).

TREATMENT: Official statement of the ATS, CDC and IDSA: Treatment of Tuberculosis (*Am J Respir Crit Care Med* 2003;167:603); http://www.cdc.gov/nchstpl/tb/pubs/mmwr/rr4720.pdf)

- **Initiation of HIV treatment:** Do not initiate treatment of both TB and HIV simultaneously due to overlapping drug toxicities, drug interactions, adherence requirements, and possible paradoxical reactions (immune reconstitution). The CDC/ATS recommendation is to: 1) continue antiretroviral therapy that was previously started; 2) avoid initiating treatment of both and always treat TB first with HAART introduced at 4-8 weeks. The possible exception is patients with advanced HIV with CD4 counts <50/mm³. WHO guidelines are:

  1. **CD4 <200/mm³:** Start ART at 2 to 8 weeks after TB treatment with EFV-based HAART; alternative "third drugs" are SQV/r and ABC; NVP

  2. **CD4 200 to 350/mm³:** Consider ART. If given, start after initial TB phase using EFV (or NVP if RIF-free continuation)

  3. **CD4 >350/mm³:** Defer ART

- **Unique issues with HIV coinfection**

  □ Atypical TB presentation with CD4 count: more non-cavitary, lower- and mid-lobe involvement and extrapulmonary disease

  □ TB incidence is increased 100-fold with HIV; HIV viral loads are higher and HIV disease progresses more rapidly with active TB (*Am J Resp Crit Care Med* 1995;151:129).

  □ Anti-TB therapy in presence of HAART is confounded by high rate of drug intolerance and drug interactions. When starting PI or NNRTI other than EFV or RTV/SQV, substitute rifabutin 2 weeks prior to PI or NNRTI to provide washout of RIF (see Table 6-2d, p.367).

  □ Immune reactivation is reported in 7% to 36% of patients who receive HAART.

- Despite differences, the treatment and response to therapy is largely the same with and without HIV.
- One report shows a high rate of morbidity and mortality in the first month of TB treatment in patients with a CD4 count <100/mm^3 at baseline (*J Infect Dis* 2004;190:1670).
- Other differences in anti-TB therapy: (1) optimal duration is unclear; (2) CD4 <100/mm^3 – continuation phase should be daily or 3x/week; (3) rifapentine is contraindicated.
- In a large trial of steroids for pleural TB in coinfected patients in Kampala showed prednisone (50 mg/d x 2 wks, then taper over 6 wks) was not associated with an increase in OIs or a decrease in CD4 cell count response (*J Infect Dis* 2004;190:869).

- **Immune reconstitution syndrome (paradoxical worsening):** May occur in absence of HIV co-infection but more common with HIV and thought to be due to immune reconstitution.

  - Characterized by worsening of symptoms and X-ray changes, with high fever, lymphadenopathy, expanding CNS lesions, large effusions (*Arch Intern Med* 2002;162:97; *Chest* 2001;120:193). Rule out other causes, especially TB treatment failure and lymphoma.
  - Severe reaction: Prednisone 1 mg/kg/day x 1 to 2 weeks, then taper. Continue TB and HIV therapy. (See above regarding corticosteroids.)
  - Mild to moderate reaction: Treat symptomatically and continue TB and HIV therapy.

6 Management of Infections

■ TABLE 6-1: **Treatment of Drug-Susceptible TB**

Drugs	Phase 1 (8 weeks) Doses, Duration	Phase 2* Regimen, Doses, Minimum Duration
	8 weeks	
INH, RIF, PZA, EMB	■ 7 d/week, 56 doses, 8 weeks or ■ 5 d/week, 40 doses, 8 weeks	■ INH/RIF 7 d/week, 126 doses or 5 d/week, 90 doses, 18 weeks ■ INH/RIF 2x/week, 36 doses, 18 weeks[†]
	2 weeks/6 week	
INH, RIF, PZA, EMB	■ 7 d/week, 14 doses x 2 weeks, then 2x/week ■ 12 doses, 6 weeks[†]	■ INH/RIF 2x/week, 36 doses, 18 weeks[†]
	8 weeks	
INH, RIF, PZA, EMB	■ 3x/week, 24 doses, 8 weeks[†]	■ INH/RIF 3x/week, 54 doses, 18 weeks[†]
	8 weeks	
INH, RIF, EMB	■ 7 d/week, 56 doses or 5 d/week, 40 doses[†]	■ INH/RIF 7 d/week, 217 doses or 5 d/week, 155 doses, 31 weeks ■ INH/RIF 2x/week, 62 doses, 31 weeks[†]

INH = Isoniaizid, RIF = rifampin or rifabutin, PZA = Pyrazinamide, EMB = Ethambutol
*Patients with cavitation at baseline, those with delayed clinical response and those with positive cultures at 2 months should receive 31-week continuation phase, for a total of 9 months (39 weeks)
[†]Patients with a CD4 count <100/mm³ should receive daily therapy during the induction phase (first 8 weeks) and receive daily or thrice weekly administration during the continuation phase. This is based on the observation of failure with rifamycin resistance in 5 of 156 participants in TBTC Study 23 who were treated twice weekly (*MMWR* 2002;51:214).

TABLE 6.2: Antituberculosis Agents

■ TABLE 6-2a: **First-line Agents: Doses**

Drug	Daily	2x/wk	3x/wk
INH	5mg/kg (300)*	15 mg/kg (900)*	15 mg/kg (900)*
RIF	10 mg/kg (600)	10 mg/kg (600)*	10 mg/kg (600)*
PZA (wt) 40-55 kg 56-75 kg 76-90 kg	 1 gm 1.5 gm 2.0	 2.0 gm 3.0 gm 4.0 gm	 1.5 gm 2.5 gm 3.0 gm
EMB (wt) 40-55 kg 56-75 kg 76-90 kg	 800 mg 1,200 mg 1,600 mg	 2,000 mg 2,800 mg 4,000 mg	 1,200 mg 2,000 mg 2,400 mg

INH (Isoniazide)	
Formulation:	50, 100, 300 mg tabs, also syrup and IV formulations
Liver:	ALT in 10% to 20%, clinical hepatitis 0.6%; INH/RIF 2.7%. Risk with ETOH, prior liver disease and postpartum; fatal hepatitis 0.02%
Peripheral neuropathy:	Dose-related, frequency 0.2%, risk with other causes of peripheral neuropathy (diabetes, HIV, drugs, ETOH, pregnancy). Prevented with pyroxidine 25 mg/day. Rare: CNS toxicity, LE syndrome, hypersensitivity reactions, monoamine poisoning – flushing with exposure to wine, cheese, etc.
Pregnancy:	Safe
Drug interaction:	Levels of phenytoin, and carbamazepine increased, but decreased by rifamycins
Monitoring:	Usually none. Monitor LFTs monthly if pre-existing liver disease or with development of abnormal LFTs that does not require D/C therapy.

RIF (Rifampin)	
Formulation:	150 mg caps
Cutaneous reactions:	Pruritis ± rash
Flu syndrome:	0.4 to 0.7%, taking RIF 2x/week
Liver:	Cholestatic hepatitis 0.6%; hepatotoxicity in 2.7% given INH/RIF
Orange discoloration of body fluids:	Warn patients that clothing and contact lenses may be stained.
Pregnancy:	Safe
Interactions:	Extensive. Reduce the following to ineffective levels: oral contra-ceptives, methadone, warfarin, protease inhibitors; see www. cdc.gov/nchstp/tb/ (Division of Tuberculosis Elimination, CDC)
Monitoring:	None

PZA (Pyrazinamide)	
Formulation:	500 mg tabs
Liver:	Dose-related hepatotoxicity; 1% at 25 mg/kg
Nongouty polyarthralgias:	Up to 40%, rarely serious enough to D/C; Rx with ASA, NSAIDs
Hyperuracemia:	Expected and not consequential; acute gout is rare.
GI intolerance:	Usually mild.
Pregnancy:	Little information; use when benefit justifies an unquantified risk.
Monitoring:	Uric acid levels are unnecessary but may be surrogate for adherence. LFTs when baseline liver disease and when given with RIF for latent TB.

(continued)

Management of Infections

6

EMB (Ethambutol)	
Formulation:	100, 400 mg tabs
Ocular:	Decreased acuity or decreased red-green discrimination. Risk is dose-related and minimal at 15 mg/kg; risk increases with daily administration and renal failure.
Pregnancy:	Safe
Monitoring:	Baseline visual acuity and Ishihara test of color discrimination. Inquire about vision changes at each monthly visit and warn patient to contact clinic immediately if change in vision. Monthly test of acuity and color discrimination with doses >15 to 20 mg/kg, duration >2 months or renal failure.

■ TABLE 6-2c: **Second-line Agents**

Rifabutin:	300 mg (half the standard rifampin dose)
Cycloserine:	10 to 15 mg/kg/day, usually 500 to 750 mg bid
Ethionamide:	15 to 20 mg/kg/day, usually 500 to 750 mg qd
Streptomycin:	15 mg/kg/day, usually 1 g qd. Age >50 years: 10 mg/kg/day, usually 750 mg qd. Streptomycin is given IM or IV 5 to 7 d/week x 2 to 4 months, then 2 to 3x/week after culture conversion.
Amikacin/kanamycin/capreomycin:	Same as streptomycin.
PAS:	8 to 12 g/day in 2 to 3 doses
Levofloxacin:	500 to 1000 mg/day
Gatifloxacin/moxifloxacin:	400 mg/day

Management of Infections

■ TABLE 6-2d: **Dose Adjustments for PI/NNRTIs When Used with Rifampin and Rifabutin (*MMWR* 2004;53:37)**

PI or NNRTI	Rifampin
EFV 800 mg hs	standard
SQV/RTV 400/400 mg bid	standard
All other PIs, boosted PIs, and NVP-combination with Rifampin is contraindicated	

PI or NNRTI	Rifabutin
IDV 1000 mg q8h; with IDV/r – standard dose	150 mg/day or 300 mg 2x to 3x/week*
NFV 1000 mg tid or 1250 mg bid	150 mg/day or 300 mg 2x to 3x/week*
FPV or FPV/r – standard dose	150 mg/day or 300 mg 2x to 3x/week*
EFV 600 mg qd (standard)	450 mg/day or 600 mg 2x to 3x/week*
RTV if sole PI or for boosting	150 mg 2x to 3x/week*
NVP – standard	300 mg/day or 300 mg 2x to 3x/week*
DLV – not recommended	
RTV/SQV – standard	150 mg 2x to 3x/week*
LPV/r – standard	150 mg 2-3x/week*
SQV – contraindicated (except RTV/SQV)	300 mg/day or 300 mg 3x/week
ATV – standard	150 mg qod or 3x/week*

* Intermittent treatment of active TB should be >3x/week with CD4 <100 cells/mm³.

TABLE 6.3: Treatment of Tuberculosis in Special Populations

■ TABLE 6-3a: **Extrapulmonary TB**

Standard 4 drug initial phase followed by INH/RIF for 4-7 months except for CNS. TB which is treated 9-12 months.

Site	Duration	Steroids
Lymph nodes	6 months	No
Bone or joint	6-9 months	No
Pleural	6 months	No
Pericarditis	6 months	Recommended
CNS TB	9-12 months	Recommended
Disseminated	6 months	No
GU TB	6 months	No
Peritoneal	6 months	No

■ TABLE 6-3b: **Pregnancy and Breastfeeding**

Regimen:	INH/RIF/EMB x 9 months or standard treatment with INH/RIF/EMB/PZA x 2 months, then INH/RIF x 4 months. The issue is safety of PZA, for which there is no evidence of adverse effects in pregnancy, but inadequate experience to assure safety. PZA is recommended in WHO guidelines but not U.S. guidelines.

6 Management of Infections

■ TABLE 6-3c: **Renal Insufficiency**

Drug	Dose with creatinine cl.<30 cc/min or hemodialysis
INH	Standard; increased risk of hepatotoxicity – monitor ALT
RIF	Standard
RZA	25-35 mg/kg 3x/week; see comment above regarding limited experience
EMB	15-25 mg/kg 3x/week
Levofloxacin	750-1000 mg 3x/week
Cycloserine	250 mg qd or 500 mg 3x/week
Ethionamide	Standard
PAS	Standard
Aminoglycosides	12-15 mg/kg 2-3x/week

■ TABLE 6-3d: **Hepatic Insufficiency**

Regimen excluding INH:	RIF/PZA/EMB x 6 months
Regimen excluding PZA:	INH/RIF/EMB x 2 months, then INH/RIF x 7 months
Regimen for severe liver disease:	■ RIF/fluoroquinolone/cycloserine/aminoglycoside x 18 months or ■ Streptomycin/EMB, fluoroquinolone/another second-line drug x 18 to 24 months

■ TABLE 6-3e: **Drug-resistant Tuberculosis**

Drug Resistance	Regimen
INH	RIF/PZA/EMB ± fluoroquinolone x 6 months
INH/RIF	Fluoroquinolone/PZA EMB aminoglycoside ± alternative agent x 18-24 months
RIF	INH/PZA/EMB ± fluoroquinolone x 9-12 months
INH/RIF and EMB	Fluoroquinolone/aminoglycoside/2 alternative agents and PZA or EMP (if active)

MONITORING

- **Baseline:** LFTs (ALT/AST, alkaline phosphotase, bilirubin), creatinine or BUN, platelet count, and CBC; PZA – uric acid, EMB – visual acuity.

- **Clinical monitoring:** Clinical assessment monthly. Warn of symptoms of hepatitis to discontinue therapy and obtain medical care – nausea, vomiting, dark urine, malaise, fever >3 days.

- **Laboratory monitoring:** LFTs with symptoms of hepatitis; some recommend routine tests at 1 and 3 months, especially if prior liver disease, older age, or alcoholism. Sputum smear and culture should be done ≤ monthly until two consecutive are negative. Some recommend chest x-ray at 2 months and at the termination of therapy.

- **Hepatotoxicity:** If ALT/AST ≥5x ULN, discontinue INH, rifampin + PZA, and give an alternative such as EMB, streptomycin + quinolone. When LFTs normal, reintroduce primary drugs one at a time (*Ann Intern Med* 1993;119:400). Options are: 1) standard therapy with more frequent monitoring; 2) RIF, EMB + PZA x 6 months; 3) INH + RIF + EMB x 2 months, then INH + RIF x 7 months. With severe liver disease consider RIF + EMB with fluoroquinolone first 2 months.
- Pregnancy

RESPONSE: Response to therapy is similar to that in patients without HIV except: 1) Drug interactions between anti-TB and HIV drugs and 2) paradoxical reactions with immune reconstitution. Most patients become afebrile within 7 to 14 days; persistence of fever beyond this time suggests resistance or another cause of fever (*Clin Infect Dis* 1992;102:797). Sputum culture becomes negative ≤2 months in 85% (*N Engl J Med* 2001;345:189). Persistence of positive cultures at ≥4 months suggests nonadherence or drug resistance. Immune reconstitution may cause the paradoxical reaction noted above; this needs to be distinguished from therapeutic failure.

TREATMENT OF LATENT TB

- **Indications:** PPD>5 mm induration, high-risk exposure, or prior positive PPD without treatment. Must rule out active disease.
- **Preferred regimens**
  - INH 300 mg/day PO + pyridoxine 50 mg/day PO x 9 months.
  - INH 900 mg 2x/week + pyridoxine 50 mg 2x/week x 9 months (DOT).
  - PZA 20 mg/kg/day plus rifabutin in place of rifampin to permit concurrent PI or NNRTI (see Table 6-2d for doses) x 2 months.
- **Comments**
  - Rifampin-containing regimens have drug interactions with PIs and NNRTIs; the preferred regimens are INH or short-course prophylaxis with PZA plus rifampin or rifabutin using dose adjustments shown in Table 6-3, p. 338-339.
  - Rifampin/PZA previously favored because it was as effective as INH for 9 months, and the probability of completing the two month course was better (*JAMA* 2000;283:1445). However, there have been subsequent reports of severe hepatotoxicity, including 6 deaths attributed to this regimen, although none of these patients had concurrent HIV infection (*MMWR* 2001;50;773). A subsequent review of case data in 1583 HIV-infected patients who participated in this trial showed no difference in rates of hepatotoxicity; AST

6 Management of Infections

>250 U/L in 12/791 (1.6%) INH recipients and in 15/792 (2.1%) RIF/PZA recipients (*Clin Infect Dis* 2004;39:561). Due to high risk of active TB, this regimen is recommended for HIV-infected patients who are not expected to complete the 9-month INH regimen, but these patients should be seen every 2 weeks and have CBC and LFTs (bilirubin and transaminase levels) monitored at baseline, 2, 4, and 6 weeks.

TREATMENT OF INH-RESISTANT STRAIN: Rifampin 600 mg/day PO + PZA 20 mg/kg x 2 months or rifabutin 150-450 mg/day (see Table 5-3, p. 147) + PZA x 2 months. The choice of rifampin or rifabutin depends on current HAART.

TREATMENT OF MULTIPLY RESISTANT STRAIN: Fluoroquinolone + PZA or EMB + PZA (Base decision on susceptibility tests and consultation with public health officials).

Mycobacterium xenopi

TREATMENT

- **Preferred regimen:** Rifampin, EMB, and SM
- **Comments:** Clinical: Pulmonary nodules (*Clin Infect Dis* 1997;25: 206)

Nocardia asteroides

PRESENTATION: Typically presents with a pulmonary nodule infiltrate or cavity that is indolent in presentation and slow to evolve. The diagnosis is based on recovery of *Nocardia* from a respiratory source. It is important to warn the laboratory to perform modified AFB stain, use appropriate media and hold the media, because 3-5 days are required for growth. Diagnosis is based on the recovery of the pathogen along with a compatible clinical syndrome.

TREATMENT

- **Preferred regimens:** Sulfadiazine or trisulfapyridine 3-12 g/day PO or IV to maintain 2 hour post-dose sulfa level at 100-150 mg/L x ≥6 months or TMP-SMX 5-15 mg/kg/day TMP PO or IV.
- **Alternative regimens**
  - □ Minocycline 100 mg PO bid x ≥6 months.
  - □ Other suggested regimens: Imipenem/amikacin; sulfonamide/ amikacin or minocycline; ceftriaxone/amikacin.
- **Comments**
  - □ Sulfonamides preferred; TMP is inactive against *Nocardia*, but TMP-SMX is often used due to the convenience of formulation.
  - □ May desensitize if hypersensitive to sulfa (see TMP-SMX, p. 290).

- Dose of sulfonamides or TMP-SMX determined by severity of illness; pulmonary or skin – low dose; CNS, severe or disseminated disease – high dose.
- Parenteral therapy is usually given 3 to 6 weeks, then oral therapy.
- Sulfa therapy – monitor sulfa level (for therapeutic level); monitor renal function (for crystalluria and azotemia) and force fluids.

RESPONSE: Most show clinical response in 5 days. Causes of failure: 1) resistance, 2) overwhelming infection, or 3) need for drainage. May need imipenem + amikacin (*Clin Infect Dis* 1996;22:891).

Penicillium marneffei
Penicilliosis
PRESENTATION: *P. marneffei* is endemic in Southeast Asia, primarily northern Thailand and southern China (*Lancet* 1994;344:110; *AIDS* 1994;8(suppl 2):35; *N Engl J Med* 1998;339:1739). The usual host has a CD4 count <50/mm³ and presents with fever, wasting, skin lesions (papular rash ± central umbilication resembling molluscum) and organ involvement: liver (hepatomegaly, abdominal pain, elevated alkaline phosphotase), marrow (cytopenias) and/or adenopathy. The diagnosis is established by evidence of pathogen in culture, smear, or histopathology; most frequent with Wright's stain of skin scraping, node biopsy, or marrow aspirate (*Lancet* 1994;344:110). Smears show elliptical yeast, some with the characteristic clear central septation (*J Med Mycol* 1993;4:195).

INITIAL TREATMENT (*N Engl J Med* 1993;339:1739)
- **Preferred regimens**
  - Severe: Amphotericin B 0.6 mg/kg/day x 2 wks, then itraconazole oral solution 200 mg PO bid x 10 wk (*Clin Infect Dis* 1998; 26:1107).
  - Mild to moderately severe: Itraconazole 200 mg PO bid.
- **Maintenance:** Itraconazole 200 mg/day for lifetime (*N Engl J Med* 1998;339:1739).
- **Comments**
  - Location: Endemic in Thailand, Hong Kong, China, Vietnam, and Indonesia (*Emerg Infect Dis* 1996;2:109; *Lancet* 1994;344:110).
  - *In vitro* sensitivity tests: Good activity with amphotericin B, ketoconazole, miconazole, and 5-FC (*J Mycol Med* 1995;5:21; *Antimicrob Agents Chemother* 1993;37:2407).
  - Itraconazole is superior to fluconazole (*Antimicrob Agents Chemother* 1993;37:2407).

RESPONSE: Response rate of 93% reported for recommended amphotericin/itraconazole regimen (*Clin Infect Dis* 1998;26:1107).

6 Management of Infections

Progressive Multifocal Leukoencephalopathy (PML), see JC Virus, p. 354

*Pneumocystis jiroveci (P. carinii)**

(*N Engl J Med* 2004;350:2487)

Pneumonia (PCP)

CLINICAL FEATURES: Subacute onset and progression of exertional dyspnea, nonproductive cough, fever and chest pain over days or weeks. P.E. typically shows fever, tachycardia, increased respiration rate ± rales.

LAB: Hypoxemia with reduced pO_2 or alveolar-arterial O_2 difference (A-a gradient), demonstrated at rest or post-exercise in mild cases. LDH is usually >500 mg/dl. X-ray usually shows bilateral, symmetrical interstitial infiltrates, but may be normal in up to 20% of cases (*Am J Roentgenol* 1997;169:967). Atypical findings include nodules, blebs and cysts. Pneumothorax is relatively common and suggests this diagnosis. Thin-section CT scan shows ground glass attenuation and a gallium scan shows increased lung uptake in patients with a negative chest X-ray. A negative thin-section CT scan does not exclude PCP.

DIAGNOSIS: Standard specimens are induced sputum; sensitivity averages 56% in meta-analysis of 7 reports (*Eur Respir J* 2002;20:982) or bronchoalveolar lavage with sensitivity of >95%. Because of low sensitivity of induced sputum, negative slides should be followed up with broncheoscopy. Standard stains for cysts and trophozoites are cresyl violet, Giemsa, Diff-Quik, Wright, and Gram-Weigert. Stains for cyst walls are Gemori-Methenamine Silver, Gram-Weigert, and toluidine blue. Some labs prefer immunofluorescent stains, which may give a higher yield (*Eur Respir J* 2002;20:982). PCR using oral wash specimens is experimental. Preliminary data show a sensitivity of 70-90% and specificity of 85%; the reduced specificity is attributed to a possible carrier state that may be corrected with a quantitative threshold (*J Infect Dis* 2004;189:1697). Positive stains and presumably other diagnostic methods remain positive for weeks after treatment (*N Engl J Med* 2004;350:2487), so treatment can be initiated before specimen collection.

* *P. carinii* has been renamed *P. jiroveci* but the eponym PCP is retained (*Emerg Infect Dis* 2002;8:891).

TREATMENT

■ Preferred regimens

- □ Trimethoprim 15-20 mg/kg/day + sulfamethoxazole 75-100 mg/kg/day PO or IV x 21 days in 3 to 4 divided doses (typical oral dose is 2 DS tid). May treat for only 14 days if mild disease and rapid response.

- □ Hypoxemia: Patients with moderately severe or severe disease (PO_2 <70mm Hg or A-a gradient >35 mm Hg) should receive corticosteroids (prednisone 40 mg PO bid x 5 days, then 40 mg qd x 5 days, then 20 mg/day to completion of treatment) starting as early as possible. IV methylprednisolone can be given as 75% of prednisone dose. Efficacy of corticosteroids for hypoxemia is established (*N Engl J Med* 1990;323:1451; *N Engl J Med* 1990;323:1500). Side effects include CNS toxicity, thrush, cryptococcosis, *H. simplex* infection, tuberculosis, and other OIs (*J Acquir Immune Defic Syndr* 1995;8:345).

- **Alternative regimens**
  - □ TMP 15 mg/kg/day PO + dapsone 100 mg/day PO x 21 days (*Ann Intern Med* 1996;124:792; *N Engl J Med* 1990;320:323:776).
  - □ Pentamidine 3-4 mg/kg/day IV infused over ≥60 min x 21 days; usually reserved for severe cases (*Ann Intern Med* 1986;105:37; *Ann Intern Med* 1990;113:203; *Ann Intern Med* 1994;121:174).
  - □ Clindamycin 600-900 mg IV q6h-q8h or 300-450 mg PO q6h + primaquine* 15-30 mg/day base PO x 21 days (*Clin Infect Dis* 1994;18:905; *Clin Infect Dis* 1998;27:524; *Arch Intern Med* 2001;161:1529).
  - □ Atovaquone 750 mg suspension PO bid with meal x 21 days (*N Engl J Med* 1993;328:1521; *Ann Int Med* 1994;121:154).
  - □ Trimetrexate 45 mg/m²/day IV plus leucovorin 20 mg/m² PO or IV q6h ± dapsone 100 mg/day; leucovorin for 3 days longer than trimetrexate (*J Infect Dis* 1994;170:165).

- **Comments**
  - □ Some recommend TMP dose of 15 mg/kg/day. The lower dose appears to be as effective and better tolerated (*N Engl J Med* 1993;328:1521; *Ann Intern Med* 1996;124:792).
  - □ ACTG 108 showed TMP-SMX, TMP-dapsone and clindamycin-primaquine to be equally effective for mild-moderate PCP (*Ann Intern Med* 1996;124:792).
  - □ Resistance of *P. jiroveci* to sulfonamides is suggested by mutations on the dihydropteroate synthase gene (*J Infect Dis* 2000;182:1192; *J Infect Dis* 1999;180:1969; *J Infect Dis* 2000;182:551), but there does not appear to be an association with treatment failure (*J Infect Dis* 2000;182:551; *JAMA* 2001;286:2450).
  - □ Adverse reactions to TMP-SMX have been noted in 25% to 50%, primarily rash (30% to 55%), fever (30% to 40%), leukopenia (30% to 40%), azotemia (1% to 5%), hepatitis (20%), thrombocytopenia (15%), and hypokalemia (TMP) (*J Infect Dis* 1995;171:1295; *Lancet*

6 Management of Infections

1991;338:431). Most can be "treated through" using antihistamines for rashes, antipyretics for fever, and antiemetics for nausea.

- Opinions vary regarding initiation of HAART during treatment of PCP. Some report better short term survival (*J Infect Dis* 2001; 183:1409); others report paradoxical worsening, due possibly to immune reconstitution (*Am J Respir Crit Care Med* 2001;164:841). Immune reconstitution with acute respiratory failure has been described (*Am J Respir Crit Care Med* 2001;164:847).

- Geographic clustering of cases suggests person-to-person spread (*Am J Respir Crit Care Med* 2000;162:1617; *Am J Respir Crit Care Med* 2000;162:1622; *N Engl J Med* 2000;19:1416; *Emerg Infect Dis* 2003;9:132). However, isolation from other vulnerable patients is not generally advocated.

- **Prophylaxis:** See p. 49

RESPONSE: Response to therapy is slow – usually 5 to 7 days. Preferred therapy (TMP-SMX) should not be changed based on an assumption of clinical failure until 4-8 days. Drug toxicity is common and may be mistaken for therapeutic non-response (*Ann Intern Med* 1996;124:972). The mortality rate of untreated PCP is 100%; for PCP with hospitalized patients given standard regimens it is 15% to 20%, and it is 60% for those requiring ventilator support (*AIDS* 2003;17:73). One meta-analysis suggested primaquine-clindamycin is the most effective salvage regimen (*Arch Int Med* 2001;161:1529).

Pseudomonas aeruginosa

DIAGNOSIS: Clinically compatible case plus recovery from a normally sterile source. Caution is necessary in interpreting growth of *P. aeruginosa* in contaminated respiratory tract specimens (sputum, bronchoscopy, etc.), especially in patients with prior antibiotics use or when the organism is recovered in low numbers.

TREATMENT

- **Preferred regimen:** Aminoglycoside + antipseudomonal beta-lactam (ceftazidime, cefoperazone, cefepime, ticarcillin, imipenem, piperacillin).

- **Alternative regimen:** Monotherapy with antipseudomonas beta-lactam, (ceftazidime, cefepime, piperacillin), carbapenem (imipenem, meropenem), ciprofloxacin, aminoglycoside.

- **Comments**
  - Antibiotic selection requires *in vitro* susceptibility data.
  - Risks: Reverse risk factors when feasible – neutropenia, corticosteroids, CD4 <50/mm^3.

- ◻ The frequently quoted adage that *P. aeruginosa* requires "double coverage" is debatable. Like other pathogens, it requires an agent active *in vitro* and, for pulmonary infections, an agent that penetrates alveolar lining fluid.

Rhodococcus equi

A review of 67 cases showed patients had a subacute pulmonary infection with infiltrate on chest X-ray, cavitation in 45 and a median CD4 count of 35/mm^3 (*Chest* 2003;123:1). *R. equi* was recovered from blood cultures in 50-80% and from sputum in 50% (*Clin Infect Dis* 2002;34:1379).

TREATMENT

- ■ **Preferred regimen:** Vancomycin 2 g/day IV or imipenem 2 g/day IV, usually combined with rifampin 600 mg/day PO or ciprofloxacin 750 mg PO bid or erythromycin PO or IV x ≥2 weeks, then oral treatment for 6 months. HAART is an important component of therapy (*Chest* 2003;123:1).

- ■ **Comments**
  - ◻ Sensitivity test guides therapy: Generally sensitive to fluoroquinolones, vancomycin, aminoglycosides (amikacin); imipenem, erythromycin, and rifampin resistant *in vitro* to penicillins and cephalosporins (*Clin Infect Dis* 2002;34:1379; *Chest* 2003;123:1).
  - ◻ Other drugs sometimes used based on *in vitro* sensitivity testing are tetracyclines, clindamycin, and TMP-SMX.
  - ◻ Duration of therapy is arbitrary, but relapses are common; most use prolonged oral maintenance therapy with macrolide or fluoroquinolone. Resistance to these agents may develop.
  - ◻ Immune reconstitution with HAART may be critical for cure.

RESPONSE: Prognosis prior to HAART era was poor (*Medicine* 1994;73:119). The prognosis with antibacterial agents plus immune reconstitution is good; the disease is chronic or fatal in 30% to 40% without HAART or with no response to HAART.

Salmonella spp.

PRESENTATION: The predominant strains in the U.S. are *S. enteriditis* and *S. typtimurium.*

TREATMENT (*Clin Infect Dis* 2001;32:331)

- ■ **Preferred regimen:** Ciprofloxacin 500-700 mg PO bid or 400 mg IV bid; total treatment is mild 7-14 day for cases that are mild and nonbacteremic; at least 4-6 weeks with advanced AIDS (CD4 <200/mm^3) ± bacteremia. Other fluoroquinolones (gatifloxacin, moxifloxacin and levofloxacin) should be equally effective.

- Maintenance for severely immunosuppressed patients with bacteremia: ciprofloxacin 500 mg PO bid.
- **Alternative regimen:** TMP 5-10 mg/kg/day/SMX IV or 1 DS bid x >2 weeks or ceftriaxone 1-2 g/day IV ≥2 weeks (see duration above).
- **Comments**
  - □ Immunocompetent hosts with salmonellosis often do well without antibiotic treatment. Most experts recommend antibiotics for all HIV-infected patients based on high rates of bacteremia (CDC/IDSA recommendations).
  - □ Relapse is common. Eradication of *Salmonella* carrier state has been demonstrated only with ciprofloxacin.
  - □ AZT is active against most *Salmonella* strains and may be effective prophylaxis (*J Infect Dis* 1999;179:1553).
  - □ Drug selection requires *in vitro* susceptibility data, especially for ampicillin. TMP-SMX preferred if sensitive. Ciprofloxacin resistance is reported (*N Engl J Med* 2001;344:1572) but is rare.
  - □ Maintenance: Some authorities recommend ciprofloxacin 500 mg PO bid x several months or TMP-SMX 5 mg/kg/day, TMP (1 DS PO bid). Need for maintenance therapy, specific regimens, and duration are not well defined.

Staphylococcus aureus

PRESENTATION: Staphylococcal infection syndromes most commonly encountered with HIV infection include:

- **Furunculosis:** There is an epidemic of infections involving "community-acquired MRSA" (USA 300 strain) which has been reported in disproportionately high numbers in MSM, but not clearly associated with HIV or IDU. This strain is clonal, global and characterized by genes for production of Panton-Valentine leukocidin (a possible virulence factor) and Mec IV (the mechanism of methicillin resistance, which is distinct from Mec I-III), found in nosocomial MRSA). The two infections most clearly associated with this strain are serious soft tissue infections, especially furuncles, and necrotizing pneumonia. Soft tissue infections account for the vast majority of infections involving MRSA (USA 300).
- **Management recommendations:** 1) Culture and sensitivity tests. Most USA 300 strains are methicillin-resistant and sensitive to many other antibiotics including TMP-SMX, macrolides, clindamycin, tetracycline and aminoglycosides. 2) Furuncles require surgical drainage. 3) If antibiotics are used, the recommendation is TMP-SMX

or doxycycline; clindamycin is appropriate if the strain is sensitive to erythromycin or the D test is negative. 4) Infection control is important, especially if the patient is hospitalized. Cover wounds and practice good hand hygiene.

- **Pyomyositis:** This is classically an infection of muscle caused by S. aureus, usually MSSA, and sometimes called "tropical pyomyositis" due to high rates in tropical countries. Most cases present with fever and focal pain; the diagnosis is usually made by CT scan (*Radiographics* 2004;24:1029) and treatment consists of drainage plus antibiotics selected by *in vitro* sensitivity tests (*Am J Med* 2004;117:420; *J Rheumatol* 2001;28:802). Some patients respond to antibiotics without surgery (*Am Surg* 2000;66:1064).

- **Staphylococcal infections associated with injection drug use** include 1) skin and soft tissue infections, 2) disc space infections, 3) sterno-clavicular joint infections and 4) endocarditis, especially tricuspid valve endocarditis. All of these were described well before the initial reports of HIV and none is notably different with HIV infection with respect to frequency or management recommendations.

TREATMENT

- **Preferred regimens**
  - □ **Parenteral:** Methicillin-sensitive *S. aureus* (MSSA): Antistaphylo-coccal betalactam (nafcillin, oxacillin, cefazolin, ceftriaxone) ± gentamicin 1 mg/kg IV q8h or rifampin 300 mg PO bid.

    Oral: Cephalexin 500 mg qid, dicloxacillin 500 mg qid, clindamycin 300 mg tid, or fluoroquinolone.

  - □ Nosocomial methicillin-resistant *S. aureus* (MRSA): Vancomycin 1 g IV q12h ± gentamicin or rifampin (above doses). Alternatives include linezolid 600 mg bid IV or PO or daptomycin 4 mg/kg/day IV.

  - □ Community-acquired MRSA: Often sensitive to TMP-SMX, clindamycin or doxycycline as well as vancomycin or linezolid. For serious infections it may be appropriate to use combinations of these or to combine with rifampin (*MMWR* 2003;52:993).

- **Comments**
  - □ Fluoroquinolones: Use of quinolone requires *in vitro* sensitivity results. Resistance is 10% for MSSA and 90% for nosocomial MRSA.

  - □ Prevalence of MRSA in community-acquired infections varies by geography but is commonly reported at 20% to 50%; these strains are resistant to all betalactams, but are sensitive to TMP-SMX, rifampin, tetracycline clindamycin, macrolides and fluoro-quinolones (*Nature* 2002;417:477; *Lancet* 2002;359:1819; *JAMA* 2000;286:1201).

6 Management of Infections

- Tricuspid valve endocarditis: nafcillin + gentamicin (MSSA) x 2 weeks (*Ann Intern Med* 1988;109:619), but abbreviated courses are generally not advocated for HIV-infected persons.
- For tricuspid valve endocarditis due to MSSA, nafcillin/oxacillin is preferred to vancomycin (*Clin Infect Dis* 2001;33:120).

Streptococcus pneumoniae

PRESENTATION: The rate of community-acquired pneumonia (CAP) is increased 8-fold with HIV infection (*Am Rev Respir Dis* 1993;148:1523) and the rate of *S. pneumoniae* is increased 150- to 300-fold (*JAMA* 1991;265:3275). A recent report from Taiwan shows a substantial decrease in rates of pneumococcal pneumonia and bacteremia in HIV-infected patients given *Pneumovax* (*Vaccine* 2004;22:2006). Rates of both CAP and pneumococcal bacteremia correlate with CD4 cell counts. Patients with pneumococcal bacteremia also have an 8-25% probability of recurrent bacteremia within 6 months (*JAMA* 1991;265:3275; *J Infect Dis* 2002;185:1364). Most of the recurrent cases involve new strains of *S. pneumoniae* and thus do not represent relapses. The clinical features of pneumococcal pneumonia and pneumococcal bacteremia are not unique in patients with HIV infection. Standard tests in CAP patients who are hospitalized include X-rays and studies for a microbial etiology including blood culture, Gram stain + culture of respiratory secretions, and urinary antigen assay for *S. pneumoniae*. HIV-infected patients with pneumococcal bacteremia respond well to antibiotic treatment. In fact, survival data show far better outcomes than in other patient populations with pneumococcal bacteremia (*Mayo Clin Proc* 2004;79:604).

TREATMENT

- **Preferred regimens:** Penicillin, amoxicillin, cefotaxime, ceftriaxone (see Comments), or fluoroquinolone (suspected or established penicillin resistance): Levofloxacin, moxifloxacin, or gatifloxacin, or telithromycin (Ketek).
- **Alternative regimens:** Macrolide.
- **Comments**
  - *In vitro* susceptibility: Susceptibility of *S. pneumoniae* based on surveillance 10,000 clinical isolates from 2000-02 in the United States: Penicillin resistance – 14%, macrolides – 25%, clindamycin – 6%, doxycycline – 6%, levofloxacin 1% (*Antimicrob Agents Chemother* 2003;47:1790).
  - Penicillin-resistant strains: Strains highly resistant to penicillin should be treated with telithromycin or fluoroquinolones quinolones (levofloxacin, gatifloxacin, or moxifloxacin). TMP-SMX is now considered inadequate for empiric use due to high rates of

resistance. Fluoroquinolone resistance is uncommon (<2%) but increasing (*N Engl J Med* 2002;346:747; *Emerg Infect Dis* 2002;8:594).

RESPONSE: Most patients respond well with clearance of bacteremia in 24 to 48 hours and clinical improvement in 1 to 3 days. Patients with pneumococcal pneumonia may transition from IV to oral antibiotics when they are clinically better, vital signs and blood gases are improved, and they can take pills.

Toxoplasma gondii
Toxoplasmic encephalitis

PRESENTATION: Toxoplasmosis in patients with HIV infection nearly always represents reactivation of latent cysts, almost always in patients with a CD4 count <100/mm³. Seroprevalence in the U.S. is about 15% but often 50-75% in some European countries and developing nations. The usual clinical presentation is fever, headache, confusion, and/or focal neurologic deficits. The diagnosis is based on 1) CNS imaging, 2) evidence of *T. gondii* by serology and PCR of CSF, and 3) response to therapy. Typical features are ≥2 ring enhancing lesions on MRI, fever, focal neurologic defect, and positive anti-*T. gondii* IgG (>90%). CSF *T. gondii* PCR is 50% sensitive and >96% specific (*Clin Infect Dis* 2002;34:103). The PCR test becomes negative post-therapy. *T. gondii* can be demonstrated by H&E stain or immunoperoxidase stain of a brain biopsy specimen, but this is rarely obtained or necessary. SPECT scans often help to distinguish CNS lymphoma and toxoplasmosis. Most patients respond to therapy with clinical and MRI improvement ≤2 weeks, which is diagnostic (*Clin Infect Dis* 2001;34:103).

TREATMENT: ACUTE INFECTION (≥6 weeks)

- **Preferred therapy:** Pyrimethamine 200 mg PO x 1, then see table:

Agent	Weight <60 kg	Weight >60 KG
Pyrimethamine	50 mg PO qd	75 mg PO qd
Leukovorin	10-20 mg PO qd	10-20 mg PO qd
Sulfadiazine	1 gm PO qid	1.5 gm PO qid
Duration: ≥6 weeks Dexamethasone 4 mg PO or IV q 6 h for mass effect.		

- **Alternative regimens**
  - Pyrimethamine + leucovorin (see preferred regimen) + clindamycin 600 mg IV or PO q6h for ≥6 weeks.

6 Management of Infections

- Pyrimethamine and leukovorin (in doses shown above) + azithromycin 900-1200 mg PO qd
- TMP-SMX (5 mg/kg TMP + 25 mg/kg SMX) IV or PO
- Atovaquone 1500 mg PO bid with meals and pyrimethamine and leukovorin (above doses)
- Atovaquone 1500 mg PO bid + sulfadiazine 1000-1500 mg PO q 6 h
- Atovaquone 1500 mg PO bid with meals

- **Comments**
  - Pyrimethamine + sulfadiazine is preferred; pyrimethamine + clindamycin is less effective but better tolerated (*Clin Infect Dis* 1996;22:268). All other regimens listed have been less well studied.
  - Clinical improvement expected within 1 week and improvement by CT scan or MRI within 2 weeks. Failure to respond and/or uncertain diagnosis is usually an indication for stereotactic brain biopsy, which yields a definitive diagnosis in 98% of cases (*Clin Infect Dis* 2000;30:49).
  - Leucovorin dose can be increased to ≥50 mg/day to reduce pyrimethamine toxicity.
  - Atovaquone regimens: May wish to confirm serum level ≥18 mcg/mL due to variable absorption.
  - Alternative regimens: Azithromycin, *AIDS* 2001;15:583; Clarithromycin, *Antimicrob Agents Chemother* 1991;35:2049; Atovaquone, *Clin Infect Dis* 2002;34:1243; TMP-SMX: *Antimicrob Agents Chemother* 1998;42:1346.

MAINTENANCE

- **Preferred regimen:** Pyrimethamine 25-50 mg/day PO + leucovorin 10-25 mg/day + sulfadiazine 500-1,000 mg PO q6h (50% acute dose).

- **Alternative regimen:** Pyrimethamine 25-50 mg/day PO + leucovorin 10-25 mg qd + clindamycin 300-400 mg PO q6h-q8h (50% acute dose); atovaquone 750 mg PO q 6-12 h ± pyrimethamine 25 mg PO qd + leukovorin 10 mg qd.

- **Comments**
  - Regimens with established efficacy: Pyrimethamine plus sulfadiazine or clindamycin.
  - PCP prophylaxis: Pyrimethamine-sulfadiazine, TMP-SMX, and atovaquone + pyrimethamine provide effective PCP prophylaxis, pyrimethamine-clindamycin does not.

IMMUNE RECONSTITUTION: Discontinue maintenance therapy when CD4 count >200 cells/mm³ x 6 months, initial therapy completed + asymptomatic.

PROPHYLAXIS: See p. 52

RESPONSE: Clinical response expected in 1 week in 60% to 80% and MRI response expected in 2 weeks. Failure to achieve these goals should prompt consideration of alternative diagnosis, especially primary CNS lymphoma, tuberculous, or brain abscess.

Treponema pallidum

Syphilis (*MMWR* 2002;51[RR-6]; *MMWR* 2004;53(RR-15):27)

PRESENTATION

- **Stages**
  - □ Primary: genital ulcer
  - □ Secondary (2 to 8 weeks): macular, papular or maculopapular rash that is generalized including palms and soles, generalized lymphadenopathy ± constitutional symptoms or aseptic meningitis
  - □ Tertiary: Cardiac, neurologic, ocular, auditory or gummatous
  - □ Latent: Early latent <1 year; late latent >1 year or duration unknown

- **Diagnosis: Primary syphilis** – darkfield and DFA test of exudate. **Late syphilis** (secondary, tertiary and latent) – non-treponemal test (VDRL or RPR) + treponemal test (FTA-ABS). Non-treponemal test titers correlate with disease activity. The RPR and VDRL responses may be atypical with HIV infection, but treponemal tests appear no different in persons with and without HIV infection. Changes in RPR or VDRL titers are significant if ≥4-fold. The diagnosis of **neurosyphilis** is made by CSF exam that shows mononuclear pleocytosis (10-200 WBC/mL), mild elevation of protein, and/or positive VDRL. The CSF VDRL is specific but not sensitive; the CSF FTA-ABS is sensitive but not specific. There is often great difficulty in establishing this diagnosis due to the high rate of false negative CSF VDRLs and the pleocytosis (5-15 monos/mL) that can be attributed to HIV, especially when the CD4 count is >500/mm³. If neurosyphilis cannot be excluded, the patient should be treated for it (*MMWR* 2004;53[RR-15]:28).

INDICATIONS FOR LP: (1) Neurologic, ocular or auditory signs or symptoms; (2) treatment failure; (3) late latent syphilis; and (4) non-penicillin treatment for VDRL/RPR titer ≥1:32. Some authorities recommend LP in all patients with HIV infection and latent syphilis.

TREATMENT: Similar to that for syphilis in patients without HIV, but closer follow-up is required to detect treatment failure or disease progression.

6 Management of Infections

- **Preferred regimens**
  - Primary, secondary, and early latent syphilis (<1 year): Benzathine penicillin G 2.4 mil units IM x 1.
  - **Late latent syphilis** (>1 year or unknown duration): Benzathine penicillin G 2.4 mil units IM weekly x 3.
  - **Neurosyphilis:** Aqueous penicillin G, 18-24 mil units/day IV x 10 to 14 days (3-4 mil units q4h) or continuous infusion ± benzathine penicillin G 3 mil units q wk x 3 after IV course.
  - **Tertiary syphilis:** Consult an expert.
- **Alternative regimens** (*MMWR* 2004;53[RR-15]:96)**:**

  Early stage: Primary, secondary and early latent – each with close clinical monitoring
  - Doxycycline 100 mg PO bid x 14 days
  - Ceftriaxone 1 gm IM or IV qd x 8-10 days
  - Azithromycin 2 gm PO x 1 dose (*N Engl J Med* 2005;353:1236)

  Late – latent without CNS involvement
  - Doxycycline 100 mg PO bid x 28 days

  Neurosyphilis:
  - Procaine penicillin 2.4M U qd + probenecid 500 mg PO qid x 10-14 days ± benzathine penicillin G 2.4M U IM weekly x 3 weeks after completion or procaine penicillin (note: probenecid is not recommended for patients with a history of sulfa allergy)
  - Penicillin allergy: Ceftriaxone 2 gm IM or IV qd x 10-14 days; desensitization to penicillin may be preferred (see Table 6-5, p.385)
- **Comment:** All patients should be evaluated for ocular and CNS involvement. If either is positive, then LP to obtain CSF is needed to rule out CNS disease.

■ TABLE 6-4: **Treatment of Syphilis in Patients with HIV Infection**

Form	Treatment	Follow-up VDRL/RPR	Expectation	Management
Primary	Benz pcu 2.4 mil IM x 1	Month 3, 6, 9, 12, and 24	1) 4x decrease by 6-12 mo; 2) sustained 4x decrease + 3) absence of clinical evidence of syphilis	Benz pen 2.4 mil IM x 3 (if LP negative)
Secondary	Benz pcu 2.4 mil IM x 1	Month 3, 6, 9, 12, and 24	1) 4x decrease by 6-12 mo; 2) sustained 4x decrease + 3) absence of clinical evidence of syphilis	As above
Early latent	Benz pcu 2.4 mil IM x 1	Month 3, 6, 9, 12, and 24	1) 4x decrease by 6-12 mo; 2) sustained 4x decrease + 3) absence of clinical evidence of syphilis	Retreat if neg LP
Late latent	Benz pcu 2.4 mil IM weekly x 3	Month 3, 6, 9, 12, and 24	4x decrease in titer in 6-12 mo	■ CSF exam if 1) clinical evidence of syphilis, 2) 4x increase in serum titer, or 3) lack of 4x decrease at 6-12 mo. ■ Retreat or treat for neurosyphilis if CSF positive*
Neuro-syphilis	Ag pcu 12-24 mil u/d x 10-14 d ± benzathine penicillin G 3 mil u/wk IM x 3	Repeat CSF exam at 3 mo and 6 mo after treatment, than q 6 mo until CSF WBC is normal and CSF-VDRL is negative.	CSF WBC ↓ at 6 months and CSF normal 12	Consider re-treatment for neurosyphilis if CSF WBC not decreased at 6 mo post-treatment* or if CSF-VDRL is positive 2 yrs post-treatment

*CSF WBC (attributed to syphilis) not decreased at 6 months; CSF changes positive at 2 years; persistent signs or symptoms of neurosyphilis; VDRL titer in CSF increased ≥4x at 6 months or titer ≥1:16 fails to decrease 2x at 6 months or 4x at 12 months.

6 Management of Infections

■ TABLE 6-5: **Penicillin Allergy Skin Test and Desensitization** (*MMWR* 2002;51[RR-6]:28)

Penicillin Skin Test:

- Reagents: Benzylpenicilloyd poly-L-lysine (*Pre-Pen*) + minor determinant if available. If minor determinants is not available, use *Pre-Pen* only.
- Positive control for epicutaneous test is commercial histamine (1 mg/mL).
- Negative control is diluent, usually saline.
- Sequence: Epicutaneous test → Positive (wheal >4 mm at 15 min) = penicillin allergy; negative histamine control + negative prick test = unreliable; positive histamine test + negative prick test = do intradermal test.
- Epicutaneous (prick) test: Drops on forearm pierced with #26 needle without blood wheal >4 mm at 15 min is positive.
- Intradermal test: 0.02 mL intradermal injection forearm with #26 or #27 needle; at 15 min a wheal >2 mm larger than negative controls and the initial wheal = positive

Desensitization:

- Indication: Positive skin test.
- Route: Oral or IV; oral is safer and easier.
- Site: Hospital setting.
- Time: Requires 4 hours.
- Schedule: Administer every 15 minutes using the following amount in 30 mL aliquots for oral administration.

Dose	Units/mL	mL	Units	Dose	Units/mL	mL	Units
1	1,000	.10	100	8	10,000	1.20	12,000
2	1,000	.20	200	9	10,000	2.40	24,000
3	1,000	.04	400	10	10,000	4.80	48,000
4	1,000	.80	800	11	80,000	1.00	80,000
5	1,000	1.60	1,600	12	80,000	2.00	160,000
6	1,000	3.20	3,200	13	80,000	4.00	320,000
7	1,000	6.40	6,400	14	80,000	8.00	640,000

7 | Systems Review
(Complications are listed by organ system)

Cardiopulmonary Complications

Dilated Cardiomyopathy (*N Engl J Med* 1998;339:1153)

CAUSE: Unknown, but hypotheses include: 1) mitochondrial toxicity from AZT (*Ann Intern Med 1992*;116:311; *Cardiovasc Res* 2003;60:147; *Clin Infect Dis* 2003;37:109; *J Acquir Immune Defic Syndr* 2004;37:S30), 2) HIV infection of myocardial cells (*N Engl J Med* 1998;339:1093), 3) L-carnitine deficiency (*AIDS* 1992;6:203), and 4) selenium deficiency (*J Parenteral Ent Nutr* 1991;15:347).

FREQUENCY: 6% to 8% for symptomatic cardiomyopathy in longitudinal studies (*Eur Heart J* 1992;13:1452; *Clin Immunol Immunopathol* 1993;68:234). Rates of left ventricular diastolic dysfunction with routine echo are much higher and correlate with stage of immunosuppression (*Heart* 1998;80:184).

SYMPTOMS: CHF, arrhythmias, cyanosis, and/or syncope

DIAGNOSIS: Echocardiogram showing ejection fraction <50% normal ± arrhythmias on EKG, not otherwise explained.

TREATMENT (*Am J Cardiol* 1999;83:1A)

- **HAART**
- **ACE inhibitor:** Enalapril 2.5 mg bid; titrate up to 20 mg bid. Alternatives: Captopril 6.25 mg tid up to 50 mg tid or lisinopril 10 mg/day titrated up to 40 mg/day
- **Persistent symptoms:** Add diuretic: hydrochlorothiazide 25-50 mg/day, furosemide 10-40 mg/day (up to 240 mg bid) or spirolactone 25 mg/day (up to 50 mg bid)
- **Refractory:** Consider digoxin 0.125-0.25 mg/day
- **Other options:** Treat hypertension, treat hyperlipidemia, discontinue EtOH, discontinue cocaine, discontinue AZT; some recommend supplemental carnitine, and/or selenium if deficient.

Cardiovascular disease associated with antiretroviral agents (See p. 106 and Table 4-25, p. 108)

Pulmonary Hypertension (see *Adv Cardiol* 2003;40:197)

CAUSE: Suspected cause is HHV-8 (*N Engl J Med* 2003;349:1113)

FREQUENCY: Infrequent, does not correlate well with CD4 count. Histology is similar to primary pulmonary hypertension.

SYMPTOMS: Major symptom is exertional dyspnea. Other symptoms are exertional chest pain, syncope, cough, hemoptysis, and fatigue.

DIAGNOSIS: X-ray shows enlarged pulmonary trunk or central pulmonary vessels (early), massive right ventricular and right atrial enlargement (late). Echo shows dilated right atrium and ventricle ± tricuspid insufficiency. Doppler echo shows pulmonary arterial systolic BP >30 mm Hg. The best test is cardiac catheterization to show increased pulmonary artery pressure, increased right atrial pressure, and normal pulmonary capillary pressure. Lung scan and pulmonary function tests are normal.

TREATMENT (usually progressive despite treatment)

- **HAART:** Some reports show improvement with HAART (*Clin Infect Dis* 2004;38:1178), but others dispute this (*Clin Infect Dis* 2004;39:1549).
- **Epoprostenol** (*Angiology* 2000;162:1846; *Am J Respir Crit Care Med* 2003;167:1433)
- **Diuretics**
- **Oral anticoagulant**
- **Sildenafil** 25 mg/day. Increase by 25 mg every 3 to 4 days up to 25 mg qid (*AIDS* 2001;15:1747; *AIDS* 2002;16:1568; *N Engl J Med* 2000;343:1342). Note drug interactions with antiretroviral agents.
- **Antiviral therapy:** HHV-8 is possible causative agent, but role of antiviral agents active against that virus (ganciclovir, foscarnet and ciclofovir) is not clear. These drugs do not appear to alter the natural history of Kaposi's sarcoma, which is also caused by HHV-8 (*J Acquir Immune Defic Syndr* 1999;20:34)

Tricuspid Valve Endocarditis

CAUSE: Risk is injection drug use (IDU) caused by *S. aureus* in 50% to 70% (see p. 32); streptococci in 20%

FREQUENCY: A longitudinal study of 2529 IDUs followed for 16,469 patient-years showed an endocarditis rate 4-fold higher with HIV infection (13.8/1000 patient-years vs 3.3/1000 patient-years) (*J Infect Dis* 2002;185:1761).

SYMPTOMS: Fever, dyspnea, weight loss

DIAGNOSIS: Duke criteria: Definite = 2 major, 1 major and 3 minor, or 5 minor. Possible = 1 major and 1 minor, or 3 minor (*Am J Med* 1994;96:200; *Clin Infect Dis* 2000;30:L33).

Systems Review

- **Major:** 1) Positive blood culture for likely agent from ≥2 sticks or persistent bacteremia and 2) Endocardial involvement by echo or new murmur of valve regurgitation.
- **Minor:** 1) IDU or other predisposing cause; 2) fever >38°C; 3) vascular phenomena; 4) immunologic phenomena; 5) bacteremia not meeting major criteria; and 6) echo positive but not diagnostic (*Am J Med* 1994;96:200).

TREATMENT

- **Nafcillin** 12 gm IV/day x 4 weeks plus tobramycin 1 mg/kg q8h x 3 to 5 days (*Ann Intern Med* 1988;109:619; *Eur J Clin Microbiol Infect Dis* 1994;13:559). Note: The 2-week nafcillin/tobramycin course is advocated for uncomplicated *S. aureus* tricuspid valve endocarditis in IDUs but should not be used for patients with HIV infection.
- **Vancomycin** 1 gm IV q12h x 4 weeks plus tobramycin 1 mg/kg q8h x 3 to 5 days. (Preferred to betalactam only for MRSA or if major contraindication to betalactams).
- **Surgery:** Valve replacement in HIV-infected patients shows low operative risk, but poor long-term outcome when associated with IDU (*Ann Thorac Surg* 2003;76:478).

DERMATOLOGIC COMPLICATIONS

Bacillary Angiomatosis (*Arch Intern Med* 1994;154:524; *Dermatology* 2000;21:326; Clin Infect Dis 2005;40:S154) (See p. 330)

CAUSE: *Bartonella henselae* and *B. quintana*. Both cause cutaneous lesions that do not differ in appearance, histopathologic findings, or treatment, although organ trophism differs.

PRESENTATION: Papular, nodular, pedunculated, and verrucous forms. Lesions usually start as red or purple papules that gradually expand to nodules or pedunculated masses. They appear vascular and may bleed extensively with trauma. There is usually one or several lesions, but there may be hundreds.

DIFFERENTIAL: Kaposi's sarcoma, cherry angioma, hemangioma, pyogenic granuloma, dermatofibroma.

DIAGNOSIS: Skin biopsy shows lobular vascular proliferation with inflammation; Warthin Starry silver stain shows typical organisms as small black clusters. Serology is available (IFA and EIA); IFA titers >1:256 usually indicates active infection.

TREATMENT (see p. 330)

Candidiasis, Cutaneous (*Clin Infect Dis* 2000;30:652)

CAUSE: Superficial infection of skin/mucous membranes, usually by *C. albicans*.

PRESENTATION (SKIN): Moist, beefy red with scaling and satellite papules. Variations: Intertrigo, balanitis, glossitis, angular cheilitis, paronychia, nail dystrophies.

DIAGNOSIS: Usually clinical; KOH prep or fresh mount shows pseudohyphae.

TREATMENT

- **Topical:** Ketoconazole, miconazole, clotrimazole, econazole, or nystatin – all bid.
- **Systemic:** Ketoconazole (200-400 mg PO qd) or fluconazole (100-200 mg PO qd).

Cryptococcosis (*Clin Infect Dis* 2000;30:652)

CAUSE: Disseminated cryptococcosis, usually from a pulmonary portal of entry

PRESENTATION: Nodular, papular, follicular, or ulcerative skin lesions; may resemble molluscum. Usual locations are face, neck, scalp.

DIAGNOSIS: Serum cryptococcal antigen assay is usually positive. Skin biopsy with Gomori methenamine silver stain shows typical encapsulated, budding yeast, and positive culture. Perform LP in any patient with a positive serum cryptococcal antigen or culture for *C. neoformans*.

TREATMENT: If negative LP, fluconazole 400 mg/day PO x 8 weeks, then 200 mg/day. If positive LP, see pp. 310-311.

Dermatophytic Infections

DEFINITION: Fungal infection of skin, hair, and nails

CAUSE: *Tinia rubrum, T. mentagrophytes, M. canis, E. floccosum, T. tonsurans, T. verrucosum, T. soudanense* (*Candida* causes typical nail and skin lesions), *Malassezia furfur* causes tinea versicolor. (Note: *Candida* and *M. furfur* are not dermatophytes.)

PRESENTATION

- ***T. pedis:*** Interdigital pruritis, scaling, fissures and maceration. Concomitant nail dystrophies seen frequently. Plantar and moccasin variants seen ± interdigital involvement. Pruritic, red lesions between toes ± interdigital fissures, extension to adjacent skin and nails, scaling is always present.

- **Onychomycosis:** Starts with discoloration and thickening, usually on distal nail at one side and spreads toward the other side and toward the cuticle, leaving heaped up keratinous debris.
- ***T. corporis:*** Circular erythematous scaling that spreads with central clearing (ringworm).
- ***T. cruris:*** Red scaly patch on inner thigh with sharply demarcated borders.

FORMS: Tinea corporis (ringworm), tinea cruris (jock itch), tinea pedis (athlete's foot), tinea unguium or onychomycosis (nail involvement), and tinea captis (ringworm of scalp)

DIAGNOSIS: Scrapings of skin lesion or discolored nail bed for KOH preparation. This may be supplemented with culture of scraping on Sabouraud's medium.

TREATMENT

- **Onychomycosis:** Topical therapy is usually not effective.
  - □ Preferred treatment: Terbinafine (*Lamisil*) 250 mg/day x 8 weeks (fingernails) or 12 weeks (toenails). Terbinafine is also hepatotoxic and is expensive but has better long term results than itraconazole (*Brit J Dermatol* 1999;141[Suppl 56]:15).
  - □ Itraconazole (*Sporanox*) "pulse therapy," 400 mg/day for 1 week/month x 2 months (fingernails) or x 3 months (toenails). Main concerns are hepatotoxicity, drug interactions, cardiotoxicity, and cost of treating a benign infection.
- ***Tinea corporis, tinea cruris, tinea pedis:*** Topical agent for 2 weeks (*T. cruris*) to 4 weeks (*T. pedis*):
  - □ Clotrimazole (*Lotrimin*)* 1% cream or lotion bid
  - □ Econazole (*Spectazole*) 1% cream qd or bid
  - □ Ketoconazole (*Nizoral*) 2% cream qd
  - □ Miconazole (*Monostat-Derm*)* 2% cream bid
  - □ Butenafine (*Mentax*) 1% cream
  - □ Terbinafine (*Lamisil*)* 1% cream or gel qd or bid
  - □ Tolnaftate (*Tinactin*)* 1% cream, gel, powder, solution, or aerosol bid

  ---
  * Available over-the-counter.

- **Refractory, chronic, or extensive disease:** Terbinafine 250 mg qd x 2 to 4 weeks; itraconazole 100-200 mg qd x 2 to 4 weeks. Griseofulvin microsized 250-500 mg bid. Griseofulvin should be last of treatment options.

Drug Eruptions

CAUSE: Most common are antibiotics, especially sulfonamides (TMP/SMX, FPV, TPV), beta-lactams, anticonvulsants, NNRTIs.

7 Systems Review

PRESENTATION: Most common – morbilliform, exanthematous, usually pruritic ± low grade fever; usually within 2 weeks of new drug and days of re-exposure. Less common and more severe forms:

- Urticaria: Intensely pruritic, edematous and circumscribed
- Anaphylaxis: Laryngeal edema, nausea, vomiting ± shock
- Hypersensitivity syndrome: Severe reaction with rash and fever ± hepatitis, arthralgias, lymphadenopathy, and hematologic changes with eosinophilia and atypical lymphocytes, usually at 2 to 6 weeks after drug is started (*N Engl J Med* 1994;331:1272). See abacavir (p. 137) and nevirapine (p. 260)
- Stevens-Johnson syndrome: Fever, erosive stomatitis, disseminated erosions ± blisters dark red macules, ocular involvement; mortality – 5%
- Toxic epidermal necrolysis: Epidermal necrosis with scalded skin appearance ± mucous membrane involvement; mortality – 50% (*N Engl J Med* 1994;331:1272)

TREATMENT: In severe and very symptomatic reactions, discontinue implicated agent (for TMP-SMX, see p. 315)

- Pruritic uncomplicated drug rashes: antihistamines, topical antipruritics, and topical corticosteroids
- Stevens-Johnson Syndrome and toxic epidermal necrolysis: Severe cases are managed as burns with supportive care; corticosteroids are not indicated (*Cutis* 1996;57:223).

Folliculitis

CAUSE: Bacterial folliculitis due to *Staphylococcus aureus* is most common. Other causes include *Pityrosporum ovale* (intrafollicular yeast), *Demodex folliculorum* (intrafollicular mite), and eosinophilic folliculitis, in which biopsy shows eosinophilic inflammation without a detectable infectious agent.

PRESENTATION: Follicular papules and pustules on face, trunk, and extremities; usually very pruritic causing excoriations; multiple exacerbations and spontaneous remissions; usually seen with CD4 counts 50-250 cells/mm³. Folliculitis may reactivate with immune reconstitution.

DIAGNOSIS: Clinical presentation and biopsy: follicular inflammation ± follicular destruction and abscess formation. Special stains such as PASD and B+B may show infectious agent. Multiple eosinophils destroying the hair follicle wall and eosinophilic abscesses are seen in eosinophilic folliculitis. Culture of pustule may grow *S. aureus*.

TREATMENT: Varies according to the etiologic agent involved.

- *S. aureus*: Topical erythromycin or clindamycin or systemic anti-staphylococcal antibiotic
- *P. ovale*: Topical or systemic antifungal agents
- *D. folliculorum*: Permethrin cream or topical metronidazole
- Eosinophilic: Topical steroids, phototherapy with UVB and/or PUVA (*N Engl J Med* 1988;318:1183; *Arch Dermatol* 1995;131:360)
- General: Antihistamines (high dose, mixed classes together) for symptomatic relief

Herpes Simplex (Clin Infect Dis 2005;40:S167) (see p. 347)

Herpes Zoster (see p. 349)

Kaposi's Sarcoma (KS) (see p. 420)

Prurigo Nodularis (*Int J Dermatol* 1999;37:401)

FREQUENCY: Common usually with CD4 <200 cells/mm^3

CAUSE: A report from Uganda based on skin biopsies concluded most were due to arthroped bites; the authors suggested a name change to "arthropod-induced) prurigo of HIV" (*JAMA* 2004;292:2614).

PRESENTATION: Hyperpigmented, hyperkeratotic, often excoriated papules and nodules up to 1 cm; 90% are above nipple line. Major symptom is severe pruritus. Usually associated with other signs of chronic pruritus or excoriations, including lichen simplex chronicus, patches of hyperpigmentation, linear erosions, ulcerations, and scars.

DIFFERENTIAL: Warts, traumatized folliculitis, deep fungal infections, perforating diseases

DIAGNOSIS: Clinical features; biopsy may be necessary. This typically shows dense perivascular and interstitial infiltrates with eosinophilis (*JAMA* 2004;292:2614).

TREATMENT: Must interrupt vicious cycle: Pruritus → scratch trauma → lichenification → increased pruritus. Treat with high-potency topical steroids under occlusive dressing. May benefit from oral anti-histamines or phototherapy. Refractory cases may benefit from 100 mg/d thalidomide (*Arch Dermatol* 2004;140:845).

Scabies (*MMWR* 2002;51[RR-6]:68)

CAUSE: *Sarcoptes scabiei* (mite)

PRESENTATION: Small red papules that are intensely pruritic, especially at night. Sometimes presentation is the "burrow," a 3- to 15-mm line which represents the superficial tunnel the female mite digs at 2 mm/day to lay eggs. Usual locations are the interdigital webs of the

7 Systems Review

fingers, volar aspect of the wrist, periumbilical area, axilla, thighs, buttocks, genitalia, feet, and breasts. Scabies crostosus (crusted or "Norwegian" scabies) is a severe form seen in compromised hosts, including AIDS patients. There is uncontrolled spread to involve large areas, sometimes the total skin surface with scales and crusts that show thousands of mites.

DIAGNOSIS: The mite is 0.4 x 0.3 mm, 8-legged, and shaped like a turtle. It is visible to the naked eye but burrowing precludes detection. Scrape infected area, place on a slide with a coverslip, and examine under 10x magnification to demonstrate mites or eggs.

TREATMENT: All family members and close contacts must be treated at the same time.

- **Permethrin cream** (5%) (*Elimite*) applied to total body, neck down, and washed off at 8 to 14 hours. Re-treat at 1 to 2 weeks. All household members must be treated simultaneously even if asymptomatic. A 30 g tube of *Elimite* is usually adequate for an adult.

- **Lindane** (1%) (*Kwell*) 1 oz lotion or 30 g cream applied as a thin layer to total body, neck down, and washed off at 8 hours is an alternative. Lindane is less expensive than *Elimite*, but there is rare resistance and more side effects.

- **Ivermectin** (*Stromectol*) 200 µg/kg PO repeated at 2 weeks (*N Engl J Med* 1995;333:26). Not recommended as first line treatment in uncomplicated cases.

- Rash and pruritus may persist up to 2 weeks post-treatment – warn patients.

- Bedding and clothing must be decontaminated; machine wash in hot water and machine dry with high heat, or dry clean.

- **Itching:** Hydroxyzine (*Atarax*) or diphenhydramine (*Benadryl*)

- **Scabies crustosus (crusted or "Norwegian" scabies):** Isolate immediately and use strict barrier precautions. Treat with ivermectin 200 µg/kg PO followed by a second dose 1 to 2 weeks later, plus permethrin topically until scales and crust have resolved. Topical karolytics such as salicylic acid gel or urea creams are also recommended.

Seborrheic Dermatitis

CAUSE: The yeast *Pityrosporum* is recovered from lesions, but it may not play a central role in HIV-associated seborrhea (*J Am Acad Dermatol* 1992;27:37).

PRESENTATION: Erythematous plaques with greasy scales and indistinct margins on scalp, central face, post auricular area, presternal, axillary, and occasionally pubic area

DIFFERENTIAL: Psoriasis and dermatophytic infections

DIAGNOSIS: Clinical features

TREATMENT

- **Topical steroid:** Mid-potency such as triamcinolone 0.1% or weaker (desonide 0.05%), hydrocortisone 2.5% for the face ± ketoconazole 2% cream applied twice per day for the duration of the flare only.
- **Shampoos:** Tar-based (*Z-tar, Pentrax, DHS tar, T-gel, Ionil T plus*), selenium sulfide (*Selsun, Exelderm*), or zinc pyrithione (*Head & Shoulders, Zincon, DHS zinc*) applied daily, or ketoconazole shampoo applied twice per week.

GASTROINTESTINAL COMPLICATIONS

Anorexia, Nausea, Vomiting

MAJOR CAUSES: Medications (especially antiretrovirals, antibiotics, opiates, and NSAIDs), depression, intracranial pathology, GI disease, hypogonadism, pregnancy, lactic acidosis, acute gastroenteritis

HAART: Nausea ± vomiting and/or abdominal pain are reported in 2% to 17% of patients given PIs (*J Acquir Immune Defic Syndr* 2004;37:1111). The most common agents, in rank order, are RTV, IDV, LPV/r, TPV/r, FPV, ATV, and SQV. The effect is dose-related. Similar symptoms are frequent with AZT.

EVALUATION: Lactic acid level, morning testosterone level, GI evaluation (endoscopy, CT scan), intracranial evaluation (head CT scan or MRI). Interruption of antiretroviral regimen or single-drug switch may be necessary.

TREATMENT: Treat underlying condition.

- **Anorexia**
  - Megestrol (*Megace*).400-800 mg qd. Weight gain is mostly fat. May decrease testosterone level or increase blood sugar. Consider megestrol + testosterone.
  - Dronabinol (*Marinol*) 2.5 mg PO bid; active ingredient of marijuana. Weight gain is mostly fat.
- **Nausea and vomiting**
  - Prochlorperazine (*Compazine*) 5-10 mg PO q6h-q8h; trimethobenzamide (*Tigan*) 250 mg PO q6h-q8h; metoclopramide (*Reglan*) 5-10 mg PO q6-8h; dimenhydrinate (*Dramamine*) 50 mg PO q6h-q8h; lorazapam (*Ativan*) 0.025-0.05 mg/kg IV or IM; haloperidol (*Haldol*) 1-5 mg bid PO or IM; dronabinol 2.5-5 mg PO bid; ondansetron (*Zofran*) 0.2 mg/kg IV or IM.
  - Note: Phenothiazines (*Compazine, Haldol, Tigan*, and *Reglan*) may cause dystonia. *Zofran* efficacy is established only for cancer chemotherapy and costs $16.64/4 mg. Metoclopramine is preferable to dimenhydrinate (ovazepam and ondansetron.

7 Systems Review

□ PEG: May require percutaneous endoscopic gastrostomy (PEG) to deliver nutrition and medications, including HAART regimen.

Aphthous Ulcers

CAUSE: Unknown

DIFFERENTIAL: HSV, CMV, drug-induced ulcers; biopsy recommended for non-healing ulcers.

CLASSIFICATION

- **Minor:** <1 cm diameter, usually self-limiting (with healing in 10 to 14 days)
- **Major:** >1 cm, deep, prolonged, heals slowly, causes pain, and may prevent oral intake (*AIDS* 1992;6:963; *Oral Surg Oral Med Oral Pathol* 1996;81:141)

TREATMENT

- **Topical treatment 2x to 4x/day**
  - □ Lidocaine solution before meals
  - □ Triamcinolone hexacetonide in *Orabase*
  - □ Fluocinonide gel (*Lidex*) 0.05% ointment mixed 1:1 with *Orabase* or covered with *Orabase*
  - □ Amlexanox (*Aphthasol*) 5% oral paste (*J Oral Maxillofac Surg* 1993;51:243)
- **Oral and intralesional therapy (refractory cases)**
  - □ Prednisone 40 mg/day PO x 1 to 2 weeks then taper (*Am J Clin Dermatol* 2003;4:669)
  - □ Colchicine 1.5 mg/day (*J Am Acad Dermatol* 1994;31:459)
  - □ Dapsone 100 mg/day
  - □ Pentoxifylline (*Trental*) 400 mg PO tid with meals
  - □ Thalidomide 200 mg/day PO x 4 to 6 weeks ± maintenance with 200 mg 2x/week. Note: Thalidomide is "experimental" for aphthous ulcers. See p. 310 for purchase instructions. Thalidomide has strict requirements for use, but is very effective (*N Engl J Med* 1997;337:1086; *Clin Infect Dis* 1995;20:250; *J Infect Dis* 1999;180:61; *Arch Dermatol* 1990;126:923).

Candidiasis, Oropharygeal (thrush) (see p. 331)

Systems Review

Diarrhea, Acute

(Acute diarrhea defined as ≥3 loose or watery stools for 3 to 10 days)

DIAGNOSTIC EVALUATION

Medication-related

- Main antiretroviral agents: All PIs, especially nelfinavir, lopinavir/ritonavir, saquinavir, and didanosine (buffered formulation)
- Management (*Clin Infect Dis* 2000;30:908)
  - □ Loperamide 4 mg, then 2 mg every loose stool, up to 16/day
  - □ Calcium 500 mg bid; psyllium 1 tsp qd-bid or 2 bars qd-bid; oat bran 1500 mg bid
  - □ Pancreatic enzymes 1-2 tabs with meals

Pathogen detection (*Clin Infect Dis* 2001;32:331; *Arch Pathol Lab Med* 2001;125:1042)

- Blood culture: MAC, *Salmonella*
- Stool culture: *Salmonella, Shigella, C. jejuni, Vibrio, Yersinia, E. coli* 0157
- Stool assay for *C. difficile* toxin A and B
- O&P examination + modified acid fast stain (*Cryptosporidia, Cyclospora, Isospora*), trichrome or other stain for microsporidia, and antigen detection (*Giardia*)

Radiology

- Plain X-rays and contrast X-ray: usually not helpful
- CT scan: most helpful with pseudomembranous colitis, CMV colitis, and lymphoma

Endoscopy: Most useful for CMV, Kaposi's sarcoma, and lymphoma

CAMPYLOBACTER JEJUNI

FREQUENCY: 4% to 8% of HIV-infected patients with acute diarrhea; rates are increased up to 39-fold in MSM (*Clin Infect Dis* 1997;24:1107; *Clin Infect Dis* 1998;26:91; *Clin Infect Dis* 2005;40:S152)

CLINICAL FEATURES: Watery diarrhea or bloody flux, fever, fecal leukocytes variable; any CD4 count

DIAGNOSIS: Stool culture; most laboratories cannot detect *C. cinaedi, C. fennelli*, etc.

TREATMENT (*Clin Infect Dis* 2001;32:331): Erythromycin 500 mg PO qid x 5 days; fluoroquinolone resistance rates are >20%.

7 Systems Review

CLOSTRIDIUM DIFFICILE

FREQUENCY: Up to 36% of HIV-infected patients with acute diarrhea (*Diag Microbiol Infect Dis* 2002;44:325)

CLINICAL FEATURES: Watery diarrhea, fecal WBCs variable; fever, hypoalbuminemia, and leukocytosis are common. Nearly all patients have recent (within 2 week of onset) exposure to antibacterial agents, especially clindamycin, ampicillin, and cephalosporins; less commonly – macrolides, fluoroquinolones, TMP-SMX, and rifampin. Antiretrovirals, antivirals, antifungals, dapsone and INH are not implicated. May occur with any CD4 count; low CD4 count is not clearly associated with increased risk of this complication or with more severe disease.

DIAGNOSIS

- Stool toxin assay: Tissue culture or EIA preferred (may need to repeat toxin assay)
- Endoscopy: pseudomembranous colitis (PMC), colitis, or normal (this procedure is not usually indicated)
- CT scan: Colitis with thickened mucosa

TREATMENT (*N Engl J Med* 2002;346:334)

- Metronidazole 250 mg PO qid or 500 mg PO tid x 10 to 14 days (preferred)
- Vancomycin 125 mg PO qid x 10 to 14 days
- Antiperistaltic agents such as loperamide (*Imodium*) or atropine/diphenoxylate (*Lomotil*) are contraindicated.

RESPONSE: Fever usually resolves within 24 hours and diarrhea resolves in an average of 5 days. About 20% to 25% have relapses at 3 to 14 days after treatment stopped. Virtually all respond to treatment unless ileus is present; relapse post therapy in 15% to 20% (*N Engl J Med* 2002;346:334).

Recent reports indicate a possibly more virulent strain of *C. difficile* that produces more severe disease, is associated with major complications (toxic megacolon, requirement for colectomy, death), and is relatively refractory to treatment (*Clin Infect Dis* 2005;40:1591; *CMAJ* 2004;171:466). There is no evidence this is more or less common with HIV infection. Oral vancomycin is preferred in severe cases.

ENTERIC VIRUSES

FREQUENCY: 15% to 30% of HIV infected patients with acute diarrhea

CLINICAL FEATURES: Watery diarrhea, acute, but one-third become chronic; any CD4 cell count

DIAGNOSIS: Major agents: adenovirus, astrovirus, picornavirus, calicivirus (*N Engl J Med* 1993;329:14); clinical laboratories cannot detect these viruses.

TREATMENT: Supportive treatment with fluids and antiperistaltic agents.

ESCHERICHIA COLI

■ TABLE 7-1: *E. coli* **Strains and Treatment**

Agent	Clinical Presentation	Treatment
Enterotoxigenic (ETEC)	Traveler's diarrhea	■ Ciprofloxacin 500 mg bid x 3 days ■ TMP-SMX DS bid x 3 days
Enterohemorrhagic 0157:H7 (EHEC)*	Bloody diarrhea	Antibiotics contraindicated
Enteroinvasive (EIEC)	Dysentery	■ Ciprofloxacin 500 mg bid x 5 days ■ TMP-SMX DS bid x 5 days
Enteropathic (EPEC)	Watery diarrhea	Usually no antibiotic or Ciprofloxacin 500 mg bid x 3 days

* Only *E. coli* that can be detected with stool analysis in most labs.

SALMONELLA (See p. 375)

FREQUENCY: 5% to 15% of HIV infected patients with acute diarrhea

CLINICAL FEATURES: Watery diarrhea, fever, fecal WBCs variable; any CD4 count

DIAGNOSIS: Stool culture, blood culture

TREATMENT (See p. 375)

SHIGELLA (*Clin Infect Dis* 2005;40:S152)

FREQUENCY: 1% to 3% of HIV infected patients with acute diarrhea. *Shigella* bacteremia is more common with HIV infection, and HIV-infected patients appear more likely to relapse after treatment (*Scand J Infect Dis* 1994;26:411).

CLINICAL FEATURES: Watery diarrhea or "bloody flux," fever, fecal WBCs common; any CD4 count

DIAGNOSIS: Stool culture

TREATMENT (*Clin Infect Dis* 2001;32:331)

■ Ciprofloxacin 500 mg PO bid x 3-7 days

■ TMP-SMX 1 DS PO bid x 3-7 days (Cases acquired internationally are often resistant to TMP-SMX, and HIV-infected patients often have reactions to this drug, so fluoroquinolones are preferred.)

■ Azithromycin 250 mg PO qd x 5 days

7 Systems Review

IDIOPATHIC

FREQUENCY: 25% to 40% of HIV infected patients with acute diarrhea

CLINICAL FEATURES: Variable noninfectious causes; rule out medications (including lactic acidosis), dietary, irritable bowel syndrome.

DIAGNOSIS: Negative studies including culture, O&P examination, and *C. difficile* toxin assay

EMPIRIC TREATMENT, SEVERE ACUTE IDIOPATHIC DIARRHEA

- Ciprofloxacin 500 mg PO bid
- Ofloxacin 200-300 mg PO bid x 5 days ± metronidazole (*Arch Intern Med* 1990;150:541; *Ann Intern Med* 1992;117:202; *Clin Infect Dis* 2001;32:331).

Diarrhea, Chronic

(AIDS-defining criteria are chronic diarrhea with >2 loose or watery stools/day for ≥30 days.)

CRYPTOSPORIDIA (see p. 339)

FREQUENCY: 10% to 30% of chronic diarrhea in AIDS patients

CLINICAL FEATURES: Enteritis; watery diarrhea; no fecal WBCs; fever variable; malabsorption; wasting; large stool volume with abdominal pain; remitting symptoms for months; CD4 cell count <100/mm³ is associated with recurrent, refractory and/or chronic course. The most important goal is immune reconstitution.

DIAGNOSIS: Modified acid-fast stain of stool to show oocyst of 4-6 µm. Several IFA stains are commercially available but not superior to modified AFB (*Clin Infect Dis* 2003;36:903).

TREATMENT (See p. 339)

CYCLOSPORA

FREQUENCY: <1% of chronic diarrhea in AIDS patients (not uniquely susceptible)

CLINICAL FEATURES: Enteritis; watery diarrhea; CD4 cell count <100/mm³

DIAGNOSIS: Stool acid-fast smear: Resembles *Cryptosporidia*

TREATMENT: TMP-SMX 1 DS bid x 3 days

CYTOMEGALOVIRUS (see p. 341)

FREQUENCY: 15% to 40% of chronic diarrhea in AIDS patients

CLINICAL FEATURES: Colitis and/or enteritis; fecal WBC and/or blood; cramps; fever; watery diarrhea ± blood; may cause perforation;

hemorrhage, toxic megacolon, ulceration; CD4 cell count <50/mm^3

DIAGNOSIS

- Biopsy to show intranuclear inclusion bodies, preferably with inflammation, vasculitis
- CT scan: segmental or pancolitis ± enteritis
- Cannot establish this diagnosis with CMV markers in blood or stool; need biopsy.

TREATMENT (See p. 344)

RESPONSE: Results of antiviral treatment variable (*Ann Intern Med* 1990;112:505; *J Infect Dis* 1993;167:278); foscarnet and ganciclovir are equally effective or ineffective (*J Infect Dis* 1995;172:622). Main result of antiviral therapy is decreased CMV shedding.

ENTAMOEBA HISTOLYTICA

FREQUENCY: 1% to 3% of chronic diarrhea in AIDS patients

CLINICAL FEATURES: Colitis; bloody stools; cramps; no fecal WBCs (bloody stools); most are asymptomatic carriers; any CD4 cell count

DIAGNOSIS: Stool O&P examination. Must distinguish from non-pathogenic *E. dispar*, which is a non-pathogen and most common in positive stool exams (*J Clin Microbiol* 2003;41:5041; *Lancet* 2003;361:1025).

TREATMENT: Metronidazole 500-750 mg PO or IV tid x 5 to 10 days, then iodoquinol 650 mg PO tid x 21 days or paromomycin 500 mg PO qid x 7 days

GIARDIA LAMBLIA

FREQUENCY: 1% to 3% of chronic diarrhea in AIDS patients (not uniquely susceptible)

CLINICAL FEATURES: Enteritis; watery diarrhea ± malabsorption, bloating; flatulence; any CD4 cell count

DIAGNOSIS: Antigen detection

TREATMENT: Metronidazole 250 mg PO tid x 10 days

ISOSPORA BELLI (see p. 353)

MICROSPORIDIA: ENTEROCYTOZOON BIENEUSI OR ENTEROCYTOZOON (SEPTATA) INTESTINALIS (see p. 355)

MYCOBACTERIUM AVIUM COMPLEX (MAC) (see p. 356)

FREQUENCY: 10% to 20% of chronic diarrhea in AIDS patients

7 Systems Review

CLINICAL FEATURES: Enteritis; watery diarrhea; no fecal WBCs; fever and wasting common; diffuse abdominal pain in late stage; CD4 cell count <50/mm^3.

DIAGNOSIS: Positive blood cultures for *M. avium* complex; biopsy may show changes typical of Whipple's disease, but with AFB; CT scan may be supportive: hepatosplenomegaly, adenopathy, and thickened small bowel.

TREATMENT (See p. 356)

RESPONSE: Slow response over several weeks

IDIOPATHIC (PATHOGEN-NEGATIVE)

FREQUENCY: 20% to 30% of chronic diarrhea in AIDS patients who undergo a full diagnostic evaluation including endoscopy

CLINICAL FEATURES: Usually low-volume diarrhea that resolves spontaneously or is controlled with antimotility agents (*Gut* 1995;36:283). Typically not associated with significant weight loss and often resolves spontaneously.

DIAGNOSIS: Biopsy shows villus atrophy, crypt hyperplasia/no identifiable cause despite endoscopy with biopsy and EM for microsporidia (*Clin Infect Dis* 1992;15:726). These histologic changes are unlikely to explain diarrhea because they are seen in symptom-free persons with HIV (*Lancet* 1996;348:379). With pathogen-negative, persistent, large volume diarrhea, must rule out KS and lymphoma.

TREATMENT: Supportive care (frequent small feedings, bland food, avoid caffeine and lactose): atropine/diphenoxylate (*Lomotil*) or loperamide (*Imodium*), nutritional support. Consider gluten-free diet.

Esophagitis

■ TABLE 7-2: **Esophageal Disease in Patients With HIV Infection**

	Candida	Cytomegalovirus (CMV)	Herpes Simplex Virus	Aphthous Ulcers
See also	p. 331	p. 344	p. 347	p. 394
Frequency	50% to 70%	10% to 20%	2% to 5%	10% to 20%
Clinical features				
Dysphagia	+++	+	+	+
Odynophagia	++	+++	+++	+++
Thrush	50% to 70%	<25%	<25%	<25%
Oral ulcers	Rare	Uncommon	Often	Uncommon
Pain	Diffuse	Focal	Focal	Focal
Fever	Infrequent	Often	Infrequent	Infrequent

	Candida	Cytomegalo-virus (CMV)	Herpes Simplex Virus	Aphthous Ulcers
Diagnosis				
Endoscopy	■ Usually treated empirically ■ Pseudo-membranous plaques; may involve entire esophagus	■ Biopsy required for treatment ■ Erythema and erosions/ulcers, single or multiple discrete lesions, often distal.	■ Biopsy required for treatment ■ Erythema and erosions/ulcers, usually small, coalescing, shallow	■ Similar in appearance and location to CMV ulcers
Micro-biology	■ Brush: Yeast and pseudo-mycelium on KOH prep or PAS ■ Culture with sensitivities may be useful with suspected resistance	■ Biopsy: Intra-cellular inclu-sions and/or positive culture. ■ Highest yield with histopath of biopsy and culture. Culture not recommended false positives.	■ Brush/biopsy: Intracyto-plasmic inclusions + multinucleate giant cells, FA stain, and/or positive culture.	■ Negative studies for *Candida*, HSV, CMV, and other diagnoses.
Treatment				
Acute	■ Fluconazole 200 mg/day PO, up to 800 mg/day. ■ Refractory cases: Caspo-fungin 70 mg/day IV x 1 then 50 mg/day or mycofungin 150 mg qd Itraconazole soln 200 mg/day or voriconazole 200 mg PO or IV bid (many drug interactions) ■ Amphotericin 0.5-0.7 mg/kg/day IV	■ Ganciclovir 5 mg/kg IV bid x 2 to 3 weeks or valganciclovir 900 mg bid x 3 weeks, then 900 mg/day (when able to swallow). ■ Foscarnet 40-60 mg/kg q8h x 2 to 3 weeks. ■ HAART ■ Efficacy of antiviral treatment is 75%.	■ Acyclovir 200-800 mg PO 5x/day or 5 mg/kg IV q8h x 2 to 3 weeks or valacyclovir 1 gm PO tid (when able to swallow).	■ Prednisone 40 mg/day PO x 7 to 14 days, then taper 10 mg/week or more slowly. ■ Thalidomide 200 mg/day PO (*BJM* 1989;298: 432; *J Infect Dis* 1999;180:61). ■ Corticosteroids by intralesional injection.
Mainten-ance	■ Fluconazole 100-200 mg/day PO for frequent or severe disease)	■ Maintenance treatment is valgancyclovir recommended with relapsing disease	■ Maintenance treatment is arbitrary; acyclovir 200-400 mg PO 3 to 5x daily.	■ None

Notes:

1. One-third of AIDS patients in pre-HAART era developed esophageal symptoms (*Gut* 1989;30:1033). Esophageal ulcers are usually due to CMV (45%), or they are

idiopathic/aphthous ulcers (40%); HSV accounts for only 5% (*Ann Intern Med* 1995;122:143).

2. With endoscopy a diagnosis is established in about 70% to 95% (*Arch Intern Med* 1991;151:1567). Response to empiric treatment often precludes need for endoscopic diagnosis of *Candida* esophagitis. Yield with barium swallow 20-30%.

3. Other diagnostic considerations: Drug-induced dysphagia (*Am J Med* 1988;88:512), including AZT (*Ann Intern Med* 1990;162:65) and ddC; infection, including *M. avium*, TB, cryptosporidia, *P. carinii*, primary HIV infection, histoplasmosis, and tumor, including KS or lymphoma (*BMJ* 1988;296:92; *Gastrointest Endosc* 1986;32:96).

4. Fluconazole is the preferred treatment for *Candida* because of established efficacy, more predictable absorption, and fewer drug interactions compared with voriconazole, ketoconazole, and itraconazole.

DIFFERENTIAL: Review for non-HIV-related cause, especially if CD4 is >200/mm^3. Most common are esophagitis that is medication- or food-related and GERD. With CD4 <200/mm^3: Common – *Candida*; Less common – HSV, CMV, idiopathic; Rare – TB, *M. avium*, histoplasmosis, PCP, cryptosporidia, Kaposi's sarcoma, lymphoma

Gingivitis

CAUSE: Anaerobic bacteria

PHASES: Linear gingival erythema $\rightarrow$ necrotizing gingivitis $\rightarrow$ necrotizing periodontitis $\rightarrow$ necrotizing stomatitis

■ TABLE 7-3: **Phases of Gingivitis**

Lesion	Location	Clinical Features
Linear gingival erythema	Gingiva	Painless, bright red at gingival margin
Necrotizing gingivitis	Gingiva	Painful, red gingiva, and ulceration
Necrotizing periodontitis	Gingiva and bone	Painful, red gingiva, and loose teeth
Necrotizing stomatitis	Gingiva, bone, and soft tissue	Painful, red gingiva, and removable teeth

TREATMENT

- **Routine dental care:** Brush and floss ± topical antiseptics: *Listerine* swish x 30-60 seconds bid, *Peridex*, etc.

- **Dental consultation:** Curettage and debridement

- **Antibiotics** (necrotizing stomatitis): Metronidazole; alternatives – clindamycin and amoxicillin-clavulanate

Systems Review

LIVER DISEASE

Differential diagnosis of abnormal LFTs in the patient with HIV infection (*JAMA* 2004;292:243)

HEPATITIS

- **HAV:** Acute infection (*Clin Infect Dis* 2001;32:297) (see p. 404)
- **HBV flare** (with HBsAg) (see p. 404):
  1. Discontinuation of TDF, 3TC, FTC (*J Hepatol* 1998;29:306; *J Infect Dis* 2002;186:23)
  2. Resistance of HBV to TDF or more commonly to FTC or 3TC
  3. Immune reconstitution
- HCV (see p. 407):

ALCOHOL TOXICITY OR OTHER SUBSTANCE ABUSE (*J Acquir Immune Defic Syndr* 2001;27:4426)

DRUG TOXICITY: Acetaminophen (*Clin Infect Dis* 2004;38:565), INH, PIs, NNRTIs, statins, etc.

OPPORTUNISTIC INFECTIONS INCLUDING MAC AND CMV (*Am J Gastroenterol* 1988;83:1)

HAART

- Immune reconstitution syndrome (*J Acquir Immune Defic Syndr* 2001;27:426; *Clin Infect Dis* 2004;38:S65) – see p. 419
- NVP hepatitis – see p. 260
- PI/NNRTI transaminitis: 15-30% rate is increased 2-fold with HCV coinfection (*Clin Infect Dis* 2002;34:831; *JAMA* 2000;283:74; *Hepatology* 2002;35:182)
- Steatosis: primarily due to d4T, also AZT and ddI, in association with lactic acidosis; see p. 103.
- Dose modifications of antiretroviral drugs with severe hepatic disease: NRTIs: none; NNRTIs: None; caution with or avoid NVP; PIs: NFV – standard; IDV/r – 200/100 mg bid; LPV/r – may need therapeutic drug monitoring; ATV – 300 mg qd (*Clin Infect Dis* 2004;40:174), but limited clinical data.

Cholangiopathy, AIDS (*Dig Dis* 1998;16:205)

CAUSE: *Cryptosporidium* is the most common identified microbial cause (see p. 295). Other causes: microsporidia, CMV, and *Cyclospora*. About 20% to 40% are idiopathic.

FREQUENCY: Relatively rare and seen primarily in late stage AIDS

PRESENTATION: Right upper quadrant pain, LFTs show cholestasis. Late stage HIV with CD4 count <100 cells/mm^3

7 Systems Review

DIAGNOSIS: ERCP (preferred); ultrasound is 75% to 95% specific

TREATMENT: Based on cause. Treat pathogen when possible – CMV and *Cyclospora*. Usual treatment is mechanical and based on lesion.

- **Papillary stenosis:** ERCP with sphincterectomy for pain relief
- **Cholangiopathy without papillary stenosis:** Ursodeoxycholic acid (*Actigall*) 300 mg PO tid (*Am J Med* 1997;103:70). Experience limited.
- **Isolated bile duct structure:** Endoscopic stenting

RESPONSE: Average survival in HAART era is 9 months, worse with alkaline phosphatase >1000 IU/L (*Am J Gastroenterol* 2003;98:2176).

Viral Hepatitis

■ TABLE 7-4: **Viral Hepatitis**

Type	Seroprevalence* Transmission	Incubation Period	Diagnosis	Course
A	Fecal-oral; food ■ Gen. population: 40% to 50% immune ■ Acute hepatitis: 50%	15 to 50 days	■ Acute: IgM ■ Prior infection: Total HAV antibody	■ Fulminant and fatal in 0.6% ■ Self limited in >99% ■ No chronic form
B	Sex and blood ■ Gen. population: 3% to 14% ■ IDU: 60% to 80% ■ MSM: 35% to 80%	45 to 160 days	■ Acute: HBsAg + anti-HBc IgM ■ Chronic: HBsAg x 6 months + anti-HBc IgG ■ Vaccinated: HBsAb	■ Fulminant and fatal in 1.4% ■ Chronic hepatitis in 6% in general population; 10% to 15% in patients with AIDS
C	Blood (primarily) ■ General population: 1.8% ■ IDU: 60% to 90% ■ Hemophilia: 60% to 90% ■ MSM: 2% to 8%	15 to 50 days	EIA Ab + quantative HCV RNA	■ Chronic hepatitis in 85% ■ Cirrhosis in 10% to 15% in 20 years but increased risk of progression with HIV coinfection or ETOH ■ HCV has little or no effect on rate of HIV infection progression

* Seroprevalence for adults in the U.S.

Hepatitis B

DIAGNOSIS: Positive serology for HBsAg for ≥20 weeks indicates chronic infection.

Systems Review

NATURAL HISTORY: Primary HBV infection in adults is usually subclinical and self-limited. About 6%-10% patients with HBV infection became chronic carriers, as indicated by persistent HBsAg (*J Acquir Immune Defic Syndr* 1991;4:416; *J Infect Dis* 1991;163:1138). Of these, about 25% develop chronic active hepatitis, which progresses to cirrhosis in 15% to 30% and confers a long-term risk of hepatic carcinoma. The risk of hepatic complications is associated with HBV replication as indicated by markers of viral replication: HBeAg and HBV DNA levels. Patients with HIV have higher rates of chronic HBV infection after acute infection. Those with HBV/HIV co-infection have higher levels of HBV DNA, and are more likely to have e antigen and higher rates of HBV-associated liver disease (*Clin Infect Dis* 2003;37:1678; *Lancet* 2002;360:1921; *J Acquir Infect Dis Syndr* 1991;4:416). It is unclear if HBV accelerates progression of HIV, but it does increase HAART-associated hepatotoxicity (*JAMA* 283;283:74; *Clin Liver Dis* 2003;7:475).

EVALUATION

- **Diagnosis:** Test for HBsAg, anti-HBc and anti-HBs. Interpretation of an isolated anti-HBc is unclear (*J Med Virol* 2000;62:450; *Clin Infect Dis* 1998;26:895).

- **Evaluation:** Chronic HBV is defined by positive HBsAg >6 months. In these cases obtain HBeAg, anti-HBeAg and HBV DNA levels. Severity of liver disease is evaluated at baseline and every 6 months with ALT, albumin, prothrombin time, platelet count, CBC and bilirubin. Some authorities recommend alfafetoprotein levels or ultrasound of the liver at 6- to 12-month intervals to monitor for hepatocellular carcinoma. It is not known if HIV coinfection increases this risk (*Clin Infect Dis* 2005;40(suppl 3):S179). Liver biopsy is the best method to determine the grade (necroinflammatory activity) and stage (degree of fibrosis).

MANAGEMENT

- **Negative screening tests:** Patients with negative HBsAg and anti-HBs should receive HBV vaccine (see p. 44).

- **Patients with chronic HBV co-infection** should 1) be advised to avoid or limit alcohol consumption; 2) receive HAV vaccine, preferably when CD4 count is >200/mm^3; 3) be evaluated for HBV treatment, 4) choose antiretroviral regimens based on anti-HBV activity of nucleoside analog components (see below), and 5) be counseled on the risks of HBV transmission, including the need for contacts to be evaluated for HBV vaccine.

- **Patients with HBV/HIV co-infection may have exacerbation of hepatitis** due to: 1) discontinuation of NRTIs with anti-HBV activity (3TC, FTC, TDF); 2) emergence of HBV NRTI resistance (especially 3TC and FTC) (*Clin Infect Dis* 1999;28:1032), 3) immune

7 Systems Review

reconstitution with HAART with or without 3TC, FTC, or TDF (*Clin Infect Dis* 2004;39:1291) or 4) hepatoxicity of antiretroviral drugs (see p. 98).

TREATMENT

- **Goals:** Stop or delay progression of fibrosis to prevent cirrhosis and hepatocellular carcinoma.
- **Indications:** Evidence of HBV replication (HBeAg+ or HBV DNA [>100,000 IU/mL) + ALT >2x ULN and/or liver biopsy showing necroinflammation
- **Recommendations** (European Consensus Conference, Feb. 2005)
  - □ HAART not indicated:
    - (1) Peg IFN is preferred, especially in HBeAg+, elevated ALT, and HBV genotype A or B. Treat ≥6 months if HBeAg+ or ≥12 months if anti-HBe. If CD4 <500 or IFN contraindicated: consider early initiation of HAART with TDF + FTC (*Truvada*) or TDF + 3TC.
    - (2) Alternative is entecavir or adefovir.
  - □ HAART indicated:
    - (1) With HBV DNA >100,000 IU/mL, include 2 agents active against HBV.
    - (2) If anti-HBe+, low HBV DNA and normal ALT: initiate HAART of choice.
    - (3) Cirrhosis: Consider treatment at lower HBV DNA threshold of 2000 IU/mL; IFN is rarely indicated.

HBV WITH 3TC RESISTANCE: Confirm resistance of HBV to 3TC; use HAART with activity against HBV.

- Monitoring:
  - □ IFN: Monitor for hematologic and psychiatric safety.
  - □ NRTI therapy: Expect HBV DNA decrease by 1 log within 1 month; monitor HBV DNA every 3 months.
- **Regimens:** See Table 7-5, next page.

406

■ TABLE 7-5: **Treatment of HBV**

Agent/Regimen	Comment
Interferon alfa 5 million units qd or 10 million units 3x/week x 12 to 24 weeks	The response rate is lower for HIV infected patients.
Pegylated interferon PegIFN alfa 2a: 180 mcg q week or PegIFN alfa 2b: 1.5 µ/kg	■ Preferred form of IFN ■ Highest cure rate
Lamivudine 300 mg/day	At 12 months most have decreased ALT and loss of HBV DNA, but HBeAg persists; YMDD mutations for lamivudine resistance emerge at a rate of 50% in 2 yrs and 90% at 4 yrs (*Clin Infect Dis* 2001;32:963; *Clin Infect Dis* 2003;37:1678) with viral rebound and increased transaminase.
Adefovir 10 mg/day	FDA-approved for HBV. Active against lamivudine-resistant strains; rate of resistance to adefovir is <3%/yr. in absence of HIV co-infection (*J Hepatol* 194;Suppl 2:182). Not active against HIV in dose used and appears to avoid promotion of HIV resistance to nucleotides (*Gastroenterology* 2003;125:292).
Tenofovir DF 300 mg qd	Similar to adefovir, but not FDA-approved for HBV. Average decrease in HBV DNA level is 4 log IU/mL, including strains with 3TC resistance; resistance rates with short term follow-up are <2% (*N Engl J Med* 2003;348:177; *J Infect Dis* 2002;186:1844). Risk of hepatitis flare if TDF is stopped.
Emtricitabine 200 mg qd	Experience is limited but it appears similar to 3TC in terms of anti-HBV activity and probability of resistance as well (*Am J Gastroenterol* 2002;97:1618)
Tenofovir + Emtricitibine	Coformulated as *Truvada*. A preferred combination when activity against both HBV + HIV desired. Risk of HBV flare if FTC is stopped.
Entecavir 0.5 mg qd or 1 mg qd (3TC refractory)	No activity against HIV. Effective and well tolerated against HBV. Must be taken on an empty stomach.

Hepatitis C (see *Ann Intern Med* 2003;138:197)

DIAGNOSIS: The standard test is anti-HCV detection by EIA with confirmation of positives by HCV RNA; the HCV RNA should be repeated if negative at 6 months because viremia may be intermittent. Unlike HIV, HCV antibody levels may also be low, especially with HIV co-infection, so HCV RNA levels are suggested when this diagnosis is suspected with negative screening serology (*Blood* 1993;82:1010; *J Infect Dis* 1994;170:433). False-negative screening serology is most common with CD4 cell counts <100/mm^3. Unlike HIV, HCV viral load does not correlate with progression.

7 Systems Review

EPIDEMIOLOGY: Co-infection is common because both viruses are transmitted by the same mechanisms: contaminated blood, sex and perinatal transmission. However, the rates of transmission in these categories are very different, as summarized below:

Transmission rates (in absence of treatment or prophylaxis)

	HIV	HCV
Needle stick injury	0.3%	3%
Discordant couples male	13%/yr	3%/yr
Perinatal transmission	20% to 30%	2% to 5%

NATURAL HISTORY: HCV progresses to cirrhosis in 5% to 25% in 20 years; after cirrhosis, the rate of progression to liver failure is 1% to 2%/year and to hepatocellular carcinoma 1% to 7%/year (*N Engl J Med* 1995;332:1463; *N Engl J Med* 1992;327:1906; *N Engl J Med* 1999; 340:1228; *Gastroenterology* 1997;112:463). Co-infection with HIV is generally associated with higher levels of HCV viral load and a 3-fold increase in rates of progression to cirrhosis, liver failure and hepatocellular carcinoma (*Clin Infect Dis* 2001;33:240; *Lancet* 1997;350:1425; *J Infect Dis* 1996;174:690; *Blood* 1994;84:1020; *J Infect Dis* 2000;181:844; *J Acquir Immune Defic Syndr* 1993;6:602; *J Infect Dis* 1999;179:1254; *Clin Infect Dis* 2001;22:562; *J Infect Dis* 2001;183:1112); *Clin Infect Dis* 2004;38:128). Other factors associated with more rapid progression of HCV are male sex, alcohol use >50 g/d, age >35 years and low CD4 count (*Clin Infect Dis* 2004;38:128). Most importantly, HCV has little or no effect on HIV-related disease progression or on HIV response to HAART (*JAMA* 2002;288:199). Multiple studies have demonstrated a significant increase in mortality with HCV coinfection compared to HIV alone, but some of this effect is due to injection drug use, which is often present (*J Acquir Immune Defic Syndr* 2003;33:365). A Veterans Administration review showed the rate of cirrhosis with HCV/HIV co-infection was increased 10-fold compared to HCV monoinfection; the rate of hepatic cancer was increased 5-fold (*Arch Intern Med* 2004;164:2349). The rate of cirrhosis was increased 19-fold in the HAART era. However another report suggests HAART has produced a substantial decrease in deaths due to hepatic disease (*Lancet* 2003;362:1708).

HAART-ASSOCIATED HEPATOTOXICITY: Antiretroviral agents, especially protease inhibitors, are associated with increased risk of asymptomatic elevations of transaminase levels with HIV-HCV co-infection (*JAMA* 2000;283:74; *AIDS* 2000;14:2895; *J Acquir Immune Defic Syndr* 2001;27:426). Nevertheless, one large cohort of co-infected patients showed that these changes were often self-limited even when the PI was continued, and there were no cases of irreversible liver failure (*JAMA* 2000;283:74). There are no clear guidelines for antiretroviral therapy with co-infection, although a common recommendation is to discontinue these agents if patients are symptomatic or have

Systems Review

transaminase levels over 5x ULN or over 3.5x baseline levels. Most patients with grade 3/4 toxicity are asymptomatic (*J Infect Dis* 2002;186:23). In these cases there should be an investigation for other causes of liver disease (hepatitis A or B, OIs, alcohol or other hepatotoxic medications) followed by discontinuation of antiretroviral agents if no reversible cause can be found. If the ALT level does not change or if it increases, consider liver biopsy and consider HCV treatment. If the ALT decreases, reinstate ART with a new drug regimen and monitor ALT closely. Nevirapine is the only antiretroviral agent that is often considered to be contraindicated with baseline hepatic disease including HCV coinfection, but there is no evidence that the hepatic necrosis seen with this drug has any association with HCV (*Lancet* 2004;363:1253; *J Acquir Immune Defic Syndr* 2004;36: 772). Use TPV/r with caution in patients with baseline hepatic disease.

MANAGEMENT

- All HCV/HIV co-infected patients should: 1) be advised to abstain from alcohol use; 2) be informed about methods to prevent transmission of both infections (use of condoms and avoid needle sharing); 3) receive vaccinations for HBV and HAV if susceptible; and 4) be evaluated for HCV disease severity and possible treatment. Patients with cirrhosis should have consideration of alfafetoprotein levels or ultrasound to detect hepatocellular cancer.

- HCV assessment: Baseline assessment should include evaluation of severity of liver disease including measurement of serum albumin, prothrombin time, platelet count, bilirubin, ALT and CBC. ALT provides limited information about severity. Liver biopsy with histology provides the best information about HCV disease activity and fibrosis stage as a guide to HCV treatment decision, to estimate prognosis and to identify other causes of live injury (*Hepatology* 2001;33:196). However, this procedure should not necessarily be a prerequisite for therapy in co-infected patients with a relatively poor prognosis. Some patients with less advanced HCV disease may elect to wait for a new HCV agent, but it may be a long wait if the goal is to avoid IFN.

- **Indications:** 1) HCV RNA levels >50 IU/mL; 2) Liver biopsy showing portal or bridging fibrosis or moderate inflammation and necrosis; 3) No contraindication (see p. 249), 4) Stable HIV infection; and 5) Preferrably with CD4 >200/mm^3 and HCV genotype 2/3. The 2005 European Consensus Conference, Feb. 2005 recommends treating all patients with genotype 2/3 if there are no contraindications.

- **Goal:** The goal of HCV treatment is a sustained virologic response (SVR) defined as undetected HCV RNA 24 weeks after treatment completion, which appears to indicate HCV viral eradication.

- **Clinical trials** in co-infected patients: Three trials show that patients with coinfection with HIV and HCV genotype 1 have a suboptimal

7 Systems Review

response to pegylated interferon + ribavirin, the currently recommended regimen as shown in Table 7.6.

■ TABLE 7-6: **Treatment of HCV**

| Trial | Regimen Duration: 48 wks | No. | SVR* by genotype | |
			1	2/3
ACTG A5071 (*N Engl J Med* 2004;352:451)	PegIFN alfa-2a 180 µg SC/wk + RBV 600-1000 mg/d	66	14%	73%
APRICOT (*N Engl J Med* 2004;351:438)	Peg IFN (as above) + RBV 800 mg/d	289	29%	62%
RIBAVIC (*JAMA* 2004; 292:2839)	As above	205	17%	44%

*SVR: Sustained virologic response as indicated by negative assay for HCV RNA at 72 weeks or 24 weeks post treatment.

1. All treatment regimens were 48 wks including those for genotypes 2/3.

2. Genotype 1, which accounted for 70% of cases, produced SVR rates that were substantially lower than the 45%-55% rates reported in the absence of HIV co-infection (*N Engl J Med* 2002;347:975; *Lancet* 2001;358:958). The rates of SVR with genotypes 2/3 were high and comparable, although the duration was 48 weeks instead of the more customary 24 weeks advocated for monoinfected patients.

3. For all three trials the median CD4 count was 400-500/mm^3. There were inadequate data for co-infected patients with CD4 counts <200/mm^3 for any conclusions. A subset analysis of 17 patients with CD4 counts <200/mm^3 in the APRICOT study showed a good response, leading the authors to conclude that a low baseline CD4 count may not contraindicate HCV treatment.

4. Ribavirin doses were generally lower (800 mg/day) than commonly advocated (1000-1200 mg.day). This may contribute to reduced SVR rates.

5. Failure to reduce HCV RNA levels to undetectable or ˉ2 log$_{10}$ IU/mL by 12 weeks predicted failure, with only 3 exceptions in 300, in the three studies summarized above.

6. Drugs that may interact with ribavirin include ddl and AZT (high rates of anemia).

7. Interferon has established antiretroviral activity in HIV, with an average VL decrease of 0.9 log$_{10}$ in patients with high baseline VLs.

RECOMMENDATIONS FOR EVALUATION AND TREATMENT

■ Pre-therapy: General evaluation

□ *Lab:* CBC, ALT, AST, creatinine

□ *Access comorbidities:* substance abuse, psychiatric disease, cardiopulmonary disease, renal disease

□ *Evaluate HIV status:* CD4 count, VL, active OIs

□ *Evaluate HCV status:* HCV genotype, HCV viral load, ALT

Consider liver biopsy; if contraindicated, unavailable or refused, may elect to give therapy without biopsy. (Liver biopsy is most important when SVR is less likely, as with genotype 1.)

▫ *Counsel patient on benefits and risks*

SEQUENCING: The sequence of treatment with a CD4 count >200/mm^3 is arbitary. Some experts advocate HCV treatment first if HIV treatment can be delayed 6 months. Some treat HIV first to assess adherence and because HCV therapy may be more effective with good control of HIV. If the CD4 count is <200/mm^3, HAART should usually be given first.

THERAPY: PegIFN alfa 2a 180 mcg SC q week + ribavirin x48 weeks. The dose of ribavarin should be 800 mg PO qd for genotype 2/3; for genotype 1 a dose of 1000-2000 mg/day is preferred, although the trials were generally done with 800 mg/day. The 48-week duration applies to all genotypes.

MONITORING

▫ *Reinforce: birth control* now and for 6 months after

▫ *Lab:* CBC, ALT at weeks 2 and 4, then at 4- to 8-week intervals

   ANC <750/mm^3 – reduce interferon or give G-CSF

        <500/mm^3 – discontinue interferon; consider G-CSF

   Hgb <10 g/dL – reduce ribavirin 200 mg/d; consider EPO

        <8 g/dL – discontinue ribavirin; consider EPO 40,000 IU/week

   HIV: VL + CD4 count at 12-week intervals

   Thyroid – TSH at 3- to 6-month intervals

▫ *Neuropsychiatry* – evaluate monthly

   Consider antidepressants (SSRI) ± consult

▫ *HCV:* quantitative HCV RNA at 12 weeks. If positive or HCV decrease of ≤2 log with genotype 1, discontinue therapy (since the probability of SVR <1%) or consider maintenance interferon. With genotype 2/3, continue to 24 wks or discontinue.

▫ *End of therapy:* HCV RNA PCR

■ Post-therapy

   ▫ *HCV RNA* PCR at 6 months

ADVERSE EFFECTS: About 10-13% of patients in the therapeutic trials discontinued treatment prematurely due to intolerance or toxicity. Side effects of interferon include flu-like symptoms, alopecia, neuropsychiatric effects, thyroid dysfunction, leucopenia and thrombocytopenia, and for ribavirin they include anemia and birth defects. With regard to antiretroviral drugs, ribavirin increases the toxicity of ddl (*Gut* 2000;47:694; *AIDS* 2000;14:1857). Fatal lactic

7 Systems Review

acidosis has been reported, and this combination is contraindicated (*Lancet* 2001;357:280; *AAC* 1987;31:1613).

Pancreatitis (*Am J Med* 1999;107:78)

MAJOR CAUSES

- **Drugs**, especially ddI or ddI + d4T ± hydroxyurea. May be complication of lactic acidosis (NRTI-associated mitochondrial toxicity) or secondary to PI-associated hypertriglyceridemia with elevated triglyceride levels – usually >1000 mg/dL. Less common drugs: d4T, 3TC (pediatrics), RTV, INH, rifampin, LPV/r, TMP-SMX, pentamidine, corticosteroids, sulfonamides, erythromycin, paromomycin.

- **Opportunistic infections:** CMV. Less common: MAC, TB, cryptosporidium, toxoplasmosis, cryptococcus

- **Conditions that cause pancreatitis in general population**, especially alcoholism. Less common: Gallstones, hypertriglyceridemia (avg level is 4500 mg/dL), post ERCP (3% to 5% of procedures), trauma. **Note:** Despite the association between hypertriglyceridemia and PIs, other medications appear to account for >90% of cases (*Pancreas* 2003;27:E1)

DIAGNOSIS

- **Amylase** >3x ULN (p-isoamylase is more specific but not usually measured [*Mayo Clin Proc* 1996;71:1138]). Other causes of hyperamylasemia: other intra-abdominal conditions, diseases of salivary gland, tumors (lung and ovary), renal failure macroamylasemia; sensitivity: 85% to 100% (*Am J Gastroenterol* 1990;85:356).

- **Other tests**
  - □ Lipase: As sensitive as amylase but more specific. Need for amylase plus lipase is arbitrary.
  - □ CT Scan: Best method to image (*Radiology* 1994;193:297). Used to: 1) exclude other serious intra-abdominal conditions, 2) stage pancreatitis, and 3) detect complications.

TREATMENT: Supportive – IV fluids, pain control and NPO

PROGNOSIS: Best predictor of outcome is APACHE II score (*Am J Gastroenterol* 2003;98:1278)

Systems Review

HEMATOLOGIC COMPLICATIONS

Anemia

■ TABLE 7-7: **Definition of Anemia**

		Men	Women
Average	Hematocrit %	46.0 ± 4.0	40.0 ± 4.0
	Hemoglobin (g/dL)	15.7 ± 1.7	13.8 ± 1.5
	Reticulocytes	1.6 ± 0.5	1.4 ± 0.5
	Mean corpuscular vol	88.0 ± 8.0	88.0 ± 8.0
Anemia	Hematocrit	<41%	<36%
	Hemoglobin (g/dL)	13.5	12.0

SYMPTOMS: Oxygen delivery becomes impaired with activity when the hemoglobin levels <8-9 g/dL and becomes impaired at rest with hemoglobin levels <5 g/dL (*JAMA* 1998;279:217). Symptoms of chronic anemia include exertional dyspnea, fatigue, and a hyperdynamic state (bounding pulses, palpitations, roaring in ears). Late complications include confusion, CHF, angina. There is a consistently observed relationship between anemia and survival with HIV infection (*J Acquir Immune Defic Syndr* 1998;19:29; *Clin Infect Dis* 2002;34:260; *J Acquir Immune Defic Syndr* 2004;37:1245). Symptoms due to acute bleeding are those of hypovolemia with postural dizziness, lethargy, postural hypotension, and shock.

CAUSES

- **HIV:** HIV infection of marrow progenitor cells (*Clin Infect Dis* 2000;30:504). Incidence correlates with immune state: 12% with CD4 count <200 /mm³, 37% with AIDS-defining OI (*Blood* 1998;91:301). Anemia predicts death independently from CD4 count and viral load (*Semin Hematol Suppl* 4;6:18; *AIDS* 1999;13:943; *AIDS Rev* 2002;4:13; *J Acquir Immune Defic Syndr* 2004;37:1245).

  □ Findings: Normocytic, normochromic, low reticulocyte count, low erythropoietin level

  □ Factors that correlate with anemia are: CD4 <200/mm³, high VL, female sex, use of AZT, reduced BMI and black race (*Clin Infect Dis* 2004;38:1454; *J Acquir Immune Defic Syndr* 2004;37:1245).

  □ Treatment: HAART. With immune reconstitution, prior reports show increases in Hgb of 1.0-2.0 gm/dL at 6 months (*J Acquir Immune Defic Syndr* 2001;28:221; *AIDS* 1999;13:943), but results are inconsistent (*Clin Infect Dis* 2000;30:504). Consider erythropoietin (EPO) (40,000 units/week) with symptomatic and refractory cases (see Figure 7-2, p. 386). Note the average wholesale price (*AWP*) cost of EPO is about $550/week.

7 Systems Review

- **Marrow-infiltrating infection or tumor** (lymphoma, especially non-cleaved cell type, or Kaposi's sarcoma, rare) or infection (MAC, tuberculosis, CMV, histoplasmosis)
  - Findings: Normocytic, normochromic, low platelet count, evidence of etiologic mechanism
  - Treat underlying cause
- **Parvovirus B19:** Infects erythroid precursors; symptoms reflect marginal reserve (sickle cell disease, etc.) and inability to eradicate infection due to immune deficiency.
  - Findings: Normocytic, normochromic anemia, without reticulocytes, positive IgG and IgM serology for parvovirus, positive serum dot blot hybridization or PCR for parvovirus B19; the diagnosis is most likely with severe anemia, i.e., hematocrit <24%, no reticulocytes and CD4 count <100 cells/mm^3 (*J Infect Dis* 1997;176:269).
  - Treatment: May eradicate pathogen with HAART (*Clin Infect Dis* 2001;32:E122). Standard treatment with persistent parvovirus B19 and immunosuppression is IVIG 400 mg/kg/day x 5 days (*Ann Intern Med* 1990;113:926)
- **Nutritional Deficiency:** Common in late stage HIV, including B12 deficiency in 20% of AIDS patients (*Eur J Haematol* 1987;38:141) and folate deficiency due to folic acid malabsorption (*J Intern Med* 1991;230:227).
  - Findings: Megaloblastic anemia (MCV >100 not ascribed to AZT or d4T) ± hypersegmented polymorphonuclear cells, low reticulocyte count with serum B12 (cobalamin) level <125-200 pg/mL (*Semin Hematol* 1999;36:75) or a serum folate level <2-4 ng/mL (<2 ng/mL is more definitive). Note: A hospital meal may improve the RBC folate level.
  - Treatment: Folate deficiency – folic acid 1-5 mg/day x 1 to 4 months. B12 deficiency – cobalamin 1 g IM qd x 7 days, then every week x 4, then every month or 1-2 g PO qd (*Blood* 1998;92:1191).
- **Iron deficiency:** Usually indicates blood loss, especially from GI tract.
  - Findings: Most studies to detect iron deficiency show the likely cause is anemia of chronic disease with decreased Fe (<60 ug/dL), low transferrin (<300 ug/dL), and normal or increased ferritin. Ferritin level <40 ng/mL suggests iron deficiency and a level <15 ng/mL is 99% sensitive for this diagnosis but only 50% specific (*J Gen Intern Med* 1992;7:145).
  - Treatment: Detect and treat source of loss + ferrous sulfate 325 mg tid.
- **Drug-induced marrow suppression ± red cell aplasia:** Most common with AZT; less common with ganciclovir, amphotericin,

ribavirin, pyrimethamine, interferon, TMP-SMX, phenytoin (also seen with HIV *per se*, parvovirus B19, and non-Hodgkin's lymphoma).

- □ Findings: Normocytic, normochromic anemia (macrocytic with AZT or d4T), low or normal reticulocyte count.
- □ Treatment: Discontinue implicated agent ± EPO (see algorithm, p. 416).

- **Drug-induced hemolytic anemia:** Most common with dapsone, primaquine, and ribavirin (hemolytic anemia is also seen with TTP). The risk with dapsone and primaquine is dose-related and most common with G6PD deficiency.

- □ Findings: Reticulocytosis, increased LDH, increased indirect bilirubin, methemoglobinemia, and reduced haptoglobin. The combination of a haptoglobin <25 mg/dL + elevated LDH is 90% specific and 92% sensitive for hemolytic anemia (*JAMA* 1980;243:1909). The peripheral smear may show spherocytes and fragmented RBCs. Note: Coombs test is commonly positive.
- □ Treatment: Consists of oxygen, packed RBC transfusions and discontinuation of implicated drug. Severe cases in absence of G6-PD deficiency are treated with IV methylene blue (l mg/kg) (*J Acquir Immune Defic Syndr* 1996;12:477). Activated charcoal may be given to reduce dapsone levels (see p. 175).

Guidelines for Use of Erythropoietin (EPO) in the Anemic HIV Patient

GOALS OF THERAPY:

- Resolution of anemia: Hgb >11-12 g/dL (men) and >10-11 g/dL women*
- Increased energy, activity, and overall quality of life for patients, prolonged survival
- Reduced need for transfusions

Patient candidate: Refractory anemia with Hgb <11-12 gm/dL in men or <10-11 gm/dL in women*

↓

Exclude other causes of anemia:

- Bleeding (guaiac stools)
- Hemolysis (serum LDH, haptoglobin, bilirubin)
- Iron deficiency (serum iron, transferrin, % saturation, ferritin)
- B12, folate deficiency (serum B12, RBC folate if macrocytic)

NO ↓   **YES** ↓

| Start EPO 40,000 units SQ/week. Consider iron supplementation. | Correct underlying cause |

↓

Monitor response: Full response will generally not be seen for at least 4 weeks.

At 4 weeks, if Hgb increases >1 g/dL, continue at this dose.

At 4 weeks, if Hgb increases <1 g/dL, increase dose to 60,000 units/week.

At 8 weeks, if Hgb increases <1 g/dL, check iron, folate, & B12 levels. If adequate, discontinue EPO.

When Hgb approaches 13 g/dL, decrease EPO by 10,000 units/week* Titrate to maintain desired hemoglobin.†

At 8 weeks, if Hgb increases >1 g/dL, continue at this dose.

---

* These Hgb targets were picked because they are EPO standards in renal failure patients. There may be substantial individual variation in tolerance of chronic anemia. Some aim higher (*Clin Infect Dis* 2004;38:1454).

† During dose adjustment phase, hemoglobin should be monitored every 2 to 4 weeks. Allow at least 4 weeks to assess full response to dose changes.

Idiopathic Thrombocytopenia Purpura (ITP)

DEFINITION: Unexplained platelet count <100,000/mL

CAUSES

- **Most cases** are ascribed to HIV infection of multi-lineage hematopoietic progenitor cells in the marrow (*Clin Infect Dis* 2000;30:504; *N Engl J Med* 1992;327:1779).

- **Drug induced:** Review of 561 reports showed the best supporting data for a causal role for drugs in patients without HIV infection were for heparin, quinidine, gold, and TMP-SMX (*Ann Intern Med* 1998;129:886). Others with "level 1 evidence" that are used in HIV infected patients: Rifampin, amphotericin, vancomycin, ethambutol, sulfisoxazole, and lithium.

TREATMENT (*Clin Infect Dis* 1995;21:415; *N Engl J Med* 1999;341:1239)

- **HAART:** Two reports showed that with viral suppression and CD4 count rebound, median platelet count increase was 18,000/mL and 45,000/mL at 3 months (*Clin Infect Dis* 2000;30:504; *N Engl J Med* 1999;341:1239).

- **Drug-induced:** Median time to recovery with discontinuation of the implicated agent is 7 days (*Ann Intern Med* 1998;129:886).

- **Standard treatments of ITP** (prednisone, IVIG, splenectomy, etc.): Response rates are 40% to 90%; the main problem is durability (*Clin Infect Dis* 1995;21:415).

■ TABLE 7-8: **Treatment of ITP by Clinical Presentation**

Clinical Status	Treatment
Asymptomatic	■ HAART ■ Discontinue implicated drug and monitor response.
Persistent symptomatic or required for procedure	■ Above ■ Prednisone 30-60 mg/day with rapid taper to 5-10 mg/day. Risk of OI. Only 10% to 20% have sustained response. ■ IVIG 400 mg/kg days 1, 2 and 14, then every 2 to 4 weeks. Raises platelet count within 4 days; median peak response time is 3 weeks. Very expensive. ■ Rho(D) immune globulin (*WinRho*) 25-50 µg/kg over 3 to 5 minutes in Rh(=) patients, repeat day 3 to 4 prn, then at 3 to 4 week intervals as needed. Similar to IVIG but rapid infusion and less expensive. ■ Splenectomy – experience is variable: some good (*Arch Surg* 1989;124:625), some bad (*Lancet* 1987;2:342).
Hemorrhage	Packed red cells/platelet transfusions plus prednisone 60-100 mg/day or IVIG 1 g/kg days l, 2, and 14.

Systems Review

7

Neutropenia

DEFINITION: Absolute neutrophil count <750/mm^3 (Some use thresholds of 500/mm^3 or 1000/mm^3)

CAUSE: Usually due to HIV *per se* or to drugs.

SYMPTOMS: Reported risk of bacterial infections is variable, but the largest review shows an increase in hospitalization with an ANC <500/mm^3 (*Arch Intern Med* 1997;157:1825). Other reviews show that few HIV infected patients have excessive neutropenia-associated infections (*Clin Infect Dis* 2001;32:469).

TREATMENT

- **HIV associated:** HAART – ANC increase with immune reconstitution is variable (*Clin Infect Dis* 2000;30:504; *J Acquir Immune Defic Syndr* 2001;28:221). Severe and persistent neutropenia may respond to G-CSF or GM-CSF.

- **Drug associated:** Most common causes are AZT, ganciclovir, or valganciclovir; other causes include flagtosine, flucytosine, amphotericin, sulfonamides, pyrimethamine, pentamidine, antineoplastic drugs, and interferon. Treatment is to discontinue the implicated drug and/or give G-CSF or GM-CSF.

- **G-CSF or GM-CSF:** Usual initial dose is 150-300 mcg/day or 3x/wk. Dose can be titrated to lowest dose necessary to maintain ANC ≥1000/mm^3. (*N Engl J Med* 1987;371:593). Monitor CBC during cytokine treatment 2x/week.

Thrombotic Thrombocytopenia Purpura (TTP)

CAUSE: Platelet thrombi in selected organs

FREQUENCY: Unclear, may be early or late in course (*Ann Intern Med* 1988;109:194)

LAB DIAGNOSIS: 1) Anemia; 2) Thrombocytopenia (platelet count 5,000-120,000/mL); 3) Peripheral smear shows fragmented RBCs (schistocytes, helmet cells) ± nucleated cells; 4) Increased creatinine; 5) Evidence of hemolysis: Increased reticulocytes, indirect bilirubin, and LDH and low haptoglobin; and 6) Normal coagulation parameters

CLINICAL FEATURES: Fever, neurologic changes, renal failure – may be acute requiring dialysis

TREATMENT: The usual course is progressive with irreversible renal failure and death. Standard treatment is plasma exchange until platelet count is normal and LDH is normal (*N Engl J Med* 1991;325:393). An average of 7 to 16 exchanges are required to induce remission. With poor response, add prednisone 60 mg/day.

IMMUNE RECONSTITUTION SYNDROME (IRS)
(*Clin Infect Dis* 2004;38:1159)

DEFINITION: Atypical inflammatory disorders associated with immune recovery.

PATHOGENESIS: Qualitative and quantitative recovery of pathogen-specific cellular and humoral responses have been noted to multiple opportunistic pathogens including MTB, MAC, CMV, EBV, HBV, HCV and *C. albicans* (*Science* 1997;277:112; *Clin Infect Dis* 2000;30:882; *AIDS* 2002;616:2129; *J Infect Dis* 2002;185:1813).

CLINICAL FEATURES: MAC accounts for one-third of reported cases in U.S. The interval from ART to IRS is 1 week to several months; most occur in the first 8 weeks. The baseline CD4 is usually <50/mm³ at initiation of HAART and increases 2- to 4-fold in year one. There are two patterns: 1) HAART given at the time of OI treatment with IRS complicating the response to treatment, and 2) HAART given to a clinically stable patient with new expression of a dormant and previously unrecognized condition.

TREATMENT PRINCIPLES: In most cases HAART and OI therapy are continued. Symptomatic treatment is commonly successful with NSAIDs. Some patients require steroids; rarely discontinuation of HAART is required.

SPECIFIC PATHOGENS

Pathogen	Expression	Treatment
CMV	Vitritis, cytoid, macular edema, uveitis, vitreomacular degeneration	ART, IVIG, steriods, vitrectomy, anti-CMV therapy
Crytococcus neoformans	Meningitis, palsy, hearing loss, abcess, mediastinitis, adenitis	ART, azoles, steroids, meningitis
HBV, HCV	Hepatitis	Interferon, D/C ART
Herpes simplex	Chronic erosive ulcers, encephalitis	ART, anti-HSV agents, steroids
Kaposi's sarcoma	Tracheal mucosal edema, obstruction	Steroids, D/C ART
M. avium complex	Skin lesions, lymphadenitis, hepatic granuloma	ART, anti-MAC agents, NSAIDs, steroids
M. tuberculosis	Pneumonitis, ARDS, lymphadenitis, hepatitis, CNS lesions, renal failure	ART, anti-TB drugs, steroids
Parvovirus	Focal encephalitis	IVIG, D/C ART
P. jiroveci	Pneumonia	ART, anti-PCP drugs, steroids
Varicella	Zoster flare	ART, anti-VZV drugs, steroids
JC virus	Flare of PML with enhancement on MRI	ART; role of steroids unclear

7 Systems Review

MALIGNANCIES

■ TABLE 7-9: **Major HIV-associated Tumors with Risk Based on CD4 Count.**

Cancer	Relative risk vs general population			
	n	Total	CD4 >200	CD4 <50
Kaposi's sarcoma	1937	258	140	309
Non-Hodgkin's lymphoma	1158	78	44	111
Lymphoblastic lymphoma	201	134	40	109
CNS lymphoma	320	175	27	330
Cervical cancer	26	9	10	8

Analysis is from cancer registries and AIDS registries in 11 U.S. regions, 1990-96 (*J Acquir Immune Defic Syndr* 2003;32:527)

Cervical Cancer (see p. 41)

The risk for cervical cancer seems modest; the WIHS study with 1,950 HIV-infected women followed 10 years showed only one case and no increased risk compared to controls (*J Acquir Immune Defic Syndr* 2004;36:978).

Kaposi's Sarcoma

CAUSE: HHV-8

FREQUENCY: Rate is up to 20,000-fold higher with HIV compared with general population and 300-fold higher than other immunosuppressed patients (*Lancet* 1990;335:123; *J Natl Cancer Inst* 2002;94:1204). The incidence is 10-20x higher in MSM, but is increased >200-fold in women as well (*J Acquir Immune Defic Syndr* 2004;36:978). The postulated mechanism is upregulation of cytokines that regulate angiogenesis and lymphangiogenesis by HIV (*Lancet* 2004;364:740). The rate has decreased in the HAART era (*JAMA* 2002;287:221) by up to 100-fold in one report; PI and NNRTI-based HAART appear equally effective (*AIDS* 2003;17:F17). Studies from Thailand show high rates of HHV-8 infection, but minimal KS or evidence of sexual transmission of HHV-8 (*Clin Infect Dis* 2004;39:1052).

PRESENTATION: Firm purple to brown-black macules, patches, nodules, papules that are usually asymptomatic – neither pruritic, nor painful, and usually on legs, face, oral cavity, and genitalia. Complications include lymphedema (especially legs, face, and genitalia) and visceral involvement (especially mouth, GI tract, and lungs). HAART reduces the frequency of KS (*J Acquir Immune Defic Syndr* 2003;33:614), and when it develops during antiretroviral therapy the course is less aggressive (*Cancer* 2003;98:2440).

Systems Review

DIFFERENTIAL: Bacillary angiomatosis (biopsy with silver stain to show organisms); hematoma, nevus, hemangioma, B-cell lymphoma, and pyogenic granuloma

■ TABLE 7-10: **Diagnosis of Kaposi's Sarcoma**

Site	Frequency*	Diagnosis
Skin	>95%	■ Appearance; biopsy if atypical
Oral	30%	■ Lesion – purple nodule usually on palate or gingiva; biopsy if atypical
GI	40%	■ Any level; screen – stool guaiac ■ Diagnosis: Endoscopy – hemorrhagic nodule (*Gastroenterology* 1985;89:102); biopsy often negative due to submucosal location
Lung	20% to 50%	■ X-ray variable – nodule(s), infiltrates, effusions, and/or mediastinal node ■ Diagnosis: Bronchoscopy shows cherry-red bronchial nodule (*Chest* 1995;105:1314)

PROGNOSIS: CD4 count plus tumor burden staging (ACTG – *J Clin Oncol* 1989;7:201). TIS: Extent of Tumor (T), Immune status (I), Severity of systemic illness (S). TIS predicts survival (*J Clin Oncol* 1997;15:385). Good prognosis – lesions confined to skin, CD4 count >150/mm^3, no "B" symptoms.

TREATMENT

- **HAART:** Associated with lesion regression, decreased incidence, and prolonged survival (*J Clin Oncol* 2001;19:3848; *J Med Virol* 1999;57:140; *AIDS* 1997;11:261; *Mayo Clin Proc* 1998;73:439; *AIDS* 2000;14:987). One report noted 12/20 patients with HIV-associated KS treated with HAART converted to undetectable HHV-8, but it is not clear whether this represents immune control or activity of antiretrovirals against both viruses (*J Acquir Immune Defic Syndr* 2002;12:218). Immune reconstitution syndrome is rare but reported, with new adenopathy, KS lesions becoming nodular and violaceous, and increased edema (*Clin Infect Dis* 2004;39:1852).

- **Antiviral therapy:** Foscarnet, cidofovir, and ganciclovir are active against HHV-8 (*J Clin Invest* 1997;99:2082); long-term use of foscarnet or ganciclovir is associated with reduced incidence of Kaposi's sarcoma (*N Engl J Med* 1999;340:1063) but does not appear to cause tumor regression (J *Acquir Immune Defic Syndr* 1999;20:34).

- **Systemic vs local therapy:** Systemic treatment is preferred with extensive tumor burden (>25 skin lesions, visceral involvement with symptoms, extensive edema, "B" symptoms, or failure to respond to local treatment) (*Lancet* 1995;346:26).

7 Systems Review

■ TABLE 7-11: **Treatment of Kaposi's Sarcoma**

Local Treatment	Comment
Vinblastine	■ Inject 0.1 mL/0.5 cm² of solution with 0.2-0.3 mg/mL and repeat every 3 to 4 weeks as needed. ■ Most frequently used; lesions usually regress but don't disappear (*J Oral Maxillofac Surg* 1996;54:583).
Panretin gel	■ Topical 9-cis retinoic acid gel.
Liquid nitrogen	■ Usually restricted to small lesions.
Radiation	■ Usually low dose, 400 rads/week x 6 weeks; well tolerated on skin; mucositis common with oral lesions, usual indication is lesions that are too extensive for local treatment.
Cryosurgery	
Laser	

Systemic Treatment	Comment
Liposomal anthracyclines	■ Two FDA-approved formulations: Pegylated liposomal doxorubicin (*Doxil*) and liposomal daunorubicin (*DaunoXome*). These are preferred over conventional chemotherapy for better response and reduced toxicity (*J Clin Oncol* 1998;16: 2445; *J Clin Oncol* 1998;16:683; *J Clin Oncol* 1996;14:2353). ■ Doses: doxorubicin liposomal (*Doxil*).20 mg/m² every 2 to 3 weeks; daunorubicin (*DaunoXome*) 40 mg/m² every 2 weeks.
Paclitaxel (*Taxol*)	■ FDA-approved for Kaposi's sarcoma. Considered second line to anthracyclines due to greater toxicity (neutropenia and thrombocytopenia) (*J Clin Oncol* 1998;16:1112). ■ Lower doses (100 mg/m² every 2 weeks) appears to preserve efficacy with reduced toxicity (*Cancer* 2002;95:147).
Interferon alfa	■ Efficacy established especially with modest disease, but toxicity is great (*J Clin Oncol* 1998;16:1736) now rarely used. ■ Dose is 1-10 million units SC qd
Conventional chemotherapy	■ Commonly used combinations include adriamycin, bleomycin plus vincristine or vinblastine (ABV); bleomycin plus vinca alkaloids or vincristine/vinblastine (alone). ■ Newer treatments (paclitaxel and anthracyclines) are usually preferred.

RESPONSE: Kaposi's sarcoma cannot be cured; goals of therapy are to reduce symptoms and prevent progression. HAART is associated with reduced tumor burden. Antiviral drugs directed against HHV-8 have no established benefit (*J Acquir Immune Defic Syndr* 1999;20:34).

■ **Local therapy:** Local injections of vinblastine cause reduced lesion size but not elimination in most patients (*Cancer* 1993;71:1722).

■ **Systemic therapy:** Liposomal anthracyclines usually show good results with few side effects. Paclitaxel is as effective but more toxic due to neutropenia and thrombocytopenia; side effects are dose related; lower doses appear as effective with less marrow suppression.

Systems Review

Non-Hodgkin's Lymphoma (NHL)

CAUSE: Immunosuppression (CD4 count <100 cells/mm³) and EBV (50% to 80%)

FREQUENCY AND TYPE: NHL is 200 to 600 times more common among HIV-infected patients compared with the general population (*Int J Cancer* 1997;73:645; *J Acquir Immune Defic Syndr* 2004;36:978). The rate is about 3% for patients with AIDS (*J Acquir Immune Defic Syndr* 2002;29:418). Most (70% to 90%) are high-grade diffuse large cell or Burkitt-like lymphomas (*Am J Med* 2001; *Brit J Haematol* 2001;112:863).

PRESENTATION: Compared with NHL in the general population, HIV infected patients have high rates of stage IV disease with "B" symptoms and sparse node involvement. Common sites of infection and forms of clinical presentation are fever of unknown origin, hepatic dysfunction, marrow involvement, lung disease (effusions, multi-nodular infiltrates, consolidation, mass lesions, or local or diffuse interstitial infiltrates, hilar adenopathy), GI involvement (any level – pain and weight loss), and CNS (aseptic meningitis, cranial nerve palsies, CNS mass lesions).

DIAGNOSIS: Diagnosis is made by biopsy (usually required), but site depends on symptoms and results of CT scan to assess nodal and extranodal sites of involvement. Fine needle aspirate (FNA) of enlarged nodes is helpful if positive, but most are falsely negative, necessitating a biopsy. Bone marrow biopsy will often yield the diagnosis. With GI tract and hepatic involvement, a CT scan is usually more useful than endoscopy. Exudative pleural effusions are frequently seen with lung involvement – bronchoscopy is usually negative unless accompanied by lung biopsy, which has a diagnostic yield of about 60% (*Chest* 1996;110:729).

TREATMENT

- **Standard:** CHOP (cyclophosphamide, doxorubicin, adriamycin, vincristine, and prednisone). Intrathecal methotrexate or cytosine arabinoside may be given for CNS prophylaxis and should be given with meningeal involvement.

- **Alternatives to CHOP**
  - ☐ M-BACOD (methotrexate, bleomycin, doxorubicin, cyclophospha-mide, vincristine, and dexamethasone + G-CSF) (*N Engl J Med* 1997;336:16)
  - ☐ EPOCH (etoposide, prednisone, vincristine, cyclophosphamide, and doxorubicin) (*J Clin Oncol* 2004;22:1491)

RESPONSE: Initial response rates are 50% to 60%, but the long-term prognosis is poor with median survival <1 year. The usual cause of death is progressive lymphoma or progressive HIV with OIs (*Semin Oncol* 1998;25:492). The prognosis is significantly better with HAART; one report showed an 84% 1 year survival with HAART + chemotherapy (*AIDS* 2001;15:1483). **Note:** the prognosis with lymphoma plus HIV infection in the HAART era is significantly worse than for lymphoma alone, but one report shows that patients who achieve complete remission with chemotherapy had a comparable 3-year survival prognosis (74%) to HIV-negative patients with NHL (*Clin Infect Dis* 2004;38:142). Another report shows HAART is associated with reduced chemotherapy-related toxicity as well as improved survival (*J Clin Oncol* 2004;22:1491).

Primary CNS Lymphoma (PCNSL) (see p. 436)

Primary Effusion Lymphoma

CAUSE: HHV-8 and EBV (*N Engl J Med* 1995;332:1186; *Clin Microbiol Rev* 2002;15:439)

FREQUENCY: Rare: tumor registries crossed with AIDS registries show a frequency of 0.004% or 0.14% of non-Hodgkin's lymphoma in patients with AIDS (*J Acquir Immune Defic Syndr* 2002;29:418)

PRESENTATION: Serous effusions (pleural, peritoneal, pericardial, joint spaces) with no masses (*Hum Pathol* 1997;28:801)

DIAGNOSIS: Effusions are serous, contain high-grade malignant lymphocytes and HHV-8.

TREATMENT

- **HAART plus CHOP** (*J Clin Oncol* 2003;21:3948)
- **Alternatives:** Pegylated liposomal doxorubicin or liposomal daunorubicin

RESPONSE: This tumor usually does not extend beyond serosal surfaces, but prognosis is poor, with median survival of 2 to 6 months (*J Acquir Immune Defic Syndr* 1996;13:215; *J Clin Oncol* 2003;21:3948). Most patients show response to therapy with decrease in effusion size. Failure to respond to two cycles of CHOP indicates additional cycles will fail, indicating a role for liposomal doxorubicin or liposomal daunorubicin. HHV-8 levels increase with relapse and do not respond to antiviral therapy (*J Med Virol* 2003;71:399). The CD4 count is the most important predictor of progression (*Clin Infect Dis* 2005;40:1022).

NEUROLOGIC COMPLICATIONS:
Peripheral nervous system

HIV-Associated Neuromuscular Weakness Syndrome (HANWS)

CAUSE: Postulated to be caused by mitochondrial toxicity attributed to deoxy NRTIs, primarily d4T (*N Engl J Med* 2002;346:811; *Clin Infect Dis* 2003; 15:131; *AIDS* 2004;18:1403).

CLINICAL FEATURES: Summary of 69 "possible" cases by review of FDA reports (AERS). Of these, 27 were "definite" and 19 "probable" (*AIDS* 2004;18:1403). Median lactic acid level was 4.9 mmol/L. Of the 69 possible cases, 61 (88%) patients had taken d4T, although 25 (36%) had stopped this drug prior to the onset of symptoms. The median duration of d4T use was 10.5 months. Of the 27 definite cases, 14 (52%) had acute symptoms (<2 weeks). Pathology studies and EMG showed involvement of peripheral nerves, muscles or both. Clinical features include ascending paresis, areflexia and cranial neuropathies. CPK levels are often elevated.

DIAGNOSIS (ACTG, 2002)

- New onset limb weakness ± sensory involvement that is acute (1 to 2 weeks) or subacute (>2 weeks) involving legs or legs and arms
- Absence of alternative confounding illnesses: Guillain-Barré syndrome, Myasthenia gravis, myelopathy, hypokalemia, stroke

TREATMENT: Discontinue d4T and/or other causative NRTIs. Supportive care. Follow-up in the cases summarized above showed improvement in only 16/44 (36%).

Cytomegalovirus radiculitis (see p. 344)

7 Systems Review

Differential Diagnosis of Lower Extremity Symptoms in Patients with HIV Infection

Syndrome	Symptoms	Clinical Features	Ancillary Studies/ Treatment
Distal sensory neuropathy (DSN)	■ Pain and numbness in toes and feet; ankles, calves, and fingers involved in more advanced cases ■ CD4 cell count <200/mm³, but can occur at higher CD4 level	■ Reduced pinprick/vibratory sensation ■ Reduced or absent ankle jerks ■ Contact allodynia (hypersensitivity) present most cases	■ Skin biopsy shows epidermal denervation ■ Electromyography/ nerve conduction velocities (EMG/NCV) show a predominantly axonal neuropathy ■ Quantitative sensory testing or thermal thresholds may be helpful
Antiretroviral toxic neuropathy (ATN)	■ Same as DSN (above), but symptoms occur after initiation of ddl, ddC, d4T. ■ Any CD4 cell count. ■ More common in older patients and patients with diabetes	■ Same as DSN (above)	■ EMG/NCVs show a predominantly axonal neuropathy ■ Discontinuation of presumed neuro- toxic medication if severe ■ Symptoms may worsen for a few weeks (coasting) before improving
Tarsal tunnel syndrome	■ Pain and numbness predominantly in anterior portion of soles of feet	■ Reduced sensation over soles of feet ■ Positive Tinel's sign at tarsal tunnel	■ Infiltration of local anesthetic in tarsal tunnel may provide symptomatic relief
HIV-associated neuromuscular weakness syndrome	■ Ascending paresis with areflexia ± cranial nerve or sensory involvement ■ Usually associated with prolonged d4T use	■ Lactate and CPK levels usually ↑ ■ EMG/nerve conduction studies – axonal neuropathy and myopathy	■ Discontinue NRTIs, especially d4T ■ Prognosis for survival is poor
HIV-associated myopathy/AZT myopathy	■ Pain and aching in muscles, usually in thighs and shoulders. ■ Weakness with difficulty when rising from a chair or reaching above shoulders ■ Any CD4 cell count	■ Mild/moderate muscle tenderness ■ Weakness, predominantly in proximal muscles (i.e., deltoids, hip flexors) ■ Normal sensory exam/normal reflexes	■ CPK ↑ ■ EMG shows irritable myopathy ■ Discontinue AZT and follow CPK every 2 weeks. Symptoms/signs/ CPK should improve within 1 month

continued on next page

Systems Review

Syndrome	Symptoms	Clinical Features	Ancillary Studies/ Treatment
Polyradiculitis	■ Rapidly evolving weakness and numbness in legs (both proximally and distally), with bowel/bladder incontinence ■ CD4 count >500/mm³ or <50/mm³	■ Diffuse weakness in legs ■ Diffuse sensory abnormalities in legs and buttocks ■ Reduced/absent reflexes at knees and ankles	■ EMG/NCV show multilevel nerve root involvement ■ Spinal fluid helpful in determining CMV or HSV as cause ■ Treat CMV polyradiculopathy with ganciclovir or foscarnet
Vacuolar myelopathy	■ Stiffness and weakness in legs with leg numbness. ■ Bowel/bladder incontinence in advanced cases ■ CD4 cell count <200/mm³	■ Weakness and spasticity, mainly in hip, knee, and ankle flexors ■ Brisk knee jerks, upgoing toes ■ If sensory neuropathy coexists, then distal sensory loss and reduced/absent jerks	■ Spinal fluid may show elevated protein 0-10 cells/mm³ ■ Exclude B-12 deficiency and HTLV-1 co-infection ■ Thoracic spinal imaging normal ■ No established therapy, but physical therapy or methionine (3 g bid) and HAART may be helpful (*Neurology* 1998;51:266)
Inflammatory demyelinating polyneuropathies	■ Predominantly weakness in arms and legs, with minor sensory symptoms. ■ CD4 count: may occur at any level	■ Diffuse weakness including facial musculature, asymmetric in early cases, with diffuse absent reflexes ■ Minor sensory signs	■ EMG/NCVs show a demyelinating polyneuropathy ■ Spinal fluid shows a very high protein with mild to moderate lymphocytic pleocytosis, but all cultures are negative ■ Treatment: Plasmapheresis. IVIG and/or HAART
Mononeuritis or mono-neuritis multiplex	■ Mix of motor and sensory defects ■ Asymmetric ■ Evolves over weeks ■ CD4 count is variable	■ EMG and nerve conduction – asymmetric and multifocal defects ■ R/O CMV (CSF or sural nerve biopsy) and HCV	■ CD4 count >200 cells/mm³ – possible steroids ■ CD4 counts <50 cells/mm³ and severe – treat for CMV

Inflammatory Demyelinating Polyneuropathy

CAUSE: Unclear; immunopathogenic mechanism with inflammation and breakdown of peripheral nerve myelin is suspected.

FREQUENCY: Uncommon

DIAGNOSIS: There are two forms: Acute demyelinating neuropathy (AIDP, Guillain-Barré Syndrome), which occurs early in the course of HIV, and a more chronic relapsing motor weakness, CIDP, which usually occurs in late-stage HIV. Both present with a progressive ascending paralysis with mild sensory involvement. CSF shows increased protein and mononuclear pleocytosis; EMG and nerve conduction studies are critical for diagnosis. Nerve biopsy may be needed and shows mononuclear, macrophage infiltrate, and internodal demyelination (*Ann Neurol* 1987;21:3240).

TREATMENT
- **AIDP**
  - Plasmapheresis: Five exchanges with maintenance as needed.
  - Alternative is IVIG 0.4 g/kg/day x 5 days (monitor renal function).
- **CIDP:** Oral prednisone (1 mg/kg/day) or intermittent plasmapheresis or IVIG; each continued until there is a therapeutic response.

RESPONSE: Treatment usually halts progression; CIDP may require prolonged courses (*Ann Neurol* 1987;21:3240).

Sensory Neuropathies (see algorithm p. 430)

Distal sensory neuropathy (DSN) and antiretroviral toxic neuropathy (ATN) (see *AIDS* 2002;16:2105)

CAUSE: HIV infection *per se*, usually with CD4 count <200 cells/mm^3 and/or dideoxy NRTIs (d-drugs): ddl, d4T, and ddC; most common with ddl + d4T (*AIDS* 2000;14:273). DSN and ATN are indistinguishable by clinical features or biopsy.

FREQUENCY: 20% with advanced HIV over 1 year and 52% over 2 years (*Neurology* 2002;58:1764)

DIFFERENTIAL: Toxic neuropathies due to drugs (metronidazole, B6 overdose, dapsone, INH, vincristine), diabetes, entrapment neuropathies, B12 deficiency, alcoholism, uremia, inflammatory demyelinating polyneuropathy, and acute neuromuscular syndrome

DIAGNOSIS: Dysesthesia and contact hypersensitivity of feet with decreased or absent ankle reflexes. Invasive neurodiagnostic tests may be useful but are usually unnecessary. Skin biopsy shows epidermal denervation. Electromyography/nerve conduction studies show predominantly axonal neuropathy. Quantitative sensory tests or thermal tests show elevated thresholds. See Table 7-12, p. 426-427.

TREATMENT

- **ATN:** Avoid d4T, ddI, and ddC; acceptable alternative agents in this class are AZT, 3TC, FTC, ABC, and TDF.
- **DSN**: Possible response reported with HAART (*Lancet* 1998;352: 1906).
- **Symptomatic treatment**
  - Gabapentin (*Neurontin*) 300-1200 mg PO tid
  - Lamotrigine (*Lamictal*) 25 mg bid increasing to 300 mg/day over 6 weeks; one of the few treatments with confirmed benefit in clinical trials (*Neurology* 2000;54:2115). Longer trial confirmed efficacy but only in patients who were receiving neurotoxic ARTs (*Neurology* 2003;60:1508-14). Generally not a first line agent due to high incidence of rash.
  - Tricyclic antidepressants nortriptyline 10 mg hs increased by 10 mg q5d to maximum 75 mg hs or 10-20 mg PO tid; other tricyclics (amitriptyline, desipramine, or imipramine) are considered comparable. One trial failed to show response to tricyclics (*JAMA* 1998;280:1590).
  - Ibuprofen 600-800 mg tid
  - Capsaicin-containing ointments (*Zostrix*, etc.); often not well tolerated.
  - Lidocaine 20% to 30% ointment (lidocaine gel 5% was not effective in a controlled trial (*J Acquir Immune Defic Syndr* 2004;37:1584))
  - Phenytoin 200-400 mg/day
  - Severe pain: Methadone – up to 20 mg qid; *Fentanyl* patch 25-100 mcg/hour q72h or morphine (note: drug interactions between fentanyl and protease inhibitors).
  - Acupuncture failed in one reported trial (*JAMA* 1998;280;1590).
  - Avoid tight footwear, limit walking, bridge at foot of the bed, use foot soaks.

RESPONSE: Sensory neuropathy due to NRTIs is usually reversible if the implicated agent is discontinued early, e.g., within 2 weeks of the onset of symptoms. If continued, the pain becomes irreversible and may be incapacitating. Response may require up to 12 weeks after discontinuing nucleosides (*Neurology* 1996;46:999). Treatment of sensory neuropathy, beyond discontinuing NRTIs, is symptomatic. Placebo-controlled trials have shown little or no benefit with amitriptyline, mexiletine, topical capsaicin and acupuncture (*JAMA* 1998;280:1590; *Neurology* 1998;51:1682; *J Acquir Infect Dis Syndr* 1998;19:367; *J Pain Sympt Manage* 2000;19:45). Many authorities use gabapentin. Best reported results from placebo-controlled trials were

7 Systems Review

with lamotrigine, but with a small sample size (*Neurology* 2003;60:1508),

■ FIGURE 7-2: **Sensory Neuropathies in Patients with AIDS**

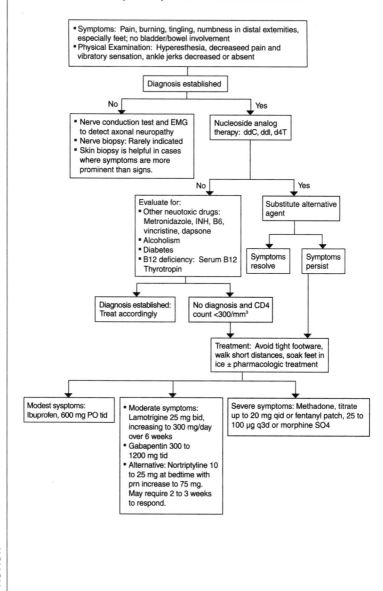

Systems Review

NEUROLOGIC COMPLICATIONS:
Central Nervous System

■ TABLE 7-13: **Central Nervous System Conditions in Patients with HIV Infection**

Agent/Condition Frequency (All AIDS Patients)	Clinical Features	CT Scan/MRI	Cerebrospinal Fluid (CSF)	Other Diagnostic Tests
Toxoplasmosis (2% to 4%) (see p. 379)	■ Fever, reduced alertness, headache,focal neurological deficits (80%), seizures (30%) ■ Evolution: <2 weeks ■ CD4 count <100/mm³	■ Location: Basal ganglia, gray-white junction ■ Sites: Usually multiple ■ Enhancement: prominent; Usually ring lesions (1 to 2 cm) ■ Edema/mass effect: Usually not as great as lymphoma	■ Normal: 20% to 30% ■ Protein: 10 to 150/mg/dL ■ WBC: 0 to 40 (monos) ■ Experimental: Toxo ag (ELISA) or PCR	■ Toxoplasmosis serology (IgG) false-negative in <5% ■ Response to empiric therapy: >85%; most respond by day 7 (*N Engl J Med* 1993;329:995) ■ MRI: Repeat at 2 weeks ■ Definitive diagnosis: Brain biopsy
Primary CNS Lymphoma (2%) (see p. 436)	■ Afebrile, headache, focal neurological findings; mental status change (60%), personality or behavioral; seizures (15%) ■ Evolution: 2 to 8 weeks ■ CD4 count <100/mm³	■ Location: Periventricular, anywhere, 2 to 6 cm ■ Sites: One or many ■ Enhancement: Prominent; usually solid, irregular ■ Edema/mass effect: Prominent	■ Normal: 30% to 50% ■ Protein: 10 to 150/mg/dL ■ WBC: 0 to 100 (monos) ■ EBV PCR in 50%	■ Suspect with negative toxo. IgG, single lesion, or failure to respond to empiric toxoplasmosis treatment (MRI and clinical evaluation at 2 weeks) ■ Thallium 201 SPECT scan (90% sensitive and specific)
Cryptococcal meningitis (8% to 10%) (see p. 336)	■ Fever, headache, alert (75%); less common are visual changes, stiff neck, cranial nerve deficits, seizures (10%); no focal neurologic deficits ■ Evolution: <2 weeks ■ CD4 count <100/mm³	■ Usually normal or shows increased intracranial pressure ■ Enhancement: Negative or meningeal enhancement ■ Edema mass effect: Ventricular enlargement/ obstructive hydrocephalus	■ Protein: 30 to 150/mg/dL ■ WBC: 0 to 100 (monos) ■ Culture positive: 95% to 100% ■ India ink pos: 60% to 80% ■ Crypt Ag: >95% sensitive and specific	■ Cryptococcal antigen in serum – sensitivity 95% ■ Definitive diagnosis: CSF antigen sensitivity and specificity >99% and/or positive culture

continued on next page

Systems Review

7

431

Agent/Condition Frequency (All AIDS Patients)	Clinical Features	CT Scan/MRI	Cerebrospinal Fluid (CSF)	Other Diagnostic Tests
CMV (>0.5%) (see p. 344)	■ Fever ±, delirium, lethargy, disorientation; headache; stiff neck, photophobia, cranial nerve deficits; no focal neurologic deficits ■ Evolution: <2 weeks ■ CD4 count <100/mm³	■ Location: Periventricular, brainstem ■ Site: Confluent ■ Enhancement: Variable, prominent to none.	■ CSF may be normal ■ Protein: 100 to 1000/mg/dL ■ WBC: 10 to 1000 (polys)/mL ■ Glucose usually decreased ■ CMV PCR positive ■ CSF cultures usually negative for CMV	■ Definitive diagnosis: Brain biopsy with histopathology and/or positive culture ■ Hyponatremia (reflects CMV adrenalitis) ■ Retinal exam for CMV retinitis
HIV Dementia (7%) (see p. 434)	■ Afebrile; triad of cognitive, motor, and behavioral dysfunction. ■ Early: Decreased memory, concentration, attention, coordination; ataxia ■ Late: Global dementia, paraplegia, mutism ■ Evolution: Weeks to months ■ CD4 count <200/mm³	■ Location: Diffuse, deep white matter hyperintensities ■ Site: Diffuse, ill-defined ■ Enhancement: Negative ■ Atrophy: Prominent ■ No mass effect	■ Normal: 30% to 50% ■ Protein: Increased in 60% ■ WBC: Increased in 5% to 10% (monos) ■ Beta-2 microglobulin elevated (>3 mg/L)	■ Neuropsychological tests show subcortical dementia ■ HIV dementia scale for screening (see p. 372)
Neurosyphilis (0.5%) (see p. 381)	■ Asymptomatic meningeal: headache, fever, photophobia, meningismus ± seizures, focal findings, cranial nerve palsies ■ Tabes dorsalis: Sharp pains, paresthesias, decreased DTRs, loss of pupil response	■ Aseptic meningitis: May show meningeal enhancement ■ General paresis: Cortical atrophy, sometimes with infarcts ■ Meningovascular syphilis: strokes	■ Protein: 45 to 200/mg/dL ■ WBC: 5 to 100 (monos) ■ VDRL positive: Sensitivity = 65%, specificity = 100% positive ■ Experimental: PCR for *T. pallidum*	■ Serum VDRL and FTA-ABS are clue in >90%; false-negative serum VDRL in 5% to 10% with tabes dorsalis or general paresis

■ TABLE 7-13: **Central Nervous System Conditions in Patients with HIV Infection** *(Continued)*

Agent/Condition Frequency (All AIDS Patients)	Clinical Features	CT Scan/MRI	Cerebrospinal Fluid (CSF)	Other Diagnostic Tests
Neurosyphilis (0.5%) – *continued* (see p. 381)	■ General paresis: Memory loss, dementia, personality changes, loss of pupil response ■ Meningovascular: Strokes, myelitis ■ Ocular: Iritis, uveitis, optic neuritis ■ Any CD4 cell count			■ Definitive diagnosis: Positive CSF VDRL (found in 60% to 70%) ■ Note: Most common forms in HIV-infected persons are ocular, meningeal, and meningovascular.
PML (1% to 2%) (see p. 354)	■ No fever; no headache; impaired speech, vision, motor function, cranial nerves ■ Late: ↓ cognition ■ Evolution: Weeks to months ■ CD4 count <100/mm³; some >200/mm³	■ Location: White matter, subcortical, multifocal ■ Sites: Variable ■ Enhancement: Negative ■ No mass effect	■ Normal CSF ■ PCR for JC virus: 80%	■ Brain biopsy: Positive DFA stain for JC virus
Tuberculosis (0.5% to 1%) (see p. 361)	■ Fever, reduced alertness, headache, meningismus, focal deficits (20%) ■ CD4 count <350/mm³	■ Intracerebral lesions in 50% to 70% (*N Engl J Med* 1992;326:668; *Am J Med* 1992;93:524)	■ Normal: 5% to 10% ■ Protein: Normal (40%) - 500/mL ■ WBC: 5 to 2000 (average is 60% to 70% monos) ■ Glucose: 4 to 0/mL ■ AFB smear positive: 20%	■ Chest x-ray: active TB in 50%; PPD positive: 20% to 30% ■ Definitive diagnosis: Positive culture CSF

Normal values: Protein: 15 to 45 mg/dL; traumatic tap: 1 mg/1000 RBCs; glucose: 40 to 80 mg % or CSF/blood glucose ratio >0.6; leukocyte counts: <5 mononuclear cells/mL, 5 to 10 is suspect, 1 PMN is suspect; bloody tap: 1 WBC/700 RBC; opening pressure: 80 to 200 mm H_2O.

CSF analysis in asymptomatic HIV infected persons shows 40% to 50% have elevated protein and/or pleocytosis (>5 mononuclear cell/mL); the frequency of pleocytosis decreases with progressive disease.

7 Systems Review

Cytomegalovirus Encephalitis (see p. 344)

CAUSE: CMV + CD4 count <50/mm^3

FREQUENCY: <0.5% of AIDS patients

PRESENTATION: Rapidly progressive delirium, cranial nerve deficits, nystagmus, ataxia, headache with fever ± CMV retinitis

DIAGNOSIS: MRI shows periventricular confluent lesions with enhancement. CMV PCR in CSF is >80% sensitive and 90% specific; and cultures of CSF for CMV are usually negative.

TREATMENT: Ganciclovir, foscarnet, or both IV (see p. 344).

RESPONSE: Trial of foscarnet plus ganciclovir showed a median survival of 94 days compared with 42 days in historic controls (*AIDS* 2000;14:517).

Dementia (HIV-Associated Dementia or HAD)

CAUSE: Chronic encephalitis with progressive or static encephalopathy due to CNS HIV infection with prominent immune activation

INCIDENCE: 7% after AIDS in pre-HAART era; 2% to 3% more recently (*Neurology* 2001;56:257). Despite a decrease in incidence, the prevalence is increasing with longer survival (*AIDS* 2003;17:1539).

PRESENTATION: Late stage HIV with CD4 count <200 cells/mm^3 and subcortical dementia. See Table 7-12 and 7-13. Early symptoms: Apathy, memory loss, cognitive slowing, depression, and withdrawal. Motor defects include gait instability and reduced hand coordination. Late stages show global loss of cognition, severe psychomotor retardation, and mutism. There may be seizures, which are usually easily controlled. The rate of progression is highly variable, but the average from first symptoms to death in the pre-HAART era was 6 months (*Medicine* 1987;66:407). Physical examination in early disease shows defective rapid eye movement, rapid limb movement, and generalized hyperreflexia. In late stages, there is tremor, clonus, and frontal release signs.

TESTING

■ TABLE 7-14: **HIV Dementia Scale (*AIDS Reader* 2002;12:29)**

Maximum Score	Test*
See below	Memory registration: 4 words given (hat, dog, green, peach) and have the patient repeat them.
6	Psychomotor speed: Record the time, in seconds, that it takes the patient to write the alphabet. Score: <21 sec = 6, 21.1-24 sec = 5, 24.1-27 sec = 4, 27.1-30 sec = 3, 30.1-33 sec = 2; 33.1-36 sec = 1, >36 = 0
4	Memory recall: Ask for the four words from above. For words not remembered give semantic clue, e.g. "animal" (dog), "color" (green), etc. 1 point for each correct answer.
2	Construction: Copy a cube and record time. Score: <25 sec = 2, 25-35 sec = 1, >35 = 0

* ≤7/12 is threshold for dementia but is non-specific requiring additional neurologic evaluation.

■ TABLE 7-15: **AIDS Dementia Complex Staging**

Stage 0	Normal
Stage 0.5	Subclinical: Minimal – equivocal symptoms; no work impairment.
Stage 1.0	Mild – minimal intellectual or motor impairment; able to do all but more demanding work or ADL.
Stage 2.0	Moderate – cannot work or perform demanding ADL; capable of self care.
Stage 3.0	Severe – major intellectual disability; unable to walk unassisted.
Stage 4.0	End stage – near vegetative stage; paraplegia or quadriplegia.

DIAGNOSIS: History, physical examination, and screening with HIV Dementia Scale as noted above. Formal testing includes: Trail Making B, Digital Symbol, Grooved Pegboard, and the HIV Dementia Scale. MRI shows cerebral atrophy (which can be present without symptoms), typically with rarefaction of white matter (*J Neurol Neurosurg Psych* 1997;62:346). CSF shows increased protein with 0-15 mononuclear cells; pleocytosis is absent in 65%. Main goal is to exclude alternative diagnosis because no test is specific for HAD.

TREATMENT: The HIV Dementia Scale (see Table 7-14) can be used to follow response to HAART. HAART has reduced the frequency of HAD, but there are sparce data to show efficacy of HAART for reversing established HAD (*J Neurovirol* 2002;8:136; *J Neurol* 2004;10:350). It is also unclear whether CNS penetration is important in the selection of agents. Antiretroviral agents with the best CNS penetration based on CSF levels are AZT, d4T, ABC, NVP, and IDV; levels are somewhat lower for EFV, ddI, 3TC, and FPV (*J Acquir Immune Defic Syndr* 1998;235:238; *AIDS* 1998;12:537). Adjunctive therapies to block immune activation are being tested in trials of NMbA receptor antagonists and antioxidants such as selegiline.

RESPONSE: HAART is associated with significant increases in survival (*AIDS* 2003;17:1539) and reduced incidence of HAD, but its role in treatment of HAD specifically is unclear (*Brain Pathol* 2003;13:104).

Primary CNS Lymphoma (PCNSL)

CAUSE: Virtually all are EBV-associated (*Lancet* 1991;337:805).

FREQUENCY: 2% to 6% in pre-HAART era – 1000 times higher than in the general population (*Lancet* 1991;338:969). The incidence has declined in the HAART but not as that of much as other HIV complications (*J Acquir Immune Defic Syndr* 2000;25:451).

PRESENTATION: Focal or non-focal signs. Symptoms include confusion, headache, memory loss, aphasia, hemiparesis, and/or seizures without fever for <3 months. CD4 count is usually <50/mm^3.

DIAGNOSIS: MRI shows single lesion or multiple lesions that are isodense or hypodense and usually homogeneous, but sometimes ring forms (*Am J Neuroradiol* 1997;18:563). With contrast, CT and MRI scans show enhancement that is usually irregular (due to rapid growth). These lesions usually involve the corpus callosum, periventricular area, or periependymal area; they are often >4 cm in diameter and usually show a mass effect (*Neurology* 1997;48:687). Major differential diagnosis is toxoplasmosis. Factors favoring CNS lymphoma are: 1) Typical neuro imaging results (above), 2) Negative anti-*Toxoplasma* IgG serology, 3) Failure to respond to empiric treatment of toxoplasmosis within 1 to 2 weeks, 4) Lack of fever, and 5) Thallium SPECT scan with early thallium uptake. CSF EBV PCR is >94% specific and 50-80% sensitive (*Clin Infect Dis* 2002;34:103; *J Natl Cancer Inst* 1998;90:364; *Lancet* 1992;342:398). Stereotactic brain biopsy is definitive and usually reserved for patients who fail to respond to toxoplasmosis treatment (*AIDS* 1995;9:1243; *Clin Infect Dis* 2002;34:103). A review of five reports with 486 AIDS patients undergoing stereotactic brain biopsy showed a 4% morbidity rate (*Clin Infect Dis* 2002;34:103).

THERAPY

- **Standard:** Radiation plus corticosteroids (*J Neuro Sci* 1999;163:32) or methotrexate (*J Clin Oncol* 2003;21:1044)
- **Chemotherapy:** May be combined with radiation plus corticosteroids. Usually reserved for patients with elevated CD4 counts.

RESPONSE: Response rates to radiation therapy plus corticosteroids is 20% to 50%, but these results are temporary, and the average duration of life following the onset of symptoms was only about 4 months in the pre-HAART era (*Crit Rev Oncol* 1998;9:199; *Semin Oncol* 1998;25:492). A trial with methotrexate showed a 74% radiographic response rate with modest toxicity (*J Clin Oncol* 2002;31:171).

Progressive Multifocal Leukoencephalopathy (PML) (see p. 54)

CAUSE: Activation of JC virus (which is ubiquitous) in patients who are immunodeficient.

FREQUENCY: 1% to 2% of AIDS patients (*J Infect Dis* 1999;180:261)

PRESENTATION: Cognitive impairment, visual field deficits, hemiparesis speech defects, incoordination with *no* fever. CD4 count is usually 35-100/mm^3, but a subset of 7% to 25% have CD4 counts >200/mm^3 (*Clin Infect Dis* 2002;34:103).

DIAGNOSIS

- MRI shows hypodense lesions of white matter without edema or enhancement.
- PCR for JCV in CSF with sensitivity of 80% and specificity of 95% (*Clin Infect Dis* 2005;40:738).

TREATMENT: None with established merit. HAART may be associated with improvement stabilization or progression (see p. 308). One report shows PML response to HAART with enhancing lesions on MRI suggesting immune reconstitution syndrome (*AIDS* 1999;13:1426). There is conflicting evidence for cidofovir (*AIDS* 2002;16:1791; *J Neurovirol* 2001;7:364; *J Neurovirol* 2001;7:374).

PROGNOSIS: Median duration of survival is 1 to 6 months. Response to HAART is possible, but some patients have developed PML while receiving HAART (*Clin Infect Dis* 2002;34:103). The most important predictor of survival is baseline CD4 cell count.

Toxoplasmosis (see p. 379)

ORAL COMPLICATIONS

Candidiasis (see p. 331)

Herpes Simplex (see p. 347)

Kaposi's Sarcoma (see p. 420)

Oral Hairy Leukoplakia (OHL) (*Clin Infect Dis* 1997;25:1392)

CAUSE: Intense replication of EBV

PRESENTATION: Unilateral or bilateral adherent white/gray patches on lingual lateral margins ± dorsal or ventral surface of tongue. Patches are irregular folds and projections.

7 Systems Review

DIFFERENTIAL: Candidiasis: OHL does not respond to azoles and cannot be scraped off, unlike *Candida*; Others: squamous cell carcinoma or traumatic leukoplakia.

DIAGNOSIS: Diagnosis is usually clinical; biopsy is rarely necessary.

IMPLICATIONS: Found almost exclusively with HIV, indicates low CD4 count, predicts AIDS, and responds to immune reconstitution with HAART.

TREATMENT (*Clin Infect Dis* 1997;25:1392): Rarely symptomatic and rarely treated, but occasional patients have pain or have concern about appearance. The options include:

- **HAART** (preferred)
- **Topical podophyllin**
- **Surgical excision**
- **Cryotherapy**
- **Anti-EBV treatment:** Acyclovir 800 mg PO 5x/day x 2 to 3 weeks, then 1.2-2 gm/day. Other effective antivirals include famciclovir, valacyclovir, foscarnet, ganciclovir, and valganciclovir. Lesions recur when treatment is discontinued.

Salivary Gland Enlargement

CAUSE: May be lymphoid proliferation due to HIV (*Ann Intern Med* 1996;125:494)

PRESENTATION: Parotid enlargement, cystic, unilateral or bilateral, non-tender, usually asymptomatic; may be painful, cosmetically disfiguring, or cause xerostomia (*Ear Nose Throat J* 1990;69:475).

DIFFERENTIAL: Must differentiate cystic from solid lesion with CT scan (*Laryngoscope* 1998;98:772) and/or fine needle aspiration (FNA). FNA useful for microbiology and cytology and decompression. May require biopsy to exclude tumor, especially lymphoma. Biopsy usually shows histology resembling Sjögren's Syndrome (*J Oral Pathol Med* 2003; 32:544) or "non-specific chronic sialadenitis" (*Oral Dis* 2003;9:55). The most common infections are mycobacteria and CMV.

TREATMENT

- FNA for decompression of fluid-filled parotid cysts; may require large-bore needle for asporation.
- **Xerostomia:** Sugarless chewing gum, artificial saliva, pilocarpine

PSYCHIATRIC COMPLICATIONS

Bipolar Disorder (Manic Depression)

FREQUENCY: 9% of AIDS patients referred for psychiatric evaluation (*JAMA* 2001;86:2849)

DIAGNOSIS: Manic episodes, depressive episodes, and mixed episodes. Differential includes familial bipolar disorder and AIDS mania (no family history, no episodes prior to late stage HIV, co-morbid cognitive impairment.

TREATMENT

- **AIDS Mania:** HAART (Acute management)
  - □ Haloperidol (*Haldol*) 0.5-5 mg bid
  - □ Fluphenazine (*Prolixin*) 0.5-5 mg bid
  - □ Risperidone (*Risperdal*) 0.5-3 mg bid
  - □ Olanzapine (*Zyprexa*) 5-20 mg hs
- One of the above ± lithium 300 mg bid titrated to level of 0.5-1.0 mEq/mL or valproic acid 20 mg/kg titrated to serum level of 50-100 ng/mL.
- **Adjunctive therapy:** Carbamazepine (*Tegretol*), gabapentin (*Neurontin*), lamotrigine (*Lamictal*)
- Care should be directed by a psychiatrist.

Delirium

DIAGNOSIS: Impaired consciousness, inability to focus or sustain interest, cognitive changes, global derangement of brain function, acute onset, altered consciousness, or disorganized thinking

TREATMENT: Correct underlying condition, which may be infection or medication related.

- **Agitation:** Neuroleptics such as haloperidol (*Haldol*) or risperidone
- **Agitation that puts others at risk:** Neuroleptics + low dose of lorazepam for sedation

Demoralization

FREQUENCY: 20% of AIDS patients referred for psychiatric evaluation

DIAGNOSIS: Exaggerated grief state, sad, hopelessness, often precipitated by life circumstances. Often mistaken for depression, but unlike depression, often can enjoy some facets of life, feels best in the mornings and does not respond to antidepressants.

TREATMENT: Psychotherapy and support

Systems Review

7

RESPONSE: Responds to psychotherapy and usually not to antidepressants

Grief (Normal state of low mood focused on loss)

Treatment is psychological rather than pharmacological (support groups, buddy systems).

Major Depression

FREQUENCY: 20% of AIDS patients referred for psychiatric evaluation (*JAMA* 2001;286:2849)

PRESENTATION: Depressed mood, loss of pleasure from activities (anhedonia), anorexia, morning insomnia or hypersomnia, difficulty concentrating, thoughts of suicide

DIFFERENTIAL: Dementia, delirium, demoralization, intoxications or withdrawal, neurologic diseases

TREATMENT: Antidepressants (Table 7-16) starting with low doses and titrating slowly ("start low and go slow") with appropriate attention to side effects and serum levels.

RESPONSE: Response rates to antidepressants is 85%; cure rate >50% (*Psychosomatic* 1997;38:423).

■ TABLE 7-16: **Depression: Drug Selection**

Agent	Advantages	Disadvantages
SSRIs	■ Relatively safe and well tolerated ■ Compared with tricyclics: Fewer drug interactions and side effects ■ Safety with overdose	■ ADRs: Sexual dysfunction, substrate and inhibitor of P450 enzymes ■ Use with PI or NNRTI may increase level of SSRI
Tricyclics	■ Equally effective compared with SSRIs ■ Also useful for neuropathy insomnia and diarrhea	■ ADRs: Anticholinergic effects, dry mouth, blurred vision, orthostasis ■ Use with PI or NNRTI may increase tricyclic level ■ Refractory arrhythmia with overdose

Obsessive-Compulsive Disorder

DIAGNOSIS: Recurrent obsessions (preoccupying thoughts that the patient finds irrational and tries to resist) and/or compulsions (actions driven by obsessions to reduce anxiety)

TREATMENT: Refer to psychiatrist or a mental health specialist.

Panic Attacks

DIAGNOSIS: Recurring anxiety attacks with fear plus somatic symptoms of excitation lasting <1 hour

TREATMENT: SSRI and refer to a psychiatrist

Sleep Disturbance

Medications with FDA approval for insomnia have potential for reinforcement and habituation. Evaluate patient for cause (major depression, mania, substance use disorder, demoralization) and refer for appropriate treatment. Insomnia temporally related to a specific stress (pre-op, grief etc.) may be treated with sedatives or hypnotics up to 1 week or with trazodone 25-150 mg hs for up to 4 weeks.

Substance Use Disorders

DIAGNOSIS: Use of substances despite clear evidence of negative consequences. Dependence: Persistent use or seeking use, withdrawal, tolerance, and physical dependence.

■ TABLE 7-17: **Detoxification**

Agent	Treatment
Sedative/hypnotic EtOH, benzodiazepines, and barbiturates	■ Long acting benzodiazepines (chlordiazepoxide – *Librium*, diazepam – *Valium*)
Alprazolam (*Xanax*)	■ Substitute clonazepam and taper
Cocaine	■ Suicidal symptoms common; may need brief hospitalization
Opioids	■ Clonidine for autonomic instability. Buprenorphine or methadone tapers; dicyclomine for GI distress

PULMONARY COMPLICATIONS

Pneumonia

PRESENTATION: Cough, dyspnea, and fever ± sputum production

CAUSE: The single major prospective study of pulmonary complications of HIV was discontinued in the pre-HAART era – 1995 (*Am J Respir Crit Care Med* 1997;155:72). Data from 3 years (1992-1995) showed 521 infections: PCP – 45%, common bacteria – 42%, tuberculosis – 5%, CMV – 4%, *Aspergillus* – 2%, and cryptococcosis – 1%. The risk of bacterial pneumonia was increased 7.8-fold compared to the general population (*Am Rev Respir Dis* 1993;148:1523). Critical factors in evaluating the HIV infected patient with suspected pneumonia are

- **HIV stage** based on CD4 count (see Table 7-19, p. 444)
- **Tempo:** Pyogenic infections and influenza evolve rapidly. PCP develops slowly in HIV infected patients, with an average duration of 3 weeks prior to presentation.
- **X-ray changes:** A negative chest X-ray generally excludes pneumonia, though 10% to 20% with PCP have a false negative x-ray (*J Acquir Immune Defic Syndr* 1994;7:39); infiltrates can be

shown in these cases with thin-section CT scan (*Am J Radiol* 1997;169:967). Rare false-negative X-rays can be seen with tuberculosis, MOTT, and cryptococcosis (see Table 7-18). Intrathoracic lymphadenopathy on chest X-ray or CT scan suggests TB, lymphoma, KS, or atypical mycobacterial infection (*J Acquir Immune Defic Syndr* 2002;31:318).

- **Injection drug use:** Associated with high rates of pneumococcal pneumonia, *S. aureus* endocarditis with septic pulmonary emboli, tuberculosis, and aspiration pneumonia.

- **Prophylaxis:** TMP-SMX (see Figure 7-3, p. 445) effectively reduces incidence of PCP, bacterial pneumonia including *S. pneumoniae, Legionella, H. influenzae*, and *S. aureus*. Influenza vaccine appears to decrease the risk of influenza (*Arch Intern Med* 2001;161:441). Pneumovax shows variable results (*Br Med J* 2002;325:292). INH substantially reduce the risk of TB.

- **Bacteria:** The most common bacterial causes of pneumonia are, in rank order: *S. pneumoniae, H. influenzae, P. aeruginosa* and *S. aureus* (*Clin Infect Dis* 1996;23:107; *Am J Respir Crit Care Med* 1995;152:1309; *N Engl J Med* 1995;333:845; *J Infect Dis* 2001;184:268; *AIDS* 2002;16:2361; *J Acquir Immune Defic Syndr* 1994;7:823; *AIDS* 2003;17:2109). The rate of pneumococcal bacteremia is increased 150- to 300-fold with HIV infection; see p. 378. *H. influenzae* pneumonia usually involves non-typeable strains (*JAMA* 1992;268:3350). *P. aeruginosa* is a cause of pneumonia in late stage HIV infection and often causes bacteremia and relapses (*J Acquir Immune Defic Syndr* 1994;7:823).

- **Atypical:** Pneumonia due to *M. pneumoniae, C. pneumoniae*, and *Legionella* appears to be relatively uncommon in patients with HIV infection (*Eur J Clin Microbiol Infect Dis* 1997;16:720; *N Engl J Med* 1997;337:682; *N Engl J Med* 1995;333:845; *Am J Resp Crit Care Med* 1995;152:1309; *Clin Infect Dis* 1996;23:107; *Am J Resp Crit Care Med* 2000;162:2063; *Clin Infect Dis* 2004;40[suppl 3]:S150).

DIAGNOSTIC SPECIMENS

- **Expectorated sputum:** Controversial, due in part to poor technique in collecting, transporting, and processing specimens.

- **Expectorated sputum for *M. tuberculosis*:** The yield with three specimens is 50% to 60% for AFB stain; and somewhat higher with PCR at 75% to 85% (*Am J Respir Crit Care Med* 2001;164:2020).

- **Induced sputum:** Recommended as an alternative to expectorated sputum for detection of AFB in patients who cannot produce an expectorated sample and as an alternative to bronchoscopy for detection of PCP. Sensitivity for detection of TB by AFB smear is about the same as it is for expectorated sputum; for PCP sensitivity is 56% (*Eur Resp J* 2002;20:982).

- **Bronchoscopy:** The yield for PCP is 95% or comparable to open-lung biopsy (*JAMA* 2001;286:2450). For *M. tuberculosis*, sensitivity is similar to that for expectorated sputum (see p. 361). For other bacteria, bronchoscopy is no better than expectorated sputum unless it is accompanied by quantitative culture.

- **Miscellaneous:** Tests to consider in atypical or nonresponsive pulmonary infections include *Legionella* urinary antigen, *H. capsulatum* serum and urinary antigen, serum cryptococcal antigen, CT scan and bronchoscopy with biopsy.

■ TABLE 7-18: **Correlation of Chest X-ray Changes and Etiology of Pneumonia**

Change	Common	Uncommon
Consolidation	Pyogenic bacteria, Kaposi's sarcoma, cryptococcosis	*Nocardia, M. tuberculosis, M. kansasii, Legionella, B. bronchiseptica*
Reticulonodular infiltrates	*P. jiroveci, M. tuberculosis,* histoplasmosis, coccidioidomycosis	Kaposi's sarcoma, toxoplasmosis, CMV, leishmania, lymphoid interstital pneumonitis
Nodules	*M. tuberculosis,* cryptococcosis	Kaposi's sarcoma, *Nocardia*
Cavity	*M. tuberculosis, S. aureus* (IDU), *Nocardia, P. aeruginosa,* cryptococcosis, coccidioidomycosis, histoplasmosis, aspergillosis, anaerobes	*M. kansasii,* MAC, *Legionella, P. carinii,* lymphoma, *Klebsiella, Rhodococcus equi*
Hilar nodes	*M. tuberculosis,* histoplasmosis, coccidioidomycosis, lymphoma, Kaposi's sarcoma	*M. kansasii,* MAC
Pleural effusion	Pyogenic bacteria, Kaposi's sarcoma, *M. tuberculosis* (congestive heart failure, hypoalbuminemia	Cryptococcosis, MAC, histoplasmosis, coccidioidomycosis, aspergillosis, anaerobes, *Nocardia,* lymphoma, toxoplasmosis, primary effusion lymphoma

7 Systems Review

CD4 count >200 cells/mm³	*S. pneumoniae, M. tuberculosis, S. aureus* (IDU), influenza
CD4 count 50-200 cells/mm³	Above + *P. jiroveci*, cryptococcosis, histoplasmosis, coccidioidomycosis, *Nocardia, M. kansasii*, Kaposi's sarcoma
CD4 count <50 cells/mm³	Above + *P. aeruginosa, Aspergillus*, MAC, CMV

RENAL COMPLICATIONS (see *Ann Intern Med* 2003;139:214; IDSA/CDC Guidelines, *Clin Infect Dis* 2005;40:1559)

DIAGNOSTIC TESTS

- **Screening:** With any proteinuria get 24-h urine protein or spot protein: creatinine; need to quantify protein

- **Patients with chronic renal disease:** imaging by ultrasound to detect stones, extrarenal and intrarenal lesions and renal size (HIVAN)

- **Miscellaneous studies:** HBV and HCV serology, complement level, ANA, serum and urine electrophoresis

- **Renal biopsy:** Indications are significant proteinuria, progressive disease, acute or subacute renal failure or nephritic syndrome with hematuria, proteinuria, hypertension and renal failure.

DIAGNOSES IN HIV-INFECTED PERSONS: HIVAN, membranous nephropathy, membranoproliferative glomerulo-nephritis, diabetic nephropathy, hypertensive nephropathy and IgA nephropathy.

Hepatitis C Co-infection (see J Am Soc Nephrol 1999;10:1566)

CAUSE: Mixed cryoglobulinemia

SYMPTOMS: Palpable purpura, decreased complement, and renal disease

DIAGNOSIS

- **Evidence of HCV** (Positive EIA + HCV RNA)

- **Renal disease** with hematuria and proteuria often in nephrotic range ± renal insufficiency

- **Low complement**

- **Renal biopsy** with evidence of HCV-related immune complexes

- **Circulating cryoglobulins** ± skin biopsy of purpuric lesion

```
                    ┌─────────────────────┐
                    │ CD4 count <250/mm³, │
                    │ prior PCP, thrush, or│
                    │ unexplained fever    │
                    └─────────────────────┘
```

* **Severe:** Urticaria, angioedema, Stevens-Johnson reaction, or fever. **Intolerance:** GI symptoms, rash/pruritis. **Mild:** Tolerable with aggressive supportive care and/or dose reduction.

TREATMENT: Pegylated interferon + ribavirin is preferred (see p. 407), but ribavirin is not recommended with creatinine clearance <50 mL/min due to increased risk of toxicity (e.g., hemolytic anemia).

Heroin Nephropathy (HAN) (*Clin Infect Dis* 2005;40:1559)

CAUSE: Unknown, possibly glomerular epithelial cell injury from toxin contaminant (*Am J Kidney Dis* 1995;25:689)

FREQUENCY: Unknown, but decreasing with increasing purity of street heroin. Frequency is increased in African Americans, who account for 94% of renal failure cases in one series of 98 patients (*JAMA* 1983;250:2935).

DIFFERENTIAL: Main differential is HIVAN. HAN shows: 1) hypertension. 2) small kidneys by echo. 3) less rapid progression to end-stage renal disease (20 to 40 months vs 1 to 4 months). 4) less proteinuria. 5) differences on renal biopsy (*Semin Nephrol* 2003; 23:117).

HIV-Associated Nephropathy (HIVAN)

CAUSE: Unknown, possibly due to HIV infection of glomerular endothelial and mesangial cells (*N Engl J Med* 2001;344:1979)

FREQUENCY: An analysis of 3,976 HIV-infected patients in Baltimore showed an incidence of 0.8/1000 patient-years. Risk factors include African-American race (RR = 7.8), AIDS (5.0) and VL >100,000 c/mL (2.0). Other risk factors are male sex, family history of renal disease (*Am J Kidney Dis* 1999;34:254; *Am J Kidney Dis* 2000;35:884) and injection drug use (*Kidney Int* 1987;31:1678; *Kidney Int* 1990;37:1325; *N Engl J Med* 1987;316:1062).

DIAGNOSIS: Baseline proteinuria is a sensitive predictor of chronic renal disease (*Clin Nephrol* 2004;61:1; *J Acquir Immune Defic Syndr* 2003;32:2003). Most patients with HIVAN present with nephrosis with proteinuria >1 gm/d, hypoalbuminemia, normal blood pressure, large echogenic kidneys and rapid progression to end stage renal disease in 1-4 months (*Kidney Int* 1995;48:311; *Am J Roentgen* 1998;171:713; *N Engl J Med* 1987;316:1062; *Sem Dialy* 2003;16:233). Renal biopsy shows a collapsing focal glomerulosclerosis with tubulo-interstitial injury. Renal biopsy is recommended to establish this diagnosis in an NIH review of HIV-associated renal disease (*Ann Intern Med* 2003;139:214). The etiology is thought to be intrarenal infection with HIV (*Nat Med* 2002;8:522; *N Engl J Med* 2001;344:1979; *J Am Soc Nephrol* 2001;12:1677).

TREATMENT

- **HAART:** Preliminary data based on biopsy results suggest benefit from HAART (*Lancet* 1998;352:783; *Clin Nephrol* 2002;57:335; *N Engl J Med* 2001;344:1979). Some show dramatic improvement with HAART (*N Engl J Med* 2001;344:1971), but this may be only temporary (*AIDS Patient Care STD* 2000;14:657).

- **Dialysis** (*Am J Kidney Dis* 1997;29:549)

- **ACE Inhibitors** (captopril 6.25-25 mg PO tid) and others show beneficial results, but most of the studies were done in the pre-HAART era, making conclusions for current management difficult (*Kidney Int* 2003;64:1462; *J Am Soc Nephrol* 1997;8:1140; *Am J Kidney Dis* 1996;28:202).

- **Corticosteroids** (60 mg/day x 2 to 11 weeks, then taper over 2 to 26 weeks) show variable results in terms of renal function and proteinuria (*Am J Med* 1994;97:145; *Kidney Int* 2000;58:1253; Semin Nephrol 1998;18:446).

- **Transplantation:** Results in 23 patients given HAART with no detectable virus and CD4 >200/mm³ showed graft survival of 87% (*Kidney Int* 2003;63:1618).

HIV-Associated Immune-Mediated Glomerulonephritides

- **COURSE:** Proliferative glomerulonephritis may be nonspecific and related to HCV, HBV, IgA nephropathy or disordered immunity. This is distinguished from HIV-associated nephropathy, seen primarily in patients of African descent (*Ann Intern Med* 2003;139:214)
- **TREATMENT:** HAART, steroids and/or ACE inhibitors

Nephrotoxic Drugs

Amphotericin, aminoglycoside, cidofovir, foscarnet, pentamidine, IV acyclovir, TMP-SMX, indinavir (see below), sulfonamides (crystal induced)

INDINAVIR: Renal calculi ± nephropathy (*Ann Intern Med* 1997;127:119)

- **Cause:** Crystallization of indinavir
- **Prevention:** Should be taken without food, but with water ≥150 mL within 3 hours post dose and ≥1500 mL/day.
- **Dose-dependent:** Especially with ritonavir in 800/100 mg bid regimen.
- **Diagnosis:** Urine shows indinavir sulfate crystals – rectangular plates of various sizes with needle-shaped crystals and pyuria (*Clin Nephrol* 2000;54:261; *N Engl J Med* 1997;336:139).
- **Symptoms:** Review of urinalysis from 140 IDV recipients showed 20% had crystalluria; 3% of these had renal colic and most of the rest had frequency plus dysuria and/or flank pain (*Ann Intern Med* 1997127:119). A prospective study of 184 IDV recipients showed 35% had albuminuria, RBCs, pyuria and crystals; those with persistent pyuria had a 25% probability of an elevated serum creatinine (*J Acquir Immune Defic Syndr* 2003;32:135).
- **Treatment**
  - □ Remove stones by ureteroscopy or by passage.
  - □ Discontinue IDV in symptomatic patients (discontinue all antiretroviral drugs or substitutes).

Thrombotic Thrombocytopenic Purpura (see p. 418)

Systems Review

7

Abbreviations

Drug Abbreviations

3TC	Lamivudine	IDV	Indinavir
5-FC	Flucytosine	INH	Isoniazid
ABC	Abacavir	LPV/r	Lopinavir/Ritonavir
APV	Amprenavir	NFV	Nelfinavir
AZT	Zidovudine	NVP	Nevirapine
d4T	Stavudine	PZA	Pyrazinamide
ddC	Zalcitabine	RIF	Rifampin
ddI	Didanosine	RTV	Ritonavir
DLV	Delavirdine	SM	Streptomycin
EFV	Efavirenz	SMX	Sulfamethoxazole
EMB	Ethambutol	SQV	Saquinavir
EPO	Erythropoietin	TDF	Tenofovir disoproxil fumarate
G-CSF	Filgrastim	TMP	Trimethoprim
HU	Hydroxyurea	TMP-SMX	Trimethoprim-sulfamethoxazole

Drug Administration Abbreviations

bid	Twice a day	m^2	Meters squared
caps	Capsules	max	Maximum
cc	Cubic centimeter	mcg	Microgram
cm	Centimeter	mEq	Milliequivalent
cm^2	Centimeters squared	mg	Milligram
d/c	Discontinue	mil	Million
dL	Deciliter	min	Minimum
DS	Double strength	mL	Milliliter
dx	Diagnosis	mm	Millimeter
g	Gram	mM	Millimole
H_2O	Water	mo	Month
Hg	Mercury	MU	Million units
hr	Hour	N	Normal (solution) or total sample size
hs	Hours of sleep		
IM	Intramuscular	ng	Nanogram
IU	International unit	OTC	Over-the-counter
IV	Intravenous	PO	By mouth
kg	Kilogram	PSI	Pounds per square inch
L	Liter	pt-yrs	Patient-years
m	Meter	q	Every

Drug Administration Abbreviations *(Continued)*

qd	Every day	VD	Volume of distribution
qhs	At bedtime	vol	Volume
qid	Four times a day	wk	Week
qod	Every other day	wgt	Weight
SQ	Subcutaneously	x	Times
sol'n	Solution	XL	Extended release
SS	Single strength	yr	Year
supp	Supply	µg	Microgram
tabs	Tablets	µL	Microliter
tid	Three times per day	µM	Micrometer
tiw	Three times per week	µmol	Micromole
U	Unit		

General Abbreviations

ACTG	AIDS Clinical Trial Group (U.S.)	C-section	Cesarean section
ADL	Activities of daily living	CSF	Cerebrospinal fluid
ADR	Adverse drug reaction	CT	Computerized tomography
AETC	AIDS Education Training Center (U.S.)	CTL	Cytotoxic T lymphocyte
AFB	Acid-fast bacillus	DEXA	Dual energy x-ray absorptiometry
AHCPR	Agency for Health Care Policy and Research (U.S.)	DFA	Direct fluorescent antibody
AI	Aluminum	DHHS	Department of Health and Human Services (U.S.)
ALT	Alanine aminotransferase	DOT	Directly observed therapy
ANC	Absolute neutrophil count	EBV	Epstein-Barr virus
anti-HAV	Hepatitis A antibody	EDTA	Ethylenediamine tetraacetic acid
anti-HBc	Hepatitis B core antibody		
anti-HBs	Hepatitis B surface antibody	EIA	Enzyme immunosorbent assay
anti-HCV	Hepatitis C antibody	EM	Electron microscopy
ART	Antiretroviral therapy	ERCP	Endoscopic retrograde cholangio-pancreatography
ASCUS	Atypical sqamous cells of undetermined significance	ETOH	Alcohol
AST	Aspartate aminotransferase	FOB	Fiberoptic bronchoscopy
AWP	Average wholesale price	FDA	Food and Drug Administration (U.S.)
BUN	Blood urea nitrogen		
Ca	Calcium	G6-PD	Glucose-6-phosphate dehydrogenase
CBC	Complete blood count		
CDC	Centers for Disease Control and Prevention (U.S.)	GFR	Glomerular filtration rate
		GI	Gastrointestinal
CF	Complement fixation	HAART	Highly active antiretroviral therapy
CMV	Cytomegalovirus		
CNS	Central nervous system	HAD	HIV-associated dementia
CPK	Creatine phosphokinase	HAV	Hepatitis A virus
CrCl	Creatine clearance	HBeAg⁻	Hepatitis B early antigen
CROI	Conference on Retroviruses and Opportunistic Infections	HBIG	Hepatitis B immune globulin
		HBV	Hepatitis B virus

General Abbreviations *(Continued)*

HCFA	Health Care Financing Administration (U.S.)	MCV	Mean corpuscular volume
		Mg	Magnesium
HCV	Hepatitis C virus	MSM	Men who have sex with men
HCW	Health care worker	MSSA	Methicillin sensitive *Staph aureus*
HDL	High density lipoprotein		
Hgb	Hemoglobin	NASBA	Nucleic acid sequence-based amplification
HPV	Human papillomavirus		
HSIL	High-grade squamous intraepithelial lesion	NCEP	National Cholesterol Education Program (U.S.)
HSV	Herpes simplex virus	NCI	National Cancer Institute (U.S.)
HSV-1	Herpes simplex virus 1	NIAID	National Institute of Allergy and Infectious Diseases (U.S.)
HSV-2	Herpes simplex virus 2		
HTLV-1	Human T-cell leukemia virus 1	NIH	National Institute of Health (U.S.)
HTLV-2	Human T-cell leukemia virus 2		
IAS	International AIDS Society	NNRTI	Non-nucleoside reverse transcriptase inhibitor
IAS-USA	International AIDS Society-U.S.A.		
		NRTI	Nucleoside reverse transcriptase inhibitor
ICAAC	Interscience Conference on Antimicrobial Agents and Chemotherapy		
		NS	Not significant
		NSAID	Nonsteroidal anti-inflammatory drug
ICL	Idiopathic CD4 lymphocytopenia		
		OHL	Oral hairy leukoplakia
IDSA	Infectious Diseases Society of America	OI	Opportunistic infection
		OP	Opening pressure
IG	Immune globulin	PAP smear	Papanicolaou smear
IgE	Immunoglobulin E		
IgG	Immunoglobulin G	PBMC	Peripheral blood mononuclear cells
IgM	Immunoglobulin M		
IL-2	Interleukin 2	PCP	*Pneumocystis carinii* pneumonia
IM	Intramuscular		
IOM	Institute of Medicine	PCR	Polymerase chain reaction
ITP	Idiopathic thrombocytopenic purpura	PEP	Postexposure prophylaxis
		PGL	Persistent generalized lymphadenopathy
ITT	Intent-to-treat (analysis)		
IVIG	Intravenous immune globulin	PHS	Public Health Service (U.S.)
JCV	JC virus	PID	Pelvic inflammatory disease
KOH	Potassium hydroxide	PI	Protease inhibitor
KS	Kaposi's sarcoma	PML	Progressive multifocal leukoencephalopathy
LDH	Lactate dehydrogenase		
LDL	Low-density lipoprotein	PMN	Polymorphonuclear leukocyte
LFT	Liver function test	PPD	Purified protein derivative of tuberculin
LP	Lumber puncture		
LSIL	Low-grade squamous intraepithelial lesion	Pr	Protease
		PUVA	Psoralen ultraviolet A-range
LVEF	Left ventricular ejection fraction	RBC	Red blood cells
		rHU EPO	Recombinant human erythropoietin
MAC	*Mycobacterium avium* complex		
MACS	Multicenter AIDS Cohort Study	RIBA	Recombinant Immunoblot assay
MAO	Monoamine oxidase		

Medical Management of HIV Infection: Abbreviations

General Abbreviations *(Continued)*

RPR	Rapid plasma regain	TLC	Total lymphocyte count
RT	Reverse transcriptase	TNF-alpha	Tumor necrosis factor-alpha
RT-PCR	Reverse transcriptase polymerase chain reaction	TSH	Thyroid stimulating hormone
		TST	Tuberculin skin test
SIL	Squamous intraepithelial lesion	ULN	Upper limit of normal
SSRI	Selective serotonin reuptake inhibitors	USPHS	Public Health Service (U.S.)
		UTI	Urinary tract infection
STD	Sexually transmitted disease	UVB	Ultraviolet B
STEPS	Systems for Thalidomide Education and Prescribing Safety	VRDL	Venereal disease research laboratory
		vs	Versus
STI	Structured treatment interruption	VZIG	Varicella zoster immune globulin
TAM	Thymidine analog mutation	VZV	Varicella zoster virus
TB	Tuberculosis	WBC	White blood count
TEN	Toxic epidermal necrolysis	WB	Western blot
THC	Tetrahydrocannabinol	WHO	World Health Organization

Index

Page numbers followed by "f" indicate figures; those followed by "t" indicate tables.

A

Medical Management of HIV Infection: Index

drug interactions with, 87t, 161
for sedative-hypnotic withdrawal, 441t
withdrawal from, 161
Bepridil, drug interactions with, 87t
Biaxin. See Clarithromycin
Bipolar disorder, 439
Blastomyces infection, 237t
Bleeding in hemophilia patients, 113
Bleomycin, for non-Hodgkin's lymphoma,
423
Blood donor screening, 6
Blood glucose testing, 38t, 105
Bone toxicity of drugs, 113, 325, 413–415
Brachial neuritis, 3t
Branched chain DNA assay, 14
Breastfeeding
antimycobacterial therapy and, 367t
antiretroviral therapy and, 120, 129
HIV transmission via, 118–119
Bronchoscopy, 443
"Buffalo hump," 100
Bupropion *(Wellbutrin, Zyban),* 162–163
Burkitt's lymphoma, 4t
Buspirone *(BuSpar),* 163–164
Butenafine *(Mentax),* for *Tinea* infections,
389
Butoconazole, for *Candida* vaginitis, 334

C

Calcium channel blockers, drug
interactions with, 87t, 95t
atazanavir, 155
Calypte **HIV-1 Urine Test,** 13, 14t
Campylobacter jejuni **infection,** 395
Candida **infection,** 4t, 331–335
cutaneous, 388
esophagitis, 2t, 333–334, 400t–401t
thrush, 2t, 3t, 331–333
treatment of, 148t, 164, 173, 208t, 237t,
267
vaginitis, 2t, 334–335
Capreomycin, for tuberculosis, 366t
Capsaicin ointment *(Zostrix),* for sensory
neuropathies, 429
Captopril
for dilated cardiomyopathy, 385
for HIV-associated nephropathy, 446
Carbamazepine *(Tegretol)*
for bipolar disorder, 439
drug interactions with, 94t–95t
for herpes zoster, 350
Cardiac drugs, interactions with, 87t
Cardiopulmonary complications,
385–387
dilated cardiomyopathy, 385
hyperlipidemia, 106–110
pulmonary hypertension, 385–386
tricuspid valve endocarditis, 378,
386–387

Caspofungin *(Cancidas),* 164
for *Aspergillus* infection, 330
for *Candida* infection, 333, 401t
CBC (complete blood count), 36–37
CD4 cell count, 19–23
in AIDS case definition, 3t
analytical variations in, 20
CD4 cell percentage, 21, 21t, 39t
complications correlated with, 2t, 58t
corticosteroid effects on, 21
factors influencing, 20–21
in HIV-2 infection, 6
in HTLV-1 co-infection, 21
in idiopathic CD4 lymphocytopenia, 23
immunologic failure and, 72
initiation of antiretroviral therapy based
on, 57–58, 58t–60t
natural history of infection and, 1f
normal values for, 20
pneumonia etiology and, 444t
prognosis and, 19
response to antiretroviral therapy, 22
seasonal and diurnal variations in,
20–21
after splenectomy, 21
technique for measurement of, 20
testing of, 39t
frequency of, 20
in pregnancy, 123
reproducibility of, 20
in therapeutic drug monitoring, 73t, 75
total lymphocyte count as surrogate for,
20, 22
treatment interruption strategies based
on, 81–82
viral load and, 1f, 15, 16, 75
CD4 repertoire, 22–23
CD8 cells, 19–20
Cefazolin, for *Staphylococcus aureus*
infection, 377
Cefepime, for *Pseudomonas* infection, 374
Cefoperazone, for *Pseudomonas* infection,
374
Cefotaxime, for *Streptococcus pneumoniae*
infection, 378
Cefoxitin, for atypical mycobacterial
infections, 359
Ceftazidime, for *Pseudomonas* infection,
374
Ceftriaxone
for *Nocardia* infection, 370
for *Salmonella* infection, 376
for *Staphylococcus aureus* infection, 377
for *Streptococcus pneumoniae* infection,
378
for syphilis, 382
Cefuroxime, for *Haemophilus influenzae*
infection, 346
Cephalexin, for *Staphylococcus aureus*

years in absence of antiretroviral
therapy, 58t
psychiatric, 439–441
pulmonary, 441–443
renal, 444–447
Controlled substances classification,
136t
Copegus. See Ribavirin
Corticosteroids
for aphthous ulcers, 394, 401t
effect on CD4 cell count, 21
for eosinophilic folliculitis, 391
for HIV-associated nephropathy,
446–447
for idiopathic thrombocytopenia purpura,
417t
for immune recovery vitritis, 344
for *M. tuberculosis* immune
reconstitution syndrome, 363
for MAC immune recovery syndrome,
359
for *P. jiroveci* pneumonia, 373
for primary central nervous system
lymphoma, 436
for prurigo nodularis, 391
for seborrheic dermatitis, 393
Cotrimoxazole. *See* Trimethoprim-
sulfamethoxazole
Counseling
of healthcare workers after occupational
HIV exposure, 128, 129
for positive result on home test kit, 10
of pregnant women, 115–116, 129
Creatinine clearance, 135
Crestor. See Rosuvastatin
Crix-belly″, 100
Crixivan. See Indinavir
Cryoglobulinemia, 444
Cryptococcus neoformans **infection,** 2t,
4t, 336–339
cutaneous, 388
immune reconstitution syndrome in, 338,
419t
meningitis, 336–338, 431t
prophylaxis for, 338
pulmonary, disseminated, or
antigenemia, 338–339
treatment of, 148t, 208t, 237t
Cryptosporidium parvum **infection,** 2t, 4t,
269–270, 339–340, 398
Cyclophosphamide
for non-Hodgkin's lymphoma, 423
for primary effusion lymphoma, 424
Cycloserine
for atypical mycobacterial infections,
361
in renal or hepatic insufficiency, 368t
for tuberculosis, 366t
Cyclospora **infection,** 398

Cytomegalovirus (CMV) infection, 2t, 4t,
341–346
activity of antivirals against, 144t
diagnostic tests for, 38t, 46
esophagitis, 344, 400t–401t
gastrointestinal, 344, 398–399
immune reconstitution syndrome in, 343,
419t
neurological, 344–345, 425, 432t, 434
pneumonitis, 346
retinitis, 217–218, 341–344
treatment of, 144t, 165–166, 217–220
Cytosine arabinoside, for non-Hodgkin's
lymphoma, 423
Cytovene. See Ganciclovir

D

d4T. *See* Stavudine
Dalmane. See Flurazepam
Dapsone, 174–176
adverse reactions to, 50, 174–175
drug interactions with, 175–176
for *P. jiroveci* pneumonia, 174t, 373
prophylaxis, 50, 174t, 445f
in pregnancy, 176
for toxoplasmosis, prophylaxis, 53, 174t
Daraprim. See Pyrimethamine
**Daunorubicin citrate liposome injection
(DaunoXome),** 176–177
for Kaposi's sarcoma, 176, 422t
for primary effusion lymphoma, 424
ddC. *See* Zalcitabine
ddl. *See* Didanosine
Delavirdine (DLV, *Rescriptor*), 83t, 86t,
177–179
advantages and disadvantages of, 64t,
177–178
adverse reactions to, 86t, 178
hepatotoxicity, 111t
clinical trials of, 178
dosing recommendations for, 86t
in renal or hepatic failure, 177, 178
drug interactions with, 178–179, 179t
clarithromycin, 171t
indinavir, 230t
lopinavir/ritonavir, 250t
methadone, 254t
nelfinavir, 259t
rifabutin, 284t, 367t
saquinavir, 294t
formulations of, 86t, 177
pharmacokinetics of, 86t, 178
for postexposure prophylaxis, 126
in pregnancy, 114t, 124t, 179
resistance to, 31t, 37t
Delirium, 439
Dementia
cytomegalovirus, 344–345
HIV-associated, 2t, 4t, 432t, 434–436,

Medical Management of HIV Infection: Index

Medical Management of HIV Infection: Index

efficiency of transmission from, 130
management resources for, 125
postexposure prophylaxis for, 130,
131t
risk of transmission from sharps
injury, 125t
transmission from healthcare worker to
patient, 129
treatment of, 112, 405–406, 407t
adefovir, 406, 407t
emtricitabine, 112, 406, 407t
entecavir, 198–200, 199t, 406, 407t
interferon, 232, 406, 407t
lamivudine, 112, 199t, 241–242,
407t
tenofovir, 112, 406, 407t
Hepatitis C virus (HCV) infection, 110,
111, 404t, 407–412
antiretroviral therapy in, 408–409
diagnosis of, 38t, 44–45, 45t, 131, 404t,
407
immune reconstitution syndrome in, 419t
occupational exposure to, 131–132
efficiency of transmission from, 131
management of infection acquired
from, 132
postexposure management of, 131
risk of transmission from sharps
injury, 125t
prognosis for, 132
renal disease and, 444–445
seroprevalence of, 131
transmission from healthcare worker to
patient, 129
treatment of, 132, 409–412, 410t, 445
interferon, 232
pegylated interferon, 270–271, 271t,
410t, 411
ribavirin, 132, 281, 410t, 411
Hepatosplenomegaly, 3t
Hepatotoxic drugs
antimycobacterial agents, 369
antiretroviral agents, 110–113
drugs associated with, 111t,
112–113, 235, 238, 244, 263–264,
278, 321, 325
grading of, 110t
hepatitis B or hepatitis C co-
infection and, 110, 111
monitoring for, 74t
in pregnancy, 121–122
Heroin nephropathy (HAN), 445–446
Herpes simplex virus (HSV) infection, 2t,
4t, 347–349
activity of antivirals against, 144t
esophagitis, 348, 400t–401t
genital, 142, 347–349
immune reconstitution syndrome in, 419t
orolabial, 142, 347

treatment of, 142–143, 143t
Herpes zoster, 2t, 143, 143t, 349–350
HHV-8 (human herpesvirus-8) infection,
activity of antivirals against, 144t
**Highly active antiretroviral therapy
(HAART).** *See* Antiretroviral therapy
Histoplasma capsulatum **infection,** 2t,
4t, 350–353
prophylaxis for, 55–56, 352
treatment of, 148t, 208t, 237t
HIV-1, 5
Circulating Recombinant Forms of, 5
subtypes of, 5
HIV-2, 5–7
antiretroviral therapy for, 67
clinical features of, 6
factors affecting management of, 6
indications to test for, 7
prevalence of, 6–7
serology of, 6, 8
transmission of, 6
HIV-associated dementia (HAD), 2t, 4t,
432t, 434–436, 435t
**HIV-associated immune-mediated
glomerulonephritis,** 447
HIV-associated nephropathy, 446–447
HIV Dementia Scale, 435, 435t
HIV RNA assays, 14–19
comparison of, 18t, 19
cost of, 15
factors not measured by, 19
frequency of, 17
indications for, 15–17
in pregnancy, 115
quality assurance for, 17
reproducibility of, 15
subtypes of, 15
techniques for, 14, 18t
for therapeutic monitoring, 16–17
HIV subtypes, 5
false-negative serology for, 8
geographic distribution of, 5, 5t
HIV vaccines, 9
Hivid. See Zalcitabine
Hodgkin's lymphoma, 2t
Home Access Express Test, 10
HPV (human papillomavirus) infection,
43
HSV. *See* Herpes simplex virus infection
HU. *See* Hydroxyurea
**Human growth hormone (somatropin,
Serostim),** 223–224
Human herpesvirus-8 (HHV-8) infection
activity of antivirals against, 144t
Kaposi's sarcoma, 420–422
primary effusion lymphoma, 424
pulmonary hypertension, 386
Human papillomavirus (HPV) infection
anal cancer and, 43

frequency of, 105
monitoring for, 74t
risks associated with, 105–106
screening for, 105
treatment of, 106
Interferon *(Infergen, Intron, Roferon)*,
231–233
drug interactions with, 233
for hepatitis B, 232, 406, 407t
for hepatitis C, 232
for Kaposi's sarcoma, 232–233, 422t
pegylated, 270–273
in pregnancy, 233
Intermittent treatment interruption (ITI),
81
Intracranial pressure elevation, in
cryptococcal meningitis, 336–338
Intravenous immune globulin (IVIG), for
idiopathic thrombocytopenia purpura, 417t
***Intron.** See* Interferon
***Invirase.** See* Saquinavir
Iodoquinol, for *Entamoeba histolytica*
infection, 399
Iron deficiency, 414
IRS (immune reconstitution syndrome),
419, 419t
Isoniazid (INH, *Laniazid, Nydrazid,*
***Teebaconin*),** 234–235
adverse reactions to, 365t
for atypical mycobacterial infections,
360
monitoring during therapy with, 52
in renal or hepatic insufficiency, 368t
resistance to, 52, 368t
for tuberculosis, 234t, 364t
latent, 369
in pregnancy, 367t
prophylaxis, 51, 234t
***Isospora belli* infection,** 4t, 315, 353
ITI (intermittent treatment interruption),
81
ITP (idiopathic thrombocytopenic
purpura), 2t, 280, 417, 417t
Itraconazole *(Sporanox)*, 236–239, 237t
for *Aspergillus* infection, 237t
for *Blastomyces* infection, 237t
for *Candida* infection, 237t, 331–334,
401t
for *Coccidioides* infection, 237t, 335
for *Cryptococcus* infection, 237t,
337–339
for dermatophyte infection, 237t
drug interactions with, 238
for *Histoplasma* infection, 237t, 351–352
prophylaxis, 56, 352
for microsporidiosis, 355–356
for onychomycosis, 237t, 389
for *Penicillium* infection, 237t, 371
in pregnancy, 239

for sporotrichosis, 237t
Ivermectin *(Stromectol)*, for scabies, 392
IVIG (intravenous immune globulin), for
idiopathic thrombocytopenia purpura, 417t

J

JC virus infection, 354–355, 419t, 433t,
437
Jock itch, 389

K

***Kaletra.** See* Lopinavir/ritonavir
Kanamycin, for tuberculosis, 366t
Kaposi's sarcoma, 2t, 4t, 420–422
diagnosis of, 421t
immune reconstitution syndrome in, 419t
treatment of, 176, 232–233, 421–422,
422t
***Ketek.** See* Telithromycin
Ketoconazole *(Nizoral)*, 239–240
for *Candida* infection, 239, 332, 333,
335, 388
drug interactions with, 92t–93t, 240,
240t
for *Penicillium* infection, 371
in pregnancy, 240
for seborrheic dermatitis, 393
for *Tinea* infections, 389
***Kwell.** See* Lindane

L

Laboratory tests, 5–47
for antiretroviral resistance, 23–36
CD4 cell count, 19–23
for *Chlamydia trachomatis,* 40
for cytomegalovirus, 46
in exposed person and source after
needle sharing or sexual contact, 134t
for glucose-6-phosphate dehydrogenase
deficiency, 46–47
for hepatitis A, 38t, 43, 404t
for hepatitis B, 38t, 44, 404.404t
for hepatitis C, 38t, 44–45, 45t, 404t,
407
for HIV diagnosis, 5–19
CLIA regulation of, 11
comparison of, 13t–14t
DNA PCR, 13
HIV-2, 6, 8
HIV RNA assays, 14–19
in newborns, 116, 122
after occupational exposure of
healthcare worker, 128
p24 antigen assay, 15
in pregnancy, 115, 116
saliva test, 12
serologic tests, 7–12 (*See also*
Serologic testing)
in source patient after occupational

Papillary stenosis, cholangiopathy with, 404
Para-aminosalicylic acid (PAS), for tuberculosis, 366t
Paregoric, 355
Paromomycin *(Humatin)*, 269–270
  for *Cryptosporidium* infection, 340
  for *Entamoeba histolytica* infection, 346, 399
Parotid gland enlargement, 438
Parvovirus B19 infection, 414, 419t
PAS (para-aminosalicylic acid), for tuberculosis, 366t
Patient assistance programs, 135. *See also specific drugs*
PBMC culture, 14t
PCNSL (primary central nervous system lymphoma), 2t, 431t, 436–437
PCP. *See Pneumocystis jiroveci* pneumonia
PEG (percutaneous endoscopic gastrostomy), 394
Pegylated interferon *(Pegasys, Peg-Intron)*, 270–273
  adverse effects of, 272–273, 272t
  for hepatitis B, 407t
  for hepatitis C, 132, 270–271, 271t, 410t, 411, 445
Peliosis hepatitis, 330–331
Penicillin
  allergy skin test and desensitization to, 382, 384t
  for *Streptococcus pneumoniae* infection, 378
  for syphilis, 382, 383t
Penicillium marneffei infection, 148t, 237t, 371
Pentamidine *(NebuPent, Pentam)*, 50, 273–275
  for *P. jiroveci* pneumonia, 273, 373
  prophylaxis, 50, 273, 445f
Pentoxifylline *(Trental)*, for aphthous ulcers, 394
PEP. *See* Postexposure prophylaxis
Percutaneous endoscopic gastrostomy (PEG), 394
Perinatal HIV transmission, 116–119. *See also* Pregnancy
  antiretroviral therapy for reduction of, 115, 116–117
    nevirapine, 117, 265–266
    zidovudine, 115, 116–117, 120–121, 326–327
  via breastfeeding, 118–119
  cesarean section for reduction of, 115, 117–118, 118t
  in developing countries, 116, 118–119, 120–121
  mechanism of, 116
  prevalence of, 116

in twin births, 116
viral load and, 116, 118
Periodontitis, necrotizing, 402t
Peripheral neuropathy, 2t, 3t, 313, 426t–427t, 428–430
  drugs associated with, 182, 235, 297–298, 308, 322
  inflammatory demyelinating polyneuropathy, 428
  sensory neuropathies, 428–430, 430f
Permethrin cream
  for *Demodex folliculorum* infection, 391
  for scabies, 392
Persistent generalized lymphadenopathy (PGL), 2t, 3t
Pharmacokinetics of antiretroviral agents. *See also specific drugs*
  food effects, 76, 84t, 86t, 88t
  NNRTIs, 86t
  nucleoside analogs, 84t–85t
  PIs, 88t–91t
Pharyngitis, 3t
Phenobarbital, drug interactions with, 94t–95t
PhenoSense, 37t
Phenotypic assays, for antiretroviral resistance, 24, 28, 29t, 37t
Phenytoin
  drug interactions with, 94t–95t
  for sensory neuropathies, 429
Pimozide, drug interactions with, 87t
Piperacillin, for *Pseudomonas* infection, 374
PIs. *See* Protease inhibitors
Pityrosporum ovale infection, 390–391
Placental transfer, of antiretroviral agents, 120, 124t
PML (progressive multifocal leukoencephalopathy), 2t, 4t, 354–355, 433t, 437
Pneumococcal vaccine *(Pneumovax)*, 54–55
Pneumocystis jiroveci (P. carinii) pneumonia, 2t, 4t, 372–374, 441–444
  immune reconstitution syndrome in, 50–51, 419t
  prophylaxis for, 49–51, 315, 442, 445f
  treatment of, 157, 171, 273, 276, 314, 315, 372–374
Pneumonia, 2t, 4t, 441–444, 443t
  Aspergillus, 329
  diagnosis of, 442–443
  etiologies of, 441–442
    CD4 cell count and, 444t
    chest X-ray changes and, 441–442, 443t
  P. jiroveci, 2t, 4t, 49–51, 372–374, 441–444
  pneumococcal, 378–379

Medical Management of HIV Infection: Index

viral load, 15–16, 18
Progressive multifocal leukoencephalopathy (PML), 2t, 4t, 354–355, 433t, 437
Prolixin. See Fluphenazine
Propafenone, drug interactions with, 87t
Protease inhibitors (PIs), 83t, 88t–91t. *See also specific drugs*
  advantages and disadvantages of, 63t–64t
  adverse reactions to, 74t, 90t–91t
    hepatotoxicity, 111t, 112–113
    increased bleeding in hemophilia patients, 113
    insulin resistance, 105–106
    lipodystrophy, 101
  dosing recommendations for, 88t–89t
    in renal or hepatic failure, 98t–99t, 100
  drug interactions with, 87t, 92t–97t
    clarithromycin, 171t
    delavirdine, 179t
    efavirenz, 193t
    indinavir, 230t
    ketoconazole, 240t
    lopinavir/ritonavir, 250t
    methadone, 254t
    nelfinavir, 259t
    nevirapine, 264t
    rifabutin, 284t, 367t
    rifampin, 367t
    ritonavir, 291t
    saquinavir, 294t
    statins, 109
    tipranavir, 311
    voriconazole, 321
  formulations of, 88t–89t
  in initial regimen, 61t–62t
  once-daily drugs, 66t
  pharmacokinetics of, 88t–91t
  poor adherence to, 77
  in pregnancy, 114t, 115, 120, 124t
  resistance to, 6, 31t–32t, 35t–37t
    changing therapy regimen due to, 77–78
  ritonavir-boosted, 63t–64t, 88t–89t, 287, 288t
    for postexposure prophylaxis, 126, 127t
  for salvage therapy, 78
  target trough levels for, 73t
  virologic failure with regimen based on, 77–78
"Protease pouch," 100
Proton pump inhibitors, drug interactions with, 87t, 95t
  atazanavir, 155
Protostat. See Metronidazole
Prurigo nodularis, 391

Pseudomonas aeruginosa **infection,** 374–375
Psychiatric complications, 3t, 439–441
  bipolar disorder, 439
  delirium, 439
  demoralization, 439–440
  grief, 440
  major depression, 440
  obsessive-compulsive disorder, 440
  panic attacks, 440
  sleep disturbance, 441
  substance use disorders, 441, 441t
Psychotropic agents, drug interactions with, 87t
Pulmonary complications, 441–443
  pneumonia, 441–444, 443t
Pulmonary hypertension, 385–386
Pyomyositis, staphylococcal, 377
Pyrazinamide (PZA), 277–278
  adverse reactions to, 365t
  for atypical mycobacterial infections, 359
  monitoring during therapy with, 52
  in renal or hepatic insufficiency, 368t
  for tuberculosis, 277, 277t, 364t
    latent, 369
    in pregnancy, 367t
    prophylaxis, 51, 52
Pyridoxine, for tuberculosis
  latent, 369
  prophylaxis, 51
Pyrimethamine *(Daraprim)* plus leucovorin, 245, 278–280
  for *Isospora* infection, 353
  prophylaxis for *P. jiroveci* pneumonia, 50, 445f
  for toxoplasmosis, 279t, 379–380, 379t
    prophylaxis, 53, 279
Pyrimethamine plus sulfadoxine *(Fansidar),* 50, 279
  for *Isospora* infection, 353
PZA. *See* Pyrazinamide

Q

Quazepam *(Doral),* 162t
Quinidine, drug interactions with, 87t

R

Rapid HIV tests, 10–12, 11t, 13t
  indications for, 12
  positive predictive value of, 12, 12t
  in pregnancy, 115
  for source patient after occupational exposure of healthcare worker, 128
Rapid plasma reagin (RPR) test, 38t, 39, 381
Rash, 3t. *See also* Dermatologic complications
  drugs associated with, 50, 121, 191, 213,

264, 308, 316–317, 321, 323
in syphilis, 381
Ravuconazole, for *Aspergillus* infection, 330
Rebetol. See Ribavirin
Rebetron. See Ribavirin
Recombivax HB, 55
Reglan. See Metoclopramide
Relenza. See Zanamivir
Renal complications, 444–447
  diagnosis of, 444
  hepatitis C and, 444–445
  heroin nephropathy, 445–446
  HIV-associated immune-mediated glomerulonephritis, 447
  HIV-associated nephropathy, 446–447
  nephrotoxic drugs, 229–230, 302–303, 447
  thrombotic thrombocytopenia purpura, 418
Renal disease
  antimycobacterial therapy in, 368t
  antiretroviral therapy in, 98t–99t (*See also specific drugs*)
Renal transplantation, 447
Rescriptor. See Delavirdine
Rescue therapy. *See* Salvage therapy
Reservoirs of HIV, 17
Resistance to antiretroviral therapy, 23–36. *See also specific drugs*
  adherence and, 68
  in HIV-2 infection, 6
  mutations causing, 30t–36t
    persistence of, 27, 76
    prevalence of, 23, 27
    treatment interruption strategies for, 80
    virologic failure without, 77
  testing for, 24–29, 76
    to assess minority species, 60–61, 76
    in chronically infected patients with virologic failure, 25–26
    in chronically infected treatment-naive patients, 27
    genotypic assays for, 24, 28, 29, 29t, 60
    indications for, 25t
    interpretation of, 24–25
    limitations of, 24
    after occupational exposure of healthcare workers, 129
    phenotypic assays for, 24, 28, 29t, 37t
    in pregnancy, 25t, 27, 120, 123
    in primary HIV infection, 26, 27t
    for salvage therapy, 24, 26
    before treatment initiation, 60
    validity after therapy is

discontinued, 76
    viral load required for, 24, 25
    Virtual Phenotype for, 28–29
Respiratory tract infections, 184
  pneumonia, 441–444, 443t
Restoril. See Temazepam
Reticulocytes, 413t
Retinal necrosis, in herpes zoster, 349
Retinitis, cytomegalovirus, 217–218, 341–344
Retrovir. See Zidovudine
Reveal G$_2$ test, 6, 11, 11t
Reyataz. See Atazanavir
Rhodococcus equi **infection,** 375
Rho(D) immune globulin (WinRho), 280–281
  for idiopathic thrombocytopenia purpura, 280, 417t
Ribavirin (Copegus, Rebetol, Rebetron, Ribasphere), 281–282
  drug interactions with, 282
    didanosine, 182, 184, 281, 282
    zidovudine, 326
  for hepatitis C, 132, 281, 410t, 411, 445
  in pregnancy, 282
Rifabutin (Mycobutin), 282–284
  for atypical mycobacterial infections, 361, 370
  drug interactions with, 87t, 92t–93t, 283–284, 284t, 367t
    atazanavir, 155
    indinavir, 231
    lopinavir/ritonavir, 249
    methadone, 254t
    nelfinavir, 259
    nevirapine, 265
    ritonavir, 290
  for *M. avium* complex infection, 282, 357–358
    prophylaxis, 53, 282, 340
  for tuberculosis, 282, 366t
    prophylaxis, 51–52
Rifadin. See Rifampin
Rifamate, 234–235, 285
Rifampin (Rifadin), 285–287
  adverse reactions to, 365t
  for atypical mycobacterial infections, 359–360
  drug interactions with, 87t, 92t–93t, 286–287, 367t, 369
    methadone, 254t
    ritonavir, 290
  in renal or hepatic insufficiency, 368t
  for *Rhodococcus equi* infection, 375
  for tuberculosis, 285, 364t
    in pregnancy, 367t
    prophylaxis, 51–52, 285
    resistance to, 368t
Rifater, 234–235, 278, 285

Rimantadine, for influenza, prophylaxis, 55
Ringworm, 389
Risperidone *(Risperdal)*, for bipolar
  disorder, 439
Ritonavir (RTV, *Norvir*), 83t, 88t, 90t,
  287–291
  advantages and disadvantages of,
    63t–64t
  adverse reactions to, 90t, 289
    hepatotoxicity, 112
    insulin resistance, 105
  clinical trials of, 288
  dosing recommendations for, 88t, 287
    in renal or hepatic failure, 98t, 289
  drug interactions with, 92t, 94t, 96t–97t,
    289–290, 291t
    clarithromycin, 171t
    delavirdine, 179t
    efavirenz, 193t
    fluoxetine, 211
    indinavir, 230t
    ketoconazole, 240t
    methadone, 254t
    nelfinavir, 259t
    nevirapine, 264t
    rifabutin or rifampin, 284t, 367t
    saquinavir, 294t
    tipranavir, 310
    voriconazole, 321
  formulations of, 88t, 287
  in initial regimen, 61t–62t
  pharmacokinetics of, 88t, 90t, 288
  for postexposure prophylaxis, 126, 127t,
    134t
  in pregnancy, 120, 124t, 291
  protease inhibitors boosted with,
    63t–64t, 287, 288t
  resistance to, 31t, 37t, 288
  target trough levels for, 73t
Roferon. See Interferon
Rosiglitazone, for lipodystrophy, 102
Rosuvastatin *(Crestor)*, 107
RPR (rapid plasma reagin) test, 38t, 39,
  381
RTV. *See* Ritonavir

S

Saliva HIV test, 12, 14t
Salivary gland enlargement, 438
Salmonella infection, 4t, 168, 315,
  375–376, 397
Salvage therapy, 78–80
  clinical trials of, 80
  mega-HAART for, 80
  protease inhibitors for, 78
  regimens for, 79, 79t, 228
  resistance testing for, 24, 26
  after three class failures, 78–80
Sandostatin. See Octreotide

Saquinavir (SQV, *Fortovase, Invirase*),
  83t, 88t, 90t, 291–295
  advantages and disadvantages of, 64t
  adverse reactions to, 90t, 293
  clinical trials of, 292–293
  dosing recommendations for, 88t
    in renal or hepatic failure, 99t, 100,
      291
  drug interactions with, 92t, 94t, 96t–97t,
    293–294, 294t
    clarithromycin, 171t
    delavirdine, 179t
    efavirenz, 193t
    indinavir, 230t
    ketoconazole, 240t
    lopinavir/ritonavir, 250t
    methadone, 254t
    nelfinavir, 259t
    nevirapine, 264t
    rifabutin or rifampin, 284t, 367t
    ritonavir, 291t
    tipranavir, 311
  food requirement for, 76, 291
  formulations of, 88t, 291
  in initial regimen, 61t, 62t
  pharmacokinetics of, 88t, 90t, 293
  for postexposure prophylaxis, 126, 127t,
    134t
  in pregnancy, 114t, 115, 124t, 295
  resistance to, 31t, 37t, 293
  ritonavir-boosted, 88t, 288t
  target trough levels for, 73t
Sargramostim (GM-CSF, *Immunex*), 221,
  418
Scabies, 391–392
Screening laboratory tests, 36–47,
  38t–39t
  chest X-ray, 40–41
  complete blood count, 36–37
  for hepatitis A, 43
  for hepatitis B, 44
  for hepatitis C, 44–45, 45t
  Pap smear, 41–43, 42t
    anal, 43
  PPD skin test, 41
  serum chemistry panel, 37
  for sexually transmitted diseases
    Chlamydia trachomatis, 40
    Neisseria gonorrhoeae, 40
    syphilis, 39–40
    trichomoniasis, 40
Sculptra. See Poly-L-lactic acid injection
Seborrheic dermatitis, 392–393
Selective serotonin reuptake inhibitors
  (SSRIs), 440t
Sensory neuropathies, 426t, 428–430,
  430f
Septra. See Trimethoprim-sulfamethoxazole
Serax. See Oxazepam

pneumococcal, 54–55
varicella, 143
Vacuolar myelopathy, 2t, 427t
Vaginal secretions, HIV detection in, 13
Vaginitis, *Candida,* 2t, 173, 208t, 237t, 267, 334–335
Valacyclovir *(Valtrex),* 141–145
  activity against herpesviruses, 144t
  for chickenpox, 350
  for cytomegalovirus infection, 343–346
  for herpes simplex virus infection, 347–348, 401t
  for herpes zoster, 349
  indications for, 142–144, 143t
  for oral hairy leukoplakia, 144
  in pregnancy, 145
Valcyte. *See* Valganciclovir
Valganciclovir *(Valcyte),* 217–220, 219t, 302
  for cytomegalovirus infection, 341, 401t
Valium. *See* Diazepam
Valtrex. *See* Valacyclovir
Vancomycin
  for *Clostridium difficile* infection, 396
  for *Rhodococcus equi* infection, 375
  for *Staphylococcus aureus* infection, 377
    tricuspid valve endocarditis, 387
Vardenafil, drug interactions with, 94t–95t
Varicella-zoster immune globulin (VZIG), 54, 350
Varicella-zoster virus (VZV) infection, 349–350
  activity of antivirals against, 144t
  immune reconstitution syndrome in, 419t
  postexposure prophylaxis for, 54
  serologic testing for, 38t
  treatment of, 143, 143t, 144t
Venereal Disease Research Laboratory (VDRL) test, 38t, 39, 40, 381
Versant HIV-1 RNA 3.0 Assay, 14, 15, 18t, 19
Versed. *See* Midazolam
Vfend. *See* Voriconazole
Vibramycin. *See* Doxycycline
Videx, Videx EC. *See* Didanosine
Vinblastine, for Kaposi's sarcoma, 422t
Vincristine
  for non-Hodgkin's lymphoma, 423
  for primary effusion lymphoma, 424
Viracept. *See* Nelfinavir
Viral load (VL)
  in acute retroviral syndrome, 15
  adherence to treatment and, 67–68, 68t
  antiretroviral therapy for reduction of, 57
  baseline, 70
  blips in, 72
  causes of increase in, 19
  CD4 cell count and, 1f, 15, 16, 75
  frequency of testing for, 17, 72

goal for suppression of, 57, 71, 74, 78
  rationale for, 72
of HIV-2, 6
HIV reservoirs and, 17
HIV RNA assays of, 14–19, 18t
HIV transmission and, 16, 116, 118, 133t
immunologic failure and, 72
initiation of antiretroviral therapy based on, 59t
interpreting changes in, 19
monitoring during pregnancy, 123
nadir of, 70
opportunistic infections related to, 16, 58t, 74
in pregnancy, 114, 115
in primary HIV infection, 3
prognosis and, 15–16, 18
rapidity of response to antiretroviral therapy, 70–71, 72
for resistance testing, 24, 25
sex differences in, 15
testing in healthcare worker after occupational exposure, 128
in therapeutic monitoring, 16–17, 73t
undetectable, 17–18
unexpectedly low, 17, 19
Viramune. *See* Nevirapine
Virco *Antivirogram,* 37t
Viread. *See* Tenofovir disoproxil fumarate
Virologic failure, 71–72, 74–76
  adherence and, 68, 68t, 75, 77
  assessment of, 75–76
  causes of, 75
  CD4 response and, 75
  convenience of therapy and, 75–76
  correlation with clinical and immunologic failure, 74–75
  discontinuation of antiretroviral therapy after, 79
  drug interactions and, 76
  with first therapy regimen, 77
  food effect and, 76
  with no resistance mutations, 77
  resistance and, 25–26, 76
    NNRTIs, 78
    NRTIs, 78
    PIs, 77–78
  salvage therapy for three class failures, 78–80, 79t
  strategies for, 77–80
  tolerability and, 76
  treatment interruption strategies for, 80
  viral load and, 17, 71–72
ViroLogic *PhenoSense,* 37t
Virtual Phenotype, 28–29
Vistide. *See* Cidofovir
Vitrasert. *See* Ganciclovir
Vitravene. *See* Fomivirsen
Vitritis

herpes zoster, 349
immune recovery, 344
VL. *See* Viral load
Voriconazole *(Vfend)*, 319–321
for *Aspergillus* infection, 329–330
for *Candida* infection, 333, 401t
for *Cryptococcus* infection, 338
drug interactions with, 87t, 92t–93t, 320–321, 329
VZIG (varicella-zoster immune globulin), 54, 350
VZV. *See* Varicella-zoster virus infection

W

Warfarin, drug interactions with, 95t
Wasting syndrome, 2t, 4t, 223–224, 251–252, 268–269, 304, 306
WB (Western blot)
for HIV-1, 7, 9, 11
for HIV-2, 6
Weight loss, 3t, 4t, 185
Wellbutrin. *See* Bupropion
***Wellcozyme* HIV-1&2 Test,** 13
Western blot (WB)
for HIV-1, 7, 9, 11
for HIV-2, 6
WinRho. *See* Rho(D) immune globulin

X

Xanax. *See* Alprazolam

Z

Zalcitabine (ddC, *Hivid*), 83t–85t, 321–323
adverse reactions to, 85t, 322–323
dosing recommendations for, 84t, 322
in renal or hepatic failure, 98t
drug interactions with, 85t, 323
formulations of, 84t, 321
pharmacokinetics of, 84t–85t, 322
for postexposure prophylaxis, 126
in pregnancy, 114t, 124t, 323
resistance to, 30t, 322
Zanamivir *(Relenza)*, for influenza, 55
ZDV. *See* Zidovudine
Zerit. *See* Stavudine
Ziagen. *See* Abacavir
Zidovudine (AZT, ZDV, *Retrovir*), 83t, 84t–85t, 323–327
advantages and disadvantages of, 64t–66t

adverse reactions to, 74t, 85t, 325–326
hepatotoxicity, 111t
hyperlactatemia, 103, 104
lipoatrophy, 101
myopathy, 426t
clinical trials of, 324
dosing recommendations for, 84t
in renal or hepatic failure, 98t, 324–325
drug interactions with, 85t, 95t, 326
ganciclovir, 220
methadone, 254t
ribavirin, 282
tipranavir, 310–311
formulations of, 84t, 323
in initial regimen, 61t–63t
for neonates, 122
pharmacokinetics of, 84t–85t, 324
for postexposure prophylaxis, 127t, 133t–134t
in pregnancy, 114t, 115, 122, 326–327
ACTG 076 protocol for, 122
for cesarean section, 117
in labor, 123t
pharmacokinetics of, 120
to reduce perinatal HIV transmission, 115, 116–117, 120–121, 326–327
safety of, 119, 120, 124t
testing for resistance to, 120
resistance to, 30t, 37t, 120, 121, 324
Zidovudine/lamivudine (AZT/3TC, *Combivir*), 83t
advantages and disadvantages of, 65t
compared with abacavir/lamivudine, 138
for postexposure prophylaxis, 126, 127t
in pregnancy, 115
in labor, 123t
to reduce perinatal HIV transmission, 120–121
Zidovudine/lamivudine/abacavir (AZT/3TC/ABC, *Trizivir*), 83t, 137
advantages and disadvantages of, 64t
clinical trials of, 138t, 139
Zithromax. *See* Azithromycin
Zocor. *See* Simvastatin
Zofran. *See* Ondansetron
Zostrix. *See* Capsaicin ointment
Zovirax. *See* Acyclovir
Zyban. *See* Bupropion
Zyprexa. *See* Olanzapine